D0908210

Essentials of
Postgraduate
Psychiatry

Essentials of Postgraduate Psychiatry

Edited by

Peter Hill
The Bethlem Royal Hospital
and the Maudsley Hospital,
London, England

Robin Murray
Institute of Psychiatry
and the Maudsley Hospital,
London, England

Anthony Thorley
St Nicholas Hospital, Gosforth,
and Newcastle University,
Newcastle upon Tyne, England

1979

ACADEMIC PRESS   London   New York   Toronto
Sydney   San Francisco
GRUNE & STRATTON   New York

ACADEMIC PRESS INC. (LONDON) LTD.
24/28 Oval Road,
London NW1

United States Edition published by
GRUNE & STRATTON INC.
111 Fifth Avenue
New York, New York 10003

British Library Cataloguing in Publication Data

Essentials of postgraduate psychiatry.
1. Psychiatry
I. Hill, Peter   II. Murray, Robin
III.Thorley, Anthony
616.8'   RC454   79–63493

ISBN (Academic Press) 0–12–791983–X
ISBN (Grune & Stratton) 0–8089–1204–6

.

Text set in 10/12 pt VIP Palatino, printed and bound
in Great Britain at W & J Mackay Limited,
Chatham

Contributors

Paul Bebbington MA, MB, B Chir, MRCP, MRCPsych, M Phil. *Lecturer, MRC Social Psychiatry Unit, Institute of Psychiatry, Denmark Hill, London SE5, England*

Sadrudin Bhanji MB, BS, MRCPsych, DPM. *Senior Lecturer in Adult Mental Illness, University of Exeter, Exeter, Devon, England*

Paul Bowden MRCS, LRCP, MRCP, MRCPsych, M Phil. *Consultant Psychiatrist, Bethlem Royal and Maudsley Hospitals, Denmark Hill, London SE5, England*

Anthony Clare MB, B Ch, BAO, MRCPI, MRCPsych, M Phil. *Honorary Consultant Psychiatrist, Bethlem Royal and Maudsley Hospitals; Senior Lecturer, Institute of Psychiatry, De Crespigny Park, Denmark Hill, London SE5, England*

John Cobb BA, BM, B Ch, MRCP, MRCPsych. *Senior Lecturer and Consultant Psychiatrist, St George's Hospital Medical School, Blackshaw Road, London SW17, England*

Joseph Connolly MB, BS, D Obst, RCOG, DCH, MRCP, MRCPsych. *Senior Lecturer and Consultant Psychiatrist, Westminster Hospital Medical School, Queen Mary's Hospital, Roehampton, London SW15, England*

Gaius Davies MB, BS, MRCGP, MRCPsych, DPM, M Phil. *Consultant Psychiatrist, King's College Hospital, London, England*

Peter Hill* MA, MB, B Chir, MRCP, MRCPsych. *Senior Registrar, Bethlem Royal and Maudsley Hospitals, Adolescent Unit Bethlem Royal Hospital, Monks Orchard Road, Beckenham, Kent, England*

Robin Jacoby BM, B Ch, MRCP, MRCPsych. *Lecturer, Institute of Psychiatry, De Crespigny Park, Denmark Hill, London SE5, England*

Peter Jefferys MB, B Chir, MRCP, MRCPsych. *Consultant Psychiatrist, Northwick Park Hospital and MRC Clinical Research Centre, Harrow, Middlesex, England*

* Present address: Senior Lecturer and Consultant Psychiatrist, St George's Hospital Medical School, Blackstow Road, London SW17, England.

Warren Kinston B Sc., MB, BS, MRCPsych.   *Research Fellow, Department of Psychiatry, Charing Cross Hospital Medical School, London W6, England*

Geoffrey Lloyd MA, MB, B Chir, MRCP, MRCPsych, M Phil.   *Consultant Psychiatrist, Royal Infirmary, Edinburgh, Scotland*

Roy McClelland MD, MRCPsych.   *Senior Lecturer and Consultant Psychiatrist, Queens University, Belfast, Northern Ireland*

Anthony Mann MA, MB, B Chir, MRCP, MRCPsych, M Phil.   *Honorary Consultant Psychiatrist, Bethlem Royal and Maudsley Hospitals; Senior Lecturer, Institute of Psychiatry, De Crespigny Park, Denmark Hill, London SE5, England*

Paul Mullen MB, BS, MRCPsych, M Phil.   *Honorary Consultant Psychiatrist, Bethlem Royal and Maudsley Hospitals; Senior Lecturer, Institute of Psychiatry, De Crespigny Park, Denmark Hill, London SE5, England*

Robin Murray MD, MRCP, MRCPsych, M Phil.   *Honorary Consultant Psychiatrist, Bethlem Royal and Maudsley Hospitals; Senior Lecturer, Institute of Psychiatry, De Crespigny Park, Denmark Hill, London SE5, England*

Maria Ron LMS (Madrid), MRCPsych, M Phil.   *Honorary Consultant Psychiatrist, Bethlem Royal and Maudsley Hospitals; Senior Lecturer, Institute of Psychiatry, De Crespigny Park, Denmark Hill, London SE5, England*

Rachel Rosser MA, MB, B Chir, MRCP, MRCPsych.   *Senior Lecturer and Consultant Psychiatrist, Charing Cross Hospital, Fulham Palace Road, London W6, England*

Richard Stern MD, MRCPsych, DPM.   *Honorary Consultant Psychiatrist, Bethlem Royal and Maudsley Hospitals; Senior Lecturer, Institute of Psychiatry, De Crespigny Park, Denmark Hill, London SE5, England*

Eric Taylor MA, MB, B Chir, MRCP, MRCPsych.   *Honorary Consultant Psychiatrist, Bethlem Royal and Maudsley Hospitals; Senior Lecturer, Institute of Psychiatry, De Crespigny Park, Denmark Hill, London SE5, England*

Anthony Thorley MA, MB, B Chir, MRCPsych.   *Clinical Lecturer in Psychological Medicine, Newcastle University; Consultant Psychiatrist, Parkwood House Alcohol and Drug Dependence Unit, St Nicholas Hospital, Gosforth, Newcastle-upon-Tyne, England*

Peter Tyrer MD, MRCP, MRCPsych, DPM.   *Senior Lecturer and Consultant Psychiatrist, University of Southampton, Southampton General Hospital, Tremona Road, Southampton, England*

Foreword

This is the first general textbook of psychiatry to emerge from the Institute of Psychiatry and the Bethlem Royal and Maudsley Hospitals—known to the world at large as 'The Maudsley'. Until now an organization which every year produces a considerable crop of monographs, books on special subjects, reviews and original articles, has eschewed such a venture. Like all exciting enterprises, it carries a certain risk—the challenge of retaining the many flavours of Maudsley teaching while reducing the whole to more amenable proportions, and of persuading a number of highly individualistic soloists to take part in an ensemble.

Henry Maudsley himself was only 23 when appointed as Superintendent to the New Cheadle Royal Hospital. By the age of 32 he had published several articles and his 'Physiology and Pathology of Mind'. It is therefore most appropriate that the challenge of producing a book based on teaching at the Maudsley should have been taken up by a younger generation of psychiatrists. I knew many of them when they worked with me as trainee psychiatrists, and have learnt much more from them than they ever did from me. Nor will it surprise the reader to learn that, during the period of the book's incubation, many of its contributors have been appointed to senior positions and have already distinguished themselves in a variety of different fields. The result of their labours is a very readable volume which provides up-to-date reviews of most of the important fields of psychiatry, with a plentiful supply of references for further reading.

The student who reads this book will find that it will illuminate many of his activities, be they clinical practice, teaching or research. He will become aware not only of important areas of knowledge, but also of areas of ignorance requiring further exploration. The latter aspect of a psychiatrist's education is often omitted, leaving a leaden lump of indigestible knowledge as an object for painful rumination. Yet it is the yeast which leavens the whole, and an essential ingredient for any serious student of psychiatry who values the Maudsley approach.

J. L. T. Birley,
Dean,
June 1979　　　　　　　　　　　　　　　　Institute of Psychiatry.

Preface

In the past two decades the scientific foundations of psychiatry have been greatly strengthened by research into such areas as the epidemiology of mental disorder, the biological understanding of the psychoses and the rational application of chemotherapy and psychotherapy. But psychiatric textbooks have seldom kept abreast of these advances and have, in particular, failed to meet the needs of the postgraduate student. This book is intended to provide the postgraduate with a portable general text that steers a middle way between unjustifiable dogmatism and obsolescent exhaustiveness, and integrates research findings into the general body of clinical knowledge. We believe that good clinical practice is grounded in and informed by the academic debate that surrounds it, and consequently have attempted not only to present the essential clinical information but also to show how it derives (or fails to derive) from rigorous scientific enquiry.

Multi-author books run the risk of inconsistency and repetition. However, since all the contributors are, or until recently have been, members of staff at the Maudsley Hospital, this volume presents a reasonably coherent point of view which emphasizes the critical approach for which that institution is renowned. This is not to say that readers should expect a narrowly uniform approach since many varieties of psychiatry are practised at the Maudsley.

From the outset we have tried to reflect the richness and variety of psychiatry as well as the need to anchor clinical practice in an objective framework. The 22 chapters are divided into four parts, the first of which places current systems of psychiatric care in historical perspective, discusses different models of mental illness, and outlines the principles of phenomenology and measurement. The second part describes the origins, presentation and course of the major clinical syndromes, while the third examines psychiatry in its social, forensic and general medical

ix

contexts. The final part includes chapters on biological and behavioural treatments and, since psychotherapy is now coming of age as a testable skill, discusses psychotherapy research as well as individual and group therapy. Throughout we have included liberal references in the expectation that readers will wish to have controversial statements supported and will feel sufficiently curious to read the originals for themselves.

In choosing to identify essentials of postgraduate psychiatry we assume a basic knowledge of such topics as routine clinical assessment, compulsory admission procedures and the ability to work within a team. We also presume multidisciplinary standards of clinical practice which we hope most psychiatrists would regard as reasonable, and levels of information which are amply sufficient for the candidate preparing for postgraduate qualifications in psychiatry. The contributors are well aware of the needs of trainee psychiatrists not only through their experience as teachers, but also because many were deeply involved in the establishment and development in Britain of the Association of Psychiatrists in Training.

Psychiatrists now represent only a small proportion of the postgraduate professionals dealing with the mentally disordered since psychologists, social workers, and nurses have all developed specialized skills indispensable to the multidisciplinary approach. But many feel that a lack of confidence in, or lack of knowledge of, the basis of clinical psychiatry hampers their response to the needs of the mentally ill. The editors believe that they will find this book valuable as will general physicians and general practitioners seeking an authoritative and yet readable account of modern psychiatry.

As editors we would like to thank the contributors for their constructive response to criticism, their patience and above all for their enthusiasm which has carried us through various drafts. We owe an immense debt to our colleagues at the Maudsley Hospital, in particular those too numerous to mention by name, who have commented on earlier drafts. The development of this book has been dependent on many untiring secretaries, and the work of Vera Seal and Doreen Blake. It could not have appeared without the able guidance of Anthony Watkinson, Ruth Gadsby and Joanna Reid of Academic Press. We thank them all.

Maudsley Hospital   Peter Hill
June 1979   Robin Murray
                                                      Anthony Thorley

Contents

xi

Part II: Clinical Disorders

Part III: Psychiatry in Special Settings

Part IV: Principles of Treatment

1 A short history of the management of the insane

Paul Bowden

The history of psychiatry is part of the social history of man. In its telling there is a tendency to oversimplify complex events, to discern purpose where probably there was none and to ascribe to people, both individually and collectively, a clarity of thought which transcends genius and a degree of foresight which is visionary. Past views on the nature of mental illness are briefly described because they provide the rationale for the way in which the insane have been treated by society. The prevalent conditions in which reform has developed contrast with more general attitudes which have usually resisted change; for this reason legislation is important because it has been used to impose a minimum of responsibility on to a reluctant community and an entrenched medical profession. A broad outline of ancient practices is presented so as to contrast customs in different cultures; their persistence into modern times is also illustrated. The development of both ideas and therapy into the Graeco-Roman era is based on schools and is therefore eponymous. This overview is, however, mostly concerned with the development of psychiatric care in institutions and illustrates the way in which their milieu depended on contemporary views of madness, which were themselves related to the prevailing social order. It is hoped that the threads of this contribution will converge on and illuminate some aspects of recent legislation and in doing so will acknowledge the way in which the insane have suffered at the hands of the ignorant and the intolerant.

Primitive healing: its legacy

In the first Chinese dynasty (c. 2600 B.C.) medicine was practised by priest-doctors and witch-doctors. By the time of the Chou dynasty, Kuan Tzu (c. 1140 B.C.) stated that there were definite institutions for the insane in which they were cared for until recovery took place (Whitwell, 1936).

The Indian Vedas are considered to be the oldest known books and the fourth book, Brahma Veda, deals exclusively with demonology, magic and sorcery, with diseases and their cure (Rao, 1975). Treatment was based on the recitation of incantations and the wearing of amulets and talismans. A particular contribution of the Vedic era was the quest for mental poise and tranquillity which Patanjali developed as the yoga system of philosophy. It laid down a system of practices which were intended to integrate the personality. There were eight stages: restraint, discipline, body posturing, breathing control, withdrawal, fixed attention, contemplation and complete tranquility. The Ayurveda, an ancient Indian system of medicine, is ascribed to divine revelation; in it a distinction is made between different dimensions of the personality, intellectual, social, emotional, spiritual and moral, which have been seen as early parallels of personality types (Varma, 1965).

The Ebers papyrus was written in about 1570 B.C. It describes the use, in Egypt, of surgical techniques, drugs and various magical and religious practices which included fumigation and purification with holy water, (Baasher, 1975). Mental disease was thought to be due to possession, and the temples were dedicated not only for worship, but also for the care of the sick. Thus, at the 'Temple of Healing' built in 2980 B.C. at Memphis, in honour of Imhotep, the chief priest was also the leading physician.

In the pre-Islamic era, life and death were seen as a continuous cycle and so great attention was paid to the afterworld. Misfortunes in life, and particularly mental illness, were thought to be due to supernatural forces although physical causes were also recognized. In the early Islamic period several causes of madness were identified: congenital, passionate, bilious and satanic. These disorders were distinguished from a group called the 'sane insane', which included defectives, and those who only demonstrated disturbances of judgement and temperament (Kaylani, 1924). In Africa, mental illness, like physical disease and personal and communal catastrophy, was thought to have a dual origin in the intrigues of the enemy and the evil influence of spirits. Traditional practices for the treatment of illness included ritual, sacrifice, public confession, free emotionality, dance, trance and incantation (Lambo, 1975).

Ellenberger (1970) has summarized the basic principles of primitive healing; in form many are still practiced in less materially advanced communities, in content they are the basis of many modern therapeutic methods. The healer, a skilled and learned man, holds a dominant position amongst his people and the patient places his confidence in the person of the healer rather than in medications or techniques. Most methods of healing are of a psychological nature and the procedure is usually a public and collective ritual. A common belief is that the soul leaves the body or is stolen and the shaman, or healer, searches for the soul and restores it to the body (Frazer, 1911). Other peoples believe that disease is caused by the presence in the body of a harmful foreign substance. The theory that illness is due to possession with evil spirits is still widely held and expulsion can be attempted mechanically, by transfer to another being, or by exorcism (Oesterreich, 1930). Healing through confession is still practised by those who hold that disease follows the infringement of a taboo and ceremonial healing continues to be an important therapeutic procedure.

Greece and Rome

Graeco-Roman philosophy and its changing views of mental illness provided a basic framework of thought and practice which was to influence Europe for almost two millennia. The Homeric school did not differentiate between mind and body and taught that mental disorder was due to external forces. To Homer the individual was part of the cycle of life in the social group to which he belonged and he was co-equal with the gods and the universe; sickness and its resolution were therefore socially defined (Simon and Weiner, 1966). A contrasting view was propounded by Hippocrates (*c.* 470–*c.* 400 B.C.) two and a half centuries later. He believed that madness arose from a disturbance of the brain and was caused by an inbalance of the elements (fire, air, earth and water) and of the humors (blood, phlegm and bile). The humors were thought to be the basis of the four temperaments: sanguineous, choleric, phlegmatic and melancholic (Simon and Ducey, 1975). Hippocrates' concept of the physician and his model of the practice of medicine has greatly influenced the emergence of medical practice in the West, but his physiological system was spurious and it impeded progress later when his teachings were uncritically followed. Perhaps the most important contribution was made by Aristotle (384–322 B.C.) who is often seen as the father of modern science; he laid the principles of the doctrine of organic evolution, developed theories of generation and heredity and founded comparative anatomy (Singer and Underwood, 1962). Aristotle taught that presence or absence of the psyche (soul) distinguished between living and non-living substances and that it was through suffering that the individual achieved self-knowledge.

At the beginning of the Christian era the popular view was that madness was caused and cured by supernatural agents which were personified by particular gods and goddesses; they acted through mortals in a state of anger or pleasure. The most important figure of this era was Galen of Pergamon (A.D. 129–199) who developed a medical system whose form was derived from Aristotle and whose substance was Hippocratic. To Galen all things were determinate; their origin lay in the heavens and was a reflection of the perfection of God. Galen sustained the belief that mental illness was due to an imbalance of humors, especially black bile and choler, and he recommended that disorders should be treated with vapors, baths, diets, emetics and cathartics.

The earliest reference to madness in the Bible (c. 1450 B.C.) is that in which it is threatened as a punishment for those who violate God's commands (Deut. xxviii:28). The Bible does not recognize insanity as an illness and records that it was customary for a person who was thought to be possessed by spirits to be stoned to death (Lev. xx:27). In contrast, the Talmud does not invoke extramundane powers, in the form of demons or evil spirits, as a cause of mental disorder; it recognizes mental abnormality and also suggests a possible classification of disorder: mental defect, confusion, acute and cyclical psychoses and disorders which result from physical illness. The text also refers to the sociolegal aspects of insanity; the insane are not considered responsible for the damage or shame they cause and they may not marry. A notably advanced view which is contained in the Talmud states that in periods of lucidity the individual is considered capable and responsible in all social and legal matters (Miller, 1975).

Britain: the influence of its conquerors

We have only limited information about British Celtic tribal society before the contemporary description of Caesar. Druids were the spiritual and intellectual leaders and, according to Pliny, they are said to have had some medical knowledge. The conquering legions had their own *medici* who practised on two levels: for the higher classes philosopher/physicians recommended treatment based on astrology and religion, while the practice for the majority was that of cruder superstition in the form of incantations and charms. The Twelve Tables was a codification of traditional customs and practice into Roman Law. The main legal principle to be applied to madness for the next nine centuries was contained in Table Five: 'If a man is raving mad, rightful authority over his person and chattels shall belong to his kinsman on his father's side or to his clansmen' (Buckland, 1932). The law distinguished insanity and mental defect from disorder due to strong passions. In the later period of the Roman Empire the responsibilities of the insane were systemized in '*Corpus Juris Civilis*' which covered the contract of marriage, the ability to testify and the subject of criminal responsibility.

The invasion of Saxons, Angles and other European groups in the fourth and fifth centuries A.D. brought with it a pagan culture which taught that mental disease was a result of demoniacal possession with the spirit *Wóden* and in fact the term *Wód* meant 'insane'. The Leech Books, the medical texts of the Anglo Saxons, were an amalgam of herbal folklore and elaborate ceremony (Bonser, 1963). When other remedies failed, violence was used in the belief that the demon could be driven out. A Celtic Welsh king, Hywel Dda (909–950 A.D.), codified his people's customs in a way which illustrated contemporary attitudes to the insane. They could not be a judge, were released from the obligations of a claim and were protected by law (Richards, 1954).

It is probable that missionaries established the first hospitals in the British Isles. They were attached to monasteries where both the physically and mentally ill were cared for. Such hospitals were founded at St Albans in 794 and at York in 937 (Dainton, 1961). The Norman conquest brought a renewed interest in Galen's humoral theories which was enhanced by the influence of travellers returning from the crusades and pilgrimages. About 1250, a Franciscan monk, Bartholomaeus Anglicus, wrote his treatise '*De proprietatibus rerum*' which recognized, 'melancholie, madness, gaurynge (staring) and forgetfulness, and frensie'. He believed that both internal events, for example anxiety and grief, and external, the bite of a mad dog, could be identified as causing mental disorder (Hunter and Macalpine, 1963). Thomas Aquinas (1225–1274) used a theological basis for his concept of the soul: since it was of divine origin it could not be sick, so he related mental disease to extraneous factors.

Institutions

Outside China the earliest forms of institutional care are thought to have been in Damascus and Basra in the post-Islamic period. In India an institution existed at Mandu in 1000 A.D. and in Turkey several were functioning by the thirteenth century (Howells, 1975). The mentally ill shared facilities with the physically ill at St John's Home in Ghent which was the oldest provision of this type in Europe; it was founded in 1191. At Elbing in Germany and at the Italian town of Bergamo shelter/hospitals were in existence before the middle of the fourteenth century. The first institution in Europe to care exclusively for the mentally ill was founded by Fray Juan Galiberto Jofré, a Mercedarian priest, and opened in 1409 in the Spanish town of Valencia. Jofré is said to have become familiar with the existence of mental hospitals during his travels in the Moslem Empire where they were places for the commitment of those regarded as anti-social: vagabonds, prostitutes and delinquents. Jofré determined that his own hospital should be solely for the protection and care of the insane (Lopez Ibor, 1975). The hospital of St Mary of Bethlehem was founded in London in 1247, and records show that in 1402 six of its 14 patients were *menti capti* or insane (O'Donoghue, 1914). Allderidge (1979) has suggested that twentieth century proclamations are reminiscent of a petition of 1414 for the reformation of hospitals in which it was emphasized that they exist, amongst other things, to maintain those who have lost their wits.

These developments were concerned primarily with the physical care of the insane, and the little knowledge that had been established about the nature of mental disorder was not to be substantially developed for several centuries. The violent were often incarcerated whereas the mildly insane were permitted to roam about the countryside. Those whose mental aberrations were manifested by religious phenomena were treated as divinely inspired saints or prophets, 'God's True Minstrels' (Langland, 1393). A common practice in continental Europe at this time was to abandon paupers, cripples and the mentally ill, in ships bound for an unknown destiny as was immortalized in Sebastian Brandt's 'The Ship of Fools' (1494). Such practices were relatively tolerant in comparison with those which prevailed later when the mentally ill were considered to be possessed by the devil, or were looked upon as sorcerers who could produce illness in others. It was a time when, 'superstitious and terror stricken, the minds of men were directed towards the miraculous and the Satanic' (Lecky, 1872). The physician was excluded from the field of mental illness which was usurped by the Inquisitors. The infamous handbook of the witch-hunter, '*Malleus Maleficarum*', which appeared in 1489, was written by two Dominican monks, Kraemer and Sprenger. Anyone who showed physical or psychological abnormality, or was the subject of natural misfortune was regarded as a witch who manifested the work of the devil. Doctors of the day did not contradict this pervading cultural attitude. Thus, Sir Thomas Browne, a prominent physician, gave expert witness against two women accused of witchcraft and was instrumental in their conviction and execution (Lloyd, 1928). In the colonies practices were similar. A law passed in Connecticut in 1642 stated, 'If any man or woman be a witch, that is hath or consulted with a familiar spirit, they shall be put to death.' At the town of Salem in New England, nineteen individuals were executed as possessed. The Middle Ages were notable for the frequency of other epidemics of mental disorder such as the flagellationist movement, dancing mania, children's crusades and the possession of whole communities, especially monastic (Ackerknecht,

1968). In 1637 a public discussion took place in Paris as to whether incubi could procreate their species; the incubus was supposed to be a male demon who attacked the chastity of girls, and the succubus, the corresponding female demon who similarly molested males (Whitwell, 1936). A more humane side of medical practice in the early seventeenth century is illustrated by Peter Turner's plea that the child of a melancholic should not be removed from her since such action might worsen her condition (Hunter and Macalpine, 1963). Similarly in 1602 the physician Jorden defended the witch Elizabeth Jackson on the grounds that her fits were natural (Rosen, 1968). A recent view (Geiss, 1978) is that these bizarre behaviours were manifestations of womens liberation which were suppressed in the witch-hunts by pious and mysogynistic men.

The Renaissance

The significance of the Renaissance for psychiatry was two-fold: first there was a rebirth of a humane attitude towards the insane, however short-lived, and second, doubts as to the supernatural causation of mental illness and other phenomena led to a search for natural causes. The views of Paracelsus (1493–1541, Phillipus von Hohenheim) typified this change; he taught that mental disorders were natural diseases and disputed the theories of the temperaments and the humors. Although much of his writing has been criticized as contradictory and inconsistent he was a humane individual; he wrote,

> The experienced doctor should not study how to exorcise the devil, but rather how to cure the insane. The insane and the sick are our brothers, let us give them treatment to cure them, for nobody knows whom among our friends or relatives this misfortune may strike.   (Zilborg, 1935)

Francis Bacon (1561–1626) also presented arguments to refute the contention that mental illness was the result of bodily disease or divine punishment.

The closure of the monasteries in the Reformation meant that physicians replaced monks in the Royal Hospitals at St Thomas's, Christ's, St Batholomew's, Bethlem and Bridewell. However, the newly established church was empowered to issue licences to physicians. The Poor Law Act was passed in 1601 and was to exert considerable influence on English social history (Leonard, 1900). It stated that unpaid overseers of the poor were to raise money in each parish for the relief of its own paupers. Initially aid was in the form of food and clothing, but later workhouses were introduced because the volume of distress made it necessary to deter the poor from seeking assistance. If an individual's mental condition reduced him to destitution he came within the remit of the Poor Law; if it led him to break the criminal law, he was judged by that law; if he wandered, he was judged by the vagrancy laws. The indigent pauper was therefore an unwelcome responsibility of the parish and was often driven out to seek help elsewhere. Shakespeare described one type of licensed beggar, the 'Tom o'Bedlam', who was privileged because he was usually exempt from the rigours of the law:

> Poor Tom, that eats the swimming frog, the toad, the tadpole, the wall newt and the water newt, that in the fury of his heart, when the foul fiend rages, eats cow-dung for pallets, swallows the old rat and the ditch dog, drinks the green mantle of the slimy pool, who is whipt from tything to tything, and stocked, punished and imprisoned.   (King Lear, III, 4)

The publication of Robert Burton's 'Anatomy of Melancholy' in 1628 gave a summary of contemporary beliefs which were clearly derived from Hippocrates and Galen. Lunacy was considered to originate in sin, and mental and moral defect were considered to be synonomous. Imbalance of the four humors was thought to contribute to illness, and their excess was relieved by blood-letting, cautery and blistering. However, two important scientific works were published in this era: in 1628 William Harvey's paper 'De Mortu Cordis' was published, and the latter half of the seventeenth century was marked by the appearance of the work of Thomas Willis who described the anatomy and physiology of the nervous system. Before long disorders formally called hysteria, hypochondria and the spleen came to be subsumed under the general name of 'nervous disorders' (Hare, 1976). The philosopher René Descartes located the soul in the pineal body, and identified it with the origin of all thought, but its essence was supernatural and immaterial. Although Descartes considered that the nature of the soul was a mystery and would remain so (Singer, 1941), he was able to identify three separate aspects: vegetative, which implied the quality by which a body is alive; sensitive, which was concerned with feeling and movement; reasoning, which was responsible for thought, will and judgement (Jefferson, 1960). McMahon (1976) has argued that Descartes' views were crucial for the development of psychiatry. In the pre-Cartesian period the biological soul served as a common substrate for both mental and physical events and therefore medicine was invariably holistic and psychosomatic. Cartesian dualism (the material body and immaterial soul) made the occurrence of any 'psychophysiological' event a biological and logical impossibility. The soul was ignored because it was supernatural and mechanistic physiopathology gained ascendancy.

Confinement

Jones (1972) has produced an excellent summary of the development of mental health services from the eighteenth century. She has described the manner in which outdoor relief was supplemented by the provision of a poorhouse which usually housed the respectable, but infirm, aged. In larger cities, the poorhouse was superseded by the workhouse. The rich, who paid for these institutions, were perennially concerned that they should be run as cheaply as possible and consequently great emphasis was placed on differentiating between those who could not work and those who would not. Bridewells, or 'Houses of Correction', received vagrants and beggars who wandered and refused to work. Unlike prisons where the inmates were responsible for their own maintenance, the Poor Law Authority maintained the pauper inmates in Bridewells. Criminal lunatics were sent to gaol where conditions were even worse than in the Bridewells. In the year 1714 lunatics were brought within the provisions of the earlier Vagrancy Act under which local magistrates were empowered to commit vagrants and those considered to be rogues, vagabonds, poachers and travelling showmen, to gaol or Bridewell. If the offender was not resident in the parish in which he was apprehended he was removed to his legal place of settlement or deposited outside the parish in which he threatened to become a burden. Affluent lunatics were boarded out with clergymen or physicians but this custom was replaced by the development of larger institutions where people could be detained at the insistence of their relatives. Their inmates had no legal protection other than by means of a writ of habeas corpus and not until the last quarter of the eighteenth century were private madhouses controlled by law. Although a source of profit for their owners, they were also the scene of brutality and neglect for their unfortunate inmates. Parry-Jones (1972) has however argued that the private madhouses provided a major public service in that they were the principal and often the only institutions to care for the insane in a specialized way, and by the mid-nineteenth century half the lunatics confined in asylums were in private licensed madhouses.

In 1646 Bethlem moved to its new site at Moorfields and unless they were paupers patients were responsible for their own maintenance. They were kept in a state of near-nakedness and outside medical practitioners were refused access, while casual visitors, who baited the inmates and enjoyed the spectacle of their degradation, were made welcome. If they were of some social standing single lunatics remained in their own house with an attendant; those from poorer families were chained in a room, kennel or cage to prevent nuisance. In 1751 St Luke's Hospital was opened in London as a result of voluntary subscription. It was a rival to the Bethlem and its staff sought to dissociate themselves from the nefarious practices at the older institution. In Manchester a Lunatic Hospital was founded in 1763; it was contiguous with the Infirmary and was to represent an important step towards creating an alliance between the treatment of physical and mental illness.

Thus whether detained in gaol, Bridewell, private madhouse, poor-house, workhouse, or in the newly developing public madhouse, the mad had entered the period of 'The Great Confinement' (Foucault, 1967). Kraeplin (1918) has described the way in which they were to be tortured,

> Blood-letting to the point of syncope, repetition of the same process, administering cold showers, douching the head after it had been shaven, putting a crown of leeches around the head, scarifying the skin and sprinkling cartharides in the open cuts, massaging with tartar salve, using tartar emetic and the rack in certain instances to control rage.

For 'diversionary' purposes abrasive ointments were rubbed into pustules on the head and genitals, incisions made and red-hot irons applied to the body. Baths, shower-baths, drenching and douching were with ice-cold or hot water and patients were confined in masks, straight-jackets or irons. Foucault (1967) describes these practices thus:

> By a curious dialectic whose movement explains all these 'inhuman' practices of confinement, the free animality of madness was tamed only by such discipline whose meaning was not to raise the bestial to the human, but to restore man to what was purely animal in him.

Restraint and non-restraint

Deutsch (1937) has stated that these barbarous practices were to be discontinued in the ensuing era of 'rational humanism'. The most significant events were the political and social revolutions in America (1776) and France (1789) which were to act as liberating agents for a multitude of reform movements. Basic to the thought and action of the period of enlightenment was an acceptance of the supreme social value of intelligence, and, as a corollary, a belief in the utility of reason in social progress (Rosen, 1958). Thus, to Thomas Paine it was the 'Age of Reason'. Later there were to be many attempts to find a material, scientific basis for mental states: for example, Lavater and Lombroso in physiognomy and Gall in phrenology. In the salons of Vienna and Paris, Anton Mesmer had dispensed with magnets and electricity; he provided a collective treatment for the rich, centring on his *baquet* which concentrated magnetic fluid. However, others were not so fortunate. After investigating the conditions at Pforzheim, Jaegerschmid, who died in 1775, proposed that less disturbed patients be given more freedom, and that restraint be employed only in the case of violent patients. Furthermore he insisted that properly trained personnel be employed to care for the patients and that the staff should report regularly to a supervising physician. These proposals were not realized but in Florence between 1774 and 1788 Vincenzo Chiarugi introduced dramatic reforms at the Hospital of St Boniface. By 1792 Pinel succeeded in obtaining permission from

Couthon, a member of the commune, to unchain the maniacs at the Bicêtre in Paris (Gardiner Hill, 1839). Three years later he was put in charge of the Salpétrière where females were imprisoned and where he introduced similar reform. Jones (1972) has distinguished two parallel and complementary movements in Britain at the end of the eighteenth century.

The first was evangelical and stemmed from an emotional appreciation of the plight of the oppressed poor. Thus, societies for the reform of particular abuses became a fashionable activity and lunacy reform was only one of the many avenues explored. Secondly, a radical philosophical school developed which was not concerned with the plight of the insane from any sense of pity; its adherents thought in terms of legal action and public institutions and reform was an inadvertent byproduct of their work. Mrs Susan Carnegie (1744–1821) founded 'The Royal Lunatic Asylum, Infirmary and Dispensary' at Montrose in 1781; she is regarded as the pioneer of mental and social welfare in Scotland (Henderson, 1964).

In 1792 a new institution was founded at York by the Quakers (Society of Friends) at the instigation of a layman, William Tuke. It was called, significantly, 'The Retreat'. Tuke was critical of medical men and their methods of mechanical restraint and the 'moral treatment' which he advocated was based on a blend of humanitarianism and Christianity. Patients were not punished if they apparently failed to control their behaviour and their milieu was pleasant and homely. Godfrey Higgins, a Yorkshire magistrate, and Edward Wakefield, a land agent and philanthropist, respectively uncovered the abuses at York Asylum and the Bethlem Hospital. Subsequently the parliamentary enquiry into madhouses of 1815 resulted in the dismissal of Thomas Monro and John Haslam from the Bethlem (Hunter and Macalpine, 1963; Masters, 1977), and William Tuke and his grandson Samuel eventually achieved the much needed reform of the pre-existing York Asylum (Tuke, 1813; Gray, 1815).

The acquittal of Hadfield who shot at King George III provided the impetus for the passing of the Criminal Lunatics Act (1800) to facilitate his disposal. It allowed for the detention of criminal lunatics 'during His Majesty's pleasure' but unfortunately it did not direct where they should be kept, nor did it provide any machinery by which they might ultimately be released. It was therefore necessary to set up a Select Committee several years later, 'to enquire into the state of Criminal and Pauper Lunatics in England'. The following recommendations were made: an asylum should be set up in each county to which both criminal and pauper lunatics could be sent; admission and discharge were to be controlled by local justices and be financed by means of a county rate.

Criminal lunatics were to be kept apart and by 1814 there was a separate ward for them at the Bethlem Hospital. This became crowded and Fisherton House, Salisbury took the overflow; fifty years later Broadmoor Hospital was opened. The County Asylum Act (1808), known as 'Wynn's Act', accepted these proposals but it did not make their implementation obligatory. The institutions which were belatedly set up were often forerunners of today's mental hospitals, some of which still occupy the same premises constructed under the original Act (Jones, 1972). Subsequently the Select Committee was to report on several existing institutions. For example, the case of the condition of William Norris at the Bethlem received much publicity. He had been held in an iron collar, with arms pinioned and feet manacled, for nine years. In addition the Committee found that at Bethlem a number of women were chained to a wall, completely naked apart from a blanket each. In the workhouses too they found the pauper lunatics to be in a state of filth, neglect and appalling brutality. A Bill was drawn up to rectify these failings by providing a competent and powerful inspectorate but it was rejected by the House of Lords in 1819. A report on the state of pauper lunatics at the 'White House', Bethnal Green, was published nearly a decade later and was to be more influential. It described how patients were placed in wooden cages which were filled with straw and where they were secured by the arms and legs.

> At weekends they were fastened at three o'clock and left there until nine o'clock on Monday. Food was brought to them and their arms were freed just sufficiently to enable them to eat. On Monday they were taken out into the yard and the accumulated excrement was washed from them with a mop dipped in cold water.   (Jones, 1972)

As a result of the individual and collective neglect and brutality which was repeatedly exposed by the London Metropolitan Commissioners the Middlesex Asylum was built at Hanwell. The Commissioners were also influential in the passing of the County Asylums Act which made visiting justices liable to send annual returns to the Secretary of State for the Home Department who was empowered to send any visitor to any asylum. The Commissioners, who were not solely medical practitioners, could grant or revoke licences and release anyone who was improperly detained. In addition, the life and illnesses of George III had a considerable effect on public opinion. Two attempts on his life resulted in changes in the law of criminal responsibility and his own five episodes of mental disorder evoked compassionate sentiments.

In France Esquirol, a disciple of Pinel, introduced a framework of psychiatric facilities whose provisions are still extant. In every *département* a lunatic asylum was opened; admissions were controlled by the local authority or, in an emergency, the *Préfet*. Voluntary admission was decided by the family who could also discharge the patient. The mental state had to be attested by several physicians and if the patient protested against the confinement a new investigation had to be instigated.

The policy of 'non-restraint' was extended by Charlesworth and later Gardner Hill at Lincoln Asylum (Gardner Hill, 1839) and in 1839 John Conolly went to Hanwell Asylum where he advocated the total abolition of restraint (Conolly, 1856). Conolly recognized that non-restraint management demanded high standards of both nursing and administrative staff and that they would be responsible for continuous surveillance and would be increasingly exposed to physical risk. Together with the asylum chaplain, Conolly organized a literacy and educational scheme as part of treatment but these plans were frustrated by the governing committee of magistrates. It was at Conolly's instigation that another asylum was built at Colney Hatch, in the parish of Friern Barnet in 1849 and he insisted that the institution should not be too large. Hunter and Macalpine (1974) have given an admirable description of the development and character of Colney Hatch asylum. Admission was determined by social criteria and depended on whether there was any alternative provision. Chronic patients were the most numerous and were considered to be incurable; cross infection with tuberculosis, typhoid and dysentery was common. The criteria of recovery were stricter for those who were legally certified as insane and community care meant return to the workhouse. Asylum medical officers did not control admissions (the parish doctor declared patients insane), or discharge (patients were released by the committee of visitors); they had no prospect of achieving consultant rank because the voluntary hospitals had no establishment for an alienist. Medical officers assisted the medical superintendents in the statutory duties, which were mainly administrative, and 'classified' patients, that is, they grouped patients with similar disabilities together. The first consultants in psychiatry later came from the ranks of the medical superintendents. At this time an important issue developed between the Poor Law authorities and the Lunacy authorities. The Board of Guardians were passing on to the county asylums the most difficult cases while retaining the less disordered, and therefore more useful, in the workhouses. It was considered that only if the county asylums could be shown to be curative institutions could their high cost be justified. If they were merely places of detention, the Poor Law authorities could rightly claim that they could do this work much more cheaply (Jones, 1972).

In the USA Dorothea Dix (1802–1887), who was born in Maine, had a considerable reformative influence on practically all the States of the Union. She gained the support of the legislatures to alleviate the conditions of the insane; she was responsible for the renovation of many old hospitals and the founding of new ones. Her influence extended to

Canada, and in Great Britain her endeavours resulted in the setting up of the Royal Commission which led to the passing of the 1857 Lunacy (Scotland) Act, which revolutionized the care and treatment of the mentally affected in that country (Henderson, 1964).

Legislation

Lord Ashley, later to become the Earl of Shaftsbury, joined the Metropolitan Lunacy Commissioners in 1828 and influenced reform for several decades thereafter. Ashley not only increased the number of commissioners but also recommended that it should be obligatory for every county to build an asylum. The Madhouse Act (1828) provided clauses which prevented collusion between the certifying doctor and the institution's proprietor, and Ashley recommended additional safeguards to prevent deceitful and lucrative cooperation between the certifying doctor and the relatives. In the Lunacy Act of 1845 the Metropolitan Commissioners were superseded by an expanded Lunacy Commission which covered the entire county and all types of institutions, including gaols, workhouses, and for the first time, the Bethlem Hospital.

In the latter part of the nineteenth century the well established legal profession controlled the social aspects of the practice of medicine with a plethora of statutes. Medical practitioners did not achieve full status until the passing of the Medical Registration Act in 1858 and the asylum doctors in particular found it necessary to organize themselves. In 1853 Dr Bucknill, Superintendent of the Devon County Asylum, founded the Asylum Journal which was to become the Asylum Journal of Mental Science, and eventually the British Journal of Psychiatry. At the same time there was a growing interest in the issue of individual and personal liberty which led to the appointment of a Select Committee of the House of Commons which was asked to study the effects of the lunacy laws on personal freedom. The Committee expressed the view, which was later to be of considerable significance in relation to the concepts of voluntary and informal status, that voluntary boarders should be allowed in small licensed institutions.

On the continent Jean-Martin Charcot was at the height of his fame and in 1885 was visited at the Salpétrière by a Moravian neurologist, Sigmund Freud. In England, the Lunacy Act (1890) consolidated all previous acts and transferred ultimate authority to the Lord Chancellor. He appointed the Lunacy Commissioners and they reported to him; they had powers of visitation and inspection over all institutions. Each county council became responsible for the building and maintaining of an asylum to which there were four methods of admission: by a reception order on petition, whereby a relative made a statement before a justice which was to be supported by two medical practitioners; by an urgency order of limited duration in which only the relatives' petition and one medical certificate were necessary; by a summary reception order, whereby a Poor Law receiving officer or the police could detain or remove pauper patients to a workhouse, a justice would be notified, and only one medical certificate was required; finally, for the aristocratic and those with property, admission by inquisition, where the Judge in Lunacy would request the Masters in Lunacy to examine an alleged lunatic. If they considered him to be of unsound mind he would be admitted to an asylum as a 'Chancery Lunatic'. In the last instance the patient had the right to contest the issue of sanity before a judge. The Lunacy Act contained detailed clauses which prevented collusion between the parties responsible for certification and the orders were valid for a limited period only, but were renewable. Medical certification was necessary to sanction the use of mechanical restraint and it could only be used as a method of treatment or to prevent the patient injuring himself or others. Letters written to certain individuals in authority were to be forwarded unopened.

Mentally abnormal offenders

Possibly the first pronouncement on the law of the plea of insanity as a defence to a grave criminal charge came from an Elizabethan, Chief Justice Coke. He ruled that a person could not commit high treason if he was in absolute madness and with a total deprivation of memory (Walker, 1968). This common law ruling was still in force in 1723 when the judge amplified on the area of criminal responsibility in Matthew Arnold's trial: 'he must not know what he is doing any more than an infant, a brute or a wild beast'.

The Criminal Lunatics Act (1800) was the first British legislation under criminal law to provide for mentally abnormal offenders. It directed that persons who were insane on arraignment and who could not be tried should be treated as criminal lunatics, and considered as 'unfit to plead'. The acquittal of McNaghten and the subsequent House of Lords ruling on his case in 1843 established the finding of 'not guilty by reason of insanity' (West and Walk, 1977). The Lords' rules reflected the prevailing idea that people are rational beings making free choices informed by conscious consideration. They neglected what was to emerge later, a dynamic understanding of man whose behaviour could be non rational, irrational and compulsive. This 'special verdict' was altered in the Trial of Lunatics Act (1883) to 'guilty but insane', allegedly to appease the indignation of Queen Victoria at the acquittal on the grounds of insanity of a man who shot at her (Binney, 1949). The Criminal Lunatics Act (1884) was the first Act which allowed for the transfer of sentenced prisoners to criminal lunatic asylums. Mental deficiency was covered by powers similar to those exercised against criminals found to be insane in the Mental Deficiency Act (1913). The gap which was left by the magistrates' courts having no express power to make findings of insanity was filled by the Criminal Justice Act (1948) which allowed magistrates to remand an individual on bail or in custody so that an enquiry would be made into his mental condition. Persons of 'unsound mind' could be detained in an institution under the provisions of the Lunacy and Mental Treatment Acts (1890 and 1930). Here there was no question of responsibility and individuals were mostly sent to ordinary mental institutions. Section 4 of the Criminal Justice Act (1948) also made it possible for magistrates to impose a probation order on individuals who required treatment for their mental condition. The 1948 Act was consolidated in the Powers of Criminal Courts Act (1973). In the Criminal Procedure (Insanity) Act (1964), the special verdict restored the terminology used in the McNaghten ruling and allowed for an acquittal on the grounds of insanity, thus amending the Trial of Lunatics Act (1883). Section 4 of The Criminal Procedure (Insanity) Act (1964) also consolidated the Criminal Lunatics Act (1800) finding of unfitness to plead. The majority of mentally abnormal offenders, however, are now dealt with under Part 5 of the Mental Health Act (1959).

In 1954 in the USA Monte Durham appealed after being found guilty of housebreaking and Judge Bazelon upheld a new test of criminal responsibility: that if a defendant's unlawful act was the product of mental disease or mental defect, he was not clinically responsible. Cognitive reasoning ceased to be recognized as the sole determinant of conduct.

Mental defect

The publication of Itard's book, 'L'Education du Savage d'Aveyron' (1799) was of singular importance in the history of mental defect. Itard wrote of his attempts to educate a wild boy who had been found by hunters in the woods. He asserted that innate defect could be minimized but not eradicated and that special training provisions were necessary. In England the first asylum for idiots was 'Park House', Highgate, which was opened in 1847. Two subscription hospitals were built in the third quarter of the nineteenth century, at Lancaster and Exeter and the first large provision by a public authority was built in 1870 by the Metropolitan Asylums Board and named 'Darenth Training Schools'. The Idiots Act (1886) laid down conditions for admission, discharge, registration and inspection which were similar to those for lunatics. Colonies were set up at the turn of the century, founded on the assumption that care would be life-long and that it was therefore better to segregate defectives from society as a whole.

Galton's work on inheritance was distorted (Blacker, 1952) but his ideas stimulated a variety of eugenic theories and it was not until the publication of Tredgold's book in 1908 that a more balanced view was restored; he identified both genetic and environmental factors in the causation of mental defect. The Report of the Royal Commission on the Care of the Feeble Minded (1908) stated that the criteria for certification should be the protection and happiness of the defective rather than the more doubtful purpose of improving racial characteristics. The Commission recognized the need to protect the feeble-minded and expressed the view that there should be no social condemnation of defectives. Local bodies should be responsible for the ascertainment of cases and for their care. The Mental Deficiency Act (1913) incorporated these recommendations. It defined idiots, imbeciles, feeble-minded and moral defectives—the latter group were thought to have some permanent mental defect coupled with marked vicious or criminal propensities. In legislative terms the moral defective was superseded by the generic term 'psychopath'. Thus the Mental Health Act (1959), in stating that the psychopath required or was susceptible to medical treatment, supported Glueck's (1954) view of the antisocial offender as a sick person needing treatment rather than punishment. These opinions have been most eloquently challenged by Wooton (1968) who believes that the expansionist school in psychiatry is simply identifying mental health with the moral or cultural ideas of its proponents.

If it was not possible for an individual to be cared for normally in society he was placed in guardianship or in an institution. A Board of Control was set up, consisting largely of the existing Lunacy Commissioners who took with them all their powers and duties. This Bill was supplemented by the Elementary Education (Defective and Epileptic Children) Act of 1914 which made it obligatory for local authorities to set up special schools for the feeble-minded. The intention was that they should provide both manual and character training for the backward child and assess educability so that those who could not be trained would be passed on to the appropriate mental deficiency authority.

Voluntary treatment

In the asylums, although treatment was largely humane in the early part of the twentieth century, the emphasis was on custodial care. Because of the size of the hospitals, there was no sense of community, and patients were isolated and care was impersonal; hospitals could at that time only take certified patients. In 1915 a Bill to 'facilitate the early treatment of mental disorder of recent origin' was introduced into the Commons but it was prematurely withdrawn. Three years later the Board of Control recommended that treatment should be available for limited periods without certification and they also expressed the hope that responsible posts in mental hospitals should be restricted to the holders of the Diploma in Psychological Medicine, which had been instituted in 1911. The Board also recommended that general hospitals should provide facilities for the early diagnosis and treatment of mental illness for both in- and out-patients. The latter development represented an important attempt to break away from the concept of the institution as the only means of treatment apart from charity and the Poor Law.

Outside Britain the framework of treatment seems to have been more enlightened. A report in the USA stated that of the first 1500 patients admitted to the Boston Psychopathic Hospital, 48% were accepted as voluntary patients: 'It is as easy and simple for the patient suffering in mind to get advice, as for another with eye or lung trouble' (Pierce, 1915). The recognition and treatment of 'shell-shock' induced by experience in the Great War demanded a change in philosophy. A contemporary publication (Elliot Smith and Pear, 1917), stated that the cornerstones of treatment in such cases should be firmness, sympathy, kindness, as well as the opportunity for unburdening of anxiety; treatment was necessarily and importantly an individual matter. Ahrenfeldt (1958) has described the manner in which the urgency of the war situation forced military medical personnel to distinguish between major and minor disorders. The second decade of the twentieth century was also marked by the development of the 'Mental Hygiene' movement spearheaded by Clifford Beers, a former patient. Protagonists based their views on several complementary ideologies: that of eugenics and the theories of degeneration (Lombroso, 1911), sex enlightenment, and the expectation of significant advances in pathology and therapeutics like those occurring at that time in somatic medicine (Odegard, 1972).

Contemporary views on the nature and treatment of mental disorder are reflected in an early Medico-Psychological Report which emphasized that,

> The present systems, which compel all persons, except those able to pay adequately for the maintenance, to apply to the Poor Law authorities in order to secure treatment, is unsatisfactory and unjust. A system which artificially creates paupers in order to obtain medical treatment necessarily acts as a deterrent, so that too frequently there is serious and even disastrous delay.

It was in this climate that, in 1907, Henry Maudsley offered a large sum of money to the London County Council for a new mental hospital. The gift depended on three conditions which ensured that only voluntary patients would be treated in the hospital: it was to deal exclusively with early and acute cases; it was to provide an out-patient clinic; there would be treatment and research on the diagnosis and treatment of mental disorder. The Maudsley Hospital was completed in 1915 and in 1924 became the first teaching school in psychiatry of the University of London. In 1948, following the National Health Service Act (1946), it was combined with the Bethlem Royal Hospital. In the same year the medical school, re-named the Institute of Psychiatry, became part of the British Postgraduate Medical Federation and was entrusted to advance psychiatry by postgraduate teaching and research.

The appointment of a Royal Commission preceded the passing of the 1930 Mental Treatment Act. The Commission drew strong parallels between physical and mental illness and emphasized the importance of prevention and treatment rather than detention. It recognized that the legal status of the majority of insane persons was that of the pauper and argued for the dismantling of the framework of lunacy legislation. It rekindled the medical model, but introduced a social flavour and emphasized the importance of community support and after-care. The Act abolished outmoded terminology which was considered to be perjorative. Admission was possible under three categories: voluntary, on written application to the person in charge of any establishment; temporary, for individuals who were considered likely to benefit from treatment, but who were unable or unwilling to make voluntary application; certified, as in the Lunacy Act (1890). The 1930 Act also encouraged the development of out-patient departments and the opening of observation wards. At about the same time the Commonwealth Fund of America sponsored the training of a small group of English social workers in the USA where such training was already taking place, and in 1929 the Board of Control recommended that an individual like the hospital almoner should be employed to help allay patients' anxieties about work and domestic problems. A year later the first English course in social work began at the London School of Economics, again financed by the Commonwealth Fund (Ashdown *et al.*, 1953).

It is extremely difficult to assess the contribution of the doctrines of psychoanalysis to these processes. Freud was developing the psychoanalytic theory, method and organization which have been described as his three great contributions (Ellenberger, 1970). In Vienna, Alfred Adler taught of the goal-directedness of the creative self as well as propounding a system of social psychology. Jung's dichotomization of the personality and his views on the collectivity of the unconscious and on the existence of archetypes were to have a profound influence on contemporary culture. Like his peers, Jung's effect outside psychiatry was primarily on academic and religious circles, but gradually psychoanalytic ideas came to influence sociologists and students of political science. To what extent these various psychodynamic models influenced the manner in which the vast majority of the mentally ill were treated in the first half of the twentieth century is less certain.

In the United Kingdom, the first forty years of the twentieth century saw many Acts passed which profoundly changed social institutions relating to the relief of destitution, conditions of work, pensions and unemployment benefit. Against this background of change, the Beveridge Report was presented to Parliament in 1942 and advocated a way to establish freedom from want through the medium of social insurance schemes, thus outlining the basis of the contemporary welfare state. There were three fundamental assumptions: provision of children's allowances, maintenance of employment, and the establishment of comprehensive health and rehabilitation services. The purpose of the health service was clearly, if idealistically, defined: 'for prevention and for cure of disease and disability by medical treatment'. This act of faith in the preventive and curative aspects of medicine was based on the premise that the provision of adequate benefits in time of sickness was contingent on a reduction in its frequency and duration. These hopes reached fruition in the National Health Service Act (1946) which made local health committees responsible for certain statutory duties: the care and removal to hospital of persons dealt with under the Lunacy and Mental Treatment Acts; the ascertainment and removal to institutions of mental defectives; the supervision, guardianship, training and occupation of those in the community; the prevention, care and after-care of all types of patient. Thus the National Health Service Act effectively devolved power from local authorities and united general and mental hospitals under new Regional Hospital Boards so that they became the responsibility of the tax-payer rather than the rate-payer.

The situation in the mental hospitals was to change rapidly in the next few years. There was a dramatic increase in the certification of old people who became in-patients in mental hospitals; from 31,000 in 1948 to 45,000 in 1954; in the same year the total residents in mental hospitals also reached a peak of 152,000. Taylor (1962) has shown how patients at this time would refuse voluntary treatment in institutions whose reputation was bad. Thus the percentages of total admissions which were voluntary varied from 45 to 50% for some of the large mental hospitals serving London, to 99% for a provincial institution. The early 1950s was the time of the introduction of phenothiazines but it also witnessed exaggerated claims on behalf of psychiatry. The Director General of the World Health Organization appeared to be fostering a questionably dangerous form of psychiatric expansionism when he wrote:

The acute need of the modern world is that modern psychological medicine shall expand its goals beyond the mere helping of individuals . . . naturally parents, educators, youth workers, social workers, politicians and many others have very important responsibilities, but the technical guidance can come only from the students of human mental and emotional development and function. (Curran, 1952)

Later in the same decade a series of articles in the *Lancet* advocated the values inherent in the active occupation of mental patients: Bickford wrote of 'The Forgotten Patient' and Martin on 'Institutionalisation', Baker described an industrial unit at Banstead Hospital and Maxwell Jones stressed the value of 'Work Therapy'. By 1955 the Lancashire Joint Mental Hospitals Board showed that in one area nearly a half of all psychiatric admissions were to small psychiatric units associated with general hospitals which altogether only accounted for a fifth of the total psychiatric beds. Clearly the newer psychiatric units had a rapid turnover of acute cases but simultaneously the 'open-door' movement in the larger mental hospitals was gaining momentum (Bowden, 1975), and influenced the type of care which they were able to provide.

In 1953 a Royal Commission was invited to investigate the law relating to mental illness and mental deficiency; it reported four years later and most of its proposals were embodied in the Mental Health Act (1959). The Act defined mental disorder and included under this rubric psychopathic disorder; the invigilatory function of the Board of Control was transferred to Regional Mental Health Review Tribunals; voluntary and temporary admissions were replaced by informal admissions: compulsory admission was to be by emergency, observation, or treatment order.

It is not intended that this contribution should examine the 1959 Act, which has been criticized and is currently under review; other chapters of this book reflect the practice of psychiatry within the Act. A historical perspective provides the background to many contemporary issues and enriches their debate. Thus, the building of the county asylums can be seen as an enlightened move away from forms of community care which were often harsh and inhumane. The contemporary move back to community based services is because asylums themselves have become less acceptable in a changed society. The workhouse selected individuals on the basis of their ability to pay their way by working, it passed on to the asylums the hopeless cases and therefore determined the character of those institutions. It was evident, however, that society would only tolerate the relatively higher cost of the asylum if it could be seen to have a curative function. A similar relationship exists today between district psychiatric units and the area mental hospital, only the criteria for transfer have changed.

This contribution has relied greatly on the apparently authoritative statements of others and has necessarily presented a somewhat polarized view of the management of the insane. This has been to clarify the issues, and because the ever present urgency for reform makes it expedient to concentrate on the defects of a system. The process of reform is typified by a few individuals pressing for change in a society which is unconcerned, and even colludes in harmful practices. Legislation is enacted but its effectiveness is reduced because it recommends the provision of facilities, or a minimum standard of care, rather than making their establishment obligatory.

At one time it was necessary to forge a link between physical disease and mental disorder so that the established authority and responsibility of the physician could be shared by the psychiatrist. While such a union was administratively and even intellectually appealing, it is arguable that the disciplines remain ideologically dissimilar and whilst the pursuit of a strict model of medicine has advantages which are evidenced throughout this book, such a model has undeniable shortcomings which make it less than satisfactory. The social and political components of the management of the insane, whether the rate-payers who maintained county asylums or the proponents of the post-Beveridge welfare state, have always made it clear that investment can only be justified if there is a discernible benefit to the community in terms of diminishing demand. Medicine and political will have not yet effected such a diminishing demand and may indeed have contributed to its converse. At the end of the day, and in spite of all the advances and reforms outlined in this chapter, the mentally ill remain perennially stigmatized and only rarely enjoy standards of care and personal opportunity which a humane and responsible society owes them.

References

Ackerknecht, E. H. (1968). 'A Short History of Psychiatry'. Trans. S. Wolff. Hafner, New York.

Ahrenfeldt, R. H. (1958). 'Psychiatry in the British Army in the Second World War'. Routledge and Kegan Paul, London.

Allderidge, P. (1979). Hospitals, madhouses and asylums. *Br. J. Psychiat.* **134**, 321–334.

Ashdown, M., Brown, S. and Clement, A. (1953). 'Social Science and Mental Health'. Routledge and Kegan Paul, London.

Baasher, T. (1975). The Arab Countries. *In* 'World History of Psychiatry' (Ed. J. G. Howells), Chapter XIII. Brunner Mazel, New York.

Beveridge, W. (1942). 'Social Insurance and Allied Services', Cmnd. 6404. HMSO, London.

Binney, C. (1949). 'Crime and Abnormality'. Oxford University Press, Oxford.

Blacker, C. P. (1952). 'Eugenics. Galton and After'. Duckworth, London.

Bonser, W. (1963). 'The Medical Background of Anglo-Saxon England'. Wellcome Historical Medical Library, London.

Bowden, P. (1975). Liberty and psychiatry. *Br. Med. J.* **4**, 94–96.

Buckland, W. W. (1932). 'A Textbook of Roman Law from Auguste to Justinian' (2nd edn). Cambridge University Press, Cambridge.

Caesar. 'De Bello Gallico'. Trans. H. J. Edwards, 1917. Heinemann, London.

Conolly, J. (1856). 'Treatment of the Insane Without Mechanical Restraint'. Reprinted 1973. Dawsons, London.

Curran, D. (1952). Quoted in 'Psychiatry Limited'. *J. Ment. Sci.* **98**, 373–381.

Dainton, C. (1961). 'The Story of England's Hospitals'. Museum Press, London.

Deutsch, A. (1937). 'The Mentally Ill in America: A History of their Care and Treatment from Colonial Times'. Doubleday Doran and Co., New York.

Ellenberger, H. F. (1970). 'The Discovery of the Unconscious. The History and Evolution of Dynamic Psychiatry'. Allen Lane, London.

Elliot Smith, E. and Pear, T. H. (1917). 'Shell-shock and its Lessons'. Manchester University Press, Manchester.

Foucault, M. (1967). 'Madness and Civilisation'. Trans. R. Howard. Tavistock Publications, London.

Frazer, J. G. (1911). 'The Golden Bough'. Vol. II, 'Taboo and the Perils of the Soul' (3rd edn). Macmillan, London.

Gardiner Hill, R. (1839). 'A Lecture on the Management of Lunatic Asylums'. Simpkin Marshall and Co., London.

Geiss, G. (1978). Lord Hale, witches and rape. *Br. J. Law Soc.* **5**, 26–44.

Glueck, B. C. (1954). Changing concepts in forensic psychiatry. *J. Crim. Law Criminol. Police Sci.* **127**.

Gray, J. (1815). 'A History of the York Lunatic Asylum'. Hargrave and Co., York.

Hare, E. (1976). Medical astrology and its relation to modern psychiatry. *Proc. Roy. Soc. Med.* **70**, 105–110.

Henderson, D. K. (1964). 'The Evolution of Psychiatry in Scotland'. Livingstone, Edinburgh.

Howells, J. G. (1975). 'World History of Psychiatry'. Brunner Mazel, New York.

Hunter, R. and Macalpine, I. (1963). 'Three Hundred Years of Psychiatry'. Oxford University Press, Oxford.

Hunter, R. and Macalpine, I. (1974). 'Psychiatry for the Poor'. Dawsons, London.

Itard, J. (1799). The wild boy of Aveyron. *In* 'The Wolf Children and the Wild Boy of Aveyron' (1972). New Left Books, London.

Jefferson, G. (1960). René Descartes on the localisation of the soul. *In* 'Selected Papers'. Spottiswoode, Ballantyne, London.

Jones, K. (1972). 'History of the Mental Health Services'. Routledge and Kegan Paul, London.

Kaylani, W. F. (1924). 'Ogala et maganeen' (The Sane Insane) by Nayszboury. Egyptian Academic Press, Cairo.

Kraepelin, E. (1918). 'One Hundred Years of Psychiatry'. Trans. W. Baskin. Owen, London.

Lambo, T. A. (1975). Mid and West Africa. *In* 'World History of Psychiatry' (Ed. J. G. Howells), Chapter XIV. Brunner Mazel, New York.

Lancet (1955). In the mental hospital. *The Lancet*, London.

Langland, W. (1393). 'The Vision of William Concerning Piers the Plowman' (Ed. R. Attwater), Everyman No. 571 (1907). Dent, London.

Lecky, W. E. H. (1872). 'History of the Rise and Influence of the Spirit of Rationalism in Europe'. Longman Green, London.

Leonard, E. M. (1900). 'The Early History of English Poor Relief'. Cambridge University Press, Cambridge.

Lloyd, J. H. (1928). Sir Thomas Brown and the witches. *Ann. Med. Hist.* **10**, 133–134.

Lombroso, C. (1911). 'Crime: Its Causes and Remedies'. Trans. H. P. Horton. London.

Lopez Ibor, J. J. (1975). Spain and Portugal. *In* 'World History of Psychiatry' (Ed. J. G. Howells), Chapter III. Brunner Mazel, New York.

Masters, A. (1977). 'Bedlam'. Michael Joseph, London.

McMahon, C. E. (1976). The role of imagination in the disease process. *Psychol. Med.* **6**, 179–184.

Miller, L. (1975). Israel and the Jews. *In* 'World History of Psychiatry' (Ed. J. G. Howells), Chapter XXII. Brunner Mazel, New York.

Odegard, O. (1972). The future of psychiatry: predictions past and present. *Br. J. Psychiat.* **121**, 579–589.

O'Donoghue, E. G. (1914). 'The Story of the Bethlem Hospital'. Unwin, London.

Oesterreich, T. K. (1930). 'Possession, Demoniacal and Other Among Primitive Races, in Antiquity, the Middle Ages, and Modern Times'. Smith, New York.

Parry-Jones, W. L. (1972). 'The Trade in Lunacy'. Routledge and Kegan Paul, London.

Pierce, B. (1915). Absence of proper facilities for the treatment of mental disorders in their early stages. *Br. Med. J.* **1**, 41–44.

Pliny. 'Natural History, XXIV'. Trans. W. H. S. Jones, 1956. Heinemann, London.

Rao, A. V. (1975). India. *In* 'World History of Psychiatry' (Ed. J. G. Howells), Chapter XXVI. Brunner Mazel, New York.

Richards, M. (1954). 'The Laws of Hywel Dda'. Liverpool University Press, Liverpool.

Rosen, G. (1958). 'A History of Public Health'. MD Publications, New York.

Rosen, G. (1968). 'Madness in Society: Changes in the Historical Sociology of Mental Illness'. Routledge and Kegan Paul, London.

Simon, B. and Ducey, C. (1975). Ancient Greece and Rome. *In* 'World History of Psychiatry' (Ed. J. G. Howells), Chapter I. Brunner Mazel, New York.

Simon, B. and Weiner, H. (1966). Models of the mind and mental illness in Ancient Greece. *J. Hist. Behav. Sci.* **2**, 303–314.

Singer, C. (1941). 'A Short History of Science to the Nineteenth Century'. Clarendon Press, Oxford.

Singer, C. and Underwood, E. A. (1962). 'A Short History of Medicine'. Clarendon Press, Oxford.

Taylor, Lord (1962). The public, Parliament and mental health. *In* 'Aspects of Psychiatric Research' (Eds D. Richter *et al.*) Chapter 2. Oxford University Press, Oxford.

Tredgold, R. F. (1908). 'Mental Deficiency'. Balliere Tindall and Cox, London.

Tuke, S. (1813). 'Descriptions of The Retreat'. Reprinted 1964. Dawsons, London.

Varma, L. P. (1965). Psychiatry in Ayurveda. *Indian J. Psychiat.* **7**, 292.

Walker, N. (1968). 'Crime and Insanity in England'. Edinburgh University Press, Edinburgh.

West, D. and Walk, A. (1977). 'Daniel McNaughton. His Trial and Aftermath'. Headley Bros, Kent.

Whitwell, J. R. (1936). 'Historical Notes on Psychiatry'. Lewis, London.

Wooton, B. (1968). Social psychiatry and psychopathology. *In* 'Social Psychiatry' (Eds J. Zubin and F. Freyhan). Grune and Stratton, New York.

Zilborg, G. (1935). 'The Medical Man and the Witch During the Renaissance'. Baltimore.

2 The phenomenology of disordered mental function

Paul Mullen

Introduction

The practice of clinical psychiatry should involve the observation and description of the patient's mental life. This is as true for those psychiatrists who seek to uncover the meaningful connections in their patient's psyche as for those whose first aim is classification and diagnosis. The initial observations of the patient should be as uncluttered by preconception as possible. Inevitably pre-existing theory to some extent directs attention towards particular facets of perceived reality. The psychiatrist, however, should constantly guard against those prior assumptions and ideological commitments which like mere prejudice form and deform in advance the very data from whence they claim to arise.

In our everyday interactions with others we come to know them through their actions and words, our concern being rarely with their mental experiences as such. Similarly in our own lives we are concerned with the objects of our experience not the mental processes themselves. The understanding we obtain from such mundane experiences inevitably generates information which is vague and difficult to communicate. A psychology which would progress cannot base itself exclusively on such subjective comprehension, however impressive and insightful it may on occasion appear. An attempt must be made to describe, define and differentiate mental phenomena if the actual specific experience of the patient is to be represented, communicated and discussed.

This chapter will attempt to delineate and describe some of the commoner phenomena of morbid mental life. In defining these phenomena the assumptions will be both as few and explicit as possible. Hopefully this may provide a language relatively free of presupposition which can act as a vocabulary for almost any system of psychopathology. A language of classification entirely innocent of prior theory is probably unobtainable and can only be striven towards as an ideal rather than as a realizable goal. This chapter will briefly outline some of the problems attendant on the description and classification of mental experience and attempt to demonstrate how a phenomenological approach offers a possible solution.

The problem of classification

The correlation of a particular word with a particular meaning derives not from any natural divisions in reality but from convention, and any vocabulary reflects established though possibly arbitrary distinctions. When attempting to classify mental functioning, which confronts us as a continuous process, there must be a splitting off and separation of certain aspects from the totality. These divisions once made tend to be seen as real entities coming from nature, not as mere creatures of convention. Though these separations facilitate comprehension, they may also place limitations on what can be observed. Colour provides an illustration of this. The human eye can respond to a given continuum within the spectrum of light and different languages have established different divisions of that spectrum into named colours. The colour terms of one particular language cannot be brought into a one-to-one correspondence with those of any other language. Thus the spectrum of light named blue in English is subsumed under several entirely distinct terms in Russian. The richness of the language available for colour will be reflected in the subtlety with which it can be spoken about and further, in everyday situations, the degrees of difference open to conscious perception may be affected. In the language used to speak of mental function the divisions made will similarly limit not only what can be spoken about, but influence what is likely to be attended to. In the example of colour, appeal may ultimately be made to the wavelength of light measured objectively, but with the mind of others there is as yet only the subjective involved instrument of the observer's own mind with which to measure. The observer is trapped like a digital computer confronting an analog reality; to speak and reason divisions must be made but those very separations will disrupt and do violence to the reality being studied.

The problem of mind as an object of study

In a science, whatever is to be studied and spoken of must become an object for the scientist. The bacteriologist, for example, has as his object the microorganism confronting him *en masse* on the culture plate, individually under the microscope and in action in pathology. The psychopathologist in contrast can never directly contemplate his object, for the mind of the other is never an object for us and can only be apprehended in its productions such as speech, actions and writing. This is not a problem entirely unique to psychopathology, for at present the tetrahedral structure of the carbon atom can no more be observed and grasped directly than can the consciousness of another. The psychopathologist differs from the chemist in always having to rely on inspection of the productions and manifestations of his object, the mind, and never the mind itself. The psychiatrist can of course observe the actions of his patient, measure performance and monitor the physical concomitants of behaviour but if we are to go beyond the purely external phenomena and try to establish a psychology which leaves a place for the psyche then the mind of our patient must become an object of study.

The very positing of a consciousness other than my own presents profound theoretical problems for, as Merleau Ponty observed, 'the very existence of other people is a difficulty and an outrage for objective thought'. If the mind of the other is to be the object of my study it must be that the consciousness I am attempting to grasp has me as an object of its consciousness, thus placing me as an object within my object. Further, I know in a very immediate and experiential sense that I am a subject not an object in the world of another and I can reasonably assume that the other person similarly experiences himself as a subject. When I observe another person grieving, his grief does not have the same significance for me as my grief, for whereas he lives through his grief for me it is an external object of observation. To do justice to a description of his grief an attempt to place myself in the position of experiencing that grief must be made while remembering that it is always an 'as if' construction however carefully I observe and listen to the account he gives of his experience. A primary assumption of other conscious minds confronting and resisting my own must be made, despite the attendant theoretical difficulties, for without such an assumption there inevitably occurs a withdrawal into the sterile absurdities of solipsism or the gross simplification of a totally mechanistic behaviourism.

Phenomenology

The phenomenological approach which largely derives from the work of Edmund Husserl (1913) attempts to carefully describe phenomena avoiding prior theoretical commitment and taking nothing for granted. An ideal phenomenological description would delineate all those essential features of an object without which it could not be truly said to be that particular object. A phenomenological description is not simply an empirical statement, for it does not derive from a process of induction based on the observation of a series of objects, nor does it necessarily produce statements which can be confirmed or falsified by further observation. Rather phenomenology attempts to grasp the essence of an object and by reflection on a particular example to reveal its necessary features.

Phenomenology assumes that it is possible to describe things themselves, not merely to discuss the uses of words, and that it is possible to relate to and know an object in the world prior to it becoming merely words and symbols in a discourse about the world. The assumption of a concrete shared reality external to the individual consciousness which is open to observation and description may seem mere common sense. Descartes, however, defined 'me' as the thought I have of myself thus converting the certainty that there is a world into a certainty of thought about the world. Kant also argued that man never perceives reality directly and things in themselves escape him, leaving only the sensory representations he termed phenomena from which the subject synthesizes his knowledge of the world. There are current schools of thought which in the same vein would claim that the world can only be known to us insofar as we study the words used to think and speak about the world. The phenomenological method attempts to return to things themselves and here we will not be concerned with its success or failure as a philosophical argument but with some of the results of its introduction into psychiatric theory, particularly since the work of the great Karl Jaspers.

The psychiatrist as observer

The psychiatrist should bring to the observation of his patient's mental state as few theoretical preconceptions and prior prejudices as possible. He must struggle for a naïvity of vision which precludes nothing and expects nothing. This requires a constant and conscious effort to free observation from the restrictions and deformations of prejudgement. The bringing together of the observations into some conceptual framework in terms of a particular theory of psychological understanding or of diagnostic formulation should await the completion of the examination lest the emerging theories contaminate the continuing observations. In practice, of course, the unprejudiced approach is an ideal to be struggled for, a project never fully realized. The direction of our questioning is constantly influenced by previous experience and our pre-existing knowledge sadly tends to direct our attention towards certain communications and away from others. Theory may inevitably predate observation but it should not be allowed to create or totally prejudice our perceptions.

The primacy of the observed over the conceptual framework should be maintained in the recording of the mental state. A bald statement by a psychiatrist that a particular patient was deluded may not be entirely valueless, but a record of the patient's actual words on which the judgement of delusion was based contains infinitely more information. The recording of the patients' utterances when describing their psychic experiences is essential. The more skilled the history-taker the more the phenomena will emerge from the free flowing communication of the assessment interview. The novice will inevitably have to rely heavily on direct questioning but this must not be allowed to degenerate into direction, nor become an excuse for indulging in a distressing cross-examination. One insensitive specimen of a psychiatrist was overheard to commence his mental state examination of an anxious but otherwise alert intelligent old lady by yelling, 'Tell us the date mother, come on now what year is it?'. Orientation always requires assessment but the crude assumption of imbecility in a patient in the onset of an interview is not only unforgivable rudeness but it will not even produce the desired information.

Form and content

This chapter is based on the assumption that it is possible to set up as a separate area of discourse a descriptive psychology concerned with apprehending phenomena, as distinct from any explanatory psychology concerned with comprehending their origins. A split is also made in the description of the phenomena themselves where a distinction is posited between the form and the content of the phenomena. An hallucination is thus an hallucination because of the form of the experience irrespective of the content. What the voices say is just not relevant to the definition of an hallucination. The precision of the distinction between form and content possible in disorders of perception is less easy to maintain in disorders of belief. A delusion is nevertheless judged to be present more from the manner in which it is adhered to and the reason for its emergence than any aspect of content. The patient is, however, understandably more concerned with the content rather than the form of his experience. The fact of being followed and in imminent danger of succumbing to a murderous plot by the combined forces of the IRA and Free Masons tends to preoccupy the deluded subject more than reflection on the degree of conviction or amenability to reason of his belief. Similarly, it is the insults heaped on his head by the disembodied voice of his persecutor which occupies the forefront of the hallucinated persons' mind, rather than any quality of reality or emanation from objective space characterizing the voice. In seeking the details of the form of a patient's experience, due consideration for the patient's understandable preoccupation with the content and import of the event must be shown. Description of the phenomena requires form and content to be recorded but classification of individual phenomena always depends more on the form, leaving the content to become largely the source of both the doctor's and the patient's theories of meaning.

This chapter is not a catalogue of all the symptoms in psychiatry but will attempt to illustrate the phenomenological approach by a discussion of perceptual disorders and of delusion. A brief mention of obsessions and disturbed emotion will be made but in view of limited space a full discussion of these areas and of other important topics such as motivation, and motor disturbance will not be possible. Thought disorder is discussed because of the peculiar difficulties it often presents and because I suspect that the phenomenological approach cannot do justice to it but, in the absence of an applied linguistics, must struggle with it.

Abnormal phenomena

Perceptual disorders

An object may be for us a perception, a conception, or an image. In perception there occurs a sensing of an object as external to us in the real world, be it by sight, hearing, touching, or smelling. Objects are usually perceived as particular things. This is especially true of visual perceptions where, for example, if I look at a cube I tend to perceive it as a cube though at most I can only immediately apprehend three of its sides and a possibility exists, until I have examined every aspect, that it is not truly a cube. Meanings tend therefore, to be imminent in perception. Conceptions are a process of thinking where if, for example, I conceive of a cube I can think of its six sides and eight angles at once, the external world placing no limitation on my conceiving as it does on my perceiving nor presenting any threat of refutation—for the cube I conceive is always my conceived and private cube. An image is also a product of thought, but is experienced figuratively as if it were a perception. An image is experienced with the mind in subjective space and, whereas a perception confronts us in the objective world having all its sensory elements full and fresh, an image tends to occur in only one sensory modality and even then lacks the vividness of true perception.

2 Phenomenology of disordered mental function   31

Perceived objects stand bodily before us resisting and infused with a quality of reality. In that we believe what we see it is done without any verification or consideration. Traditional theories of perception introduce into perception itself intellectual operations and a critical examination of the evidence of the senses to which we in fact resort only when direct observation founders in ambiguity. Be that as it may, when examining the mental state we deal not with perceptions but in accounts of perceptions after the event, into which inevitably uncertainty, justification, and judgement have crept.

The perceptions of psychiatric patients may be altered in their intensity and quality but here the concern will be with false perceptions.

False perceptions are actual sense deceptions and imply that the experience involved is of sensing something not just believing something. The outside observer finally confirms what is or is not there. The distinction between illusions and hallucinations dates from Esquirol (1833), who held that

> a person labours under an hallucination who has a thorough conviction of a sensation when no external object suited to excite this sensation has impressed his senses, whereas it is an illusion if the senses are deceived respecting the qualities, relations, and causes of impressions actually received and cause them to form false judgements respecting their internal and external sensations.

Illusions are, therefore, distortions of real perceptions, whereas hallucinations arise without any external stimulus.

Hallucinations proper have the following characteristics:
(1) They are actual false perceptions not distortions of real perceptions.
(2) They are perceived as being in the world and as inhabiting objective space.
(3) They are perceived as having the qualities of normal perceptions being just as vivid, whole and immediate.
(4) They are experienced alongside and simultaneously with normal perceptions.
(5) They are as independent of our will as is any normal perception in that they can not be conjured up or dismissed.

The hallucination may actually show a greater independence of our will and action than a normal perception for, though I can turn away from looking at the page before me or cease attending to the droning voice of a lecturer, my hallucinations will continue to force themselves to my attention. A hallucinated voice will usually penetrate the most efficient ear muffs and one patient continued to be plagued by hallucinated voices even after he had destroyed his ear drums with needles thus reducing the rest of the world to silence.

Hallucinations do not yield to argument for the immediateness of the experience like that of normal perception permits of no doubt. This having been said, patients frequently find no difficulty in discriminating between their hallucinations and true perceptions. Hallucinations are usually confined to a single sensory modality and this or some other subtle difference from normal perception may lead the patient to awareness of the false nature of the perceptions. The ease with which hallucinations are distinguished from real perceptions in some patients is illustrated by a telephonist who, despite being troubled by constant auditory hallucinations, continued to work efficiently, unerringly distinguishing them from the disembodied voices of callers. A particular patient may, of course, suffer simultaneously from hallucinations in the modalities of touch hearing, and olfaction but they will rarely be perceived as emanating from a single entity. In fact, if a patient reports a vision which also speaks, particularly if it answers back, the most likely diagnoses are malingering or hysteria, though a temporal lobe phenomena is just possible.

Illusions differ from hallucinations in being distortions of the perception of actual objects. The perceptual stimulus arises from an actual object and the illusion is formed by the perception's transformation. The other characteristics are identical with those listed for hallucination. Illusions do, however, usually exhibit a more transient existence than hallucinations and often vanish when attention is drawn to them.

A common illusion occurs in the overwrought individual whose vision on a dark night distorts the branches blowing in the wind into a perception of an attacker moving towards them. A depressed patient out driving reported being frozen in horror at the sound of a child screaming in pain only to realize later she had misperceived the squeaking of the brakes of her own car. The patient with delirium tremens is often accosted by the transpositions of the articles around him into terrifying apparitions and illusions.

Misinterpretations are distinct from illusion for they consist of a correct perception, the import of which is incorrectly deduced. Thus shiny metal may be mistaken by the weary prospector for gold, the perception of glitter being correct, its interpretation over-hopeful. Misinterpretations frequently arise in paranoid patients where, for example, every creak and bang, though correctly perceived, may be misinterpreted as the approaching footsteps of the persecutor.

Functional hallucinations may also be confused with illusions—these are somewhat rare phenomena where an hallucination occurs simultaneously and in association with a real perception. Thus hallucinatory voices may only be heard against the background of a running and dripping tap, and when the water is turned off this will abolish the hallucination for the moment. The noise of running water in this example is not transformed or distorted into an hallucinatory voice, nor is it misinterpreted as such, for the functional hallucination is heard alongside and separable from the accompanying real perception. A colleague brought to my attention the case of a man who presented with the complaint that when out driving he was assailed by insulting voices. These voices were only to be heard at traffic lights and were confined to periods when the amber signal was on. When the lights changed to red or green the voices ceased.

Pseudohallucinations are a form of imagery distinct from hallucinations and illusions which are perceptual phenomena. Pseudohallucinations are experienced as emanating from the mind, they are seen in the mind's eye, heard with the inner ear, not perceived by the actual eyes and ears. Pseudohallucinations inhabit subjective inner space not the outside world of objects. Pseudohallucinations are the patient's own thoughts and there is a feeling of responsibility for them. Unlike the images of normal mental life the morbid pseudohallucination is not under voluntary control and though it confronts the patient as within his mind it is not there at his behest, nor will it evaporate in answer to his wishes. Inner voices are the most commonly encountered examples, often being described as voices in the head or the voice of conscience. The patient with a pseudohalluci-nation of, for example, a voice, never expects others to hear it, unlike those with true hallucinations who are often surprised nobody else can perceive them. On occasions patients are encountered with both pseudohallucinations and true hallucinations or in whom one progresses from the other, and they will often be able to distinguish the two types of phenomena, experiencing one as inhabiting their private internal world, the other the shared public world.

A patient when first seen complained that she occasionally experienced a voice which said clearly 'work' or 'pull yourself together'. This she experienced as in her mind, in the subjective world of her imagining, and she attributed it to the voice of her conscience. They were thus pseudohal-lucinations. Some time later she described voices whispering to her at night from beneath the bed and behind the curtains and though the voices were now indistinct and she could not be sure exactly what they said, she was sure they were not in her mind but were coming to her from particular locations in the outside world. In this case the patient would readily accept that the now hallucinated voices were due to something having gone wrong with her mind but nevertheless experienced them as true perceptions. In this particular case the hallucinations became pro-gressively more prominent and clearly enunciated and she was finally assailed by voices emanating from various points around her room laugh-ing, talking about her and instructing her on how she should behave.

In the literature there is an unfortunate tendency to classify all halluci-nated voices which are experienced as coming from some part of the patient's own body as pseudohallucinations. This arises from a confusion between the subjective internal space of the mind and the space internal to the body, and though our own bodies can at times be perceived as both part of subjective space and as objects confronting us in the world, these two elements are not identical. A voice emanating from a patient's kneecap with all the characteristics of a true perception is a hallucination not a pseudohallucination in just the same way as a burb or a borborigma is an auditory perception not an image in the mind of its embarrassed originator. Thoughts experienced as being read aloud are similarly not pseudohallucinations if the thoughts are alienated from the individual and become an auditory perception confronting him as part of the external reality.

A problem is created by patients like the one cited earlier who say they know the voices or visions are in their mind thus indicating that they have insight into the morbid nature of their experience. In such a case it is important to distinguish whether the phenomena was experienced as a perception from objective space or really was an image within subjective space. It is absurd from a phenomenological point of view to call hallucinations pseudohallucinations simply because the patient has insight into their morbid nature, for this is to make the classification of a perceptual disorder dependent on the patient's judgement at the moment of being interviewed and not on the nature of the experiences themselves. Further, the argument that judgement is part of perception does not accord with experience where we know by what we perceive and only in the rare event of perception floundering in ambiguity is perception questioned and judged. The problem in practice is that the hallucinated patient is often doing just this by questioning and doubting his own perceptions. Further, the account of the experience is normally long after the event, by which time judgement has in fact crept in.

The relatively detailed discussion of pseudohallucinations is necessary because it is at the boundary between image and perception that many of the essential features of hallucinations as well as pseudohallucinations can be grasped. The clinical significance of such a distinction is a strictly empirical question, not a phenomenological one.

There are other forms of imagery which deserve a brief mention. *Eidetic images*, which are perfectly normal phenomena most frequently encountered in children, are images of something once perceived which can be conjured up with almost all the original details intact. Thus a page of a book previously read may be recalled as an image so vivid that the eidetic person can read out the text as from the original. *After images* are simply the persistence of a retinal impression after the subject looks away from the object. The commonest example is the persistence of a perception of a light after looking away. (Note—image here refers strictly to a perception, not a product of thought, and is only sanctioned by common usage.) *Pareidolia*, another common and normal phenomena, are the images conjured up by ill-defined sense impressions such as those which occur when staring into the dying embers of an open fire.

Perceptual disorders occur in all forms of psychotic disturbance, in disturbed states of consciousness and in normal individuals. During that phase which intervenes between the waking state and sleep many people are particularly vulnerable to experiencing illusions and hallucinations. The hallucinations on falling asleep are termed hypnogogic, and those on awakening hypnopompic. In the grief which follows a bereavement, hallucinations and pseudohallucinations of the lost one are a common and normal phenomena. In situations of extreme stress, be it physical or emotional, where high levels of general arousal pertain perceptual disturbances tend to become more frequent, albeit fleetingly. Sensory deprivation procedures have produced a wide variety of perceptual abnormalities including organized hallucinatory experiences in experimental subjects. A variety of organic states are associated with perceptual disturbance and any major disruption of cerebral function can produce such phenomena usually in association with the clouded consciousness of a confusional state. Meaningful auditory and visual hallucinations are particularly associated with temporal lobe dysfunction and it has been claimed that they may actually be produced in some subjects by direct stimulation at or near the temporal lobe. Hallucinogenic drugs induce a wide range of perceptual disturbance, the form and content of which tend to be in constant flux unlike the hallucinatory disturbances of schizophrenia, and in distinction to those of the functional psychosis they are predominantly visual in character. Dreams are obviously a related phenomena but they will not be considered here for reasons of space and because their significance as phenomena as opposed to repositories of meaning have been little considered by psychopathologists.

Certain modes of hearing voices were held by Kurt Schneider to be of special diagnostic importance in schizophrenia. The hearing of one's own thoughts read aloud, voices talking one with another and voices that maintain a running commentary on the patient's thoughts and actions were considered first rank symptoms.

Hallucinations of a somatic type need careful attention. If the patient has a somatic hallucination such as a strange tingling he may say it is due to rays directed upon him or 'as if' there were some electrical current. The sufferer from disseminated sclerosis may similarly describe a true paraesthesia as if it were an electrical current (Lhermitte's Sign). Care must therefore always be exercised to distinguish odd ways of expressing true sensory disturbances from the delusional elaborations of false perceptions. Further, it is wise not to forget that a bizarre interpretation particularly of a somatic sensation in a schizophrenic may mask the symptom of a physical disorder. The distinction between somatic hallucinations and somatic illusions raises considerable problems as to the status of perceptions arising from excitation within the central nervous system. Somatic hallucinations may occur on the basis of localized brain dysfunction as in the aura of epilepsy. In one epileptic patient the strange abdominal sensations which preceded the fit were perceived by him as writhing movements which he delusionally misinterpreted as snakes squirming around in his belly.

Delusions

A delusion is an abnormal belief. Delusions arise from disturbed judgements in which the experience of reality becomes a source of new and false meanings.

Delusions usually have attributed to them the following characteristics:

(1) they are held with absolute conviction;
(2) they are experienced as self-evident truths usually of great personal significance;
(3) they are not amenable to reason or modifiable by experience;
(4) their content is often fantastic or at best inherently unlikely;
(5) the beliefs are not shared by those of a common social and cultural background.

These characteristics are not, however, sufficient in themselves to entirely separate delusions as a class of phenomena from non-pathological beliefs and convictions.

The absolute conviction in the truth of one's beliefs is clearly not confined to the deluded subject. Further, the deluded patient may on occasion paradoxically combine an apparent total certainty with, at another level, an awareness of the delusional nature of his beliefs. This double book-keeping is illustrated by the patients who of their own volition come to psychiatrists to tell of their divine mission rather than to the relevant ecclesiastical body.

The imperviousness of a delusion to modification by reason or experience in no way distinguishes it from much common error and opinion. Logical error is not the exclusive hallmark of delusion nor sadly is the failure to expose beliefs to the test of critical appraisal confined to the mad. The errors of most normal individuals, however, are those common to their social group and take their origin from shared misconceptions. The errors of the deluded patient tend to be idiosyncratic in the extreme. Their origin is often to be sought in some as yet little-understood disruption and change of mental function which fundamentally alters the patient's knowledge of the world. The failure of the deluded subject to change his opinion when faced by contrary argument should perhaps occasion no surprise for our own mistaken beliefs recede more before the changing structure of our environment, wrought by the slow passage of time, than they do before mere reason.

The subject's delusions often appear to have great personal significance but the extent to which they direct actions is extremely variable. The grandiose delusions in the sufferer with GPI or the extensive system of beliefs to be found in many chronic schizophrenics seem often to effect the patient's behaviour not a whit. The delusions in affective psychoses perhaps somewhat more often call forth behaviour consistent with the beliefs. The manic, for example, may well act on his convictions, spending money he does not have, entering into impossibly ambitious projects and offering his unsolicited advice to all.

The content of delusions is often fantastic but then inherently unlikely notions are not unknown even among psychiatrists. The beliefs shared by those of a similar social and cultural background, particularly in the areas of theology, are excluded from the rubric of delusions however extraordinary their content.

Delusions may on rare occasion, perhaps largely by virtue of the play of chance, be true. The potentially correct delusion is most commonly encountered in morbid jealousy. A patient, for example, had the infidelity of his wife conclusively revealed to him one Christmas Eve when he returned home from work and noted that the lights on the festive tree in his front window were flashing on and off in synchrony with those of his neighbour's tree. The actual nature of the wife's relationship to this particular neighbour is not critical to the phenomenological analysis of this belief as a delusion, though it may, of course, be relevant to speculations about meaning. The way in which a belief emerges and the reasons for its acceptance are therefore part of its characterization as a delusion.

Delusions are not dependent on any defect in the patient's intelligence nor simple disruption of the faculties for reason and logical thought. An intelligent and articulate individual who becomes deluded will put these abilities to the service of the delusion and a luxuriant growth of bizarre ideas may result which are argued and defended with all the subject's usual mental agility. The memoirs of Schreber provide an excellent example of this.

Delusions are pathologically falsified judgements. They can be divided into those judgements that arise in an understandable way from particular interactions or experiences and those which appear *de novo* like sudden intuitions or brain waves. Those delusions where no connection can be comprehended between the emergence of the belief and a discernible event and which confront the observer as something absolute and irreducible are termed primary or occasionally autochthonous* delusions.

Jaspers observes that in these primary delusions there occurs an experience radically alien to the healthy person which comes before thought, although it becomes clear to itself only in thought. The primary delusion thus emerges in the context of a radical change or break in the normal mental function and is indicative of a process at work. The primary delusion is thus assumed to be an eruption of an extra conscious process into the normal flow of intentional mental life. The primary delusion cannot be fully explained by an appeal to the meaningful connections which usually govern the stream of consciousness. On the contrary it is an ultimately irreducible phenomena not amenable to psychological understanding and only explicable finally in terms of the causal connections governing the presumed organic changes in brain. Clearly this is an untestable hypothesis at present. It does not, of course, imply that the content of a primary delusion has no connection with the patient's past life or present situation; it merely claims that the emergence of the belief and part at least of its initial content will not be amenable to such an analysis. Once the primary delusion is established, the further elaboration of the delusional system will in principle be open to an analysis in terms of its meaningful connections.

An example of a primary delusion is a patient who, on asking a friend for a light for his cigarette, was passed a box of matches on which appeared the slogan 'the greatest match in the world'. This revealed to the patient in a moment of intensely experienced insight that he was the light of the world. This delusional brainwave made sense for the patient of many of his recent experiences and much of his prior life; he realized his failures had been trials, his rejections, persecutions and his sexual inadequacy part of divine inspiration. A totally new perspective on the world overthrowing most of his previous concepts came with this revelation.

Secondary delusions or delusion-like ideas emerge understandably from other psychic events or the subject's interaction with the world. Their origin can be traced to affects, drives, fears or some devastating personal experience. They are, therefore, amenable at least theoretically to analysis in terms of the meaningful connections of psychic life. A morbid alteration in a subject's mood may, for example, if it is towards elation, precede the emergence of delusions of grandeur or, conversely, a depressive swing may be followed by delusions of poverty or guilt. The hallucinated subject's perverted senses may be the starting point of a delusional development as may some real experience of injustice in a

---

* Autochthonous—original; springing new from the land itself.

paranoid personality. A suspicious prickly individual with a propensity to self-reference was exposed to a series of personal disasters including loss of job, loss of money and loss of his home following mortgage foreclosure. The events (partly self-induced) were explained by him initially as due to a generally ill-disposed world towards a man of his obvious but unrecognized talents. As he continued to ruminate on the events, a pattern became more and more obvious to him. Slowly over a period of many months a delusional system involving a complex plot by members of his family in league with the local constabulary and public health officials emerged. This delusional system became the focal point of his life, dominating from then onwards his thoughts and actions. The slow emergence of this secondary delusional system was in the context of immense personal stress, probably associated with an unrecognized depressive mood swing occurring in a person with a paranoid personality structure.

Overvalued ideas form an intermediary group on the borders of normal beliefs and secondary delusions. They are isolated convictions understandable in the context of the person's personality and life experiences which, because of a strongly associated affect, become intensely identified with and are persisted in despite what to others appears overwhelming evidence of their falsity. A man became convinced he had lost his job because he had become privy to a fraud occurring in a government department. For years afterwards he attempted to obtain redress for his wrongful dismissal and to bring to attention the supposed financial scandal. This idea, initially plausible, was pursued long after it was demonstrated to be incorrect, his actions having actually brought about extensive investigations to no avail. Although the idea was never generalized to involve and explain other areas of his life it remained an intense preoccupation and an object of immense emotional investment. He led a perfectly normal life, held conventional views on the ideas of the day, himself and his surroundings, and it was only this one idea which if touched on, however indirectly, brought forth an outpouring of anger and complex accusation. He accepted the possibility of his being mistaken but when confronted with actual evidence of his error, would resort to convoluted arguments why this particular information could be disregarded. His overvalued idea remained, therefore, for him a virtual certainty never an absolute conviction.

Primary delusions may on occasion emerge against the background of the so-called delusional atmosphere or delusional mood. The delusional mood encountered typically in the early stages of an acute schizophrenic break, is characterized by an altered experience of the world where in some intangible way events take on an odd quality and an uncanny tension. Perceptions seem to hint at personal significance, the nature of which remains just out of grasp. There is usually a sense of foreboding or even frank fear, though just occasionally the patient may be in an ecstatic state. The delusional mood may progress to a state where the objects and events around the subject become infused with a deep personal significance, the world becoming replete with meaning. In this latter stage ideas or delusions of reference abound. An idea of reference occurs where objects or events are experienced as having some direct message or import, this meaning coming as an immediate experience indissolubly linked to the perception, not as part of some subsequent interpretation.

Ideas of reference have a formal similarity to the primary delusional experience, but whereas the primary delusion ushers in a global modification of the patient's view of the world, the idea of reference is a far more circumscribed event. Occasionally the reader may come across reference to a delusional perception; this is closely akin to a primary delusion but with a more clearly defined two-stage structure. In the true delusional perception there is a true perception from which there follows as a second stage a delusional insight into the nature of reality. Here again it is the extent of the restructuring of the patient's beliefs and the depth of the scandal of logic which differentiates it from the more modest idea of reference.

Delusion is often regarded as the basic characteristic of madness. The immediate and intrusive knowledge of meaning is central to the experience of a primary delusion. The attribution of meaning in both primary and secondary delusion is not confined to any particular area of psychic function but may arise in association with perceptions, ideas, memories or even the general awareness of the world. Delusion represents a profound and complex disorganization of mental life stretching way beyond mere false ideas and mistaken beliefs.

Passivity phenomena

Passivity experiences are a group of phenomena disparate in many ways but having in common the patient's experience of some alien control or interference with his thinking, feeling, acting or perceiving. They are connected with a disturbed sense of the integrity of the self and a belief in having fallen under outside influences. They are sometimes referred to as disturbances of ego boundaries because of the associated experience of the unity of the self being broken down or violated.

Thought withdrawal and thought insertion are passivity phenomena where the patient experiences an interference with his thinking such that thoughts are put into or taken from his mind by some alien force. A patient said, 'It [a machine] keeps putting these thoughts in my mind;

they're not mine, it makes me think them', and another that, 'They steal my thoughts—I can't do anything because they keep taking the ideas out of my mind'. The patient may also experience the breaking down of the boundaries between self and others with the experience of his mind being read or his thoughts broadcast. One patient complained his innermost thoughts and fantasies were known by everyone and that the BBC was publicizing them without his permission; another said he could not see the point in talking to me because he knew that when he thought something, everyone knew about it. Yet another had the conviction that his thoughts were shared simultaneously by everyone around him. The patient may also be convinced he can read others' minds and is privy to everyone's innermost secrets.

Actions may be experienced as made or caused by outside forces. A patient who believed herself to be the victim of persecution by a race of malevolent aliens she called 'fantasias' explained that they caused her arms and legs to twitch and made her carry out silly actions like kicking her legs in the air and jumping up and down; this she claimed was accomplished by rays which controlled her brain by 'dementing' it.

Emotional states are less frequently experienced as imposed by external agencies, and in this area it is perhaps more usual for the patient to complain of being robbed of feeling or to have had his affective responses blocked by alien influence than to have new emotions imposed.

Obsessional and compulsive phenomena

An obsessional phenomena is a thought, feeling or urge arising from within the individual which persistently intrudes into consciousness despite the subject's resistance to it and the awareness that it is senseless or at the very least senselessly insistent. This definition as it stands does not distinguish obsessional phenomena from impulses and desires which though persistent may be resisted by an individual because they offend, for example, his moral sensibilities. Rejected impulses and resisted desires are, after all, the trivia of everyday life. Obsessional and compulsive phenomena are morbid only in their abnormal intensity and persistence. In the obsessional patient there is a ubiquitous consciousness of the intrusive phenomena and though the sufferer recognizes the groundlessness of the anxiety it remains an incessant preoccupation.

The term 'compulsion' is traditionally confined to motor acts and obsessions to impulses and thoughts. This distinction is often not adhered to and is of no great import.

Obsessional thinking may involve ideas or take a more concrete form in haunting images and persistent tunes. An example is provided by a patient who every time he drove his car became obsessed with the fear that he had knocked down a child and although he knew rationally no such event had occurred and tried desperately to resist the idea, it continually intruded into his thinking. He could not prevent himself carrying out the associated compulsion to check with police and hospitals and even walk back over the route looking for evidence of an accident. The compulsive act is, as here, usually secondary to the obsessional thought. Similarly compulsive hand-washing often arises from an obsessional thought of contamination. Obsessional ruminations are ideas or images which repeatedly enter consciousness despite the attempt to concentrate on something else to prevent their dominance of the thinking.

An obsession or compulsion, however repugnant or absurd it may appear to the sufferer, is always recognized as a subjective event and though unchosen is 'of them'. This is in contrast to a true passivity phenomena which is experienced as totally alien and imposed from outside. The patient's resistance to the obsession and recognition of its morbid nature is frequently put forward as the essential feature of this group of phenomena. This is true to the extent that a false belief considered by the patient to be true and self-evident and which, far from being resisted, was made part of the patient's view of reality, would be more like a delusional than an obsessional belief. In some patients, however, the resistance to an obsession fluctuates and on occasion they may appear to be convinced of the truth of the obsessional belief or of the necessity for the compulsive act. This should not lead the phenomena to be considered other than an obsession unless the loss of resistance becomes not an occasional but the constant feature of the experience.

The performance of compulsive urges often takes on highly ritualized forms. The complexity may increase until it disrupts the actual performance and this may in itself lead to anxiety and repetition. The doing and undoing aspect of the performance of compulsive rituals is often prominent with, for example, an intricate manoeuvre being carried out in one direction and then equally carefully carried out in reverse. The speech of some obsessional patients and those with marked obsessional personality traits may show a statement followed by partial retraction followed by retraction of part of the first retraction, etc., the curious to-ing and fro-ing continuing endlessly.

Emotion

The descriptive phenomenology of emotions tends to be somewhat confused and unsatisfactory. Strings of more or less appropriate adjectives are all too often substituted for description of the concrete experience.

Emotions are often conceived as psychic events with an intangible elusive quality which infuse our experiences. They are described in terms of subjective ineffable agitations, a flux of inexpressible qualities occurring independently and prior to the world of things. Emotions are, in short, presented as without objects, being that which orientates and directs judgements and perceptions rather than arising from those experiences. Satre (1966) called this approach a solipsism of affectivity and he insisted that there are no affective states which attach themselves to objects but always feelings about objects. Without the experience of some perception, conception or image, there are no emotions, for they are the 'inseparable accidents' of other mental events. If I have an emotion of love, it is love of someone or something and it is the charms of the beloved which I am aware of, not the dissociated experience of being in love. An emotional state such as sadness could, of course, become an object for consciousness, an abstraction on which it is possible to reflect, but as soon as it becomes an experience of sadness it is sadness about something.

There is a problem which arises when confronted by the pathological emotional states. The individual in the throes of a depressive illness presents the appearance of a morbid mood state occurring as a primary event which apparently forms, deforms and creates his awareness of himself and his world. It is perhaps on this very element of mood preceding experience that the concept of a morbid emotion rests. This dissociation between an emotional response and any sufficient precipitating experience is often what is said to characterize affective illness. The morbid emotional state colours the sufferer's experience of the world and in depression, for example, events however intrinsically cheering often become the source of further gloom and self-recrimination.

The terminology used to speak of the emotions is complicated as several common usages often attach to each word and every psychopathologist seems bent on introducing his own personal and technical meaning. Feelings, for example, in common parlance can refer to sensations, beliefs, presentiments, consideration for others, as well as emotional states. Depression is commonly used synonomously with sadness but some psychiatrists would confine its use to a morbid process. Affect usually refers to an intensive emotional process but in the term affective illness for a sustained and complex disturbance of mood. Mood tends to refer to the emotional tone predominating at a given moment and a mood state suggests a more lasting disposition. These kinds of distinctions are at best somewhat blurred, perhaps reflecting the phenomena themselves.

In classifying abnormal emotional states a distinction is often made between those which emerge in a comprehensible fashion from some experience and those which defeat understanding, appearing to arise as irreducible primary phenomena. The criteria of understandability is always a difficult one, particularly as some psychiatrists seem quite convinced that their own psychological understanding stretches into the innermost depths of all experiences to which man is heir. The distinction thus depends on a certain modesty in claims to understanding.

Emotional states may be profoundly affected by physical illness as in the general *malaise* of fever or the fear associated with anginal pain or bronchospasm. Mood disorders on the other hand may be accompanied by, or even present as, complaints about disturbed body function. Kurt Schneider considered that misery referred to some part of the body, as when patients complain of sadness like a pressure in the chest, or loneliness like a gnawing emptiness of the stomach, was particularly characteristic of depressive illness. In hypochondria an underlying disturbance of mood is common and in the elderly depressive preoccupations and even delusions about bodily disturbance are frequent. The type of delusion to the effect that their insides are blocked up, their brain is rotting away or their blood has dried up is often referred to as a nihilistic delusion. Strictly, however, this term should be confined to those beliefs involving a total denial of particular aspects of the world, as in a conviction of having no body or being already dead.

In depression the feelings of misery are often demonstrated by facial expression and bodily attitude as well as verbally. The characteristic physiognomy of the melancholic has the facial lines running down and outwards from the furrowed brow to the drooping mouth. The body may be generally flexed and the hands are often wrung. In some patients there is a state of purposeless agitation while in others there occurs a slowing, sometimes to the point of immobility. Occasionally the severe depressive may sit bent forward on a chair rocking to and fro for hours like a deprived infant. Weeping, sighing and brief expostulations of distress such as 'Oh dear' or 'God help me', are not uncommon in depression. It is always worth remembering that the degree to which the misery of depression is given overt expression is very variable between different cultures, classes and even individuals within particular social groupings. The expression of even profound depression may be contained and emerge only in behavioural changes, for example, decreased coping or increased drinking, or may be hidden under a fixed mask of shallow gaiety as in the smiling depressive.

Apathy is a passive indifference to the world where the subject evinces no emotional response. A dullness and loss of interest is complained of and the sufferer is in a state where nothing pleases and little even distresses. A superficially similar but distinct phenomenon is exhibited by the individual who complains of having lost all feeling. Here there is an active distress at the experiencing of the self as without the capacity to respond emotionally.

There sometimes appears to be unattached or free-floating emotions as if feelings were in search of an object. Anxiety may confront us as a primary phenomenon colouring all the patient's thoughts and actions with no clear precipitants or attachments but the semblance of existing prior to any object. Anxiety, it must be remembered, is a common and normal response when connected to a feared situation. It may also be part of a phobia, for example where the response to it is out of all proportion to the danger presented but remains connected to the phobic object or situation. Happiness may also on occasion present as an apparently primary phenomenon dissociated from any casual experience or object as with the exulted and ebullient mood state encountered in some manics. Ecstatic states may also occur in mania and other psychotic states and are often associated with some sense of spiritual revelation, though ecstasy in the normal individual is more likely to be strictly carnal.

Disturbance of language and thought

Thought can never be directly observed. The attempt to study it must, therefore, rely on language in the form of speech, writing or other symbolic creation. The entrenched tradition of speaking of thought disorder when actually confronted with disturbed language rests on the assumption that language directly mirrors thought.

Speech disorder is usually separated from language and thought disorder. It is confined to disturbance in the actual articulation due to a disruption with the mechanics of speaking. Stuttering is a typical example and the lalling speech of cerebellar dysfunction would be another. A distinction between language as a system of symbol and sign formation and thought as the content and import of those symbols and signs is occasionally made. Thus, employing this division, thought disorder would include delusions and other disturbances of the content of thought. In this section we will be concerned with disturbance of language.

The structure of language can be analysed in terms of semantics, which concerns itself with meaning, and of syntax, which is the rules governing the combination of words to form sentences. In most of the language disorders observed clinically by the psychiatrist, the disorder is in the area of meaning, the semantics rather than the syntax—the latter only being significantly disrupted in the most florid forms of psychotic speech. Meaning lies not only in the words used but just as importantly in the situational context of the utterances. Statements occur in particular spatiotemporal situations, which include speaker and hearer, the actions they are performing and various external objects and events. Further, a shared knowledge of what has been said earlier and its relationship to current statements is assumed.

In an ideal language one word or sign would exist for one meaning. In practice there are many synonyms where a particular meaning is designated by several distinct words (e.g. hide, conceal, secrete) and frequent homonyms where single words signify more than one meaning (bank of river, Bank of England, trunk of elephant, trunk—a piece of luggage). Words may also be used literally or metaphorically (a man's head, the head of a company, a glaring light, a glaring error). In the language disorders encountered by psychiatrists there may be semantic disruption arising from a confusion of homonym, synonym and metaphor. A patient at a ward round, for example, when asked if the pills were making him better, replied: 'Healed? I have no heels' (glancing at the bottom of his slippers) 'I'm only brought to heel'. The word healed is employed as a synonym for getting better, then confused with its homonym, the heel of a shoe, and in this example the metaphorical use of heel is employed to produce a nice resolution which allows the patient to comment on his resentment at being compulsorily detained. Bleuler reports a patient who, when asked if anything was weighing heavily on his mind replied: 'Yes, iron is heavy'. A patient in a group asked if he was down, immediately left saying: 'Yes, he needed to lie down'. This taking of the literal rather than the metaphorical use of words was referred to by Goldstein as concrete thinking, though whether it is truly a preference for the concrete sense or just a tendency to associate to the commonest usage of a particular word is uncertain.

A word may be chosen in language disorder not because of its relationship to the meaning of the utterance but because of an association of sound to a previous word or phrase. Thus, 'I feel like going out, stout, a drink would be nice, ice, I suppose I'll stay, lay down for a while', or, 'Everybody seems to revolve around me, involve and resolve around me.' This is termed clang association and occurs in the flight of ideas of the manic and in schizophrenic speech disorder.

Words may be invented in language disorders. These idiosyncratic words of no generally agreed significance are termed neologisms. They may consist of entirely new words, which even the patient may be hard pressed to explain, or be created by compressing or running together existing words. A patient referred to a 'mongery ridicule', and although he could spell the word, the only definition he offered was that it 'wasn't quite nice'. In this example the phonetic or sound structure is acceptable for a word in English. On occasion sounds entirely foreign to English phonetics will be emitted apparently as words. An example of a word created by condensing existing terms is 'amisachrist', which was used by a patient to describe a psychiatrist who misunderstood him (a mistaken psychiatrist). Jaspers suggested neologisms may arise from the patient's struggle to express unique and essentially incommunicable experiences.

Idiosyncratic similes and metaphors may be encountered. A schizophrenic patient of Bleuler announced her forthcoming pregnancy with 'I hear a stork clapping in my body'. A patient of mine replied to the enquiry about his religious views with 'I'm for the elected by a puff of smoke from the chimney', referring obliquely to the process which heralds the election of a new Pope in the Roman Catholic Church.

Words, phrases and occasionally syllables seem to recur far more frequently in the language of the schizophrenic than in normals. This is in part connected to the phenomena of stereotypy and perseveration. It is usually easily distinguished from the perseveration of coarse organic brain disease where identical words and phrases tend to be simply repeated. In the schizophrenic it manifests as a repeated use of similar words and phrases in different contexts. An extreme example is provided by a patient who, when asked if he understood a question, replied: 'I see something like I might be wrong like but there like the rules and I don't like the rules turned upside-down and I don't know like and I was like as though the bed turned over.' A patient reported by Kraeplin would, when writing home to relatives, fill pages with similar words or phrases presented in varying orders interminably. A more restricted vocabulary is also said to be found in the language-disordered schizophrenic than in normals of a similar educational and intellectual background. The frequent repetition involves syllables and phrases as well as words, so the problem is more likely to stem from a tendency for the same speech elements to intrude repeatedly into the language rather than just a restricted repertoire of words.

The meaning of language depends not only on the particular words but, as has been mentioned, the context of the utterance. In normal speech there is a tacit acceptance by speaker and hearer of all relevant conventions, beliefs and presuppositions of the common speech community. The disruption of context and the lack of sufficient connection between successive phrases is shown by a patient who wrote: 'I want to leave the trees are beautiful if only the food too long love.' In a single sentence the desire for discharge, the gardens, the food and a greeting are all combined. There is a failure to keep separate ideas which are unconnected and the patient's preoccupations are all jumbled together into a single statement. A patient replying to an enquiry as to how he felt, included the following:

> It doesn't really matter if you eat refined sugar as long as you can balance it by doing something else you or using your energy expending your energy in the best manner possible and I would really like to become a DJ you know I have a high sort of ambition this is why I would like a cigarette now. That's all.

Here preoccupation with diet, physical fitness, job ambitions and the desire for a cigarette become included in a response to a routine enquiry about health. This tendency was described as over-inclusion by Cameron (see Kasamin, 1944) because the patient is unable to prevent subsidiary and peripheral thoughts intruding and becoming included in the statement. A young librarian in the early stages of a psychotic episode was asked to reorganize the Divinity section of the library's filing system. This resulted in a total restructuring of the index with everything re-catalogued under Divinity. The young man had included all topics under Divinity, not from some insight into the ubiquitous nature of God, but from an inability to separate any category from any other, thus including all in one. Here over-inclusion was demonstrated in action, not speech.

The concept of redundancy has been borrowed from information theory and applied specifically to schizophrenic language disorder. Redundancy used in this technical sense refers to the likelihood that a particular word or letter will occur. The more predictable the word or letter is, the greater the redundancy, in that it conveys less information. (Information is being used here for a new unit of information irrespective of its utility or even meaning.) Normal language has a high degree of redundancy in that many of the words and phrases are predictable to a high level of certainty from the context. In the schizophrenic the disruption of the context of the language and the reduced consistency and coherence within the expression of ideas leads to a decreased predictability of the words and thus to decreased redundancy. A word salad, for example, where there is a total breakdown in the contextual restraints and words follow each other apparently at random has no redundancy, for no given word can be predicted in advance from any preceding word or phrase; each word comes as total surprise, free of the limitations of semantics or syntax. Experiments based on the redundancy concept have demonstrated that observers provided with transcripts of normal speech and schizophrenic speech with every fifth word deleted, can correctly fill in the missing word significantly more often from the normal speech confirming the decreased redundancy in the schizophrenic utterances. In related experiments it was suggested that speech disordered schizophrenics are themselves less able to utilize contextual clues and redundancy in learning written passages.

Thought-blocking is evinced by a sudden stopping in mid-sentence, despite the subject's desire to continue speaking; after a pause the flow of speech may recommence, perhaps on some unrelated topic. There may be a perplexed silence and a complaint that their thoughts have been removed, stolen, blocked or have disappeared. This phenomena can be quite dramatic in some schizophrenic patients and may be accompanied by considerable subjective distress. Blocking in the context of other signs of schizophrenic speech disorder is of diagnostic importance. When it occurs as an isolated event, however, it is easily confused with the non-specific phenomena of losing the train of one's thoughts which occurs in normals particularly when tired or under stress and as part of the speech retardation of depressive states. The presence of schizophrenic language disorder should not be assumed on the basis of thought-blocking alone.

The clinical psychiatrist most frequently observes disturbance of language in the flight of ideas of the manic and the schizophrenic language disorder, often referred to as formal thought disorder. This being so, this section will continue by discussing these two specific symptom complexes.

Flight of ideas is encountered in disturbances characterized by the elevation of mood, hypomania, mania and delirious mania, but is also mimicked by some organic brain syndromes, by one's more loquatious or intoxicated companions, and it can even appear in relatively pure form in some subjects, who on other criteria would be considered undoubtedly schizophrenic. There is an accelerated tempo of speech often referred to as 'pressure of talk'. In addition to the increased rate of delivery, the language employed is characterized by a wealth of associations, many of which seem to be evoked by more or less accidental connections. The relationship between statements is disrupted by this chaos of association and the progress of speech ceases to be guided by the unfolding of a train of thought and comes under the influence of this plethora of new connections. The excited speech wanders off the point following the arbitrary connections, and the coherent progress of ideas tends to become obscured. The somewhat haphazard verbal associations become governed by sound, rhyme, associations to peripheral concepts, double entendre, etc. In classical flight of ideas, although the connections and associations are accidental or peripheral to the general sense of the statement, they are usually in themselves fairly obvious and unremarkable and would individually be acceptable in other situations. This is in stark contrast to schizophrenic language disorder where the individual connections are often so opaque and personalized as to defy comprehension in any situation. Clang associations and puns are frequent. One manic patient I encountered attempted to speak exclusively in blank verse interspersed with long recitals from nineteenth century poets.

In flight of ideas a wide range of unusual connections drive on the rapid speech and the listener is often borne along by the flow and may even share in the amusement and pleasure the patient derives from the novel associations. The patient exhibiting flight of ideas often expresses a subjective sense of his thoughts racing and of new ideas forcing themselves on his attention.

In schizophrenic language disorder the most striking disturbances lie in the area of semantics, though in advanced forms the syntax may also be disrupted. Bleuler (1950) considered the disturbance of association to be a fundamental symptom of schizophrenia which led to a disruption of the threads which guide thinking. He considered that ideas fortuitously encountered were combined in a manner dependent on incidental circumstance rather than any train of thought. The associations between one phrase and the next, though comprehensible, may be guided not by a coherent stream of thought but by trivial or almost totally irrelevant connections. A patient when asked where she lived, replied: 'I come from Somerset. Somerset is a lovely place, everyone stops up that way, you know, before they go back home for the weekend. I'm home on my weekends but I was never really satisfied with myself nor my schoolwork.'

Clang associations, condensations and stereotypy, evinced by a tendency to return again and again to a single theme, characterize the language of schizophrenics. Bleuler considered that the language disorder of schizophrenia could vary from a barely detectable disturbance to a high degree of associational disturbance manifesting as a total confusion of words. In schizophrenia he noted:

> Thinking operates with ideas and concepts which have no, or a completely insufficient connection with the main idea and should therefore be excluded from the thought process; the result is that thinking becomes confused, bizarre, incorrect and abrupt.

Kurt Schneider considered that disjointed, fragmented and inconsequential thought was not uncommonly manifested in the speech of schizophrenics. However, he pointed out that milder degrees of such disturbance were not uncommon in normal people and this being so, however important these thought disorders might be for the theoretical definition of schizophrenia, they could not, in practice, hold much weight as diagnostic features. In ambiguous cases he held it was too difficult to pin down such phenomena as unmistakable schizophrenic symptoms, and in florid examples other more reliable diagnostic signs would be present.

Karl Schneider, in contrast, gave considerable attention to these phenomena in his 'Psychologie der Schizophrenen' (1930). He considered schizophrenic language to be characterized by:

(1) an interweaving or bringing together of heterogenous elements (fusion);
(2) a mixing and muddling up of actual definite but heterogenous elements (substitution);
(3) a snapping-off of the chain of thought (omission);

(4) the disruption of the thought content with insertion of other thought contents in place of the true chain of thought (derailment).

These disturbances can give rise to various types of thought disorder. Transitory thinking is characterized by derailments and omissions in the train of thought by which both the semantics and syntax may be disrupted. A patient, asked about whether she had trouble with her thinking replied:

> Well I'm just [long pause] No. I feel at ease but there's too many people and too many [pause] car accidents and it's too overcrowded here and I can't [pause]. This is going on all around the world, you know, it's [pause] It [pause]. A lot of bad smoke along this [laughs].

Drivelling thinking occurs where there is a mixing and muddling of the thoughts (substitution) which obscures the meaning. In drivelling, the listener may obtain an initial impression that something meaningful is being said but soon realizes that it is a flow of words and high-sounding phrases signifying little or nothing. A patient who talked at great length with slow ponderous and heavily accentuated speech included the following in a monologue:

> In other words you said that you were coming and I said to myself and I dismissed it from my thoughts. I suppose it wasn't exactly forgetting that she would be appearing but not to stress this all the time that he just wanted to come home and I was foolish over money and what have you, and you see now I could talk to him about that.

In desultory thinking the syntax is preserved but ideas force their way into the main theme, bringing together heterogenous elements (fusion) which expressed separately would have been quite acceptable.

The language of schizophrenics may be weighed down with unnecessary detail and circumstantiality in much the same way, perhaps, as writers on the subject. Complex and intricate forms of expression may serve to obscure the train of thought and platitudes and proverbs may come to totally dominate their speech.

An individual patient may be aware of the disruption of his thinking even though it is not obvious to the observer. Some patients become very concerned with words and the potential meanings hidden within these signs and symbols. The language disorder of one patient expressed itself in an extensive series of written productions about words, an extract of which is provided.

> RAYMOND = RAY-MOUND = hill of the ray = tower of the telepathic waves. Also it = RAY-MONDE, ray and world (French, Le Monde). The Germanic name which gives the modern Raymond was Regimund. Regin = strong, powerful; mund = protection. Thus my telepathy is a powerful protection. Mund = protection was often used with a word 'beorg' = him to

mean fortress. Regin is nearly the same word as the Anglo-Saxon regn = rain. Thus one has Regn = rain and mund = fortress = fortress from which comes the rain, i.e. rain = telepathic waves.

This section has been concerned with language productions but it is worth remembering that a number of reports have pointed out that in schizophrenia there occur abnormalities in the perception of speech and of short-term verbal memory. Such receptive defects could contribute to the language abnormalities.

A final point that needs emphasizing is that a variety of brain lesions produce dysphasic speech which may have superficial resemblances to formal thought disorder.

Conclusion

The purpose of the phenomenological approach in psychiatry is to orientate the clinician towards the precise observation and description of the mental state of his patients. Phenomenological description can in addition form the basis for later empirical studies and provide data for operational definitions, though the author has reservations about the latter.

Careful observation and classification is the starting point for good clinical psychiatry and above all it provides the best protection for the patient from being wrongfully labelled as mentally ill and treated as such or, conversely, from being denied care when in fact needing it.

This brief and overly selective introduction will hopefully encourage the reader to pursue the topic further.

In conclusion a final caveat from Henry Maudsley (1895):

> The indistinct and shadowy relations which some minds perceive, or feel vaguely rather than perceive, are not necessarily proofs of superfine insights into things; they certainly often betray the visionary vagrancy of the indolent and self-indulgent mind which, shirking the labour of clear and precise thinking, delights to drift in a vagabondage of misty feeling and shadowy thought.

References

Aggernaes, A. (1972). The experienced reality of hallucinations and other psychological phenomena. *Acta Psychiat. Scand.* **48**, 220–238.

Anderson, E. W., Trethowan, W. H. and Kenna, J. C. (1959). An experimental investigation of simulation and pseudodementia. *Acta Psychiat. Scand.*, Suppl. 132.

Arthur, A. Z. (1964). Theories and explanations of delusions. A review. *Am. J. Psychiat.* **121**, 105–115.

Bleuler, Eugen. 'Dementia Praecox or the Group of Schizophrenias'. Trans. A. Zinkin, I.U.P.N.Y., 1950.

Esquirol, J. E. D. (1833). 'Observations of the Illusions of the Insane'. Renshaw and Rush, London.

Ey, Henri (1969). Outline of an organo-dynamic conception of the structure, nosography and pathogenesis of mental disease. *In* 'Psychiatry and Philosophy' (Ed. M. Natanson). Springer Verlag, Heidelberg, New York and London.

Fish, F. J. (1962). 'Schizophrenia'. J. Wright, Bristol.

Fish, F. J. (1974). *In* 'Clinical Psychopathology' (Ed. M. Hamilton) (revised edn). J. Wright, Bristol.

Flor-Henry, P. (1976). Lateralized temporal limbic dysfunction and psychopathology. *Ann. N.Y. Acad. Sci.* **280**, 777–795.

Hare, E. H. (1973). A short note on pseudo-hallucinations. *Br. J. Psychiat.* **122**, 469–476.

Hirsch, S. R. and Shepherd, M. (1974). 'Themes and Variations in European Psychiatry'. J. Wright, Bristol.

Hoch, P. H. and Zubin, J. (Eds) (1966). 'Psychopathology of Schizophrenia'. Grune and Stratton, New York.

Husserl, E. (1913). 'Ideas. General Introduction to Pure Phenomenology'. Trans. W. R. Boyce Givson. Allen and Unwin, London.

Husserl, E. (1970). 'Logical Investigations'. Trans. J. N. Findlay. Routledge and Kegan Paul, London.

Jaspers, Karl (1968a). 'General Psychopathology'. Trans. from 7th edn by J. Hoenig and M. W. Hamilton. Manchester University Press, Manchester.

Jaspers, Karl (1968b). The phenomenological approach in psychopathology. *Br. J. Psychiat.* **114**, 1313–1323.

Kasanin, J. (Ed.) (1944). 'Language and Thought in Schizophrenia'. University of California Press, California.

Kraupl Taylor, F. (1966). 'Psychopathology, its Causes and Symptoms'. Butterworth, London.

Kraeplin, E. (1919). 'Dementia Praecox and Paraphrenia'. Trans. M. Barclay. Livingstone, Edinburgh.

Landis, C. and Mettler, F. A. (1964). 'Varieties of Psychopathological Experience'. Holt Rinehart and Winston, New York.

Leff, J. P. (1968). Perceptual phenomena and personality in sensory deprivation. *Br. J. Psychiat.* **114**, 1499–1508.

Lewis, A. (1967). 'Inquiries in Psychiatry'. Routledge and Kegan Paul, London.

Lewis, A. (1976). A note on classifying phobia. *Psychol. Med.* **6**, 21–22.

Lyons, J. (1969). Introduction to theoretical linguistics. Cambridge University Press, Cambridge.

Maudsley, Henry (1895). 'The Pathology of Mind'. Macmillan, London.

Maher, Brendan (1972). The language of schizophrenia: a review and interpretation. *Br. J. Psychiat.* **120**, 3–17.

May, Rollo, Angel, E. and Ellenberger, H. F. (Eds) (1956). 'Existence: a New Dimension in Psychiatry and Psychology'. Basic Books, New York.

Merleau Ponty, M. (1963). 'The Structure of Behaviour'. Trans. A. L. Fisher. Beacon Press, New York.

Merleau Ponty, M. (1962). 'Phenomenology of Perception'. Trans. Colin Smith. Routledge and Kegan Paul, London.

Pribram, K. H. (1976). Language in a sociobiological frame. *Ann. N.Y. Acad. Sci.* **280**, 798–812.

Roth, M. (1959). The phobic anxiety depersonalisation syndrome. *Proc. Roy. Soc. Med.* **52**, 587–595.

Sartre, J. P. (1966). 'The Psychology of Imagination'. Trans. B. Frechtman. Washington Square Press, Washington.

Schmitt, R. (1970). Phenomenology. *In* 'The Encyclopaedia of Philosophy' (Ed. Paul Edwards) Vol. 6, pp. 135–151. Macmillan and Free Press, London.

Schneider, Karl (1930). 'Psychologie der Schizophrenen'. Thieme, Leipzig.

Schneider, Kurt (1958). 'Psychopathic Personalities'. Trans. M. Hamilton. Cassell, London.

Schneider, Kurt (1959). 'Clinical Psychopathology'. Trans. M. Hamilton. Grune and Stratton, New York.

Schreber, D. P. (1955). 'Memoirs of my Nervous Illness', translated and edited by I. MacAlpine and R. A. Hunter. R. A. Dawson, London.

Sedman, G. (1966). A phenomenological study of pseudohallucinations and related experiences. *Acta Psychiat. Scand.* **42**, 35–70.

Shepherd, M. (1961). Morbid jealousy: some clinical and social aspects of a psychiatric syndrome. *J. Ment. Sci.* **107**, 687–704.

Slade, P. (1976). Hallucinations. *Psychol. Med.* **6**, 7–13.

Straus, E. W. (1966). 'Phenomenological Psychology'. Tavistock, London.

Straus, E. W. (1948). 'On Obsession'. Nervous and Mental Disease Monographs, No. 73.

Tuke, D. Hack (1892). 'A Dictionary of Psychological Medicine', 2 vols. Churchill, London.

3 The disease concept in psychiatry

Anthony Clare

At the present time there is a tendency, most notable among certain psychologists, psychoanalysts and sociologists, to disparage the concept of disease and challenge the appropriateness of its application in psychiatry. Attempts have been made to eliminate the concept altogether (Szasz, 1960; Albee, 1970) by declaring that the concept does not exist, that mental illnesses are ideological constructs (Leifer, 1971) or political expedients (de Monterice, 1970; Basaglia, 1970). A sociological perspective on psychopathology has developed with as its main focus the effects of 'labelling' (Becker, 1953; Scheff, 1966; Erikson, 1964). In place of the mental disease concept, it is recommended that one speaks instead of problems of living, faulty learning, maladaptation, communication disorders, social disturbances and identity crises. Other arguments concerning the applicability of the disease concept owe more to a dissatisfaction with the current reliability and validity of psychiatric diagnoses (Termelin, 1968; Scharfetter, 1971; Scheff, 1974) than to the more philosophical doubts concerning the possible non-existence of the concept itself. A related controversy concerns the so-called 'medical model' (Siegler and Osmond, 1966; Lazare, 1973), a controversy whose ultimate resolution is hardly advanced by the fact that it is not at all clear what the term means to its critics and supporters alike. Finally, there is the question of the social implications of the application of the disease concept in psychiatry.

The concept of disease

The difficulty of defining disease is implicit in the very structure of the word itself (Dubos, 1968). So many different kinds of disturbance can make a person feel not at ease and provoke him to seek the advice of a physician that it is hardly surprising that the word sometimes appears to encompass most of the difficulties inherent in the human condition. Two views of disease, major and contrasting, have wrestled with each other down through the centuries of western medicine from the time of the Greeks, and to this day elements of both can be detected in current formulations of physical as well as psychiatric disease. One view, that of Hippocrates and his disciples, envisages disease as a combination of signs and symptoms observed to occur together so frequently and so characteristically as to constitute a recognizable and typical clinical picture. Diseases were not the malignant creations of capricious gods or irrational forces but were regarded as natural phenomena developing in accordance with natural laws. The Hippocratic view of disease laid great emphasis on the need to base medicine on the natural sciences, on a profound knowledge of the biological phenomena of life in health and disease, on a recognition of the influence, beneficient and malign, of environmental factors and on a realization of close interdependence between body and mind. Hippocratic writings on the subject of health and disease have retained a universal appeal to this day:

> The scientist recognizes in them the first known systematic attempt to explain the phenomena of disease in terms of natural laws; he shares the interest of the Greek physicians in precise observations objectively made and carefully recorded. The clinician admires Hippocrates for his shrewd observation of signs and symptoms characteristic of each disease, for his knowledge of prognosis based on clinical experience, and for his penetrating concern with the patient as a complex human being integrated in his community. The student of public health points to Hippocratic emphasis on the roles of environment and ways of life in the occurrence of disease. . . . Much of modern medicine consists in the unfolding and elaboration of Hippocratic concepts.   (Dubos, 1968)

Such a *clinical-descriptive* or *syndromal* definition of disease was imaginatively implemented by Thomas Sydenham, the English physician of the late seventeenth century, who on the basis of precise and methodical recording of signs and symptoms succeeded in differentiating a remarkable array of diseases including scarlet fever, measles, gout, smallpox and malaria. Yet Sydenham belonged to the contrasting tradition, sometimes termed Platonic, which envisaged diseases as specific and separate entities and he argued that they could be reduced to 'certain and determinate kinds with the same exactness as we see it done by botanic writers in their treatises on plants' (Taylor, 1972). As one plant differs from another in some crucial manner, so do diseases differ. Diseases, from this vantage point, were conceived of having some form of autonomous existence with natural histories of their own, as beings invading the body from without or as parasites growing within it. Such a reification of disease persists to this day despite the fact that it rests on a confusion of cause with its effect.

In Taylor's words, 'the cause of a disease may be a concrete object entering the body of a human being but the disease so caused is an attribute of the human being involved'. Shades of such confusion can be detected in a phrase such as 'the incidence of a particular disease' when what is actually meant is the incidence of *patients* with a particular disease.

One vigorous opponent of the concept of disease as extraneous pathology attacking normal life from outside was Rudolf Virchow, the precociously brilliant German pathologist who insisted on locating disease inside the body:

> diseases are neither self-subsistent, circumscribed, autonomous organisms, nor entities which have forced their way into the body, nor parasites rooted on it . . . they represent only the course of physiological phenomena under altered conditions.   (Virchow, 1847)

Virchow was to modify such a view many years later but his original conception persisted and laid the foundation for the *disease-as-lesion* view which came to dominate medical thinking. Diseased organs became the focus of serious study and pathological anatomy flourished (Foucault, 1973). Spectacular triumphs were to follow. Indeed it is only now that the shortcomings of such an approach, always obvious in psychiatry where few organic lesions have been demonstrated, have become manifest. The idea of an abnormality or a lesion is relatively straightforward as long as one is concerned with a departure from a recognized and standard pattern. The problem is that it is not always apparent what constitutes a lesion or where normal variation ends and abnormality begins. Conditions such as hypertension, diabetes, congenital abnormalities and anaemia are examples of disturbances which pose difficulties for the disease-as-lesion view. An even more serious shortcoming of this idea of disease is that symptoms and signs, whose physicochemical foundation has yet to be demonstrated, strictly speaking cannot be acknowledged as diseases. Thus migraine, Meniere's disease, trigeminal neuralgia and obesity are among a host of conditions which would have to be conceptualized in some alternative fashion.

Some critics have exploited what seems to be a serious, even fatal flaw in the defence of the concept of mental disease by insisting on the demonstration of a physical lesion as pathognomonic evidence of the existence of disease. Szasz puts this case with characteristic bluntness:

> Disease means bodily disease. Gould's Medical Dictionary defines disease as a disturbance of the function or structure of an organ or part of the body. The mind (whatever it is) is not an organ or part of the body. Hence it cannot be diseased in the same sense as the body can.   (Szasz, 1974)

The relationship of the mind to the body, a problem with an ancient history going back to Aristotle and further, cannot be dismissed so cavalierly.

We do not know how mind and body interact but, as Popper and Eccles (1977) point out, 'this is not surprising since we have really no definite idea how physical things interact'. Few psychiatrists are philosophers however and most have replied to Szasz's argument either by pointing out that many physical disorders lack an established physical pathology (Kety, 1974; Roth, 1976) or by insisting that at the heart of every psychiatric disorder is a specific pathological abnormality waiting to be uncovered. This latter view envisages mental symptoms and abnormal mental states not as diseases in their own right but as the epiphenomena of underlying physical disturbances. The basic premise of such a view is stated with some pungency by Macalpine and Hunter (1974):

> The lesson of the history of psychiatry is that progress is inevitable and irrevocable from psychology to neurology, from mind to brain, never the other way round. Every medical advance adds to the list of diseases which may cause mental derangement. The abnormal mental state is not disease, nor its essence or determinant, but an epiphenomenon. That is why psychological theories and therapies which held out such promise at the turn of the century when so much less was known of localization of function of the brain, have added so little to the understanding and treatment of mental illness, despite all the time and effort devoted to them.

The biologically inclined psychiatrist takes satisfaction in the fact that the list of conditions in which psychological disturbances appear to be symptomatic of underlying physical pathology continues to expand. Such confidence has led to suggestions that psychiatry should split, retaining certain mental conditions assumed to arise from 'natural' rather than psychological, interpersonal or social causes ('natural' in this case being defined as 'biological brain dysfunctions, either biochemical or neurophysiological in nature') and discarding such disorders as dependency syndromes, existential depressions and various social deviancies 'since these disorders arise in individuals with presumably intact neurophysiological functioning and are produced primarily by psychosocial variables' (Ludwig, 1975). Such disorders are not properly the concern of the physician-psychiatrist and are more appropriately handled by non-medical professionals.

Engel (1977) has expressed harsh criticisms of those he terms 'reductionist' who argue that all behavioural phenomena of disease must be and eventually will be conceptualized in terms of physicochemical principles and those who are 'exclusionist' and argue that whatever is not capable of being so explained must be excluded from the category of disease. 'Among physicians and psychiatrists today, the reductionists are the true believers, the exclusionists are the apostates, while both condemn as heretics those who dare to question the ultimate truth of the biomedical model and advocate a more useful model.' Engel is one who questions, articulating arguments propounded by others (Illich, 1974; Comfort, 1972; Mahler, 1975) critical of current medical trends in the identification and treatment of disease. He suggests the replacement of the defective biomedical model by a 'biopsychosocial model' of disease which would take into greater account environmental determinants, the patient's social context and the complementary system devised by society to deal with the disruptive effects of illness, namely the physician's role and the health care system.

Behind such views lies a conviction that the emphasis on the biological basis of disease results in a neglect of the wider psychosocial implications. The fact that environmental factors such as nutritional excess, insufficient exercise, emotional tension, smoking and other deleterious habits can provoke vascular disease in persons with abnormal lipid and cholesterol metabolism is one which critics such as Engel tend to emphasize to illustrate the extent to which the simple disease-as-lesion argument has been abandoned in general medicine itself. Indeed, there are those such as Sedgwick (1973) who have gone further and insisted that all disease, physical and mental, might more accurately be described as 'social constructions', that disease is a human notion, a pragmatic concept applied by man on the basis of social and personal values that can and do change.

Such ideas bear more than a passing resemblance to the concept of disease as 'adaptation to stress' which is associated with the name of Adolph Meyer, professor of psychiatry at Johns Hopkins at the turn of the century. Meyer based his concept on a 'psychobiology' which made no sharp division between physiological and psychological data but emphasized that many if not all diseases are the expressions of both organic and psychic factors. Disease, in this view, is a 'reaction' of the whole organism to its environment. The individual being unique, his disease is unique. Such a formulation makes it difficult to construct a classification system wherein diseases can be classed in general. Nor is it easy to distinguish between those reactions of the organism which qualify as diseases and those which can be seen as natural and normal. What it does do is re-emphasize the individual and personal aspects of disease and the role of environmental factors in its genesis and manifestations.

Disease can also be defined in terms of a *deviation from normal*, that is to say as a statistical concept. Such a formulation derives support from demonstrations such as that of Pickering and his colleagues (Oldham *et al.*, 1960) that essential hypertension is a graded characteristic depending, like height and intelligence, on polygenic inheritance and shading gradually into normality. Other physical disorders which can be conceptualized usefully in this way include cervical cancer, diabetes mellitus and sickle cell anaemia. However, as Kendell (1975) points out, such a statistical definition of normality and abnormality fails to distinguish between those deviations which are harmful, such as high blood pressure, from those which are not, indeed which might actually be beneficial, such as superior intelligence. Scadding's attempt to meet this objection (Scadding, 1967) has merited much attention but it too leaves some major problems unresolved. Confronted by the shortcomings inherent in the various definitions of disease, Scadding proposes one of his own:

> A disease is the sum of abnormal phenomena displayed by a group of living organisms in association with a specified common characteristic or set of characteristics by which they differ from the norm for their species in such a way as to place them at a biological disadvantage.   (Scadding, 1967)

Such a definition indicates the need to establish normal standards for relevant populations, no easy matter when psychological and behavioural standards are under scrutiny, and implies a statistical basis for the concept of abnormality. The definition of mental illness as a deviation from psychological norms is also contained in the views put forward by Lewis (1955) in his influential paper 'Health as a Social Concept'. In physical disease, the diagnosis rests on establishing a deviation from agreed physical norms such as those relating to cardiac size, respiratory flow, glomerular filtration rate or whatever. Environmental and psychological factors, including social and cultural ones, play an often crucial role but the diagnosis of physical disease rests on a demonstration of a disturbance in an organ or bodily system. In mental illnesses, argues Lewis, such a part-function disturbance occurs in one or more of the recognized psychological functions, functions such as perception, learning, remembering, feeling, thinking, motivation, impulse control, etc. Disturbances in perception or memory are the psychiatric equivalent of disturbances in, say, the liver or the lymphatic system. Deviant, maladapted, non-conformist behaviour, on the other hand, is only pathological if it is accompanied by a manifest disturbance in one or more such psychological part-functions. For mental disease to be inferred in Lewis's view,

> disorder of function must be detectable at a discrete or differentiated level that is hardly conceivable when mental activity as a whole is taken as an irreducible datum. If non-conformity can be detected only in total behaviour, while all the particular psychological functions seem unimpaired, health will be presumed not illness.   (Lewis, 1955)

The problem here is that there are a number of areas, such as the personality disorders and the so-called sexual perversions, in which the presence or absence of a disturbance in psychological part-functions such as impulse control or learning is not at present clear. In addition, we know considerably less about psychological functions at the present time than we do about physiological ones. Lewis's insistence that social norms should not become a criterion of normality represents, in one critic's eyes, little more than an aspiration. 'In many areas if we are determined not to resort to social criteria, all we can do is defer judgement' (Kendell, 1975). In practice of course deferring judgement is precisely what many psychiatrists do. In those conditions, such as the major psychotic ill-nesses in which there are grounds for supposing the existence of some underlying somatic process and in which there is relatively clear-cut evidence of disturbed psychological functioning, most psychiatrists appear reasonably agreed as to the legitimacy of conceptualizing such conditions as diseases. In other conditions, and most notabably the personality disorders, in which evidence of psychological part-function is conspicuously lacking and in which no underlying physiological distur-bance is likely psychiatrists and psychologists adopt profoundly con-tradictory positions (Asubel, 1961; Szasz, 1972) while the more cautious among them refrain from committing themselves one way or the other.

An illustrative case in point is alcoholism. Several prominent experts argue for its retention as a disease state (Blume, 1977; Keller, 1960; Winokur et al., 1971). Others believe that the concept may be applied to some forms of alcohol abuse but not to others (Chafetz, 1966; Davies, 1974). Still others reject the notion of alcoholism as disease altogether (Steiner, 1969; Szasz, 1972; Mulford, 1970). Davies (1974) wryly sums up the degree of confusion in this area by observing that since there are more than 30 definitions of alcoholism currently available and at least three definitions of disease, 'one would need to assemble about 90 doctors to debate the present topic to make it likely that at least two would under-stand each other' (Davies, 1974). (See Chapter 10.)

In practice, the formulation of a named disease may be founded on little more than an isolated symptom or symptoms (e.g. tension headache, rheumatism) in which case only a *symptomatic diagnosis* can be made. It may rest on no more than a combination of clinical signs and symptoms observed to cluster together frequently and distinctively as a *syndrome* (e.g. migraine, phobic anxiety). It may depend on *morbid pathological* changes (e.g. an inflamed appendix, gallstones), *biochemical abnormalities* (e.g. porphyria, diabetes), specific *deficiencies* (e.g. pernicious anaemia, pellagra) or measurable *disorders of function* (e.g. respiratory emphysema). It may even be defined on the basis of some *chromosomal abnormality* or *change* (e.g. Down's syndrome, Turner's syndrome). Depending on the stage to which a disease has evolved, the formulation of a diagnosis can end in very different sorts of conclusions. One major purpose of diag-nosis, however, is that it should permit reasonably accurate predictions to be made concerning aetiology, prognosis and response to treatment.

Taken together, these aspects of the disease concept constitute some if not all of the elements of the so-called 'medical model'.

The medical model

The notion of the medical model is by no means unequivocal but is subject to much uncertainty and confusion. A number of definitions, some contradictory, some overlapping, are in current use. They have been admirably summarized by Macklin (1973). She has identified four main versions. The first is a relatively neutral statement to the effect that according to the medical model psychological ailments are held to be analogous to physical ones in so far as both sorts of ailments have ascertainable causes and the disease state is manifested in symptoms. No specification of the types of causes is provided (Sahakian, 1970). The second is similar but adds the important addendum that the medical model characteristically focuses on the causes of abnormal or maladaptive behaviours rather than the behaviours themselves and construes the 'real' disorder in terms of an underlying disease state of the organism (Ullman and Krasner, 1965). In this view, the medical model involves not merely a conceptual characterization of the nature of emotional disorder but also entails a certain sort of procedural process of diagnosis and treatment on the part of the clinician. The third version emphasizes the view that the medical model, in attempting to explain the origins of neurotic and psychotic behaviour, alcohol addiction, delinquency, marital difficulties and school learning difficulties as 'sicknesses inside the person', make them 'discontinuous with normal behaviour'. The medical model, in other words, suggests that these conditions are among a number of discrete mental illnesses, each with a separate cause, prognosis and potential treatment (Albee, 1969). Finally, there is the mdedical model as described by Szasz and mentioned earlier. This differs from the preceding three in that whereas Szasz attributes to the medical model the assumption of neurological and/or physicochemical causes, the first three definitions are neutral with respect to the types of causes presupposed by medical model theorists.

As Macklin (1973) notes, with the exception of the first definition, which is the most neutral and general of all those cited, each characterization of the medical model 'is propounded by a writer who is attempting to reject the model'. Thus the second definition is proposed by behaviourists who regard neurotic symptoms as simple learned habits. According to this *behavioural model*, eliminating the symptoms eliminates the neurosis. There is no underlying disease. There are symptoms. In this formulation, psychoses possibly, and neuroses and personality disorder certainly are examples of abnormal behaviour that has been learned and is being maintained either because it leads to positive effects or avoids negative ones. The typical therapeutic response includes establishing the behaviour to be modified, the conditions under which it occurs, the factors responsible for the persistence of the behaviour, a set of appropriate treatment conditions and a schedule of retraining (Lazarus, 1968; Liberman and Raskin, 1971; Eysenck, 1975).

The third definition of the medical model proposed above is that of one whose concerns are primarily related to social and institutional reform and whose criticisms of the medical model relate to its impact on the nature of the institutions developed for intervention and prevention and the kind of manpower used to deliver care. The so-called *social model* highlights the manner in which the individual functions in the social system. The mind–body dichotomy is regarded as spurious or irrelevant and the individual viewed as a unit, the condition, form and destiny of which are moulded primarily by environmental forces. Mental illnesses are seen as evolving processes, reactions to socially disruptive events such as bereavement, poverty, overcrowding, pollution and marital breakdown (Weiss and Bergen, 1968). Treatment consists of reorganizing the patient's relation to the social system or of reorganizing the social system itself. Having a mental illness in the words of one social psychiatrist is 'a social project' and it is seen to concern not only the patient himself but

> his friends and relations, neighbours, work mates and employers. The local authority and the Department of Social Security and Health may be involved. If he goes to hospital, psychiatrists, nurses, social workers, psychologists, occupational therapists and welfare organizations of various kinds all come into the situation. So something essentially very private and personal, something which may seem a very inferior affair, now becomes of obvious public concern. (Shoenberg, 1972)

As a generalization, the social and behavioural models of psychiatric disturbance have grown up in contrast to the biological or medical model. The *psychoanalytical model*, on the other hand, has historical roots as deeply embedded in antiquity as those of the biological standpoint. In the view of one eminent psychiatric historian, 'modern dynamic psychotherapy derives from primitive medicine and an uninterrupted continuity can be demonstrated between exorcism and magnetism, magnetism and hypnotism and hypnotism and the modern dynamic schools' (Ellenberger, 1970). According to this model, adult neuroses and vulnerabilities to stress are the consequence of early childhood deprivation, developmental fixations at certain crucial stages of maturation, distortions in early relationships and confused communications between parent and child. Therapy consists in clarifying the meaning of events, feelings, impulses and behaviour in the context of past and often forgotten or repressed events and experiences. A crucial aspect of this model is the doctor–patient relationship, the therapeutic alliance, which enables the patient to work through the disturbance and abandon familiar but destructive methods of coping with reality.

Other models have been described (Siegler and Osmond, 1974) including the *conspiratorial*, in which psychiatric illness exists only in the eye of the observer, the so-called patient being the victim of labelling, the *family interaction* model, wherein the entire family is deemed 'sick' and is brought for help by the 'index patient' who may well be the healthiest member, and the *moral* model which portrays mental illness as identical with deviance and the mentally ill as responsible, autonomous, self-willed individuals to be held responsible for their anti-social activities. There is also the *psychedelic model* in which mental illness is viewed as a metaphorical 'trip', the patient proceeding through a state of 'super-sanity' and, if properly guided, emerging on the far side in a more enlightened and sensitive condition. This last view, popularized by the imaginative writings of Ronald Laing (Laing, 1967), bears remarkable similarities to the highly romanticized view of tuberculosis which held sway during parts of the last century and which has recently been examined by Sontag (1978). Those afflicted with TB were often portrayed as highly imaginative, sensitive and artistic individuals, too cultured and cultivated to bear the horrors of a vulgar, coarse and brutal world. The illness itself was often seen as a pretext for leisure, a way of retiring from the world without having to take responsibility for the decision. So well entrenched was the idea that TB and artistic creativity were connected that at the end of the century one critic suggested that it was the progressive disappearance of TB which accounted for the current decline of literature and the arts (Dubos and Dubos, 1952). It is worth noting that Sontag dates the destruction of the TB myth from the time when proper treatment for the condition was developed, with the discovery of streptomycin in 1944 and the introduction of isoniazid in 1952. The implications for the romantic metaphor of mental illness and its eventual decline are obvious.

These are some of the models formulated to explain the phenomena subsumed under the term mental illness. Some of them are relatively discrete but the majority overlap one with the other. In practice, a clinician may well borrow ideas and practices from many of them when handling particular patients or problems. But, given the dominance of the medical model, it is necessary to return to the discussion of what exactly it is. Hornstra (1962) has identified as its particular characteristics the following: a specific aetiology, a predictable course, manifestations describable in signs and symptoms and a predictable outcome modifiable by certain describable manoeuvres. Lazare's definition (Lazare, 1973), which he derives from Slater and Roth (1969), is similar apart from the fact that it includes the proposition that 'there eventually will be found a specific cause related to the functional anatomy of the brain' for each abnormal mental condition. However, few proponents of the medical model believe that unicausation is an essential feature of the medical model. There are very few doctors who now hold that cigarettes are the sole cause of cancer, excess blood lipids of arteriosclerosis and deficient insulin of diabetes. Multiple causation, including genetic, familial, somatic, psychological, social and cultural 'causes', has long been accepted in medicine though this has not prevented those, like Milton and Wahler (1969), from arguing that the locus of the disease process as postulated by the medical model is 'inside the person'.

A more serious criticism of the applicability of the medical model to psychiatry relates to the relative unreliability of psychiatric diagnoses. Diagnoses are of questionable value if useful predictions cannot be made from them. If the diagnoses themselves are subject to disagreement and discrepancy, the accuracy and hence the value of these predictions will be correspondingly reduced. Kendell (1975) summarizes the issue when he declares 'the accuracy of the prognostic and therapeutic inferences derived from a diagnosis can never be higher than the accuracy with which, in any given situation, that diagnosis can itself be made'. Diagnostic unreliability can result from inconsistency on the part of the diagnostician (Ward *et al.*, 1962), differences in diagnostic significance attributed to elicited symptoms (Beck *et al.*, 1962; Katz *et al.*, 1969), inadequacies of the nomenclature (Cooper *et al.*, 1972), the influence of diagnostic 'set' and suggestion (Termelin, 1968; Rosenhan, 1973), lack of psychiatric experience on the part of the diagnostician (Schmidt and Fonda, 1956) and international variation in the way diagnostic categories are implemented (Pichot *et al.*, 1966; Rawnsley, 1967; Cooper *et al.*, 1972; Kendell *et al.*, 1974). Impressed by these diagnostic deficiencies, a variety of experts have suggested that the conventional descriptive diagnostic categories should be discarded altogether (Masserman and Carmichael, 1936; Colby, 1960; Menninger, 1963; Mannoni, 1973). However, others argue that with special efforts to control inter-observer variation, appropriate training, adequate acquaintance with an agreed rating scale or internationally accepted glossary of terms and the use of standardized psychiatric assessments, significant improvements in diagnostic reliability can be achieved (Wilson and Meyer, 1962; Wing *et al.*, 1967; Cooper *et al.*, 1972; WHO, 1973).

When attempts have been made to improve reliability in this way, relatively high levels of diagnostic agreement between psychiatrists have been reported. Using an early version of the Present State Examination,

Wing and his colleagues (Wing *et al.*, 1967) reported a concordance rate of 92% between two psychiatrists rating patients diagnosed as schizo-phrenic. Kendell (1973) found an average level of diagnostic agreement of 77% between Maudsley-trained psychiatrists asked to rate an unselected series of new in-patients with five minutes to spare for each interview and no additional information provided. Kreitman and his colleagues obtained a level of agreement of 75% for organic diagnoses and 61% for functional psychoses but only 28% for neurotic disorders (Kreitman *et al.*, 1961), a finding which supports the general view that organic states produce higher concordance rates than functional states, and psychotic illnesses higher rates than neurotic illnesses and personality disorders.

Documented disagreement in diagnosis and diagnostic test interpreta-tion is not limited to psychiatry (Clare, 1976) but exists in relation to, among other fields, radiology (Etter *et al.*, 1960), cardiology (Butterworth and Rappert, 1960), paediatrics (Derryberry, 1938) and laboratory testing (Belk and Sunderman, 1947). Beck and his colleagues (1962) drew atten-tion to the significant inter-observer errors reported in the assessment of such conditions as chest disorders and the degree of pathological inflammation of the tonsils (Beck *et al.*, 1962). There are good grounds for believing that all varieties of the diagnostic process are at times subject to significant inter-observer (and, to a lesser extent, intra-observer) varia-tion. It is the particularly vulnerable state of psychiatric classification which has led psychiatrists to devote more attention perhaps than their medical colleagues to analysing such variations with a view to reducing them further. Recent work (Leroy and Mellegard, 1971; Kellett *et al.*, 1975) has helped clarify what kinds of information contribute to and detract from reliability and what categories are particularly sensitive to diagnostic disagreement. Another important development has been the construc-tion of revised versions of standard classifications in which the diagnostic rules are made explicit (Feighner *et al.*, 1972; Fischer, 1974; Spitzer *et al.*, 1974), revisions which can lead to impressive increases in inter-diagnostician agreement (Zubin *et al.*, 1975).

Classification

The shortcomings inherent in the concept of psychiatric disease and in psychiatric diagnostic practice contribute, in large part, to the inability of psychiatrists to produce an acceptable internationally agreed classification of psychiatric diseases. Some critics, as a result, have sug-gested the abolition of psychiatric diagnoses altogether, while Menninger (1963) has argued that it is a pointless exercise to classify either patients or diseases since every individual patient is unique and so is his illness.

However, Shepherd (1976) has sharply attacked such a view. 'To discard classification', Shepherd declares, 'is to discard scientific thinking' and he quotes, with approval, the statement of Gerhard Wasserman to the effect that 'scientific theories, apart from introducing hypotheses, deal with characteristics of classes of phenomena and systems and with relations between classes of phenomena. A scientist's initial task is to classify publicly observable properties of systems' (Wasserman, 1974). Stengel (1959) attributed some of the resistance to classification exhibited by psychiatrists to the fact that many diagnostic terms carry aetiological implications and that the theoretical objections of different schools of psychiatry to each other's aetiological assumptions thwart attempts to arrive at an agreed classification. Such assumptions are quite explicit with diagnostic terms such as psychogenic psychosis and reactive depression. Stengel's solution, which was that all diagnoses should be stripped of their aetiological implications and regarded simply as 'operational' definitions, represents an aspiration rather than a feasible policy. Another solution is a classificatory system with separate axes for symptomatology and aetiology (Essen-Moller, 1971). Others have pressed for the use of additional axes relating to premorbid personality (Zeh, 1962) and physical and psychosocial factors (Rutter et al., 1973) while Ottosson and Perris (1973) have argued for a multiaxial classification of mental disorders with separate axes for symptomatology, severity, aetiology and course. Such an approach is useful but certain problems remain. For example, methods of classifying personality are at present clearly inadequate and the advantages of employing an axis for personality are correspondingly limited.

Nevertheless, the arguments for the development of a multiaxial classification have grown and specific proposals for such a scheme in the field of child psychiatry were proposed at the Third WHO Seminar (Rutter et al., 1969) and were later elaborated at the Fifth Seminar (Tarjan et al., 1972). Four axes are represented. The first describes 'clinical psychiatric syndromes'; the second, the child's intellectual level; the third, associated or aetiological physical disorders; and the fourth concerns psychosocial factors. The main theoretical advantage of such a system is that when a case involves several types of abnormal functioning it ensures uniformity of practice in the aspects of the case which are coded, the number of codes used and the order in which the codings are placed. In this respect it has been found to be superior to the more orthodox ICD coding system (Rutter et al., 1973).

Another solution, and one strengthened by the fact that there is not one functional psychiatric disorder which has been convincingly shown to be separated from other neighbouring syndromes by points of rarity or where the relevant distribution curve has been shown to be bimodal, is that the representation of mental disorders as separate and distinct categories be discarded and replaced by a dimensional approach to disorder. The most persistent proponent of the view has been Eysenck. His criticisms can be summarized as follows. Factor analytic studies have revealed no evidence of the clustering assumed by the categorical disease model. Factor score distributions are almost always continuous and individuals tend to score on all factors and not just on one. Using criterion analysis, there is evidence that both psychosis and neurosis are graded traits present to greater or lesser extent in the whole population but distinct from each other. Finally, a dimensional system, based on the three dimensions of psychoticism, neuroticism and interversion/extroversion is regarded as necessary for theoretical and clinical purposes.

It is true that factor analytic studies have failed to confirm the existence of disease clusters but hardly surprising since this statistical approach is only capable of producing dimensions in the first place. With regard to the question of criterion analysis, Eysenck claims to have demonstrated a continuity between his psychotic and normal populations (Eysenck, 1951) but the battery of tests on which such a finding rests bears little resemblance to any of the methods used by clinicians to distinguish between psychosis and normality, nor have these tests been shown to be more effective discriminators than traditional methods. It is true that 'psychoticism' is a graded trait on which several populations of psychotics have been shown to score significantly higher than normals. But proof is lacking that 'psychoticism' has much to do with any clinical psychosis and Kendell (1975) has queried whether the psychoticism factor items on the PEN questionnaire might not be more accurately described as representing a personality trait of callousness than as measuring psychosis.

The evidence in favour of a categorical classification is hardly persuasive either however. There is little solidity about the boundaries of any of the major disease categories and intermediate conditions, such as schizoaffective psychosis and borderline psychosis, abound. Persistent searches for evidence of discontinuities in the distribution of symptom patterns have resulted in conflicting results. Genuine discontinuities have been reported between psychotic and neurotic depressions (Carney et al., 1965) and denied (Kendell and Gourlay, 1970). However, cluster analyses (Everitt et al., 1971) have produced four separate clusters identifiable with the manic and depressive phases of manic-depressive illness, with acute paranoid schizophrenia and, to a lesser extent, with chronic schizophrenia. In this same study, however, the analyses failed to yield any clusters identifiable with neuroses, personality disorder or with alcoholism. At the present time, neither the dimensional nor the categorical approach is clearly superior to the other and in principle both are available.

Another approach to the problem of classification which stands somewhat apart from the others is that of Foulds (1976). Foulds uses the term 'personal illness' to emphasize that what has changed for the worse in psychiatric illness are those characteristics which pertain uniquely to the person. He proposes a hierarchy of personal illness. The lowest class in his hierarchy, Dysthymic States, contains patients suffering from anxiety, depression and/or elation but not from symptoms and signs characteristic of the classes higher in the hierarchy. The second class, Neurotic Symptoms, contains patients suffering from conversion, phobic, dissociative, compulsive or ruminative symptoms in addition to one or more of the Dysthymic States. The third class, Integrated Delusions, contains patients suffering from delusions of persecution, grandeur and/or contrition in addition to one or more of the groups of Neurotic Symptoms and one or more of the groups of Dysthymic States. The class highest in the hierarchy, Delusions of Disintegration, contains patients suffering from hallucinations and delusions of passivity and influence in addition to one or more symptoms from each of the classes below. In practice, most clinicians, on empirical grounds, observe a somewhat similar hierarchy in which the organic psychoses come first, followed by the functional psychoses, with schizophrenia preceding manic-depressive psychosis, and neurotic illness coming at the bottom. In general, any given diagnosis excludes the presence of symptoms of conditions higher in the hierarchy and includes some or all of the symptoms of lower conditions.

Despite its strengths, Foulds' classificatory system remains largely private and hence to date has not been used in any extensive research effort. The need for an agreed system of classification for research purposes has been outlined in a number of reports, one of which has proposed three types of solution (WHO, 1970). The first, 'which appeals to computerised neo-Kraepelinians' (Shepherd, 1976), reads as follows:

If it is possible to obtain an accurate detailed description of the patient's behaviour and present state and of changes in these factors over a period of time, it would appear to be unnecessary to insist on obtaining rigid agreement among different investigators on a precise diagnostic classification. The main requirement is that collaborating investigators in different centres should establish empirically that, despite theoretical differences, they can use the same clinical measuring instruments and arrive at similar quantitative conclusions concerning aspects of a patient's present state, such as pressure of speech, agitation, presence of delusions and hallucinatory activity. Given a sufficient number of reliable indices of this kind, correlations can be sought between individual clinical symptoms and syndromes and biological data. Agreement on a system of clinical diagnosis can then become a goal rather than a pre-condition . . .

Such an approach has been adopted by the WHO International Pilot Study of Schizophrenia. That the combination of clinical data, computer-derived syndromes, numerical taxonomy and factor analysis can help increase the reliability of data-collection is rarely in dispute. It may even generate novel hypotheses concerning correlations between biological and psychosocial data. It can certainly indicate the variable borders between the major psychoses. However, it is doubtful whether it can do much to resolve the problem of where these borders should be drawn since 'the major constraints on further developments in computerised diagnosis appear to lie in limitations in the standard nomenclature itself' (Spitzer and Endicott, 1975).

A second approach is based on the assumption that experienced psychiatrists can agree on the diagnosis of certain illnesses such as schizophrenia and that the major problem in the diagnosis of a condition such as schizophrenia involves the limits within which a patient can be regarded as schizophrenic and beyond which he is not. A panel of psychiatrists from different backgrounds and theoretical vantage points is drawn and only when there is unanimity between them is a patient accepted as suffering from the disease in question. A similar criterion, namely unanimity concerning the absence of the disorder, can provide an adequate control group. The problem is that the inclusive and exclusive criteria may not be clear or may actually result in important subgroups being excluded from study.

The third approach involves techniques, such as cluster and factor analyses, which dispense with the need for some degree of homogeneity in the patient population under scrutiny and which aim instead to establish significant relationships through correlational analysis of patients believed to represent a diagnostic continuum (see above).

While the need for a system of disease classification, a nosology, is obvious from the viewpoint of the researcher, it is no less obvious from that of the clinician. Perhaps the most important function of a diagnosis for clinical psychiatry is its power to predict treatment response. It is often advanced as an argument for the value of a diagnostic approach in psychiatry that differences in response to therapeutic agents such as ECT, tricyclic antidepressants, mono-amine oxidase inhibitors, phenothiazines and lithium do occur to a significant extent. However, there is much overlap between treatments, particularly in neurotic conditions but also in the psychoses (Murphy et al., 1978). The phenothiazines are used for their 'anti-psychotic' actions in schizophrenia, their tranquillizing effects in mania and to sedate in agitated depressions. Lithium has been advocated for aggressive conditions and alcoholism as well as for affective psychoses. Electroconvulsive therapy, while classically recommended for seriously depressed patients, has enthusiastic advocates for its use in catatonic schizophrenia and severe mania. At the present time, psychiatry clearly lacks treatments of such specificity as is possessed by substances such as cyanocobalamin or thyroxine in physical medicine. The most appropriate analogy between psychiatric drugs and physical ones is with the steroids, a group of drugs exerting a wide variety of effects and used in a remarkable array of conditions. It is worth noting, too, that many of the conditions in which the steroids are used, such as multiple sclerosis, ulcerative colitis and the auto-immune disorders, are at a similar stage of development as diseases as most psychiatric disorders, namely the syndrome stage.

The sick role

The last aspect of the 'medical model' to be considered concerns the so-called '*sick role*'. This idea is largely derived from the writings of the sociologist, Talcott Parsons. Parsons (1951) described four features of the sick role which help distinguish it from orthodox deviancy. Firstly, there is the exemption from normal social role responsibilities. This exemption requires legitimization by the physician. People are sometimes reluctant to accept that they may be sick and the physician may serve as a court of appeal. This is particularly true of psychiatric ill-health. Secondly, the sick person cannot be expected to get better by an act of decision or will. He is in a condition that must 'be taken care of'. Of course the process of recovery may be spontaneous but while the illness lasts the patient cannot help it; his condition must be changed not merely his attitude. Thirdly, implicit in the definition of the state of being ill is the view that illness is undesirable and the patient has an obligation to want to get well. Fourthly, there is the related obligation, proportional to the severity of the condition, to seek technically competent help, namely in the most usual sense that of a physician and to co-operate with him in the process of getting well.

The extent to which a mentally ill person is responsible for his actions is a question which crops up in a number of guises and most often in forensic situations. The extent to which a mentally ill person is responsible for his illness is as difficult a question to answer. Only two models answer unequivocally—the 'moral' model that the patient is primarily responsible and an 'organic' model, which as we have seen tends to be confused with the medical approach, that declares he is not responsible at all. The actual answer probably varies depending on individual circumstances, psychological and social factors and the nature of the condition itself. What is clear, however, is that at the heart of the medical approach and the corresponding sick role is the belief that the psychiatrically ill person, in common with the physically ill one, is not fully responsible for his being sick and, once sick, is unable without some form of professional advice and/or treatment to return to a state of health save in exceptional circumstances.

Summary

Psychiatrically ill patients suffer from illnesses whose aetiology and pathogenesis at the biological, psychological, behavioural and social levels remain obscure. In Kety's words, 'we have only unsubstantiated hypotheses of how to prevent them' (Kety, 1974). What is required is extensive research but research, to be fruitful, needs to be based on firm foundations. Psychiatry lacks an accepted nomenclature or list of approved terms for describing and recording clinical observations. It also lacks a reliable system of classification. Nevertheless, the broad consensus within psychiatry at the present time is that the advantages of the disease approach, the diagnostic exercise and the present rudimentary classification system outweigh the disadvantages and that the early results of attempts to improve the situation are encouraging.

References

Albee, G. (1969). Emerging concepts of mental illness and models of treatment: the psychological point of view. *Am. J. Psychiat.* **125**, 870.

Albee, G. (1970). The emperor's model. *Int. J. Psychiat.* **9**, 29–31.

Asubel, D. (1961). Personality disorder is disease. *Amer. Psychologist* **16**, 69–74.

Basaglia, F. (1970). 'L'institution en negation. Rapport sur l'Hôpital Psychiatrique Gorizia'. Editions du Seuil, Paris.

Beck, A. T., Ward, C. H., Mendelson, M., Mock, J. E. and Erbaugh, J. K. (1962). Reliability of psychiatric diagnoses: 11. A study of consistency of clinical judgement ratings. *Am. J. Psychiat.* **119**, 351–357.

Becker, H. (1963). 'Outsider: Studies in the Sociology of Deviance'. The Free Press, New York.

Belk, W. P. and Sunderman, F. W. (1947). A survey of the accuracy of chemical analyses in clinical labs. *Am. J. Clin. Path.* **19**, 853–861.

Blume, S. (1977). The 'Rand' Report. Some comments and a response. *J. Stud. Alc.* **38**, 1, 163–168.

Butterworth, J. S. and Rappert, E. H. (1960). Auscultatory acumen in the general medical population. *J.A.M.A.* **174**, 32–34.

Carney, M. W. P., Roth, M. and Garside, R. F. (1965). The diagnosis of depressive syndromes and the prediction of E.C.T. response. *Br. J. Psychiat.* **111**, 659–674.

Chafetz, M. E. (1966). Alcohol excess. *Ann. N.Y. Acad. Sci.* **133**, 808–813.

Clare, A. W. (1976). 'Psychiatry in Dissent'. Tavistock Publications, London.

Colby, K. M. (1960). 'An Introduction to Psychoanalytic Research'. Basic Books, New York.
Comfort, A. (1972). What is a Doctor? *Lancet* **7758**, 1, 971–974.
Cooper, J. E., Kendell, R. E., Gurland, B. J., Sharpe, L., Copeland, J. R. M. and Simon, R. (1972). 'Psychiatric Diagnosis in New York and London'. Maudsley Monograph, no. 20. Oxford University Press, London.
Davies, D. L. (1974). Editorial: alcoholism as a disease. *Psychol. Med.* **4**, 130–132.
Derryberry, M. (1938). Reliability of medical judgements on malnutrition. *Pub. Hlth. Rpt.* **53**, 263–268.
Dubos, R. (1968). Man, medicine and environment. Pall Mall Press, London.
Dubos, R. and Dubos, J. (1952). Consumption and the Romantic Age. *In* 'The White Plague'. Little, Brown and Co, Boston.
Ellenberger, H. (1970). 'The Discovery of the Unconscious'. Allen Lane and Penguin, London.
Engel, G. L. (1977). The need for a new medical model: a challenge for biomedicine. *Science* **196**, 4286, 129–136.
Erikson, K. (1964). Notes on the sociology of deviance. *In* 'The Other Side' (Ed. H. Becker). The Free Press, New York.
Essen-Moller, E. (1971). Suggestions for further improvement of the international classification of mental disorders. *Psychol. Med.* **1**, 308–311.
Etter, L. E., Dunn, J. P., Kammer, A. G., Osmond, L. A. and Reese, L. C. (1960). Gastroduodenal X-ray diagnosis: a comparison of radiographic techniques and interpretations. *Radiol.* **74**, 766–70.
Everitt, B. S., Gourlay, A. J. and Kendell, R. E. (1971). An attempt at validation of traditional psychiatric syndromes by cluster analysis. *Br. J. Psychiat.* **199**, 319–412.
Eysenck, H. J. (1951). Schizothymia—cyclothymia as a dimension of personality. *J. Personal.* **20**, 345–384.
Eysenck, H. J. (1975). 'The Future of Psychiatry'. Methuen, London.
Feighner, J. P., Robins, E., Guze, S. B., Woodruff, R. A., Winokur, G. and Munoz, R. (1972). Diagnostic criteria for use in psychiatric research. *Arch. Gen. Psychiat.* **26**, 57–63.
Fischer, M. (1974). Development and validity of a computerized method for diagnosis of functional psychoses. *Acta Psychiat. Scand.* **50**, 243–288.
Foucault, M. (1973). 'The Birth of the Clinic'. Tavistock Publications, London.
Foulds, G. A. (1976). 'The Hierarchical Nature of Personal Illness'. Academic Press, London and New York.
Hornstra, R. A. (1962). The psychiatric hospital and the community. Paper read at the Annual Workshop in Community Mental Health, Candler, N. Carolina.
Illich, I. (1974). Medical Nemesis. *Lancet* **1**, 918–922.
Katz, M., Cole, J. O. and Lowery, H. A. (1969). Studies of the diagnostic process: the influence of symptom perception, past experience and ethnic background on diagnostic decisions. *Am. J. Psychiat.* **125**, 937–947.
Keller, M. (1960). Definition of alcoholism. *Quart. J. Stud. Alc.* **21**, 125–134.
Kellett, J. M., Copeland, J. R. M. and Kelleher, M. J. (1975). Information leading to accurate diagnosis in the elderly. *Br. J. Psychiat.* **126**, 423–430.
Kendell, R. E. (1973). Psychiatric diagnoses: a study of how they are made. *Br. J. Psychiat.* **122**, 437–445.
Kendell, R. E. (1975). 'The Role of Diagnosis in Psychiatry'. Blackwell, Oxford.
Kendell, R. E. and Gourlay, J. (1970). The clinical distinction between psychotic and neurotic depression. *Br. J. Psychiat.* **117**, 257–260.

74 A. Clare

Kendell, R. E., Pichot, P. and von Cranach, M. (1974). Diagnostic criteria of English, French and German psychiatrists. *Psychol. Med.* **4**, 187–195.
Kety, S. S. (1974). From rationalization to reason. *Am. J. Psychiat.* **131**, 957–963.
Kreitman, N., Sainsbury, P., Morrissey, J., Towers, J. and Scrivener, J. (1961). The reliability of psychiatric assessment: an analysis. *J. Ment. Sci.* **107**, 887–908.
Laing, R. D. (1967). 'The Politics of Experience'. Penguin, Harmondsworth.
Lazare, A. (1973). Hidden conceptual models in clinical psychiatry. *N. Eng. J. Med.* **288**, 7, 345–351.
Lazarus, A. A. (1968). Learning theory and the treatment of depression. *Behav. Res. Ther.* **6**, 83–89.
Leifer, R. (1971). The medical model as ideology. *Int. J. Psychiat.* **9**, 13–21.
Leroy, A. and Mellgard, M. (1971). The use of information in diagnostic decisions. *Acta Psychiat. Scand.* **108**, 609–616.
Lewis, A. (1955). Health as a social concept. *Br. J. Sociol.* **4**, 109–124.
Liberman, R. P. and Raskin, D. E. (1971). Depression: a behavioral formulation. *Arch. Gen. Psychiat.* **24**, 515–523.
Ludwig, A. M. (1975). The psychiatrist as physician. *J.A.M.A.* **234**, 6, 603–604.
Macalpine, I. and Hunter, R. (1974). The pathography of the past. *Times Literary Supplement*, 15 March, 256–257.
Macklin, R. (1973). The medical model in psychoanalysis and psychotherapy. *Compr. Psychiat.* **14**, 1, 49–69.
Mahler, H. (1975). Health—a demystification of medical technology. *Lancet* **1**, 829–834.
Mannoni, O. (1973). The antipsychiatric movement(s). *Int. Soc. Sci. J.* **XXV** (4), 489–503.
Masserman, J. and Carmichael, H. T. (1938). Diagnosis and prognosis in psychiatry. *J. Ment. Sci.* **84**, 893–946.
Menninger, K. (1963). 'The Vital Balance: the Life Process in Mental Health and Illness'. Viking Press, New York.
Milton, O. and Wahler, R. G. (1969). Perspectives and trends. In 'Behaviour Disorders' (Eds O. Milton and R. G. Wahler). Lippincott, New York.
de Monterice, B. (1971). Practical radicalism. *Int. J. Psychiat.* **9**, 676–687.
Mulford, H. A. (1970). Meeting the problems of alcohol abuse: a testable action plan for Iowa. Iowa Alcoholism Foundation, Cedar Rapids, Iowa.
Murphy, D. L., Shiling, D. J. and Murray, R. M. (1978). Psychoactive drug responder subgroups: possible contributions to psychiatric classification. In 'Psychopharmacology, A Generation of Progress' (Ed. M. A. Lipton et al.). Raven Press, New York.
Oldham, P. D., Pickering, G., Fraser Roberts, J. A. and Sowry, G. S. C. (1960). The nature of essential hypertension. *Lancet* **1**, 1085–1093.
Ottosson, J. O. and Perris, C. (1973). Multidimensional classification of mental disorders. *Psychol. Med.* **3**, 238–243.
Parsons, T. (1951). 'The Social System'. The Free Press, Glencoe, Ill.
Pichot, P., Bailly, R. and Overall, J. E. (1966). Les stéréotypes diagnostiques des psychoses chez les psychiatres Français. Comparison avec les stéréotypes Americains. Proceedings of the fifth International Congress of the Collegium Internationale Neuropsychopharmacologicum. Excerpta Medica International Congress Series No. 129.
Popper, K. R. and Eccles, J. C. (1977). 'The Self and Its Brain: An Argument for Interactionism'. Springer International, London.
Rawnsley, K. (1967). An international diagnostic exercise. In 'Proceedings of the

Fourth World Congress of Psychiatry', **4**, 2683–2686. Excerpta Medica Foundation, Amsterdam.
Rosenhan, D. L. (1973). On being sane in insane places. *Science* **179**, 250–258.
Roth, M. (1976). Schizophrenia and the theories of Thomas Szasz. *Br. J. Psychiat.* **129**, 317–326.
Rutter, M., Lebovici, S., Eisenberg, L., Sneznevskij, A. J., Sadoun, R., Brooke, E. and Lin, T. (1969). A triaxial classification of mental disorders in childhood. *J. Child Psychol. Psychiat.* **10**, 41–62.
Rutter, M., Schaffer, D. and Shepherd, M. (1973). An evaluation of the proposal for a multiaxial classification of child psychiatric disorders. *Psychol. Med.* **3**, 244–250.
Sahakian, W. S. (1970). 'Psychopathology Today' (Ed. W. S. Sahakian). Peacock, Itasca, Ill.
Scadding, J. G. (1967). Diagnosis: the clinician and the computer. *Lancet* **2**, 877–882.
Scharfetter, C. (1971). Die Zuverlässigkeit psychiatrischer Diagnostik: Schwierigkeiten und Wege zu ihrer Lösung. *Schweizer Archiv fur Neurologie, Neurochirugie und Psychiatrie* **109**, 419–426.
Scheff, T. (1966). 'Being Mentally Ill'. Aldine, Chicago.
Scheff, T. (1974). The labelling theory of mental illness. *Am. Sociol. Rev.* **39**, 3, 444–452.
Schmidt, H. O. and Fonda, C. P. (1956). The reliability of psychiatric diagnosis: a new look. *J. Abnorm. Soc. Psychol.* **52**, 262–267.
Sedgwick, P. (1973). Illness—mental and otherwise. *Studies* **1**, 3, 19–40. The Hastings Center—Institute of Society, Ethics and the Life Sciences, Hastings-on-Hudson, New York.
Shepherd, M. (1976). Definition, classification and nomenclature: a clinical overview. *In* 'Schizophrenia Today' (Eds D. Kemali, A. Bartholini and D. Richter) Pergamon Press, Oxford.
Shoenberg, E. (1972). The anti-therapeutic team in psychiatry. *In* 'A Hospital Looks at Itself' (Ed. E. Shoenberg). London, Cassirer.
Siegler, M. and Osmond, H. (1966). Models of madness. *Br. J. Psychiat.* **112**, 1193–1203.
Siegler, M. and Osmond, H. (1974). 'Models of Madness, Models of Medicine'. Collier Macmillan, London.
Slater, E. and Roth, M. (1969). 'Clinical Psychiatry'. Bailliere, Tindall and Cassell, London.
Spitzer, R. L. and Endicott, J. (1975). Attempts to improve psychiatric diagnosis. *In* 'Annual Review of Psychology' (Eds M. R. Rosenweig and L. N. Porter) **26**, 643.
Spitzer, R. L., Endicott, J. and Robins, E. (1974). 'Research Diagnostic Criteria'. Biometrics Research, New York State Department of Mental Hygiene, New York.
Steiner, C. (1969). The alcoholic game. *Quart. J. Stud. Alc.* **30**, 920–938.
Stengel, E. (1959). Classification of mental disorders. *Bull. W.H.O.* **21**, 601–663.
Sontag, S. (1978). Illness as metaphor. *New York Review of Books* **XXIV**, 22, 10–16.
Szasz, T. S. (1960). The myth of mental illness. *Am. Psychol.* **15**, 113–118.
Szasz, T. S. (1972). Bad habits are not diseases. *Lancet* **ii**, 83–84.
Szasz, T. S. (1974). 'The Second Sin'. Routledge and Kegan Paul, London.
Tarjan, G., Tizard, J., Rutter, M., Begab, M., Brooke, E. M., de la Cruz, F., Lin, T-Y., Montenegro, H., Strotzka, H. and Sartorius, N. (1972). Classification and

mental retardation: issues arising in the Fifth WHO Seminar on Psychiatric Diagnosis. Classification and Statistics. *Am. J. Psychiat.* **128**, No. 11, May Suppl., 34–45.

Taylor, F. Kraupl (1972). Part 2. A logical analysis of the medico-psychological concept of disease. *Psychol. Med.* **2**, 1, 7–16.

Termelin, M. K. (1968). Suggestion effects in psychiatric diagnosis. *J. Nerv. Ment. Dis.* **147**, 349–353.

Ullmann, L. P. and Krasner, L. (1975). 'A Psychological Approach to Abnormal Behavior' (2nd edn). Prentice-Hall, Englewood Cliffs.

Virchow, R. (1847). Standpoints in scientific medicine. *In* 'Diseases, Life and Man. Selected Essays by Rudolf Virchow'. Trans. L. J. Rather, 1958. Stanford University Press, Palo Alto.

Ward, C. H., Beck, A. T., Mendelson, M., Mock, J. E. and Erbaugh, J. K. (1962). The psychiatric nomenclature. *Arch. Gen. Psychiat.* **7**, 198–205.

Weiss, R. J. and Bergen, B. J. (1968). Social supports and the reduction of psychiatric disability. *Psychiatry* **31**, 107–115.

Wilson, M. S. and Meyer, E. (1962). Diagnostic consistency in a psychiatric liason service. *Am. J. Psychiat.* **119**, 207–209.

Wing, J. K., Birley, J. L. T., Cooper, J. E., Graham, P. and Isaacs, A. D. (1967). Reliability of a procedure for measuring and classifying 'Present Psychiatric State'. *Br. J. Psychiat.* **113**, 499–515.

Winokur, G., Rimmer, J. and Reich, T. (1971). Alcoholism IV. Is there more than one type of alcoholism? *Br. J. Psychiat.* **118**, 525–531.

World Health Organization (1973). Report of the Eighth Seminar on Standardisation of Psychiatric Diagnosis, Classification and Statistics. WHO, Geneva.

World Health Organization (1970). Biological research in schizophrenia. *Wld Hlth Org. Techn. Rep. Ser.* No. 450.

Zeh, W. (1962). Bemerkungen zu einem Klassifikationsverschlag der psychischen Störungen von Erik Essen-Möller, Lund. *Nervenarzt* **33**, 404–410.

Zubin, J., Salzinger, K., Fleiss, J. L., Gurland, B., Spitzer, R. L., Endicott, J. and Sutton, S. (1975). Biometric approach to psychopathology. *Ann. Rev. Psychol.* **26**, 621–671.

4 Measurement in psychiatry

Anthony Mann and *Robin Murray*

Historical development

Psychiatry was later in adopting methods of scientific reasoning and clinical observation than the rest of medicine, and many of the early pertinent measures of men's behaviour and mental function were developed by psychologists rather than psychiatrists (Hill, 1966). Two historical hypotheses formed the basis for much of this work. The first, which originated with John Locke (1632–1704) views man as a blank sheet claiming that what he becomes is determined by his experience. This hypothesis necessitated the study of external stimuli and the response of the individual. It was soon evident that the human response has both a physical component such as the avoiding of a noxious stimulus, and an emotional component such as fear. Investigation of the relationship between these two components led to the development of psychological and physical measures, and to that field of endeavour relating behavioural psychology with psychophysiological measures.

Meanwhile, Francis Galton (1822–1911) originated the tradition in which variations in man are accepted and made the object of study in order that they be delineated and quantified. Differences in intelligence were first assessed by Binet in 1905 and the psychological correlates of different body builds by Kretschmer in 1921, while differences in personality were quantified by Cattell in 1946. The most successfully developed have been measures of intelligence which have now reached such scientific accuracy and sophistication that despite the absence of an agreed definition of intelligence or any material component to it, the IQ is widely accepted as an index of human development.

The two psychological traditions stemming from Locke and Galton respectively are not incompatible. For instance, psychophysiological measures have been studied in conjunction with measures of individual differences in personality, and some relationships between them found (Eysenck, 1967). But, instruments developed by psychologists have generally been more useful in establishing constitutional features such as personality, IQ, or autonomic reactivity than in assessing psychiatric disorder *per se*. An exception has been the recent and fruitful application of the tenets of behavioural psychology to certain neuroses (Chapter 21).

Progress in physical medicine during the last fifty years has followed discovery of the pathology of diseases previously described only as syndromes. Once these discoveries were made accurate techniques of detecting and quantifying pathology developed allowing the recognition of illness and the assessment of its severity to move from the realm of the physician's intuition. The aetiology of the major psychiatric disorders remains largely unknown, so the psychiatrist cannot call upon the radiologist or pathologist to help in diagnosis or assessment of the effect of therapy. Electroencephalography has not yet fulfilled its early promise as an instrument for use in clinical psychiatry, and laboratory tests, while often quite precise, are not clearly relevant to the clinical state of the patient (Hollister and Overall, 1974). Recently developed biological measures have yet to make a major impact on the assessment of functional psychiatric disorders. Some progress has been made in relating the galvanic skin response and forearm blood flow to psychopathology (Bond *et al.*, 1974), and also with the average evoked response in psychosis (Buchsbaumn *et al.*, 1975), and with eye tracking dysfunction in schizophrenia (Holzman *et al.;* 1976). In addition, serum creatine phosphokinese appears to be elevated in acute psychosis (Meltzer, 1976), and low platelet monoamine oxidase has been reported as predisposing to psychiatric disorder (Murphy, 1977).

However, with respect to measurement, psychiatry has lagged behind. On the one hand the psychologists have developed sophisticated measures of human difference and begun to quantify elements of behaviour, but this work has seldom been applicable to clinical problems. On the other hand the physicians have developed therapies that can be adequately assessed, based upon knowledge of the underlying pathology and its accurate measurement. Yet, in the last thirty years many psychiatrists have devised methods of measurement for their own work. The absence of satisfactory biological markers for psychiatric disorders has meant that the instruments consist of rating schedules, questionnaires and standard interviews. Their use has increased so much that as Hamilton (1976) states 'it is scarcely possible to look through any copy of a general psychiatric journal without finding at least one paper which involves the use of a scale of some sort'.

The impetus behind the attempts to measure psychiatric phenomena have come from three sources. The first has been the attempt to improve the quality of observation, making the psychiatrist's work more scientific, objective and less intuitive in keeping with the other medical sciences, and allowing scientific hypotheses to be tested. The second has been the increasing interest in the epidemiology of mental disorder. Shepherd and Cooper (1964) have reviewed the historical development of this method of study which proved its value in 1914 with the demonstration of the cause of pellagra psychosis by Goldberger. Finally, the development of psychopharmacology since 1952 has necessitated the elaboration of instruments intended to assess change in the severity of mental illness (Pichot, 1974).

Before describing some of these instruments it is worth remembering that they are only devices for recording information about a patient, the data obtained being no better than its source. Inadequate, misleading or incorrect information is not changed by recording it on a rating scale. A free and full psychiatric history and examination still yields more information than any standardized instrument. Furthermore, the fundamental method of assessing progress in psychiatry remains the clinical judgement of whether a patient is worse, unchanged or improved. Such judgements are often denigrated but when made by experienced clinicians who take into account the information provided by other observers—psychologists, nurses, and social workers—they can be very accurate. The value of measuring instruments is that they are uniform for all patients and all occasions, and standard in their significance because the items, their grades and manner of use have been previously defined. They, therefore, permit comparison between individuals and between the same individual on different occasions, but at a cost of flexibility.

The principles underlying instruments measuring psychiatric disorder

Instruments designed for use in clinical psychiatry serve three main functions, namely:

(1) to identify psychiatric cases in a population at risk;
(2) to standardize psychiatric interviews thereby improving the accuracy of assessment and diagnosis;
(3) to measure the severity of psychiatric symptomatology, thereby allowing change and the effects of treatment to be assessed.

These three principal functions together with some examples of instruments designed for each of them will be elaborated later but first the principles which should underly any measuring instrument will be described.

The purpose of the instrument

Although sometimes capable of fulfilling all of the three functions outlined above, most instruments have one primary function. This should be made clear, as should the sensitivity of the instrument to the various conditions in the psychiatric spectrum. Most clinicians recognize a distinction in this spectrum between personality traits and symptoms, the latter being manifestations of neurotic, psychotic or psychosomatic disorders. It is feasible for an instrument to assess both traits and states, or several different disorders, but many concentrate on one clinical category. A clear understanding of an instrument's purpose is essential to prevent its misapplication.

The administration of the instrument

The purpose of an instrument will usually determine where and by whom it is administered. Thus, one intended for psychosomatic disorders might best be administered in a general hospital and one for neurotic patients in general practice. The length of an instrument and its content will be influenced by the setting in which it is to be used.

An instrument can be completed in three ways. The patient can report about himself, or observations and inferences about his behaviour and emotional functioning can be made by professional or non-professional interviewers. The self-report questionnaire is economic of professional time, and records directly the response of the individual experiencing the phenomena—the patient himself. Such questionnaires are amenable to actuarial methods of scoring, and are highly sensitive to drug-induced changes (Kellner, 1971). On the other hand, they require that the patient should be able to concentrate, be literate and ideally be familiar with the terms used to describe emotions. This last point is important because patients and psychiatrist do not interpret words in the same way. Pinard and Tetrault (1974) found that patients could not distinguish clearly between sadness, fatigue and anxiety because they experienced them simultaneously.

The alternative to the self-administered questionnaire—the observer rated schedule—can be administrated by an individual who is skilled (e.g. a psychiatrist), or semi-skilled (e.g. a nursing aide) or unskilled such as a relative. The use of family members to provide data about patients is, however, comparatively untested and subject to considerable bias. Scales designed to be used by the non-professional interviewer should not require the observer to interpret the subject's response, but rather concentrate on recording behaviour. A schedule to be given by a psychiatrist can allow the observer considerable opportunity for judgement and discrimination, but special training in its application and interpretation will increase reliability (Wing *et al.*, 1967).

The composition of the instrument

Many instruments conform to a basic structure in which a large number of items are grouped into a number of scales on which a score may be obtained; in some such as the depression inventories (p. 91) the scale scores may be summated to give a global score, while in others such as the descriptive schedules (p. 87) the scores are represented separately. The items can be formulated as statements or questions to which the responder must agree or disagree, e.g. the Eysenck Personality Inventory. As an alternative to this forced choice, the responder can be offered a number of gradations to each item so that the strength of the response can be assessed. Thus the adverbs 'Mildly', 'Moderately', and 'Extremely' can stretch the meaning of adjectives like anxious, dejected or suspicious (Cliff, 1959).

The choice of words in an item is extremely important. Pinard and Tetrault (1974) gave a list of adjectives describing various affects such as sadness or anxiety to doctors, nurses and patients. The 'communication gap' demonstrated between the different classes of subjects was so great that the authors concluded that 'the communication of feelings by words is imprecise and inaccurate', and that 'prudence and awareness are the more necessary when assessing mood in a research situation'. Problems of instrument design are discussed by Oppenheim (1966).

Lorr (1974) has recently summarized the desirable characteristics of scales. They should be unidimensional so that a scale should cover one component only such as depression or paranoia, and not be combined as in depressed-paranoid. Furthermore, they should be unipolar and in this they may not mirror clinical concepts. For example, depression and mania are better represented by two scales starting from zero, than a scale with depression at one end and mania at the other since, for example, a patient with a mixed affective psychosis will require an independent rating for both these aspects. Another desirable objective is that scores on the scale should be graded in equal steps so that a score of two is half the strength of a score of four. This can be difficult to achieve. How, for instance, should a patient with constant depressive ruminations be assessed on a depression scale in comparison to another with fluctuating affect but who has attempted suicide? A partial solution to this dilemma can be reached if items take account of both the severity and duration of a symptom.

Sources of error

Attention needs to be paid to sources of bias which may be general to all forms of instrument or dependent on its method of administration. Common to all forms are errors from *response set* and the *bias towards the middle*. The former implies that some responders are inclined to either agree or disagree with propositions excessively. This error can be countered by phrasing certain questions so that agreement is signified by the negative. Bias towards the middle indicates the reluctance of some responders to rate an extreme response, thus producing an excess of middle responses. This tendency can be countered by giving the subject only two or four choices thus eliminating the middle position or by incorporating extra categories of severity so that responders will be encouraged to move their responses towards the extremes.

Some errors are specific to self-administered questionnaires. These are *social desirability* and *defensiveness*. The former implies that subjects will rate what they consider acceptable rather than what is accurate (Edwards, 1957). This error can be important when questionnaires are used to assess the effect of therapy as some patients may try to please the doctor. Characteristic defensiveness is the attribute of responders who give an inaccurate response to avoid giving away information about themselves. Both these sources of bias can be reduced by careful wording of questions and, if necessary, by the incorporation of certain questions which will detect those subjects concerned(with social desirability. The Eysenck Personality Inventory, for instance, contains a Lie Scale.

The observer, scoring a schedule, is an important new source of errors of which two are the *halo effect* and *proximity*. The former means that an observer, having obtained a general impression of the presence or absence of pathology, is inclined to rate items in accordance with this preconception. Thus having ascertained that the subject has one biological symptom of depression such as diurnal variation he may be more likely to rate others such as early morning wakening. The latter implies that contiguous ratings have an effect on each other. Both these observer errors can be minimized by interspersing the items of the various scales, so that, for example, in a mental state schedule an observer does not complete all the items on depression consecutively.

Reliability

Reliability concerns the accuracy with which measurement is performed. To the extent that an instrument possesses reliability measurement using it will have precision. Poor reliability in ratings may derive from the subject, the observer or the instrument itself. The subject will contribute a measure of error by the unpredictability of his responses and by fluctuation in the manifestation of his condition. Observers influence the material obtained for rating by variations in their administration of the instrument and by differences in the relationship each observer forms with the subject (Salzinger, 1977). Their rating of the obtained material is affected by differences in experience and preconceptions. Finally, faulty instrument design particularly for self-administered questionnaires contributes to the error as outlined previously.

Reliability can be checked by three methods. The first is *inter-rater reliability* where ratings of the same material by different observers either simultaneously or consecutively are compared. Second is *test-retest reliability*, which if the condition of the subject remains constant, allows observer and instrument error to be checked by testing the same individual on several occasions. Because the subject rarely remains in a static condition this method is less useful in clinical psychiatry than in other fields. The third method is to assess *split half reliability*. This involves dividing the whole instrument into two equal halves, and comparing a subject's score on each half. If all items are of equal importance the two halves should have a similar score. Difference in the score of the two halves suggests that the scale score in the original instrument is an aggregate of divergent and possibly unrelated items. In general the reliability of self-administered questionnaires depends on the clarity of the questions and the care of the design, and that of observer rated schedules on having clear accompanying instructions together with a period when different raters work together to obtain standardization. Although reliable methodology is now accepted as necessary to a scientific psychiatry, the appropriate use of statistically sound measures of reliability is less appreciated. Bartko and Carpenter (1976) have recently reviewed the most frequently used and misused reliability measures.

Validity

An instrument must show that it measures what it was intended to do, i.e. has validity. The practical demonstration of *criterion validity* includes checking that the items relate to the phenomena being assessed (content validity) and that the instrument can distinguish between a population possessing the condition to which it is supposed to be sensitive and one that does not (external validity). A further useful demonstration is that the instrument accords in its results with other instruments purporting the same function (concurrent validity). *Construct validity* means that the results obtained from the instrument relate to the hypotheses underlying its design. Items on a scale that measure the same variable should correlate well together (convergent validity) and items that measure different variables should have a low correlation (discriminant validity). Validation is not a once only procedure, but should be re-examined when the instrument is used for new populations, particularly those with fresh attributes such as being part of a different culture.

Instruments in common use in psychiatry

The remainder of this chapter is devoted to a discussion of some of the measuring instruments commonly used in psychiatry. More lengthy and inclusive discussions are available elsewhere (National Institute of Mental Health, 1966; Buros, 1972; ECDEU, 1976). Two criteria have determined inclusion in this chapter, namely frequent appearance in the psychiatric literature (Buros, 1972), and scientific value (as judged by the authors). Tests of intellectual or cognitive ability, some of which are discussed in Chapter 13, are not included. Only those personality tests widely used in psychiatric research are described and projective tests such as the Rorschach or Thematic Apperception Tests are not. The interested reader is referred to Murstern (1965) and Singer (1977) or Jensen (1958). Techniques for the assessment of change in the attitudes of an individual, such as the repertory grid and semantic differential, have been well reviewed by Fransella (1975).

Case finding

The purposes of epidemiological investigations are manifold, but include assessing the prevalence of disorder in a population, searching for aetiological clues to psychiatric disorders, and estimating individual risks of acquiring a disease by studying its distribution on a large scale. Mechanic (1970) has written of the poor standard of case identification in many surveys, and in particular of the folly of accepting such inadequate data as numbers of admissions as indicative of incidence. The major problem in surveys is that most populations contain subjects with symptoms ranging from the transient and minor to the gross and chronic, making it difficult to agree what constitutes a psychiatric case.

As a diagnostic interview is impractical for large-scale surveys, investigators have tried to find alternatives. These have included employing unskilled interviewers, using questionnaires that purport to provide a psychiatric diagnosis, or using screening questionnaires to identify potential cases who can then be diagnosed by interview. The importance of accurate case identification is emphasized by Mechanic (1974) who writes 'like a ship that begins on the wrong course, an epidemiological investigation that uses weak and unreliable measures of its dependent variable is unlikely to reach its required destination'. It remains difficult for psychiatric research workers to be confident that they have satisfactory measures for case finding. This fact together with doubt that the identification and treatment of a patient greatly alters the course of an illness means that, as Eastwood (1971) states, 'screening for psychiatric disorders must remain at the experimental phase and is not ready for inclusion in the medical services'.

(i) The Cornell Medical Index (CMI) was one of the first questionnaires employed as a screening instrument (Brodman *et al.*, 1949). It is designed to be filled in by patients before seeing their doctor, thus providing him with useful information about their health, and is based on the traditional medical review of systems with special emphasis on the psychiatric. In the two decades following its introduction the CMI was used by many investigators including Shepherd *et al.* (1966). This group reported CMI results on 2245 patients seen in general practice and 1485 out-patients, but concluded that although the CMI detected severe disorders, many neurotics were misclassified as normal. There is now general agreement that the CMI is old-fashioned and naïve in design with no place as an instrument for psychiatric evaluation although it continues to have some use as a conserver of a physician's time (Buros, 1972).

(ii) The General Health Questionnaire (GHQ) was developed by Goldberg (1972) as a self-administered questionnaire that would 'identify respondents with a non psychotic illness, by assessing the severity of their psychiatric disturbance'. The GHQ consists of 60 items, with a shorter version of 30 to which the patient can reply on a four point scale from 'much more than usual' to 'less so than usual'. The instrument asks the respondent for perception of recent change in himself, thus detecting symptoms rather than personality traits. Goldberg states that 'a patient's score on the GHQ is in many ways analogous to the ESR in general medicine. A high score indicates that there is probably something wrong but it does not reveal the diagnosis'. The instrument is thus a screening device detecting likely psychiatric cases who should then undergo a diagnostic interview.

Since its publication, the GHQ has been widely used. In addition to Goldberg's own studies in general practice, Sims and Salmons (1975) compared the responses of consecutive new psychiatric out-patients with those of a matched sample attending a general practitioner. Examination of those of the psychiatric referrals who scored below the cut-off point showed that many had improved since referral, while the proportion of those scoring above the cut-off point attending the practitioner's surgery appeared to represent the hidden morbidity of the general population. Recently Mann (1977) had used this instrument to screen all those attending a number of centres for the detection of hypertension. Over 12,000 questionnaires were completed, attesting to the GHQs acceptability to the general population, its ease of administration and therefore its suitability for community surveys.

(iii) The Hopkins Symptom Checklist (HSCL) was not initially designed as a screening test but evolved from an instrument produced to evaluate change in psychotherapy, and was subsequently used with considerable success as a measure of symptomatic improvement in drug trials. Its extensive use in North America has provided large-scale normative data as well as scores for patient groups. Derogatis and his colleagues (1974) are substantially correct in claiming that there is 'adequate confirmation of it as a reliable, valid, psychological measurement scale'.

The HSCL consists of 58 questions concerning psychophysiological and affective symptoms to which the respondent is required to answer on a four-point scale from 'not at all' to 'always'. Factor analysis of the items produced five major factors—somatization, obsessive-compulsive, interpersonal sensitivity, depression and anxiety. These formed the basis of a 35-item version intended for use as a screening instrument (the Lipman-Rickels Scale) whose efficacy has been compared with that of the General Health Questionnaire. The two tests performed very similarly, but the GHQ was more inclined to miss the psychiatrically disturbed individuals who were characteristically defensive or had their symptoms for a long time, while the Lipman-Rickels Scale appeared unduly sensitive to those who had a subclinical disturbance or a purely physical illness (Goldberg et al., 1976).

Description and diagnosis

A number of studies have shown if two psychiatrists independently interview and diagnose patients with functional disorders they are likely to make the same diagnosis only 30–40% of the time, and even when both are experienced and share the same orientation the agreement is rarely better than 60% (Kreitman, 1961; Beck *et al.*, 1961). This lack of diagnostic agreement has been a major handicap to psychiatric research particularly when comparisons are being made between studies carried out in different countries (p. 358). The reasons for diagnostic disparity were analysed in a study by Ward *et al.* (1962) in which 153 patients were examined by two psychiatrists: 62·5% of the diagnostic disagreement was attributed to the inadequacies of the classification system used in psychiatry, 32·5% to inconsistency on the part of the psychiatrists, and only 5% to variation in the history given by the patients. These findings prompted a great deal of research into how diagnoses are made (Kendell, 1975), and into ways of describing phenomena with greater reliability.

These attempts at standardization have three purposes. The first is to control the interview setting and the questions asked of the subject so that similar information is likely to be forthcoming to different interviewers. The second is to train the observer so that standardization of judgement can be obtained on the information elicited. The third is to provide clear definitions of the descriptive categories to be employed thereby reducing some of the nosological difficulties, leading to a number of attempts to provide operational definitions of different mental illnesses. The best known are the Feighner criteria (Feighner *et al.*, 1972) which have become widely accepted among American research workers in the modified form known as the Research Diagnostic Criteria (Spitzer *et al.*, 1975).

Standardized interview schedules can be divided into two types: (a) Descriptive Schedules which simply bring the variables of the interview under control to produce information that can be subjected to statistical analysis, and (b) Diagnostic Schedules which aim to match the clinical process so that a diagnosis can be made.

(i) The Wittenborn Psychiatric Rating Scale (WPRS) was originally developed to provide a means whereby a trained observer could interview a psychiatric in-patient, score the ratings and prepare a symptom profile. The best known version employs 72 scales and can be used to describe both acute and chronic patients. The WPRS has been widely used for psychopharmacological research and for inter-hospital comparisons (Wittenborn, 1974; ECDEU, 1976). It has the advantage that great attention has been paid to its standardization, but it is rather cumbersome and concentrates on observed behaviour to the exclusion of the reported experience of the patient.

(ii) The Inpatient Multidimensional Scale (IMPS) has a history somewhat similar to the Wittenborn Scale and the two have often been compared. It contains 89 items mostly rated on nine-point scales, and the need for definitions is circumvented by a careful avoidance of all technical terms. The first item, for instance, is phrased so that the observer must state not whether the patient displays verbal retardation but whether, compared to the normal person, his speech is 'slowed, deliberate or laboured'. The IMPS is designed for use with patients suffering from functional psychoses and severe neurotic disorders, and ordinarily it can be completed following a 30 to 45 minute semi-structured interview (Lorr and Klett, 1967).

In addition to its use in typing patients, the IMPS has been widely used as a criterion of change in therapeutic trials (Lorr, 1974). It is both reliable and valid, but suffers from the disadvantage that the 12 'elementary syndromes' and four 'major disorders' which it determines are the product of statistical analysis and do not accord with clinical concept. Thus, in their account of the use of the IMPS in six different countries Lorr and Klett (1969) noted that for many of the collaborators some of the psychotic syndromes had no meaning.

(iii) The Brief Psychiatric Rating Scale (BPRS) covers a similar field to the two previous scales, but as its name implies it is shorter. It was originally developed to provide an efficient and clinically valid means of assessing efficacy in psychopharmacological research (Overall and Gorham, 1962), but later research demonstrated its utility for the descriptive classification of psychiatric patients (Overall, 1974). The BPRS now consists of 18 symptom constructs each to be rated on a seven-point scale of severity ranging from 'not present' to 'extremely severe'. These rating constructs cover the full range of psychopathology usually shown by in-patients but do not distinguish adequately between different neuroses, so that the BPRS is less suitable for out-patient use.

The BPRS has become the most widely used rating scale in psychopharmacological research, being used not only to evaluate the extent but also the nature of drug effects; for example, whether a particular phenothiazine has more effect on paranoid symptoms or hallucinations. BPRS ratings can also be used to classify patients into phenomenologically homogeneous sub-types: empirical cluster analysis of BPRS profiles have repeatedly identified six phenomenological patterns, and computer programs are now available for classifying patients (ECDEU, 1976).

(iv) The Psychiatric Status Schedule (PSS) was published to provide 'an easily learned technique of simultaneously examining, recording and calculating the mental status of a psychiatric patient' (Spitzer et al., 1970). It is concerned with the symptoms experienced by the patient during the preceding seven days, and consists of an interview schedule and a matching inventory of 321 dichotomous items. The exact form of words for each question is stipulated, and the corresponding ratings are closely tied to the wording of the patient's reply; limited further probing is allowed if his reply is incomplete or ambiguous.

The PSS requires training but can be used by non-psychiatrists, and because it is so highly structured produces high reliability. It has, however, been criticized as being scanty in its coverage of psychotic symptomatology and not effective for alcoholism and psychopathy. Cooper and his colleagues (1972) also claim that it wastes psychiatric skill as it allows so little scope for the interviewer to probe for better information.

Spitzer and Endicott (1968) used this schedule as the basis for a computer programme, Diagno I, in which the computer allocated each patient to one of 27 diagnostic categories. For the same material, the computer always matches same conclusion thus eliminating one of the major sources of variability in diagnosis—the psychiatrist himself. This was soon followed by Diagno II, a more complex programme using history data as well as current mental status, and generating a wider range of diagnoses. The authors were able to show that agreement between the diagnoses made by this programme and those made by clinicians were as good as that between two groups of clinicians, thus demonstrating that the computer's diagnoses possessed adequate face validity.

(v) The Present State Examination (PSE) which was first published in 1967 has now reached its ninth edition (Wing *et al.*, 1974). It is more flexible than the PSS in that the interviewer can omit detailed questioning of areas of possible psychopathology should a probe question for that area be answered negatively. Thus although the PSE's 140 items cover all the information usually gained from a clinical interview, the questioning can be tailored to the pathology present. The ratings on certain groups of items are summed to produce a score on 38 'syndromes' such as 'auditory hallucinations' or 'situational anxiety', and the 'syndromes' are then processed by a computer programme named CATEGO to give a standardized diagnostic grouping. CATEGO follows a clinician's logic without his idiosyncrasies.

The PSE is designed for use by psychiatrists after a specified period of training, so that inter-rater reliability is high. Unfortunately, it is not yet satisfactory for all psychiatric conditions. It is excellent for the diagnosis of schizophrenia, but there is less agreement with clinical judgement in the diagnosis of the neuroses and personality disorder, and organic psychosis cannot be adequately assessed. Nevertheless, the PSE has enabled great strides to be made in comparing psychiatric diagnosis throughout the world (p. 358). It has also been used as a measure of psychopathology in studies of the biochemistry of psychosis (Rodnight *et al.*, 1976), the effect of phenothiazines on schizophrenia (Hirsch *et al.*,

1973), and of differences of pathology in long and short stay hospital patients (Mann, 1972). The use of the PSE in community studies is more questionable and has prompted Wing (1976) to differentiate between individuals with no symptoms, those with borderline symptoms and those with specific disorders.

(vi) The Standard Psychiatric Interview (SPI) complements the PSE since it is intended for use with subjects who may not consider themselves psychiatrically disturbed (Goldberg *et al.*, 1970). It covers medical history, present and past psychiatric history, and family history, and also includes a section on abnormalities observed during the interview. The SPI produces a score representing the extent and severity of the symptomatology, and the interviewer is able to determine whether the subject is a psychiatric case and name a diagnosis. A high degree of reliability can be obtained among interviewers if they have undergone a period of training. The SPI is economical of time and appropriate for use in community surveys since it is more sensitive to affective and psychosomatic disorders than to the psychoses. An example of its use is an evaluation by Cooper *et al.* (1975) of the efficacy of a social worker in treating patients in general practice.

The assessment of specific disorders

The instruments described in this section are designed for individual psychiatric disorders, and many claim to be sensitive to change in severity thus allowing the effects of treatment to be assessed. These instruments are constructed on the twin assumptions that a score representing the number and severity of the symptoms elicited will fluctuate as the intensity of the condition does, and that this score is a more precise estimate of the severity of the condition than is clinical judgement. Unfortunately, Noble and Lader's (1971) attempt to correlate rating scale scores with psychophysiological measures did not provide much corroborative evidence for these assumptions.

To maximize sensitivity to change, preference is often given in these instruments to items concerning symptoms which are not only common in the condition under study, but are also likely to vary in the short-term. For instance, the clinical assessment of anxiety includes an evaluation of the subject's anxiety proneness, but since this trait is unlikely to alter with treatment to the extent that peripheral autonomic symptoms are, the inclusion of items on anxiety proneness would reduce an instrument's sensitivity to change. Preference is also given in many instruments to items that are conceived as representing the severity rather than the form of the illness. Thus, a scale measuring depression might include an item on weight loss since it is considered indicative of severity rather than one on diurnal variation which tends to be used to delineate the type of a depressive illness.

A final caveat in the interpretation of instruments measuring disorders other than depression is that made by Cooper (1970) who notes that unhappy people tend to say yes to questions about psychopathology to an excessive extent. So an instrument purporting to measure anxiety might, in fact, reflect the extent of depression present.

Affective disorders

Not only are there many scales specifically for assessing depression, but general rating schedules such as the BPRS and IMPS (p. 88) can be used although they are less sensitive (Raskin and Crook, 1976). Global clinical judgements are still employed while self-rating forms come into their own when assessments have to be repeated frequently (Hamilton, 1976). The profusion of possible measures for affective disorders means that each research worker can select the one most appropriate to his purpose, but limits comparison of different studies. Perhaps a solution for the individual research worker is to use one of the well standardized and widely accepted measures discussed below in addition to one more individually tailored to his particular investigation.

(i) The Hamilton Rating Scale (HRS) was one of the first rating scales primarily designed for depressive illness, and has become highly popular for drug trials, and as both a basis and a standard for other scales (Hamilton, 1967; ECDEU, 1976). It is intended for use in the course of an ordinary psychiatric interview, is highly reliable and correlates well with clinical judgement. Factor analysis of the HRS has been reported twice (Hamilton, 1967; Mowbray, 1972) and both studies found a major factor representing the severity of depression plus five lesser factors. The structure of the scale makes it score highly when somatic symptomatology is present, but underestimate the severity of depression in patients with few somatic symptoms or concerns. Its other major disadvantage is that it is difficult to use frequently on the same subject.

(ii) The Beck Depression Inventory (BDI) consists of 21 categories of symptoms and attitudes with four or five statements of severity for each; the patient picks the statement which most closely matches his current experience (Beck *et al.*, 1961). The BDI has been validated against independent psychiatric judgement, and by testing hypotheses about the behaviour of depressed patients; for instance, high scorers on the inventory become extremely pessimistic after experimentally induced failure on a task, as was predicted. The BDI correlates well with the HRS and has the advantage that it need not be administered by an observer with psychiatric training. An abridged version has been devised as a screening test in general practice (Beck and Beamsderfer, 1974).

(iii) The Zung Self Rating Depression Scale (SDS) comprises 20 sentences which the patient rates in one of four quantitative terms Zung (1965). The items are based on 'those clinical diagnostic criteria most commonly used to characterize depressive disorders' and consequently the SDS correlates well with clinical ratings. So as to be able to distinguish between primary depression and depression occurring as part of other psychiatric conditions Zung (1974) developed a companion observer-rated Depression Status Inventory.

(iv) The Manic State Scale. In contrast to the large number of rating scales for depression, there were until recently no satisfactory measures of mania. Thus, although some general scales such as the WPRS and IMPS (p. 87) include items yielding a mania factor most studies assessing mania have relied on global estimates. To remedy this Beigel and his colleagues (1971) designed a manic state scale with 26 items, each one of which is rated on separate five-point scales for 'frequency' and 'intensity'. This scale is for use by trained nursing staff to take advantage of the fact that they have the most extensive contact with hospitalized manic patients. High inter-rater reliability has been observed and a close correspondence found between the total scores, two psychiatrists' global ratings of the severity of manic symptoms and check list scores of manic symptoms (Murphy *et al.*, 1974). Although this scale has yet to be used extensively it offers promise both in quantifying manic behaviour and in delineating clinical and biological differences in manic-depressive patients.

(v) The Taylor Manifest Anxiety Scale (TMAS: Taylor, 1953). Anxiety scales are generally divided into those which measure anxiety proneness as a personality trait, and those which purport to measure anxiety as a symptomatic disorder. But, de Bonis (1974) analysed a large number of anxiety scales and found their content to be remarkably similar suggesting that scales invented to measure state anxiety are often contaminated by items reflecting trait anxiety.

The TMAS has achieved a remarkably wide usage considering the simplicity of the original report. It is based upon 50 items, culled from a personality inventory, which a panel of clinical psychologists considered useful in the assessment of chronic anxiety reactions. Not surprisingly many of the items are concerned with enduring trait anxiety, and a study by Kellner and Scheffield (1968) showed the TMAS to be the worst measure of change in levels of anxiety state.

(vi) The Hamilton Anxiety Scale (HRAS) was designed for the rating of anxiety as part of anxiety neuroses rather than for the rating of anxiety symptoms occurring in other psychiatric disorders or trait anxiety (Hamilton, 1959, 1960). Assessment is made during a clinical interview on the severity of abnormality in 12 symptoms items and one behaviour item, and good reliability can be obtained by psychiatrists experienced in its use. Hamilton's correlation matrices identified a general factor of anxiety and bipolar factor of psychic versus somatic symptoms; this fits the clinical view of anxiety as comprising both a feeling state and alterations in physiological function.

(vii) The Self-Rating Anxiety Scale (SAS) and its counterpart the Anxiety Status Inventory (ASI) which is scored by a clinician employ 20 items to be rated on four-point scales (Zung, 1974; ECDEU, 1976). The correlation between the two scales for patients with anxiety neurosis is 0·74.

(viii) The Leyton Obsessional Inventory (LOI). When Cooper (1970) attempted to study obsessionality among houseproud housewives he discovered that there was no satisfactory measuring instrument. He, therefore, developed the Leyton Obsessional Inventory which consists of 69 questions each printed on a separate card for the respondent to put into either the 'yes' or 'no' slots of an answer box. The LOI provides a measure of both obsessional symptoms and traits, as well as the extent to which the symptoms interfere with the subject's life and how much they are resisted. It distinguishes satisfactorily between obsessional patients and normal individuals (Murray *et al.*, 1979) and a principal components analysis on the replies of 302 normal subjects revealed three distinct components called 'clean and tidy', 'incompleteness', and 'checking'. The LOI has proved its worth in a number of studies, but its length and rather cumbersome application have restricted its use.

(ix) Analogue Scales. In recent years there has been a revival of interest in very simple line indicators. The rater is asked to locate the variable in question by marking a point along a line which runs between two extremes (Zealley and Aitken, 1969). For instance in a scale for fear one end would represent no fear at all and the other very severe fear. Such scales can be completed either by patients and observers and high inter-rater reliability can be obtained (Lader and Marks, 1971). A scale can be constructed for each of patient's target symptoms and thus individual clinical change can be monitored. Since these scales are personally tailored they are of less value for large-scale studies.

Personality

(i) The Minnesota Multiphasic Personality Inventory (MMPI) is the most widely used of all inventories being especially valued in North America (Buros, 1972). It was originally developed as an aid to psychiatric diagnosis and consists of 550 statements covering a variety of areas from physical health to social attitudes (Hathaway and McKinley, 1943). These statements are grouped into nine scales some of which are clinical, e.g. 'depression', 'hysteria', 'paranoid', and some of which are personality factors, e.g. 'ego strength'. Each scale has been worked out empirically on groups of patients diagnosed as depressive, hysteric, paranoid, etc. The test results are plotted as a profile which can be compared with that obtained in normal people and in different types of patient. The disadvantages of the MMPI are that it is cumbersome, time consuming, and that it does not assess personality function within the normal range of adjustment: it is illogical to use psychiatric patients as a criterion group for normal personality dimensions and to mix psychiatric states like 'depression' with personality traits like 'ego strength'. Nevertheless, the MMPI can be used as a legitimate aid to psychiatric description rather than a personality test. The fact that it has been so widely used means that extensive normative data is available (Buros, 1972).

(ii) The Eysenck Personality Inventory (EPI) is the personality questionnaire most widely used in Britain (Eysenck and Eysenck, 1964). Its 48 questions measure two major factors, extraversion–introversion and neuroticism. The use of these orthogonal (independent) dimensions permits the specification of an individual by placing him within a two-dimensional space. The test also incorporates a 'Lie Scale' which enables the tester to assess the extent to which the subject has 'faked good'. Eysenck and his co-workers have produced a vast amount of research based on his inventory and have attempted to put his personality dimensions on a firmer biological footing by adducing evidence from genetic, psychophysiological and even endocrinological sources. Eysenck and Eysenck (1969) developed a new form of the test which incorporates a scale for measuring a third major orthogonal dimension of personality called psychoticism. This dimension has not been widely accepted by clinicians who claim that it could equally well have been called psychopathy.

(iii) The Middlesex Hospital Questionnaire (MHQ) aims to provide 'a rapid quantification of common symptoms and traits relevant to the conventional diagnostic categories of psychoneurotic illness'. It covers six areas—free floating anxiety, obsessions, phobias, somatic anxiety, depression and hysteria—to yield a profile of six scores (Crown and Crisp, 1966). The MHQ has been used for the study of special groups such as the middle aged, and those with rheumatoid arthritis (Crown, 1974) and recently a large community survey has been completed (Crisp *et al.*, 1977). The MHQ lacks statistical refinement, and validation can be criticized (Goldberg, 1972) but as its results are readily understood by clinicians, the instrument has become a popular one.

References

Barkto, J. T. and Carpenter, W. T. (1976). On methods and theory of reliability. *J. Nerv. Ment. Dis.* **163**, 307–316.

Beck, A. T., and Beamesderfer (1974). Assessment of depression. *In* 'Psychological Measures in Psychopharmacology' (Ed. P. Pichot). Karger, Basel.

Beck, A. T., Ward, C. H., Mendelson, M., Mock, J. and Erbaugh, J. (1961). An inventory for measuring depression. *Arch. Gen. Psychiat.* **4**, 561–571.

Beigel, A., Murphy, D. and Bunney, W. E. (1971). The manic-state rating scale. *Arch. Gen. Psychiat.* **25**, 256–262.

Bond, A. J., James, D. C. and Lader, M. H. (1974). Physiological and psychological measures in anxious patients. *Psychol. Med.* **4**, 365–373.

Brodman, K., Erdnan, A. J., Lorge, I., Wolff, G. and Broadbent, T. H. (1949). The Cornell Medical Index. *J.A.M.A.* **140**, 530–540.

Buchsbaumn, M. (1975). Average evoked response in schizophrenia and affective disorder. *In* 'The Biology of Major Mental Psychoses' (Ed. D. Freedman), Vol. 54. Raven Press, New York.

Buros, O. K. (1972). 'The Seventh Mental Measurements Yearbook'. Gryphon Press, New Jersey.

Cliff, N. (1959). Adverbs as Multipliers. *Psychol. Rev.* **66**, 27–43.

Cooper, B., Harwin, B. G., Depla, C. and Shepherd, M. (1975). Mental health care in the community. *Psychol. Med.* **5**, 372–380.

Cooper, J. E. (1970). The Leyton Obsessional Inventory. *Psychol. Med.* **1**, 48–64.

Cooper, J. E., Kendell, R. E., Gurland, B. J., Sharpe, L., Copeland, J. and Simon, R. (1972). 'Psychiatric Diagnosis in London and New York'. Maudsley Monograph 20. Oxford University Press, Oxford.

Crisp, A. H., Ralph, P. C., McGuinness, B. and Harris, G. (1978). Psychoneurotic profiles in the adult population. *Br. J. Med. Psychol.* **51**, 293–301.

Crown, S. and Crisp, A. H. (1966) A short clinical diagnostic self-rating scale for psychoneurotic patients. *Br. J. Psychiat.* **112**, 917–923.

Crown, S. and Crown, J. M. (1973). Personality in early rheumatoid disease. *J. Psychosom. Res.* **17**, 189–196.

de Bonis, M. (1974). Content analysis of 27 anxiety inventories and rating scales. *In* 'Psychological Measures in Psychopharmacology' (Ed. P. Pichot). Karger, Basel.

Derogatis, L. R. (1974). The Hopkins Symptom Checklist. In 'Psychological Measures in Psychopharmacology' (Ed. P. Pichot). Karger, Basel.
Early Clinical Drug Evaluation Unit (1976). 'ECDEU Assessment Manual'. H.E.W. Rockville, Maryland.
Eastwood, M. R. (1971). Screening for psychiatric disorder. Psychol. Med. 1, 199–208.
Edwards, A. L. (1957). 'The Social Desirability Variable in Personality Assessment and Research'. Holt, New York.
Eysenck, H. J. (1967). 'Biological Basis of Personality'. C. Thomas, Springfield.
Eysenck, H. J. and Eysenck, S. B. G. (1964). 'Manual of Eysenck Personality Inventory'. University of London Press, London.
Fransella, F. (1975). In 'Methods of Psychiatric Research' (Eds P. Sainsbury and N. Kreitman). Oxford University Press, Oxford.
Feighener, J. P., Robins, E., Guze, S. B. (1972). Diagnostic criteria for use in psychiatric research. Arch. Gen. Psychiat. 26, 57–63.
Goldberg, D. (1972). 'Detecting Psychiatric Illness by Questionnaire'. Maudsley Monograph 22. Oxford University Press, Oxford.
Goldberg, D. P., Cooper, B., Eastwood, M. R., Kedward, H. B. and Shepherd, M. (1970). A standardized interview for use in community studies. Br. J. Prev. Soc. Med. 24, 18–23.
Goldberg, D. P., Rickels, K., Downing, R. and Hebacher, P. (1976). A comparison of two psychiatric screening tests. Br. J. Psychiat. 129, 61–68.
Hamilton, M. (1959). A rating scale for anxiety. Br. J. Med. Psychol. 32, 50–55.
Hamilton, M. (1960). A rating scale for depression. J. Neurol. Neurosurg. Psych. 23, 56–62.
Hamilton, M. (1967). Development of a rating scale for primary depressive illness. Br. J. Soc. Clin. Psychol. 6, 278–296.
Hamilton, M. (1976). The role of rating scales in psychiatry. Psychol. Med. 6, 347–349.
Hathaway, S. R. and McKinley, J. C. (1943). 'The Minnesota Multiphasic Personality Inventory'. University of Minnesota Press, Minneapolis.
Hill, D. (1966). Measurement in psychiatry. Proc. Roy. Soc. Med. 59, 1025–1028.
Hirsch, S., Gaind, R., Rohde, P., Steven, B. C. and Wing, J. K. (1973). Outpatient maintenance of chronic schizophrenic patients with long-acting fluphenazine. Br. Med. J. i, 633–637.
Hollister, L. and Overall, J. E. (1974). Evaluations of pharmacotherapy in co-operative studies. In 'Psychological Measures in Psychopharmacology' (Ed. P. Pichot). Karger, Basel.
Holzman, P., Levy, D. and Proctor, L. (1976). Smooth pursuit eye movements, attention, and schizophrenia. Arch. Gen. Psychiat. 33, 1415–1420.
Jensen, A. R. (1959). Reliability of Protective Techniques. Acta Psychol. 16, 108–136.
Kellner, R. (1971). Improvement criteria in drug trials with neurotic patients. Psychol. Med. 1, 416–425.
Kellner, R., Kelly, A. V. and Smithfield, B. F. (1968). The assessment of changes in anxiety in a drug trial. Br. J. Psychiat. 114, 863–869.
Kendell, R. E. (1975). 'The Role of Diagnosis in Psychiatry'. Blackwell, Oxford.
Kreitman, N. (1961). The reliability of psychiatric diagnosis. J. Ment. Sci. 107, 876–886.
Lader, M. and Marks, I. (1971). 'Clinical Anxiety'. Grune and Stratton, New York.
Lorr, M. (1974). Assessing psychotic behaviour by the IMPS. In 'Psychological Measures in Psychopharmacology' (Ed. P. Pichot), Karger, Basel.

Lorr, M. and Klett, C. J. (1967). 'Inpatients Multidimensional Psychiatric Scale'. Palo Alto Psychologists Publication.

Lorr, M. and Klett, C. J. (1969). Cross-cultural comparison of psychotic syndromes. *J. Abnorm. Soc. Psychol.* **74**, 531–543.

Mann, A. H. (1977). Psychiatric morbidity and hostility in hypertension. *Psychol. Med.* **7**, 653–659.

Mann, S. A. (1972). *In* 'Evaluating a Community Service' (Eds J. K. Wing and A. M. Hailey). Oxford University Press, Oxford.

Mechanic, D. (1970). Problems and prospects in psychiatric epidemiology. *In* 'Psychiatric Epidemiology' (Eds E. H. Hare and J. K. Wing). Oxford University Press, Oxford.

Meltzer, H. Y. (1976). Serum creatine phosphokinase in schizophrenia. *Am. J. Psychiat.* **133**, 192–196.

Mowbray, R. M. (1972). The Hamilton Rating Scale for depression: a factor analysis. *Psychol. Med.* **2**, 272–280.

Murphy, D. L. (1977). Neurotransmitter-related enzymes and psychiatric diagnosis. *In* 'Current Issues in Psychiatric Diagnosis' (Ed. R. Spitzer). Raven Press, New York.

Murphy, D. L. *et al.* (1974). The quantification of manic behaviour. *In* 'Modern Problems in Pharmacopsychiatry' (Ed. P. Pichot), Vol. 7. S. Karger, Basel.

Murray, R. M., Cooper, J. E. and Smith, A. (In press). The Leyton Obsessional Inventory: the responses of 73 obsessional patients. *Psychol. Med*.

Murstern, B. I. (1965). 'Handbook of Protective Techniques'. Basic Books, New York.

National Institute Mental Health (1966). 'Handbook of Psychiatric rating Scales' (Eds S.Lyerly and P. S. Abbott). U.S. Govt Printing Office, Washington D.C.

Noble, P. and Lader, M. (1971). The symptomatic correlates of the skin conductance changes in depression. *J. Psych. Res.* **9**, 61–69.

Oppenheim, A. N. (1966). 'Questionnaire Design and Attitude Measurement'. New York, Basic Books.

Overall, J. E. (1974). The brief psychiatric rating scale in psychopharmacology research. *In* 'Psychological Measures in Psychopharmacology' (Ed. P. Pichot). Karger, Basel.

Overall, J. E. and Gorham, D. R. (1962). The brief psychiatric rating scale. *Psychol. Rep.* **10**, 799–812.

Pinard, G. and Tetrault, L. (1974). Concerning semantic problems in psychological evaluation. *In* 'Psychological Measures in Psychopharmacology' (Ed. P. Pichot). Karger, Basel.

Pichot, P. (1974). Introduction. *In* 'Psychological Measures in Psychopharmacology' (Ed. P. Pichot). Karger, Basel.

Raskin, H. and Crook, T. H. (1976). Sensitivity of rating scales completed by psychiatrists, nurses and patients to antidepressant drug effects. *J. Psych. Res.* **13**, 31–41.

Rodnight, R., Murray, R. M., Oon, M. C. H., Brockington, I. F., Nicholls, P. and Birley, J. L. T. (1976). Urinary dimethyltryptamine and psychiatric symptomatology and classification. *Psychol. Med.* **6**, 649–657.

Salsinger, K. (1977). Sources of bias in psychiatric interviews. *In* 'Current Issues in Psychiatric Diagnosis' (Ed. R. Spitzer). Raven Press, New York.

Shepherd, M. and Cooper, B. (1964). Epidemiology and Mental Disorder. *J. Neurol. Neurosurg. and Psych.* **27**, 277–290.

Shepherd, M., Cooper, B., Brown, A. G. and Kalton, G. W. (1966). 'Psychiatric Illness in General Practice'. Oxford University Press, Oxford.

Singer, M. (1977). Psychological tests and psychiatric diagnosis. *In* 'Current Issues on Psychiatric Diagnosis' (Ed. R. Spitzer). Raven Press, New York.

Sims, A. C. and Salmons, P. H. (1975). Severity of symptoms of psychiatric outpatients. *Psychol. Med.* **5**, 62–66.

Spitzer, R. L. and Endicott, J. (1968). Diagno. *Arch. Gen. Psych.* **18**, 746–756.

Spitzer, R. L., Endicott, J., Fleiss, J. L. and Cohen, J. (1970). The Psychiatric Status Schedule. *Arch. Gen. Psych.* **23**, 41–55.

Spitzer, R. L., Endicott, J. and Robins, E. (1975). Research Diagnostic Criteria. *Biometrics Research.* N.Y. State, Dept. Ment. Hyg.

Taylor, J. A. (1953). A personality scale of manifest anxiety. *J. Abnorm. Psychol.* **48**, 285–290.

Ward, C. H., Beck, A. T., Mendelson, M., Mock, J. E. and Erbaugh, J. K. (1962). The psychiatric nomenclature. *Arch. Gen. Psych.* **7**, 198–205.

Wing, J. K. (1974). 'Measurement and Classification of Psychiatric Symptoms'. Oxford University Press, Oxford.

Wing, J. K. (1976). A technique for studying psychiatric morbidity. *Psychol. Med.* **6**, 665–671.

Wing, J. K., Birley, J. L. T., Cooper, J. E., Graham, P. and Isaacs, A. D. (1967). Reliability of a procedure for measuring and classifying present psychiatric state. *Br. J. Psychiat.* **113**, 499–515.

Wittenborn, J. R. (1974). The W.P.R.S. A quantification of observable psychopathology. *In* 'Psychological Measures in Psychopharmacology' (Ed. P. Pichot). Karger, Basel.

Zealley, A. K. and Aitken, R. C. B. (1969). Measurement of mood. *Proc. Roy. Soc. Med.* **62**, 993–996.

Zung, W. (1965). A self-rating depression scale. *Arch. Gen. Psych.* **12**, 63–70.

Zung, W. (1974). The measurement of affects. *In* 'Psychological Measures in Psychopharmacology' (Ed. P. Pichot). Karger, Basel.

5 Child psychiatry

Peter Hill

Child psychiatry is concerned with the child who suffers emotionally, whose individual development is distorted, or whose behaviour causes distress to his family or similar caring adults. Such a child is colloquially considered 'disturbed' when he manifests symptoms which seem inappropriate, and which persist in spite of simple measures taken to alleviate them. Much of childhood psychiatric disorder is best seen as *quantitative* deviation from accepted norms, multifactorially determined and falling largely into two groups: conduct disorders and emotional disorders, each of which may be differentiated from the other on a variety of counts—family background, prognosis etc. The traditional disease model finds application in only a handful of disorders such as infantile autism.

Epidemiology

There is an important distinction to be made between the prevalence of *symptoms* and the prevalence of child psychiatric *disorder*. Disorder implies *multiple* symptoms and a *measure of distress or handicap*; in other words there is an adverse influence on the child's satisfactory functioning as an individual or on his development. Consideration must also be given to whether such symptoms are *abnormal*. Particular symptoms or behaviours may be normal at one age and abnormal at another (e.g. enuresis). These variations are documented in epidemiological studies: Lapouse and Monk (1958), the Buckinghamshire Child Survey (Shepherd *et al.*, 1971), the Isle of Wight Survey (q.v.), etc. which also testify to the extensive prevalence of single psychiatric symptoms in the general child population. Account needs to be taken of the severity and persistence of symptoms as well as their setting in terms of demands made on the child (e.g. by first attendance at school) and the prevailing cultural norms and expectations.

No single symptom is pathognomonic of psychiatric disorder. Although the presence of some—antisocial behaviour, peer group difficulties, poor concentration—are more likely than others to indicate the presence of psychiatric disorder, they may still occur in isolation without indicating more general maladjustment. Thumb sucking, nail biting and other 'comfort' habits are so common as to predict psychiatric pathology only rarely, the same being true of disorders of sleep and food intake in young children when these occur as single items of behaviour.

An important point is that disturbed behaviour at school is not necessarily accompanied by disturbed behaviour at home and vice versa. Situation specificity is not uncommon in childhood symptomatology and should not be taken as evidence against the presence of disorder.

The epidemiological studies carried out by Rutter and his colleagues are the most thorough and extensive yet performed. Initially all (2199) 10- and 11-year-old children living on the Isle of Wight (an island off the south coast of England, population 96,000) were screened for educational, intellectual, psychiatric and physical handicaps. Children identified in the screening questionnaires were individually assessed, as were a number of non-responders, 'normals' and children aged five to 15 with neurological disorders. The findings, documented mainly in Rutter et al. (1970a, b) are extensive but attention may be drawn selectively to certain conclusions relevant to childhood psychiatric disorder within this population:

(a) a prevalence amounting to 6·8% of the childhood population sampled (4·0% conduct disorder, 2·5% emotional disorder);
(b) an absence of significant relationship with social class;
(c) an overall two-fold excess of boys, though if emotional disorders were taken individually these contained a small excess of girls;
(d) an increase in prevalence as IQ progressively falls;
(e) a marked association between reading retardation and conduct disorder;
(f) an increase in the rate of psychiatric disorder to 10·4% if physical handicap not involving the brain was present (asthma etc.);
(g) a five-fold increase in rate (though age ranges differ in extent) if brain disorder present (34·3%). In both this and the previous group no association of particular symptoms with particular brain disorder was found and the increased rate was true for all disorders.

(h) Only a one in 10 likelihood of receiving psychiatric help.

The age cohort has been followed up into adolescence where a somewhat higher rate has been found to prevail. Just what that rate is depends on criteria that did not apply to the younger group. If handicapping psychiatric disorder is considered the rate is 7·5% (Rutter *et al.*, 1976). However, Leslie (1974) found rates of psychiatric disorder among 13- and 14-year-olds in Blackburn to be 21% of boys and 14% of girls, and Henderson *et al.* (1971) found an overall prevalence of 16% among the adolescents of an Australian town, suggesting that more general agreement as to prevalence could in fact be found around 10–15%. Within the group of disordered adolescents it is noteworthy that the proportion diagnosed as emotional disorder rises to equal that diagnosed as conduct disorder and that the sex ratio becomes virtually equal.

Application of the same instruments to the 10-year-olds in a London Borough revealed a doubling of the rate of psychiatric disorder (all types) and specific reading retardation (Rutter *et al.*, 1975b). This could readily be related to such variables as family discord, parental deviance, social disadvantage and certain school characteristics, all of which were more frequent in London, though why such factors *should* be more common remains unanswered. At the other end of the age range Richman *et al.* (1975) found a 7% prevalence of moderate or marked behaviour disorders among a general population random sample of three-year-olds. Most children so identified were active, disobedient, difficult to manage; relatively few showing a 'neurotic' picture. At this age the male predominance was a mere trend and statistically non-significant.

Classification

A classification is a means of ordering knowledge and conveying information between people. For clinical use the information available for placing a disorder within a classification system is potentially rich if that system has previously been used for clinical and research documentation. It would follow that one purpose of classification is to promote reliable communication between workers, whether clinicians or researchers. A second would be the provision of a framework wherein concepts of separate disorders may be refined. Lastly, the planning and administration of services may be more discriminatory if a meaningful classificatory system can be developed.

The structure of a classificatory system reflects its purpose. For clinical work the information required is that pertinent to associated disability, prognosis and treatment response. It would be convenient for aetiology to be included and indeed much medical classification *is* aetiological; it is often said that this is the preferred model. However, it is equally true that there are numerous instances where classification by form, as in renal disease or leukaemia, is of greater value. What is more, no universally accepted system of aetiology exists in child psychiatry, though systems utilizing psychoanalytic concepts have had some currency. In that these rely upon inferred constructs and dynamics their reliability is weak. Furthermore, many analysts eschew classification, arguing that it is reductionist, ignoring the unique character of the individual child. This is a confusion of classification with formulation; placing a disorder within a scheme is not meant to be a complete summary of the individual's situation. Nevertheless, an effective classificatory system must reflect the fact that most child psychiatric disorder is multifactorially determined, not just by a coincidence of adverse factors and specific vulnerabilities but by the interweaving of elements that cause disorder to *arise* and those which cause it to *persist*.

Leaving aetiology aside, it is still necessary to classify and to erect a system of categories 'mutually exclusive and jointly exhaustive' (Stengel, 1959), valid, meaningful, reliable, practical and acceptable to would-be users. There is no natural system and such systems as exist draw upon both traditional and empirical findings. Rutter (1965, 1977b) has discussed the validity of distinguishing categories similar to those in Table I in terms of social and family background, prognosis, associated cognitive factors, sex and age incidence etc. and it would seem reasonable to place some confidence in a system of this kind. Obviously there are disorders more typically 'adult', such as schizophrenia or obsessive-compulsive disorder, which may be diagnosed in childhood, making it necessary that a classification of childhood disorder be subsumed into a total classificatory system for psychiatric disorder at all ages.

There exist in any one child various aspects of his disorder which may combine in various patterns and which vary independently of each other (or nearly so), each containing relevant information. For example, mental retardation, infantile autism and epilepsy may co-exist in one child. A simple list of categories begs the question as to which aspect of the disorder is selected, or, if other aspects are also to be listed, in what order? Clearly information must be coded on several parameters when several types of abnormal functioning are present. If these parameters are defined and rules established to ensure a uniform number of codings in a given order, a *multiaxial* classification system results.

In its efforts to standardize psychiatric classification and prepare ICD 9 the WHO has sponsored seminars which have spawned studies that evaluate a multiaxial approach. One of these described by Rutter *et al*. (1969) involves three axes: (1) clinical psychiatric syndrome; (2) intellectual level; (3) associated or aetiological physical conditions. To these have

Table I   *Clinical syndromes*

(A) *Psychoses specific to childhood*
   infantile autism
   disintegrative psychosis
   atypical

(B) *Emotional disorders specific to childhood*
   with anxiety and fearfulness
   with misery and unhappiness
   with sensitivity, shyness and social withdrawal
   relationship problems (sibling jealousy etc.)

(C) *Conduct disorder*
   unsocialized
   socialized
   mixed disturbance of conduct and emotions

(D) *Specific developmental delays*
   reading
   arithmetic
   speech/language
   developmental dyspraxia

(E) *Hyperkinetic syndrome*

(F) *Symptomatic*
   tics and Gilles de la Tourette's syndrome
   specific disorder of sleep
   specific disorder of eating
   encopresis
   enuresis

(G) *Mental subnormality*
   mild
   moderate
   severe and profound

---

been added in subsequent studies similar axes, such as 'developmental delays' and 'associated psychosocial factors'. For each child, coding is made on each axis. If no abnormality is present on a particular axis this information is indicated by a zero code for that axis. A descriptive glossary enables the system to be used by clinicians of differing theoretical persuasions.

Categories on the first axis are descriptive (i.e. as in A, B, C, E, F in Table I) and reflect as far as possible available information from research studies, discriminating between, for example, neurotic and conduct disorders in terms of symptom cluster, response to treatment, prognosis, etc. Coding on the second axis reflects the intellectual performance (i.e. IQ), not the nature or cause, such as Down's syndrome. The biological and specific developmental delay axes are self-explanatory. There are, predictably, reliability difficulties with a psychosocial axis where theoretical bias and inferential judgements cloud descriptive assessment. It has been established that experienced child psychiatrists find the use of a multiaxial scheme to be easier and more reliable than a multi-category system such as ICD 8 (Rutter *et al.*, 1975a).

Disturbed children and their families

Children are dependent upon caring adults, most obviously their parents, to meet their physical and psychological needs during maturation. In order to understand a child's symptoms and behaviour it is necessary to appraise those elements in the family which provoke, foster, maintain, or otherwise precipitate and modify the signs of distress and deviance in the child. There is extensive testimony among the more anecdotal literature to the effect that parental expectations have a powerful determining factor upon the development of a particular child and the way in which he responds to stress. Similarly, it is a touchstone of clinical practice that the parents' own childhood experience finds resonance in their parenting practice. It is possible to specify the tasks that a family involved in child-rearing must perform: the provision of attachments, a secure base for exploration, adequate and appropriate sensory and social experience, supplemented by instruction and example, opportunities for identification, consistent discipline and a stable value system, an unambiguous communication network and the fostering of age-appropriate autonomy. Because of space limitations, only a sample of the more objective findings on family pathology can be referred to here. Some additional discussion is presented in the following section on maternal deprivation and in the section on juvenile delinquency in Chapter 16.

Statistical studies of parent–child relationships provide two main dimensions of parental attitudes which may be correlated with characteristics in the child (Becker, 1964), as in Fig. 1. It should be emphasized that such schemes are highly simplified abstractions and most particularly do not separately represent the contributions of the child as a frequent initiator of parent–child interactions and as a possessor of physically specifically individual characteristics which are likely to influence parental attitudes. To pursue this latter point further, the particular temperamental characteristics observed in infancy by the New York Longitudinal Study (e.g. Thomas *et al.*, 1968) which predicted the later development of behaviour in that child were:

(a) a tendency to withdraw in the face of novelty;

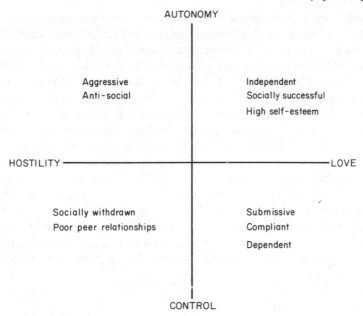

Fig. 1 Dimensions of parental attitudes.

(b) slow adaptability to change;

(c) high intensity of emotional reactions;

(d) irregularity of biological function (sleep, elimination, etc.);

(e) predominant negative mood (crying, fussy).

These, at face value, would seem to result in a 'difficult' child, likely to exasperate otherwise tolerant parents, and thus modify their attitudes towards him. Similar examples of the way in which individual differences, such as sex and IQ, predispose to psychiatric disorder have been mentioned in the epidemiological section. No child is a *tabula rasa*.

Specific infant-rearing practices have been widely studied with repeated confirmation of the finding that NO particular 'maladjustment' or personality traits arise from the use of specific measures—for example, demand feeding rather than scheduled feeding. It is the *parental attitudes* which are important rather than the individual methods employed although often the two can be very difficult to disentangle.

The relevance of marital discord and disharmony between the members of the whole family are well documented in studies of antisocial behaviour (q.v. Chapter 16). Typically it is the presence of an infantilizing, anxiously over-protective parent who displays an apprehensive solicitude towards the child which is particularly associated with 'neurotic' symptoms (Jenkins, 1968).

Parental illness, both psychiatric and to a lesser extent physical, is associated with an increased risk of psychiatric disorder in the child, probably mainly through its impact on family life. In Rutter's (1966) study there were three times as many psychiatrically ill parents among the families of children with psychiatric disorder than among the families of children attending dental and paediatric clinics. Children were particularly susceptible if there was psychiatric illness in the mother rather than the father, if there were affective symptoms in that illness, and if the child were involved in the parent's symptoms (e.g. obsessional fears of harming the child). Little relationship was found between the specific type of illness in the parent and the type of disorder in the child, though the child of a chronically neurotic or personality-disordered parent was more at risk for the development of psychiatric disorder (of any type) than the child of a psychotic parent.

Little stress has been placed here on the effect of family dynamics as understood in terms of content and meaning rather than form. Some mention is made in the section on family therapy in Chapter 22.

'Maternal deprivation'

During the second half year of life the child forms *attachments* and *bonds* to specific figures. The definition of 'attachment' is difficult without provoking controversy but, following the work of Bowlby (e.g. 1969), the following characteristics are now generally accepted:

(a) Behaviours exhibited differentially by the child in order to gain or maintain proximity to the attachment figure, e.g. following, clinging, crying, etc.

(b) An emotional need for such proximity which, if denied, results in distress. Brief separations may be tolerated without distress, suggesting the presence of 'psychological' (or 'affectional') bonds which endure during the physical absence of the attachment figure and which probably depend on some internal representation of that figure.

(c) The facilitation of some behaviours (e.g. exploration) by the physical presence of the attachment figure.

(d) A 'developmental' origin independent of feeding, care-taking, etc. provided by the attachment figure, though apparently requiring a certain intensity and duration of social interaction between child and attachment figure.

In Schaffer and Emerson's (1964) study 71% of infants formed their initial attachment to one person only: the mother in 95% of all cases. The remaining 29% formed their first specific attachments with several individuals. Within one month the father was also selected as an attachment figure by 27% of the sample infants and by 18 months of age most (87%) of the infants had developed multiple attachments—not only to mother and father but also to grandparents, siblings, second-degree relatives and neighbours. Attachments may be ranked in a hierarchy of intensity but there is no evidence that the first attachment is qualitatively different from the others. The mother is usually the person who is best placed to become the child's principal attachment figure but to concentrate specifically on the mother–child attachment at the expense of the other interactive behaviour of the child is artificial. Mothers do not only provide themselves as attachment figures but also, for example, feed, protect, and play with their children. Adequate 'mothering' additionally implies a warm, stable relationship with the child and the provision of a satisfactory behavioural model. None of these functions is the prerogative of mothers alone. It remains to be established that there is any component of maternal care that cannot be provided by other caretakers under suitable circumstances. For this reason, the term 'maternal deprivation' must remain imprecise unless to specify just what aspect of 'mothering' is absent.

The development of *psychological bonds* appears to allow *attachment behaviours* to subside, thus freeing the child from separation anxiety and the required proximity of attachment figures, particularly in the face of stress. It is generally assumed that the quality of future social relationships depends on the establishment of secure bonds with attachment figures and it is traditionally held that formation of such bonds is most likely to occur in infancy, between six months and four years, and unlikely to be achieved in later life. Such assumptions about the irreversibility of bonding failure have recently been challenged (Clarke and Clarke, 1976).

In a critique of the topic, Rutter (1972) differentiates between long- and short-term 'deprivation'. *Short-term maternal deprivation* refers to a reaction commonly noted in pre-school children separated from their mothers by admission to a residential nursery or paediatric ward. Obviously this involves a change of environment and methods of care and separation from other relatives as well as mother. Characteristically, the child's reaction progresses through stages of:

(1) protest (tears, etc.)
(2) despair (apathy and misery)
(3) detachment (apparent contentment with a striking indifference to the mother on her return)

This distress may be mitigated by introducing the child to his caretakers before the separation date, by their preservation of an active memory of the mother (by talking about her to the child), by the presence of other familiar figures and by the availability of an affectionate and active

involvement with a stable caretaker. Taken as a whole the evidence suggests that, notwithstanding the importance of a strange environment, it is separation from a person to whom an attachment has been formed that is the key variable. This may be compounded by an absence of suitable conditions under which new attachments may be formed, for example being surrounded by nurses who work on a task-orientated system and who work to an unpredictable roster. The reaction is analogous to bereavement and involves *bond disruption*. Following the reunion of child and mother a readjustment follows the initial indifference or rejection displayed by the child. This may result in apprehensive clinging when the mother, for example, tries to leave the room, but has almost always disappeared after a few months. It is difficult to demonstrate any long-term effects of single brief separations but repeated admissions into residential care may be indicators of family discord and thus be superficially associated with psychiatric disturbance in the child.

Long-term maternal deprivation traditionally refers to the various experiences (or lack of them) pertinent to an upbringing in a poor quality residential institution, the consequences of a 'broken-home' or even of lack of warmth in mother–child interaction. It is clear that what is loosely termed 'deprivation' is really 'privation' and that several experiences and mechanisms are involved. The long-term consequences are usually listed as:

(1) antisocial behaviour
(2) poor development of IQ and language
(3) poor physical growth ('deprivation dwarfism')
(4) 'affectionless psychopathy'.

Broken homes appear to function as an indicator of marital discord as it is families broken by divorce and desertion that produce antisocial children, rather than those broken by parental death (see Chapter 16). Lack of warmth in parent–child relationships is known to be associated with antisocial behaviour in the child and it seems likely that components such as stealing and unsocialized aggression relate to a failure to discover a secure relationship with an adult in which identificatory social learning can occur.

Poor cognitive development is apparently a consequence of the low intensity and poor quality of social, perceptual and linguistic stimulation that is particularly common in low-quality residential institutions rather than a privation of any indefinable component of mothering. Similarly, poor growth seems related to inadequate food intake rather than a *direct* result of emotional factors; it would be inaccurate to state that 'mother love' is essential for adequate growth, though possible to hypothesize that misery reduces food intake. 'Affectionless psychopathy' is a somewhat dated term referring to a syndrome characterized by: (a) an inability to form lasting relationships; (b) indiscriminate friendliness and social disinhibition, apparently analogous to the approach component of infantile attachment behaviour; (c) a lack of guilt, often with aggressive or antisocial behaviour. As a *syndrome* this is now uncommon among children in residential care (Wolkind, 1974) though the *individual* clinical features comprising the syndrome continue to be common in such children. The social components are generally assumed to be irreversible after the age of three years and seem to be a consequence of a failure to form bonds because of an absence of opportunities for stable relationships with caring staff. It needs to be added, however, that many residential homes actively discourage intense relationships between staff and children. Thus, one has to consider not only the effect of privations in early life but also the quality of ongoing staff–child relationships.

Phobias

Fears are common amongst otherwise normal children; probably nine out of every 10 children at some stage in their development will develop a fear of, for example, dogs, spiders, the dark, ghosts or burglars (MacFarlane *et al.*, 1954). Fears of this type are 'unrealistic', non-adaptive, and cannot easily be explained away by an appeal to rationality. When they are handicapping and persistent the term 'phobia' is applicable.

There is some relationship with age (see Berecz, 1968). Fearful reactions to strangers or separation from a parent are virtually universal 'phases' of infancy and are regarded as part of normal development when manifest at that time. Between ages two and five, fears of certain animals or objects are especially common but by middle childhood fears of anticipated or imaginary dangers and of the supernatural are predominant. With increasing maturity the number of fears declines throughout middle childhood but at age 11 there is a small resurgence. This, in part, is due to the fact that school refusal is commonest at this age and may be classified as a phobia. By the age of 12, fears of natural events have begun to abate and, with adolescence, social anxieties and agoraphobic symptoms may first be seen in affected individuals.

In an extensive review, Miller *et al.* (1974) conclude that no single type of personality or parent–child relationship is associated with or specific to phobias. Furthermore, they draw attention to the fact that childhood phobias are only rarely invariant responses to simple, discrete stimuli. In most instances the phobic stimulus is complex and the phobic response less predictable accordingly. The situation is complicated by the difficulty of rating the severity of the fear in view of the poor reliability existing between physiological, subjective and observational assessments.

Furthermore, the complaint of fear may be used by the child for manipulative ends.

The aetiology of childhood fears is speculative, though it seems eminently reasonable to assume that when such fears are handicapping this may represent a failure of parents, teachers or peers to promote sufficient confrontation with the stimulus and teach or display adequate coping behaviour. This may reflect parental psychopathology—for example, the presence in a parent of similar phobic reactions—or reflect a disturbance of family function (q.v. school refusal).

The comparative results of various treatment methods have been inadequately demonstrated. Success is claimed for both psychotherapy and behaviour therapy, though in all likelihood a positive result requires *both* a trusting relationship and eventual confrontation with the feared object or stimulus. Interpretations made within a psychotherapeutic setting often highlight relationships with parents though should not necessarily be confined to the traditional pattern of illuminating displaced oedipal fears of parental punishment according to the 'little Hans' paradigm. The classical desensitization package is difficult to apply to children; many of them do not provide stable hierarchies, become bored, or refuse to relax or fantasize. Graded exposure in which anxiety is allowed to rise but not to unmanageable levels, or vicarious extinction by viewing modelled approaches to the phobic object (Bandura *et al.*, 1967) are alternative, considerate, behavioural approaches.

It is generally believed that childhood fears appear and disappear rapidly. Certainly the prognosis of treated phobic children appears good. Hampe *et al.* (1973) found that two years after treatment only 7% of 62 children still had severe phobic symptoms.

School refusal

The distinction between school refusal and school truancy is real, though not universally accepted, probably because of the comparative rarity of school refusal. Hersov (1960a, b) was able to demonstrate important differences between school refusers and truants seen at a psychiatric clinic. Truancy is associated with antisocial behaviour, poor academic attainments, and a family background marred by disharmony and disciplinary inconsistency. Conversely, school refusal was typically manifested by children who were dependent, inhibited and timid. Their academic attainments were appropriate or even superior, their school behaviour exemplary. Quite unlike the truants they came from families characterized by over-protection and with a history of neurotic disorders.

Most children at some time or other show some reluctance to attend primary school (Moore, 1966) but nearly always do attend—parental pressure winning the day. The clinical picture of school refusal is based on those attending for treatment and accounts for rather less than 3% of all child psychiatric referrals. Amongst these the sex incidence is equal and the age at presentation is most commonly 11 years (Smith, 1970).

In addition to a refusal to go to or remain in school in the face of parental pressure, entreaty or threat, the child may display overt panic at the time to leave for school. Alternatively he may later run home from school in panic. Various reasons may be offered by the child: complaints of fear of exams, games, bullying, vomiting or fainting in assembly, or of a particular teacher. In some instances there may be only somatic complaints (vomiting, headaches, abdominal pain), restricted to term-time weekday mornings, which disappear when he is allowed to stay at home. In young children an acute onset is characteristic in contrast to the more insidious development often seen in adolescents. Precipitating events often include changes of teacher or school, illness or bereavement in the family, a new house or the departure of a close friend.

Such behaviour may be a symptom of various psychiatric disorders and reflect differing mechanisms. Smith's (1970) findings based on a group of clinic attenders suggested three categories:

(1) separation anxiety, mainly in young children;
(2) true phobia of aspects of school itself without previous difficulties in attendance;
(3) fears of failure or rejection, typically in older children with high standards but fragile self-esteem (well described by Leventhal and Sills, 1964) and not uncommonly associated with depressive symptomatology.

For many years, separation anxiety was held to be the fundamental pathology (Johnson *et al.*, 1941). It remains true that this is a frequent underlying pathology, especially in younger children, though certainly not universal (Hersov, 1977; Smith, 1970). Eisenberg's (1958) description of the contribution of parental anxieties and unresolved dependency needs to separation fears in the child is particularly lucid. Skynner (1974) has extended the concept of school refusal arising in the context of disturbed relationship between a child and a mother who is immature and insecure in her maternal role to an approach which takes into account passivity and dependency on the part of the father who is unable to assert himself appropriately as husband and parent. Parents who have never achieved satisfactory separation from their families of origin or who had unfortunate school experiences themselves find corresponding difficulties promoting their children's separation and school attendance in the face of protest by the child.

Children with a separation anxiety frequently express fears of harm befalling a parent. This should not be glibly attributed to unconscious hostility before finding out whether there have been overt parental threats of suicide or departure—whether expressed directly to the child or heard in a quarrel between the parents. When separation anxiety is mooted as fundamental it should be demonstrated in other separation situations and be relieved by the presence of attachment figures.

In contrast to the group of children in whom separation anxiety dominates the clinical picture, older children often display a slowly developing school refusal in the setting of a more widespread disturbance of individual personality and seriously disturbed family function. Coolidge *et al*. (1957) referred to the distinction between these two groups as 'neurotic crisis' or 'way of life' (types I and II respectively) an oft-repeated catch phrase. Type II children have, for years, been timid, fearful of challenges to their precarious self-image, and experience difficulties establishing themselves in the out-of-family peer group. The increasing demands of school life, both educational and social, are met by maladaptive responses characterized by withdrawal into the bosom of the family, though this is often at the expense of a worsening in parent–child relationships with acrimonious recrimination, stubbornness and wilful protestation by the child replacing earlier compliance.

Treatment

Management usually involves *recognition* (thus avoiding multiple, unnecessary physical investigations or prolonged convalescence where somatic symptoms exist) and *correction* of inappropriate class or school, unnecessary games, etc. For acute cases (usually under age 11) conforming to Coolidge's type I picture, most authorities agree on an early return to school on a decided date with firm, consistent action involving both parents with support from the psychiatric team and liaison with the school. This is sometimes termed a 'Kennedy' approach after the author of a well-known paper describing the complete remission of symptoms in all of 50 type I cases subjected to a prompt return to school on the above lines (Kennedy, 1965).

Where there is a longer history, the initial assessment dictates the specific involvement of particular techniques—psychotherapeutic (individual or family based) pharmacological, behavioural—and the way in which these may be interwoven with a programme of *graded return* to the school with successive brief trips to the vicinity of the school and the completion of school work at home, collecting books from school, going to the classroom for non-threatening activities, progressively. The essential aim is to hand over to the parents all responsibility for maintaining the child's attendance. Thus, at the same time as this programme for the child, the parents will need guidance in their handling of the re-entry to school, particularly an encouragement of firmness in the face of attempts by the child to remain at home. Hersov (1977) in a seminal review provides an exhaustive discussion of treatment approaches.

In the most severe cases admission to an in-patient unit will allow milieu therapy, separation from parents, intensive treatment of underlying disorders, and ensures continued education. This may need to be followed by boarding school placement if adverse family factors are not correctable. A home tutor should be regarded as a last resort.

The outcome of treatment is generally favourable; overall about two-thirds successfully return to school. Good prognosis is not only related to younger age (adolescents seem to have more serious individual and family pathology) but also to the stability of the home and the psychological sophistication of the parents.

Tyrer and Tyrer (1974) in a retrospective study, suggest that one in three of all school refusers later present as adult neurotics, not with any particular type of neurosis, though Pittman *et al.* (1968) note that nine out of a series of 11 cases of work phobia had a childhood history of school refusal.

Obsessions

Superficially 'obsessional' behaviour is common in children and is in fact an adherence to ritual (touching lamp-posts, etc.) performed as a component of a solitary game, unaccompanied by severe anxiety or an inability to refrain. True obsessive-compulsive neurosis is rare. Onset is nearly always after the age of seven and is often sudden. Hand-washing, touching and bed-time rituals are common and often extend to include other members of the family in their performance. At this stage they may acquire additional significance to the child as they may represent the acquisition of control over others. Clearly, this may perpetuate matters as power corrupts and anxiety remains unconfronted.

Adolescents may display obsessive-compulsive symptoms in the context of depression or as a transient phenomenon accompanying other neurotic symptoms in an adjustment reaction. There is no unequivocal evidence to support the traditional notion that obsessional symptoms in the adolescent presage schizophrenia.

The attachment to unusual objects and the 'preservation of sameness' found in autistic and some mentally retarded children must not be confused with an obsessional neurosis.

Hysteria

As with adults, the diagnosis of hysteria in children does not imply the absence of organic pathology. The elaboration of the symptoms or handicaps of organic disease may ensure that the gains of the sick role are perpetuated, that conflict-engendering situations may be avoided, or that the challenge of developmental tasks is evaded by procrastinatory illness behaviour. Slater's (1965) well-known demonstration that organic disease was subsequently discovered in one-third of a group of adult patients diagnosed as hysteria is echoed by Caplan's (1970) finding that 13 out of 28 pre-pubertal children originally diagnosed as having hysteria were found later to have an organic basis for the presenting symptoms. That this is not merely a function of inaccurate diagnosis is suggested by Dubowitz and Hersov's (1976) review of five children with hysterical disturbance of motor function. In each instance the hysterical symptoms followed an 'undoubtedly organic but relatively mild illness'. Such cases as these respond well to a cessation of physical investigations and a programme of physical rehabilitation (with or without operant reinforcement schedules) and firm reassurance. The purpose of such an approach is to help the child give up his maladaptive sick-role behaviour and help him and his family cope with any stress that has precipitated the reaction. Children whose hysterical symptoms appear to develop as symbolic representations of unconscious conflicts (the traditional conversion symptom) will require more weight to be given to a psychotherapeutic approach to the individual or family.

The diagnosis of hysterical personality disorder should not be made in childhood or early adolescence as the traits of theatricality, egocentricity or emotional lability are to be found singly or combined in most, if not all, children during normal development.

Depression

Depressive symptoms (misery, weepiness, etc.) commonly occur in emotionally disturbed children but whether they represent adult-type depressive illness is controversial.

Frommer (1968) argued that a quarter of her child patients suffered from depression, often presenting with somatic symptoms, antisocial behaviour or elimination disorders and claimed that they benefited from antidepressant drugs. The weakness of an argument that extends from treatment to cause is well known; headaches, for example, may be attributed to aspirin deficiency. One further difficulty is that the female predominance in adult depressive populations is not seen in her sample. Pearce (1974) applying a discriminant function analysis to 126 cases characterized by a depressive syndrome of 'morbid depression, sadness, unhappiness, tearfulness' found no association with 'depressive equivalents' of aggression, stealing, or enuresis.

Examining the links between depressive illness in adults and 'depression' in children we find no correlation between depressive symptoms in a psychiatrically disturbed child and depression in the parent (Rutter, 1966). Neither does depression in children seem to persist or occur when those children become adults. Robins' (1966) follow-up was unable to demonstrate that clinic children diagnosed as neurotic had a higher rate of depression in adult life than control children.

A possible hypothesis is that depression takes a different form in children than its adult counterpart. It is known that manic-depressive illness in its usual adult form is exceptionally rare before puberty (Anthony and Scott, 1960) and some people have suggested that its pre-pubertal manifestation is, for example, hyperactivity. The child psychiatric population, however, produces no more adult manic-depressives than the general population (Dahl, 1971) which apparently refutes the hypothesis.

Graham (1974) has pointed out that 'to question whether children get depressive illness in the same way that adults do implies a belief in the concept that adult depression is an illness, a concept of which one can remain suspicious'. In his discussion of childhood depression he considers that pure depressive illnesses are rare before puberty and suggests that, when sadness and misery present as the major features of a disorder of childhood, such disorders should best be viewed as reaction to environmental circumstances rather than illness. The existence of expressed unhappiness does not by itself warrant a diagnosis of depression. In the Isle of Wight Survey (Rutter *et al.*, 1970b) the occurrence rate of sadness and misery within the three groups of emotional disorder, conduct disorder, and mixed emotional and conduct disorder was remarkably similar. Furthermore, there was poor agreement between teachers and parents as to whether the child was miserable or not, illustrating the rarity of an unremitting mood change unmodified by situation. Tearfulness is a ready response to stress in pre-school children and, of course, in early infancy is virtually the only available negative affective response. In middle childhood, apathy, social withdrawal, a wish to run away, anorexia, psychogenic pain, and psychomotor retardation may present as symptoms of depressive mood. With the advent of puberty, developing cognitive maturity allows the expression of complaints of hopelessness and guilt and the psychopathological picture begins to represent adult-type depression.

It is perhaps justifiable to suggest that a child may be considered depressed when the overall picture is dominated by depressive symptoms which have persisted longer or have become more intense than the appropriate response to an original putative precipitant. The lability of mood in children means that one would not necessarily expect *unremitting* sadness, rather a too-ready tendency to slip into sadness. Treatment approaches will depend on whether the depression is seen as relatively autonomous, when antidepressants would be indicated, or relatively reactive, in which case alleviation of the prevailing stressful situation would be the logical approach. Where stresses occur in relation to school or various physical illnesses, a direct attack on the situation producing stress in combination with supportive psychotherapy for the child may suffice. As always, rational provision of treatment is dependent upon precise formulation.

Suicide

Before puberty, suicide is exceptionally rare. Shaffer (1974) found no UK suicides younger than 12 in the years 1962–1968. The incidence subsequently increased during adolescence. Possible explanations of the rare occurrence before puberty include an immature and distorted concept of death (e.g. reversibility), a lack of ability to plan or obtain the means for committing suicide, and the absence of adult-type depressive symptomatology (hopelessness, etc.).

According to Shaffer's study, suicide is typically committed by a child with several of the following characteristics:

(a) above average intelligence with conceptual and physical maturity;
(b) a family background disturbed by divorce, non-communication or rejection;
(c) recent involvement in antisocial behaviour (theft, etc.) and non-attendance at school;
(d) close experience of suicidal behaviour in peers or relatives;
(e) an apparently depressed mental state with marked guilt;
(f) recent humiliation or imminent disciplinary action, e.g. Court appearance, parents to be informed of misbehaviour by the school;
(g) feeling abandoned socially or within an incomprehending family.

In nearly half of all adolescent suicides, previous suicidal talk, threats or attempts have been noted. Contrary to common assumptions, actual suicide in childhood and adolescence is rarely impulsive (though threats and token attempts may be), successful suicides showing evidence of planning, even ingenuity.

Conduct disorders

Many children are seen by child psychiatrists because their behaviour excites social disapproval. When such behaviour forms the principal component of a psychiatric disorder the term conduct disorder is applied, this being the most prevalent child psychiatric disorder by virtue of the high incidence and relatively poor prognosis of the condition. Children so designated persistently and excessively lie, steal, disobey, truant, fight, set fires or display unacceptably aggressive behaviour. Promiscuity in girls, though not in boys, is similarly included (Cowie *et al.*, 1968). For the psychiatric diagnosis to be made it must be shown that the child's anti-social behaviour is associated with disturbances of personal functioning or impairment of the pursuit of personal happiness and satisfaction. In other words, not only is the behaviour excessive, as judged by age-related norms, but the child is also either suffering or his personal development is being seriously impeded.

The distinction from delinquency is important. In that the term delin-quent can be applied to anyone who breaks the law, the number of juvenile delinquents is likely to exceed the number of children with conduct disorders; infringements of the law are extremely common in adolescence (q.v. Chapter 16). Even if the number of convicted adoles-cents is taken as a measure of the prevalence of delinquency it is clear that, as one boy in five will be convicted of an offence before the age of 21, one is dealing with a much more frequent phenomenon than the presence of conduct disorder which has an approximate point prevalence of 5% with a male/female ratio of 4:1 in middle childhood (i.e. roughly one boy in 12 at any point in time). Delinquency is a sociolegal label and defines a larger group than the socio-psychological label of conduct disorder. There is a large but incomplete overlap. Most convicted adolescents do not reoffend and do not show evidence of psychiatric disorder. Conversely, not all children with conduct disorders will come before the Courts, because, for example, their truancy may be insufficient to warrant legal action or their mendacity may be beyond the interest of the Courts. Nevertheless, there are a number of children and adolescents who persistently offend and, as with adult offenders, it can be shown that persistent offenders are very likely to be psychologically abnormal (Stott and Wilson, 1977).

It is, perhaps, obvious that antisocial behaviour is far from homogen-eous and a measure of sub-classification becomes inevitable. The most familiar scheme applied to conduct disorder is an adaptation of Hewitt and Jenkins' classification of delinquency:

(1) *Socialized* in which the antisocial behaviour is seen as normal for a particular sub-cultural group and the child is espousing standards appropriate for that group as a whole. Mays (1954), in particular, has stressed the essential normality of the personality. Oft-cited examples are truancy and gang membership.

(2) *Unsocialized* in which the behaviour is antisocial by any standards, often associated with abnormalities in the personality.

(3) *Mixed Disorder* in which antisocial behaviour is accompanied by marked neurotic symptoms.

The scheme is not without its critics. Elizabeth Field (1967) has demonstrated its shortcomings with respect to the prediction of family characteristics. The Isle of Wight study demonstrated that neurotic symptoms were common in conduct disorder and that the distinction between the mixed group and the remainder of conduct disordered children was based to a considerable degree on the severity of the antisocial symptoms. Scott's scheme (q.v. Chapter 16) has evident appeal, particularly when applied to the formulation of an individual case but has not been empirically tested on a large scale.

Aetiology

The aetiology of conduct disorders will naturally overlap that of delinquency and it is advisable to read this section in conjunction with the sub-section on juvenile delinquency in Chapter 16. There are likely to be some differences because children with conduct disorders may be of any age, whereas delinquency is a term applicable to those over the age of criminal responsibility (10 in the UK). One factor explored in the sparse literature on conduct disorder (as opposed to delinquency) is reading retardation. On the Isle of Wight one-third of the 10- and 11-year-old children who were severely retarded in reading exhibited antisocial behaviour and one-third of the antisocial children were severely retarded in their reading (after IQ had been partialled out). Both these rates are way above general population norms after taking account of sex differences. Reading delay was equally common in pure conduct disorders and mixed conduct disorders; there was no significant increase in the rate among emotionally disordered children. After inspecting the developmental characteristics and background features of the children involved, Rutter *et al.* (1970b) argued that both reading difficulties and antisocial behaviour may arise from a shared temperamental basis or that antisocial behaviour may represent a maladaptive response to the frustration of educational failure with a consequent repudiation of social values expressed by the school.

Treatment

Treatment approaches are difficult to summarize. A rational approach would combine measures to reverse or counteract aetiological factors with a combined educational and therapeutic attitude towards the establishment of satisfactory social development and the amelioration of subjectively distressing symptoms. Thus, for example, conjoint family therapy aimed at reducing covert identifications and vicarious satisfactions may allow for a more consistent disciplinary attitude within the family and be combined with the provision of a classroom-based operant programme at school. For another child the family focus may be that of marital therapy with a view to minimizing overt discord (or covert scape-goating) in conjunction with group psychotherapy for the child. Alternatively, remedial reading and individual counselling of the child by a teacher or social worker may be indicated. The permutations are numerous and generally unevaluated. Because of this, accurate formulation is essential as a prerequisite for the construction of a rational treatment scheme and should be phrased so as to predict treatment strategies. Is the family atmosphere one of irreversible rejection, necessitating the removal of the child into care, or one of, say, discord unmitigated by warmth to an extent where a boarding school for maladjusted children is appropriate? Is there reading delay as a consequence of established truancy or has reading disability led to a rejection of school? Is there overactivity to an extent requiring medication before educational measures can be effective? The range of treatment and appropriate measures extends beyond the psychiatric repertoire. It may well be argued that the essentially psychiatric task is one of formulation.

The prognosis for conduct disorders of childhood is not encouraging. Graham and Rutter (1973) found that in the medium term (four to five years) about three-quarters of conduct disordered children remain so and about half of children with mixed disorders remain disturbed true to initial diagnostic type. Robins (1966), looking at the long-term prognosis of seriously antisocial boys seen in a Child Guidance Clinic, found that about half of them were seriously antisocial adults thirty years later.

The impact of available contemporary treatments on this gloomy course of events is usually held to be negligible but in fact it is unexplored.

Tics

These are quick, sudden, purposeless, coordinated movements, which frequently occur in the same form at the same place in the body, can be suppressed voluntarily at the expense of mounting tension, increase with anxiety, and can be imitated.

Perhaps one in 10 normal children show tic-like movements at some stage but these do not usually persist. The usual age of onset of tics in clinic attenders is between five and 10 and there is a three-fold male predominance. Most commonly facial (blink, grimace), motor tics may spread down and distally, disappearing in reverse order. Vocal tics include grunts and, notoriously, coprolalia in Gilles de la Tourette's syndrome. Associations between tics and both developmental and psychiatric disorders are described in most studies but it must be remembered that these have drawn their samples from clinic populations. There seems to be a high order of parental psychiatric illness and a sizeable minority of cases have a family history of tics which is sometimes extensive. IQ is normally distributed among tiqueurs who, as a group, probably display no excess of definite neurological abnormalities. Studies which report a high incidence of soft neurological signs in Tourette's syndrome (e.g. Shapiro et al., 1973) are methodologically insecure though suggest a significant neurophysiological component. The differential diagnosis includes torsion dystonia and spasmodic torticollis, myoclonus, chorea, and orofacial dyskinesia.

Aetiology

The male predominance, association with other developmental disorders, age of onset and good prognosis argue for a developmental origin. Perhaps interaction with psychiatric disorder, temperament or stress acts as an additional factor promoting the persistence of the movement. The suggestions that tics either represent a symbolic expression of aggression or anxiety or act as conditioned avoidance responses evoked by stress and reinforced by anxiety reduction are, of course, not mutually exclusive hypotheses. Corbett (1977) has suggested that tics derive from the startle reflex of babies, components of which are perpetuated by learning mechanisms. Not all abnormal movements in a tiqueur are tics. Some may represent an attempt to ward off or socially justify the tic by converting it into a purposive movement. It seems likely that coprolalia is a response to a given tic as the obscenities used vary according to person and culture. Rarely, tics are the result of encephalitis lethargica or medication with phenothiazines or butyrophenones.

Treatment

Some psychological management is mandatory, to explain, reassure and minimize stress. Minor tranquillizers or relaxation training are widely used. Haloperidol is superior to placebo (Connell et al., 1967) but side-effects limit its use as a drug of first choice. Initial dosage should be 0·5 mg t.d.s., higher doses often being required for multiple tics.

The evidence for the efficacy of massed practice, whereby the repeated voluntary performance of a tic is held to increase reactive inhibition according to Hull's learning theory is anecdotal (e.g. Yates, 1958). Corbett (1977) reports that successful abolition by massed practice of an eye blink tic may be effective in extinguishing multiple tics; it is hypothesized this tic acts as a trigger to a chain of tic movements extending down the body.

Prognosis

At eight year follow-up 40% of Corbett *et al.*'s (1969) tiqueurs had completely recovered and a further 53% improved though as a group they showed an increased rate of anxiety and depressive symptoms. Traditionally, coprolalia worsens the outlook though the prognosis for Gilles de la Tourette's syndrome is not as bad as originally believed in that although persistence into adult life is likely, organic or psychotic deterioration is exceptionally rare.

Enuresis

Nine out of 10 UK children are dry by night at age 10. Whether this achievement results from formal training, social learning, or the emergence of an inherent behaviour pattern is controversial. After age five the prevalence diminishes slowly with age to 2% at age 15, long persistence tending to be particularly related to low IQ. The subject is thoroughly reviewed in Kolvin *et al.* (1973).

Aetiology

Most hypotheses propose an interaction between maturation and experience. Some assert that maturation alone is responsible for noctural continence, this representing the emergence of an inherent behaviour pattern. Enuresis, therefore, results if the maturation of behaviour is disrupted by anxiety. Others add training as a second factor which explains the influence of certain environmental factors, such as family disorganization, which do not necessarily mediate their effects through anxiety. Shaffer (1977) has argued for a view that enuresis is a response that has persisted because of interference by biological and social factors acting to inhibit normal social learning. The following factors (see Kolvin *et al.*, 1973) are associated with enuresis and require explanation by any aetiological hypothesis:

- greater concordance in MZ than DZ twins (Bakwin, 1961)
- higher incidence in relatives
- socio-economic classes 4 and 5 over-represented
- large families
- institutional upbringing
- male predominance
- tendency for IQ to be below average
- excess of stress events during early childhood (maternal death, hospital admission) (Douglas, 1973)

small functional bladder capacity (Starfield, 1967)

Enuresis always occurs in non-REM sleep, though there is no good evidence that enuretic children are hard to rouse (Graham, 1973).

There are two important associations:

(1) Urinary tract infections (UTI):
>   5% of enuretics (usually girls) have significant bacteriuria;
>   15% of children with UTI are enuretic in consequence;
>   treating the UTI cures enuresis in 30%.

(2) Psychiatric disorder (see below).

Classification

Distinctions are often made between (a) primary (never dry) (b) secondary (interim dry period, i.e. an *onset*), and the presence/absence of daytime wetting.

The validity of these distinctions is not established beyond doubt, though tradition assumes a general predominance of biological or maturational factors in primary enuresis and psychogenic or stress-related factors in secondary enuresis. No difference in the rate of psychiatric disorder between the two groups has in fact been demonstrated.

Psychiatric disorder

Most enuretics are psychiatrically normal, but psychiatric disorder is at least twice as common as in the general child population (Shaffer, 1973a), particularly so in girls and daytime wetters. No specific association exists with any particular psychiatric syndrome or individual item of behaviour except encopresis. There are three possible mechanisms (Shaffer, 1973a):

(1) enuresis secondary to psychiatric disorder;

(2) psychiatric disorder reactive to shame and parental disapproval of the enuresis;

(3) family factors (disorganization etc.) and early childhood stress which contribute to both enuresis and psychiatric disorder.

Management

Initial assessment includes a history and examination with particular attention to the back and lower limb neurology, as well as sending urine for microscopy, bacteriology, protein and glucose screening. Individual interviews with parents and child, consideration of sleeping arrangements and parental attitudes towards child and treatment approach, reassurance and explanation are always needed. A star chart should be employed to achieve a baseline record and is often sufficient treatment in its own right. Tricyclic antidepressants are the only drugs shown to be superior to placebo (Shaffer *et al.*, 1968). Their administration results in dryness within a few days in a majority but most of these will relapse on discontinuation thus restricting their use to 'first aid' measures—holidays, or pending rearrangement of bedrooms to enable the use of an alarm. The 'bell and pad' enuresis alarm is the most effective treatment, 80–90% achieving dryness, failures usually ascribed to faulty technique. About one-third of patients relapse but can be successfully treated. It has been shown that 'overlearning' by giving the newly continent child a fluid load at bed-time will reduce the likelihood of relapse (Young and Morgan, 1972). In understanding the rationale of the alarm one presumably needs to invoke a non-specific 'gadget' effect as well as acknowledging the manner in which the family's approval becomes focused on dry nights. In addition it may well be that the efficacy of the actual alarm is best understood in terms of avoidance learning or a punishment paradigm, rather than a classical conditioning paradigm, as the end result of treatment is a continent child who sleeps through the night rather than one who wakes to micturate.

The practical aspects of alarm treatment require meticulous attention to ensure that the child is woken adequately, does not interfere with the apparatus, does not suffer false alarms, and co-operates with the parent in changing the sheets and re-setting the alarm after he has passed water in a bedside pot. Careful demonstration and child–parent co-operation are vital. Any associated psychiatric disturbance or bacteriuria requires attention in its own right.

Daytime wetting

About three-quarters of day-time wetters are also incontinent at night. Combined day and night wetting is associated with a higher rate of psychiatric disturbance. The following types need to be considered:
   (1) Disorganized children from chaotic families with no habit training;
   (2) Practically mute, shy girls at school who are frightened to go or ask to go to the lavatory;
   (3) 'Giggle micturition' (urine passed during laughter);
   (4) Urinary tract infections and the urethral syndrome;
   (5) Ectopic ureter opening into urethra, neurogenic bladder.

Encopresis

Nearly all children achieve faecal continence by the age of four years. Subsequently the rate of faecal soiling is about 1%, more commonly in boys. 'True' encopresis is properly defined as 'the deposition of fully formed faeces in inappropriate places', and typically follows a clean period ('discontinuous soiling'). The term is also loosely used to cover other types of soiling such as:

    (a) lack of training ('continuous soiling') defaecating in pants, bed etc. as though in nappies, without very much anxiety or shame;

    (b) constipation with overflow or leakage due to
        Hirschprung's disease, fissure or drugs, particularly tricyclic antidepressants,
        psychological inhibition of defaecation leading to dyschezia;

    (c) diarrhoea as a result of
        organic disease,
        fear;

    (d) anal 'masturbation' (digital insertion for pleasure or comfort, not necessarily sexual).

'True' encopresis seems to result as a consequence of anxiety-tinged or coercive toilet training (Anthony, 1957) which results in precarious continence, likely to break down. The child associates the pot or toilet with fear or anxiety at the possibility of not being able to defaecate to parental order and the consequent escalation of parental anxiety or anger. Once away from the anxiety-creating situation and relaxed he will defaecate either in his pants or secretively in a private receptacle, such as a cupboard or secluded corner: 'respite defaecation' (Woodmansey, 1967).

There is a clinical impression that children who defaecate in inappropriate receptacles not infrequently exploit the practice. Stools may be deposited in the parental bed or in wrapped parcels in cupboards. Sometimes these are a clumsy attempt at shamed concealment but often seem to express hostility to parents, particularly when accompanied by smearing, and especially where such parents have obsessional standards of cleanliness. No single group of characteristics define the encopretic child or his family though many observers comment on the prevalence of discord and rejection within the family and of covert aggressiveness and denial as features of the child's psychopathology. The selectivity of situation and the normal consistency (ripe bananas) of the stool argue for a measure of faecal continence achieved and then lost in the face of acute or chronic stress. Certainly it seems reasonable to assume that the factors which led to the establishment of the encopretic habit may not be the same as those which ensure its persistence.

Treatment involves 'de-training' parents as well as the child in an attempt to lower the tensions and hostility which have accumulated. A combination of a psychotherapeutic approach to the child and parents in conjunction with a star chart with tangible back-up reinforcers is usually appropriate to encourage appropriate defaecation *as well as* continence. If constipation has occurred this requires simple investigation and appropriate laxatives. Severe cases often require admission to a psychiatric in-patient unit.

Dyslexia

Traditionally, *'dyslexia'* refers to a specific, constitutional, genetically determined difficulty in learning to read despite conventional instruction, adequate intelligence and socio-cultural opportunity. It is distinguished from other forms of reading disability by its gravity and purity, and associated with:
   (a) a family history of reading difficulties;
   (b) spelling difficulties;
   (c) speech delay;
   (d) clumsiness;
   (e) poor left/right differentiation (NOT crossed laterality in which e.g. right-handedness and left-eye dominance are combined).
By analogy with acquired dyslexia in adults it is conceived of as being secondary to a localized cortical immaturity (Critchley, 1964).

This concept of a specific disease entity arises from the study of clinic-based samples, and as such has been criticized by e.g. Rutter and Yule (1975) who review epidemiological surveys. They prefer the term *'specific reading retardation'* (SRR) which applies to children whose reading ability falls, say, two standard errors below the level which age, IQ and schooling would predict. This concept is broader than 'dyslexia' and does not imply a discrete neurological entity. Its epidemiological characteristics include a prevalence of 4–10% (depending on whether a semi-rural or inner-urban area is considered), and a male predominance of 3 or 4 to 1. Associations described for dyslexia, to which may be added large family size, low socio-economic status, and poor concentration with short attention-span, are statistically valid but hardly ever occur all in one child, and are seen in children without SRR. There is no specific pattern of neurodevelopmental abnormalities to suggest a *single* dyslexia syndrome. This is not to say that SRR does not exist as an entity: the prevalence is above that predicted by a normal distribution of reading skills (i.e. there is a hump on the distribution curve), and the associations are statistically significant, differentiating SRR from 'reading backwardness' due to low IQ.

There is an increased prevalence of SRR in neuro-epileptic children, but their numbers are so small that, overall, there is no increased prevalence of neurological abnormality in SRR, apart from the developmental abnormalities listed above. The aetiology of SRR seems, therefore, to be multifactorial with developmental, neurological, temperamental and family variables combining with educational influences. Emotional disturbance does *not* seem to be an aetiological factor (Rutter *et al.*, 1970b).

There is a marked association with antisocial behaviour in middle childhood, possibly arising out of classroom frustration and boredom (Rutter *et al.*, 1970b). Roughly one-third of 10-year-old children with reading retardation were diagnosed as conduct disorder in the Isle of Wight survey and, conversely, one-third of conduct disorder children were more than 28 months retarded in their reading compared with the level predicted from IQ.

Remedial education is mandatory, with consideration as to whether counselling may alleviate disillusionment and demoralization. Special dispensations are available for examination candidates. The prognosis is poor even when remedial help is offered, spelling difficulties being especially persistent.

Infantile autism

This, the commonest form of 'childhood psychosis' is best understood as a syndrome rather than a single medical condition. A suitable review of the development of the concept is Rutter (1974) and the original description by Kanner (1943) has hardly been bettered, though it is restricted to autistic children of normal intelligence.

Epidemiology

The Middlesex survey (Lotter, 1966) showed a prevalence of 0·02% for nuclear autism with a nearly three-fold male predominance. A real bias towards social classes 1 and 2 exists.

Aetiology

An organic bias is suggested by the presence of neurological abnormalities in about a quarter of all cases, the development of fits during adolescence in a third (Rutter, 1970) and an association with phenylketonuria, rubella embryopathy, neurolipidoses, infantile spasms and encephalitis. Moreover, in 12 out of 17 twin pairs discordant for autism the presence of autism was associated with a biological hazard likely to have caused brain injury (Folstein and Rutter, 1977). Hauser *et al.* (1975) have demonstrated an enlargement of the left temporal horn in some autistics. Most autistic children, however, show no neurological abnormality. A disorder of language may be decisive, as sequencing skills, coding capacity and meaning concepts can be shown to be radically impaired and would affect thought and comprehension in addition to speech (Hermelin and O'Connor, 1970). Furthermore, an important prognostic indicator is speech development by age five. It is possible that defective cognitive processes in addition to language abnormalities are involved; most autistic children are of limited intelligence (three-quarters have IQ under 70) and IQ is the most potent prognostic guide (Lockyer and Rutter, 1969).

The importance of environmental and emotional factors is controversial. The original 'refrigerator parents' concept has been unsubstantiated by controlled studies (e.g. Cox *et al.*, 1975) which show the parents to be normal people, though professional classes tend to be over-represented. Improvement of interpersonal behaviour in the child is not a predictor of improvement in other areas of behaviour.

Folstein and Rutter's (1977) finding of the 36% concordance in MZ twin pairs (c.f. 0% in DZ pairs) indicates that a genetic propensity sometimes operates. Disorders of special sense organs seem also relevant (Wing, 1969), particularly in the genesis of autistic traits in otherwise handicapped children.

Total picture

Kanner's (1943) original description should be read. Wing (1970) provides a wider account. For brevity the clinical abnormalities are summarized in Table II.

Cognitive picture

IQ is stable and does not increase with improving socialization. Performance subtest scores characteristically exceed verbal scores. This is a real cognitive deficit, not a motivational problem.

Differential diagnosis

There is a longstanding confusion between infantile autism and *schizophrenia* presenting in childhood. It is now apparent from the work of Kolvin's group (Kolvin, 1971) that these are two separate conditions

Table II   A classification of behavioural abnormalities

(A) *Abnormalities of language:*
   abnormal response to sounds
   very poor comprehension of gesture and speech
   no imaginative play
   poor or absent gesture
   restricted social imitation
   abnormal speech: absence or delayed acquisition
                    immediate echolalia
                    delayed echolalia with pronoun reversal
                    immature syntax, often telegrammatic
                    neologisms
                    concrete, pedantic content and expression
                    unusual delivery or modulation

(B) *Social abnormalities:*
   aloof and indifferent to people
   poor gaze contact
   no cooperative play (though may relish rough and tumble)
   no persisting friendships, weak parental attachments, no discrimination
      between people
   indifference to social conventions, insensitivity to others' feelings

(C) *Rituals and routines:*
   rigid play (lining up 'toys') or preoccupation with sterile topics (bus routes etc.)
   resistance to change with 'preservation of sameness' of environment (time-
      tables, furniture placement, etc.)
   attachments to particular, often unusual, objects or collections
   tantrums when frustrated by denial of above

All the above three categories should be represented with an onset before 30
months for the full diagnosis to be made.

(D) *Additional abnormalities may be present and include:*
   a lack of curiosity and unresponsiveness to people in infancy (deafness is often
      queried)
   unpredictable fears, screaming or laughter
   abnormal movements (finger stereotypies, spinning self or objects, toe-walking
      etc.)
   difficulties learning manipulative tasks (doorknobs) and orientations (up-
      down)
   hyperkinesis
   self-destructive behaviour and rocking
   isolated skills (jigsaws, music, computation, rote memory)

differing in their symptomatology, epidemiology, age of onset, family history, cognitive characteristics and prognosis. Schizophrenia in children hardly ever occurs before age seven and resembles adult schizophrenia in its psychopathology, genetics and epidemiology. Most of its victims are of normal intelligence.

Real difficulties arise in the differentiation of infantile autism from *disintegrative psychosis*—a profound regression in speech and language associated with vague illness at about age three or four with subsequent overactivity, dementia, impoverished social behaviour, mannerisms and stereotypies (see Corbett *et al.*, 1977). Similarly, *dysphasia* of developmental or acquired origin requires recognition; it appears that there may be children with behaviour patterns apparently intermediate in form between dysphasia and infantile autism, though the cognitive deficits and language handicaps of the two conditions are quite distinct (Bartak *et al.*, 1975).

Autistic behavioural traits are not uncommon in severe mental retardation and in blind or deaf children. It is wise to describe them as such rather than blithely applying a label of infantile autism which may raise parents' hopes with regard to educational opportunities.

Management

Although no specific 'treatment' is available, various approaches offer help. *Educational placement* in a special school is mandatory if IQ permits. The parents will always need *support, information and guidance*; to this end the National Society for Autistic Children is invaluable. More specifically, parents have been involved in a variety of experimental programmes based on *behaviour modification* which aim to teach social behaviour, improve language, and minimize unacceptable or self-destructive behaviour (Howlin *et al.*, 1973; Schopler and Reichler, 1971). *Medication* is of only occasional use in the control of hyperkinesis, aggressive outbursts or screaming at night. There is no evidence in favour of a psychotherapeutic insight-directed approach; certainly in the school setting an educational attitude based on regressive techniques has shown to be inferior to specific skills training within a structured programme (Rutter and Bartak, 1973).

Prognosis

Autistic children do not develop into adult schizophrenics, they become autistic adults. Although some improvement in social behaviour and rituals is likely to occur during middle childhood, most adult autistics remain severely handicapped in institutions, families or sheltered employment. Half of all autistic children remain mute and only one in six can manage ordinary school and work (Rutter, 1970). The overall prognosis is poor if no speech is acquired by age five and if the IQ is below, say, 50 (Lockyer and Rutter, 1969).

Hyperkinetic syndrome

Considerable confusion, not to say acrimony, surrounds this topic, not least because of the tendency for some North American paediatricians to over-prescribe stimulants in an attempt to control overactive and destructive children. It is argued elsewhere that the assumption that severely overactive children are necessarily brain damaged is false and that 'minimal brain dysfunction'—often taken as synonymous with hyperkinesis—is a misleading and obsolete term, best forgotten.

There remain considerable differences in the use of the term 'hyperkinetic syndrome'. In the UK it is applied to children who are persistently and incorrigibly overactive irrespective of situation. Ounsted (1955) provides the classic account and comments upon an apparent association with temporal lobe epilepsy. It seems likely that many such children are intellectually retarded; some are autistic or obviously brain-damaged with hard signs evident on neurological examination. Stimulants are sometimes beneficial but not uncommonly produce a tearful, withdrawn reaction; an apparent depression necessitating withdrawal of the drug. With the passing of the years overactivity becomes underactivity and apathy. The diagnosis is not made very commonly and is not further discussed here.

In North America there is a readiness to describe a child as hyperactive or hyperkinetic on the basis of criteria well summarized by Cantwell (1975). The disorder begins early in life and is characterized by four core symptoms:

(1) hyperactivity (energetic, fidgety child 'always into things', most evident in the classroom and *not* always present at interview);
(2) impulsivity (impetuous recklessness);
(3) distractibility (short attention span, distracted by extraneous stimuli);
(4) excitability (low tolerance of frustration, easily over-excited, tantrums).

Most accounts include reference to antisocial behaviour, learning disabilities, and the presence of soft neurological signs. Taken in turn, it seems true that a significant number of such children behave antisocially and that the extent of this increases with the passage of time, presumably as a reaction to disillusionment with school failure and peer group difficulties or rejection by the family of origin. Learning disabilities, perhaps related to the attentional and impulse-control deficits, are common in hyperactive children who under-achieve in the classroom even when IQ is taken into account (Minde *et al.*, 1971).

The association with soft neurological signs is problematic. Werry *et al.* (1972) in a carefully standardized procedure found an excess of minor neurological abnormalities suggestive of developmental delays and coordination difficulties, but no excess of hard signs, EEG abnormalities or histories of insults to the brain. Perhaps a half of all hyperactive children display such soft signs. Waldrop *et al.* (1968) described an association between minor physical anomalies (as found in Down's syndrome) and overactive behaviour in some pre-school children. There has been some positive replication of her findings in the USA but negative findings in a UK study (Sandberg *et al.*, 1978).

Aetiological considerations are somewhat speculative. It should be noted that hyperkinetic children (in the American sense) are not necessarily overactive; they may, in fact, differ in the *type* of activity displayed (Cantwell, 1977). Nevertheless, it remains a popular postulate that such children, who are usually boys, have under-aroused central nervous systems with insufficient cortical inhibitory control over sensory input and motor activity. Some neurophysiological studies support this notion (Satterfield *et al.*, 1974) which also provides a model for the use of stimulants which are believed to stimulate the mid-brain reticular activating system and thus cause cortical inhibition.

Cantwell (1976) has reviewed the evidence for genetic factors. It would appear that the biological, though not the adoptive, parents of hyperactive children show increased prevalence rates of alcoholism, sociopathy and (St. Louis) hysteria. The biological fathers were likely to be overactive children.

Treatment

A host of studies have confirmed the beneficial effects of stimulant drugs—mainly *d*-amphetamine and methylphenidate—on hyperactivity (see e.g. Conners, 1972). Various other agents (pemoline, thioridazine, imipramine etc.) have beneficial effects but for various reasons are less convenient. No one drug is best for all patients but methylphenidate, in that it appears to have less effect on height gain than amphetamine, is a suitable first choice. The principal risks are suppression of growth, insomnia and tearfulness. Administration during the mornings of school days only, with careful monitoring of weight and height is mandatory. Fortunately, drug abuse is rare.

Operant schedules for improving classroom behaviour have independent benefit but the most effective treatment approach is likely to be a combination package wherein medication, behaviour modification, remedial education and counselling of the child and his family combine and mutually facilitate each other.

No long-term benefits have been shown to definitely accrue from any single treatment measure. Follow-ups performed by those such as Minde *et al.* (1971) show a depressing picture of educational failure, low self-esteem, and antisocial activity in adolescence. The symptom of high activity itself diminishes with age but the attentional difficulties persist.

Cantwell (1975) is at pains to point out that what is described is a syndrome with various aetiologies and subgroups. In view of Shaffer *et al.*'s (1974) suggestion that overactivity is a non-specific symptom of psychiatric disorder, the question remains as to how far the hyperkinetic syndrome as defined in America is separate from such diagnoses as conduct disorder used in the UK.

Brain damage

Taken as a group, brain-damaged children show a higher prevalence of psychiatric disorder—five-fold in the Isle of Wight study (Rutter *et al.*, 1970a). Clearly this is a result of various associated factors such as low IQ having a high prevalence among such a group. Furthermore, Shaffer *et al.* (1975) found that children who had sustained severe head injuries were likely to come from socially disadvantaged families. Nevertheless, a persisting excessive rate of childhood psychiatric disorder obtains when IQ (Rutter *et al.*, 1970a), physical handicap (Seidel *et al.*, 1975) and social disadvantage (Shaffer *et al.*, 1975) are controlled for. Brain damage itself has a specific effect but it is important not to overstate the case.

Notions of a 'continuum of reproductive casualty' (Knobloch and Pasamanick, 1966) extending from, for example, spontaneous abortion of an embryo to behaviour disorder, arise from the observation that children with behaviour problems, usually antisocial, have experienced an increased incidence of obstetric difficulties. However, such apparent excess dwindles away if social disadvantage is controlled for, as obstetric complications and conduct disorder are both associated with low socioeconomic status. Shaffer (1977) considers the effect of neonatal asphyxia and finds only minimal consequences when behaviour, intelligence and educational difficulties are considered. Various authorities have followed Strauss' (1947) claim that a behaviour disorder characterized by overactivity, inattentiveness, impulsivity and particular perceptual or learning difficulties allowed one to infer brain damage even in the absence of hard neurological signs. Children who behaved in this way frequently displayed 'soft' signs (minor choreoathetoid movements, poor laterality differentiation, dysdiadochokinesis) which led to the application of the label 'Minimal Brain Dysfunction' (or 'Damage'). There seems to be an assumption that this is common and an indication for drug treatment (Wender, 1972).

The logical problem of assuming damage to the brain in the absence of hard evidence is obvious. 'Soft' signs are for soft minds when taken out of the context of a full neurological examination as not only are they extremely common but also reflect developmental delay when they do not reflect unreliability in their detection. Whether any particular pattern of behavioural symptoms suggests brain injury deserves further investigation.

Most brain-damaged children in the Isle of Wight study showed the usual mix of conduct disorders and emotional disorders. Certainly there was no uniform clinical picture. Nevertheless, there is an association between brain damage and certain *rare* psychiatric disorders: disintegrative psychosis, confusional states, petit mal status, and some cases of infantile autism (most autistic children show no evidence of brain damage). Turning to an examination of the relative prevalence of symptoms, both Rutter *et al.* (1970a) and Shaffer *et al.* (1974) found no excess of overactivity or impulsivity in brain-damaged children (psychiatrically disordered and otherwise) over controls, though both symptoms are a common accompaniment of conduct disorder (with or without brain damage). The conclusion is unavoidable: no behavioural stereotype characteristic of brain damage exists.

Just how brain damage exerts its influence on the prevalence of psychiatric disorder is unresolved. With respect to the type of damage, Shaffer (1973b) concluded that the following factors increased the risk of psychiatric disorder:

(a) bilateral lesions
(b) electrically active lesions (fits)
(c) presence of psychomotor fits
(d) IQ under 80
(e) adverse home environment.

Curiously enough, male sex does not appear to increase the risk and it is noteworthy that psychiatric disorder within a population of children with brain damage does not show the usual predilection for boys (Rutter *et al.*, 1970a). Surprisingly too, neither age when sustained, severity, or locus of cortical injury was associated with psychiatric outcome in Shaffer *et al.* (1975). This is not to say that such factors are irrelevant to the loss or acquisition of particular *skills*: dominant hemisphere injury has increasingly poor prognosis for speech recovery after the age of four (Basser, 1962).

Harrington and Letemendia (1958) found that children seen at a Child Guidance Clinic were distinguishable from other children with head injury by their pre-traumatic adjustment or family adjustment at the time of referral, rather than by the severity of the injury. This is confirmed in the Isle of Wight work and the studies of Seidel *et al.* (1975) and Shaffer *et al.* (1975). The parallels with Gruenberg and Pond's (1957) findings in epilepsy are evident. As in children with normal brains, marital discord, parental mental illness, repeated separations, parental criminality etc., are epidemiologically associated with psychiatric disorder.

Rutter (1977a) has performed a series of exercises to attempt to elicit the nature of the mechanism whereby brain damage increases the prevalence of disorder. He finds no evidence for an interactional effect whereby brain damage increases the vulnerability of the child to psychosocial stress and asserts that brain injury and psychosocial stress act independently. He draws attention to the adverse effect on cognitive skills, citing the higher rate of reading retardation among brain-injured controls, and to the possible adverse effects on behaviour of anticonvulsants (Stores, 1975) or repeated admission to hospital (Douglas, 1975). He does not explicitly consider the notion that the threshold for the appearance of psychiatric disorder may be lowered by such factors and pays surprisingly little attention to the family's perception of the child's injury and handicap.

In the assessment of the individual child it is important to note that there are no psychological tests specific for brain damage (Herbert, 1964). A WISC verbal-performance discrepancy is a very poor indicator of damage in the individual case.

Anorexia nervosa

Characteristically a disorder of adolescent and young adult women, the typical manifestations of this otherwise mysterious condition are well known. Comment here is restricted to two areas of debate: the essential nature of the disorder, and treatment.

There is an important problem of definition. Whereas the usual approach has been to specify the readily observable aspects, food avoidance, weight loss, amenorrhoea, overactivity etc., various voices have been raised in favour of specifically psychological criteria. Part of the reason for this is a need to isolate a nuclear syndrome from other causes of food refusal or weight loss such as depression. Bruch (1974a) has posed a persuasive hypothesis wherein the 'relentless pursuit of thinness' is 'a desperate struggle for a self-respecting identity' associated with a disturbance of body image and misinterpretations of proprioceptive stimuli coupled with a paralysing sense of personal ineffectiveness. The sources of such disability lie within the family interactions and rearing practices so that the child never fully learns the significance of her own bodily feelings and is confused about her own hunger sensations since these have always been anticipated or negated by parents who 'know better'. The similarities between this model and Kohut's (1972) views on narcissism and the development of a satisfactory sense of self are to be noted in passing. Dieting during adolescence provides the girl with an experience of exerting power over her body and a satisfying sense of accomplishment otherwise unavailable to her. The familiar stubbornness and negativism of the anorexic represent an indiscriminate rejection of help—a desperate defence against inner feelings of helplessness and impotence. As opposed to a conforming manner during childhood when remarkable compliance and anxiety to please were prominent, individuation during adolescence and the necessity to develop autonomy arouses serious psychic conflict to which the pursuit of thinness provides a solution. Control of weight and eating assumes overwhelming importance for the patient and becomes the metaphor by which personal worth is secretly described. Food, weight and eating totally preoccupy the girl's daily life (as in externally imposed starvation) but the all-important control may break down with gorging followed by subsequent guilt, even suicide.

Support for the hypothesis comes from Bruch's own (uncontrolled) studies, from studies such as that of Slade and Russell (1973) which systematically demonstrate anorexics' tendency to perceive themselves as fatter than they are and 'deny' their emaciation, and from Silverstone and Russell (1967) who showed that although anorexics could detect their own gastric hunger contractions they were often unable to interpret them as hunger pains.

Crisp (1967) has suggested that the primary nuclear form of anorexia nervosa is characterized by a central symptom of phobia of normal adolescent weight following the growth changes of puberty. Dieting in response to a dislike of being 'fat' becomes a headlong pursuit of security and comfort in physiological childhood with a freedom from the demands, particularly sexual, of adolescence. An equation is made by the anorexic of weight with growth, hence growth is avoided by weight loss. Like Bruch the emphasis is on a phenomenological distinction of a nuclear, true anorexia nervosa from anorexia secondary to other psychiatric conditions. Slade and Welbourne (1976) have made a similar point by suggesting that there is a characteristic attitude which may be elicited by naming a very small quantity of carbohydrate food that the girl avoids eating and asking what would happen if she did eat it. A response along the lines of 'I'd immediately put on too much weight' or 'I'd never stop if I started' should make one, they suggest, diagnose incipient anorexia nervosa if some weight has already been lost.

Russell has recently (1977) reviewed the evidence for a primary disturbance of hypothalamic function. Most of the physiological abnormalities are corrected by regaining weight but cyclical fluctuations in gonadotrophins and the expected release of LH after a course of oestrogen are not re-established, suggesting a persistent and possibly primary defect of hypothalamic functioning. Although he suggests an aetiological model incorporating both psychological and physical factors he does not refute the possibilities that weight loss may irreversibly damage some hypothalamic functions or that recovery of weight in the experimental subjects was unaccompanied by attainment of emotional equilibrium or even regular eating habits, both of which might disturb hypothalamic activity.

Using psychological criteria it is obvious that a higher prevalence figure would obtain than that indicated by case register studies which rely on a medical diagnosis having been made, usually only when amenorrhoea and serious weight loss supervene. Such registers yield an incidence rate of roughly 1/100,000 population per year (range 0·37–1·6; Kendell *et al.*, 1973). A bias towards a higher rate among middle-class families exists in some, but not all, areas or countries. Whatever criteria are used, most workers agree that a female predominance of about 15 to one exists and there is some evidence that the condition is becoming more common. Amongst a vulnerable population of largely middle-class, late adolescent girls, Crisp *et al.* (1976) discovered a prevalence rate of severe cases of one in 100 girls.

The issue of treatment is clouded by polemic. Most clinicians combine supervised re-feeding with some sort of individual or family psychotherapy. Eminent authorities (e.g. Tolstrup, 1975; Bruch, 1974b) have dismissed behaviour modification techniques as not validated by sufficient follow-up. However, Kellerman (1977), with only a limited literature search, was able to find nine studies of behaviour modification in anorexia nervosa which incorporated follow-ups ranging from four to 30 months and indicated positive gains more extensive than mere weight correction, sufficient for him to consider behaviour modification the treatment of choice. Anecdotal clinical experience suggests that some anorexic patients merely 'play the game' as far as supervised weight gain goes and have no commitment to personal, attitudinal change, thus relapsing rapidly after weight correction. It would seem advisable, particularly in view of a 5% death rate (Morgan and Russell, 1975), to combine individual or family psychotherapy *and* behavioural techniques. One might reasonably expect nearly three-quarters of all hospitalized anorexia cases to remit or substantially improve with treatment (see e.g. Morgan and Russell, 1975).

Adolescence

This period of rapid cognitive, emotional and social change extends from the onset of puberty to an indefinite end-point in the late teens when physical development is complete and sufficient independence achieved for the assumption of adult roles. The latter require the individual to have developed his own identity and to have achieved an emotionally secure autonomy. Dependence upon the family of origin must, therefore, be relinquished, social roles explored, genital sexuality mastered and peer group standards adopted in such a way that sufficient integration of personality is maintained throughout. Given that rate of development in adolescence is governed by physical and cognitive growth, family expectations, and by the standards demanded by school and peer group, it is not surprising that the pace is uneven and largely beyond the control of the individual. Moreover, the precise demands of, say, parents and peer group are often at variance.

It is generally supposed, therefore, that adolescence is a period of inevitable psychological upheaval, much psychiatric disorder in this age group being regarded as 'adolescent turmoil'. This concept implies that psychiatric disorder is due to difficulties inherent at this developmental stage and that the prognosis is good.

The traditional psychoanalytic view is that adolescents are transiently maladjusted as a result of a resurgence of oedipal conflicts with consequent excessive, crippling, defences. A smooth passage through adolescence is thus deviant. This is linked with the development of secure identity, accompanied by its negative counterpart of role diffusion, which results in 'experimentation' with deviant behaviour indicative in adults of major psychopathology but normal in adolescents. However, various studies have demonstrated the freedom from psychopathology with good adjustment in the majority of adolescents (e.g. Offer, 1969). There seems to be reasonable agreement that about 10–20% of adolescents display psychiatric disorders (Masterson, 1967; Leslie, 1974) which, on follow-up, have prognoses no different from any other age group. Overall, two-thirds of Masterson's adolescents were still handicapped five years later. The roots of adolescent disorder lay apparently within childhood and within the family rather than in a primarily developmental crisis, and the bland assumption, 'he'll grow out of it' seems dangerously optimistic.

Whether adolescent turmoil exists in any case without prompting major pathology is a separate issue. Non-handicapping symptoms of anxiety, misery, sensitivity, and altercations with parents are found in perhaps as many as one in two adolescents at some time (Masterson, 1967; Rutter *et al.*, 1976), and would thus indicate that inner turmoil is common though not universal, may lie undetected, and does not produce major psychopathology, impaired function, or alienation from parents for the great majority of adolescents. Moreover, many such symptoms are eminently understandable in developmental terms. For example, the characteristic of rebellious non-conformity may represent a rejection of parental values enabling separation from the parents to be facilitated, the symptoms of anxiety may be seen as the natural consequence of conflicting role demands, the depressive mood swings as a consequence of a sense of loss at an earlier dependent security. What needs to be stressed is that most adolescents sustain a smooth transition from childhood to maturity and that such symptoms, although common, are neither universal or necessary. Whether they predispose to the increased prevalence of handicapping psychiatric disorder at this age (q.v. Epidemiology) remains conjectural. The overall conclusion is that those adolescents who have poor adjustment with their families and show handicapping psychiatric disorder arising *de novo* in adolescence merit as much psychiatric concern as, and have a corresponding prognosis to, individuals in any other age group.

The variety of psychiatric disorder occurring in adolescence reflects the transitional nature of the developmental stage of adolescence. Firstly, disorders with their roots in childhood: conduct disorder, emotional disorder, tics etc. Secondly, disorders similar to those in adult populations: adult-type neuroses such as agoraphobia, suicidal depression, anorexia nervosa, schizophrenia, etc. In addition the emergence of social and sexual demands produces management difficulties of chronic handicaps such as infantile autism. It has not been established that there are any psychiatric disorders specific to adolescence; those adolescents who manifest psychiatric pathology require similar approaches to diagnosis and prognosis as children and adults with similar symptomatology.

Approaches to treatment

It is exceptionally difficult to summarize the available therapeutic measures in the child psychiatrist's repertoire as these include interference with the child's family, school, and even where he may live to an extent which is beyond the medical concept of therapy. Such activities as advising parents, teachers or social workers are, of necessity, more extensive than similar activities in adult psychiatry. From the wide range of treatment manoeuvres employed in child psychiatry only three topics are briefly considered.

1 Psychotherapy

This is the most commonly used approach to the individual child, though the form it takes varies from play-centred with younger children to a verbal, conversational mode with older patients. The therapist's style and interventions may be analytically derived (Freud, 1966; Klein, 1932; Sandler *et al.*, 1973) or assume a client-centred, Rogerian stance (e.g. Reisman, 1973). Probably because of these various techniques and styles little has been done to evaluate the relative efficacy of different therapeutic methods either in individual therapy, casework with parents, or groups. Only one methodologically valid demonstration of comparative efficacy exists: Eisenberg *et al.*'s (1965) study of brief individual psychotherapy with emotionally disordered children, which demonstrated a significant clinical improvement compared with assessment-only controls.

It may well be, however, that the hard-headed approach that demands statistical proof is missing the point that the child psychiatrist is heavily involved with palliation and the alleviation of distress, and that, for many of his treatments, these are the aims, rather than an insistence on 'cure'. Furthermore, many child psychotherapists are markedly less discriminating than their adult counterparts concerning the characteristics of the patients that they take on for treatment and this may limit their therapeutic success.

The practice of conjoint family therapy (q.v. Chapter 22) is in vogue at present, though its efficacy in the alleviation of childhood psychiatric disorder relies almost exclusively on testimony.

2 Behaviour therapy

Potentially this has a wide range of application and there are various reports of its success. With the exception of enuresis alarms, it cannot be said that many such claims are based on sufficiently large samples to enable one to say with any confidence that it is a 'preferable' model to psychotherapy.

Bell and Pad is of proven benefit in enuresis. Similar alarms may be worn in pants for the treatment of day time wetting.

Desensitization (usually *in vivo*) is now widely regarded as the treatment of choice in monosymptomatic phobias. It has also been found useful in conjunction with *response prevention* and *modelling* in a few obsessive-compulsive children. *Stimulus fading* is a variant commonly employed with elective mutes.

Flooding is rarely practised with children, though the restraints applied in school to keep a child with school refusal from escaping home may be viewed according to a flooding paradigm. Yule *et al.* (1974) cite the case of an 11-year-old with whom flooding succeeded where desensitization had failed to alleviate a phobia of bursting balloons.

Operant techniques may be used in modifying classroom or ward behaviour, controlling hyperkinesis, speech training, and may be combined with a shaping technique or extinction programme. The reinforcements may be inferred from analysis of behavioural data obtained but those commonly used include praise, sweets, the freedom to perform other pleasurable activities, or tokens that may be exchanged at a later date for rewards. A star chart is a simple form of operant training. Extension of the practice to the families of disturbed children with parents as co-therapists along the lines suggested by Patterson (e.g. 1971) and including reciprocal contracts between parents and child have found considerable application.

Time out (from positive reinforcement) is a particularly severe form of extinction training whereby undesirable or antisocial behaviour is immediately followed by social isolation such as placement in a featureless room, alone, for a given period. McAuley and McAuley (1977) have described the usefulness of time out with close limit-setting in the outpatient management of conduct disorders.

Modelling by therapists directly or using doll-play may be used in the treatment of phobias, feminized behaviour in boys, or in social skills training. Particularly in the latter, video feedback has been used when self-esteem allows.

Massed practice has been used in the treatment of tics, the tic movement being repeated without rest to encourage the accumulation of reactive inhibition.

Graded change has been used to eliminate the rituals or bizarre attachments displayed by autistic children. For example, the blanket which an autistic child insisted on carrying everywhere was progressively trimmed until only a minute fragment remained which was spontaneously discarded (see Marchant *et al.*, 1974).

3   Drugs

These have been mentioned in the context of respective disorders. To recapitulate, the following are of accepted benefit:

(1) *Methylphenidate* and *dexamphetamine* in the hyperkinetic syndrome (Connors, 1972).
(2) *Phenothiazines* in aggressive behaviour disorders, the hyperkinetic syndrome (Werry *et al.*, 1966) and in schizophrenia.

(3) *Tricyclic antidepressants* in enuresis (Shaffer *et al.*, 1968), school refusal (Gittelman-Klein and Klein, 1971) and persistent depressive symptoms in older children and adolescents (Weinberg*et al.*, 1973).

(4) *Haloperidol* in tics (Connell *et al.*, 1967) and hyperkinesis (Barker and Frazer, 1968).

(5) *Benzodiazepines* in anxiety in adolescents, though note the likely adverse effect in younger children (Lucas and Pasley, 1969).

(6) *Sulthiame* for behaviour disorders in subnormal children (Al-Kaisi and McGuire, 1974).

At an anecdotal level, lithium has been advocated for affective illnesses in older children (Annell, 1969) and MAOIs for depressive symptoms (Frommer, 1968).

The outcome of childhood psychiatric disorder

Infantile autism has a generally poor prognosis. IQ above 50 and speech acquisition by age five predict more favourably (q.v.). It does not develop into schizophrenia in adult life.

Schizophrenia in childhood has a poor prognosis, except perhaps for some acute psychotic 'shifts' in adolescents. Schizophrenics who present in adult life may have shown a childhood pattern of low IQ, under-achievement at school, CNS disorder, social withdrawal and eccentricity with poor peer relationships (Offord and Cross, 1969). If children show pre-schizophrenic psychiatric disorder it is commonly of mixed neurotic and antisocial type. Most schizophrenics have experienced no significant childhood difficulties. The majority of shy, withdrawn children seen at clinics have an excellent prognosis.

Depression in children is controversial (q.v.). Depressive symptoms in children do not predict adult depression and are not especially common as a symptom group in the children of parents who have a history of depression. Manic-depressive illness, which hardly ever occurs before puberty, is likely to recur in adult life.

Aggressive or antisocial conduct disorders have a poor outlook, severe examples presenting as adult psychopaths with marital difficulties, poor work records, worse social relationships, more psychiatric disorder ('schizophrenia' and 'hysteria' in Robins' (1966) study), alcoholism and crime. Nearly all adult psychopaths were antisocial children. The prediction of adult psychopathy apparently correlates with the severity of the childhood disorder.

Neurotic disorders in childhood are not usually predictive of adult neurosis. In Robins' (1966) study, neurosis in adult life was no more common in the clinic patients than in the controls; the majority of childhood neurotics were not neurotic adults. However, *if* neurotic children present to psychiatrists in adult life it is usually with a neurotic disorder (Pritchard and Graham, 1966). Retrospective studies of adult neurotics (Tyrer and Tyrer, 1974) show that 10–20% displayed symptoms of school refusal as children. There does not seem to be any specific link between school refusal and any particular adult neurosis. This suggests a life-long neurotic predisposition applicable, perhaps, to one in three school refusers. The so-called neurotic traits of childhood (thumb-sucking, nail-biting, enuresis, food fads, stammering, fears) do not in themselves predict either childhood or adult neurosis. Specific object phobias nearly always begin in childhood, quite unlike agoraphobia or social phobia.

The hyperkinetic syndrome may remit in terms of overactivity, but leave underactivity, attention defects and emotional maladjustment in its wake which may predispose to later antisocial behaviour.

Mental retardation persists, though changes of IQ of ± 15 points may occur. School provides the toughest test in the lives of many mildly retarded children whose social adjustment improves after leaving school.

'Adolescent turmoil' is often applied as a label to psychiatric disorder during adolescence and the benign prognosis implied is frequently mis-leading (q.v.).

Specific reading retardation is known to have a poor medium-term prognosis and probably persists into adult life (with spelling the major difficulty) unless remedial help is provided.

Bereavement in childhood is mildly associated with adult psychiatric disorder, more particularly so with severe depression and suicidal behaviour in women who lost their father during adolescence (Hill, 1972).

References

Al-Kaisi, A. H. and McGuire, R. J. (1974). The effect of sulthiame on disturbed behaviour in mentally subnormal patients. *Br. J. Psychiat.* **124**, 45–49.

Annell, A. L. (1969). Lithium in the treatment of children and adolescents. *Acta Psychiat. Scand. Suppl.* **207**, 19–30.

Anthony, E. J. (1957). An experimental approach to the psychopathology of childhood: encopresis. *Br. J. Med. Psychol.* **30**, 146–175.

Anthony, E. J. and Scott, P. D. (1960). Manic-depressive psychosis in childhood. *J. Child Psychol. Psychiat.* **1**, 53–72.

Bakwin, H. (1961). Enuresis in children. *J. Pediat.* **58**, 806–819.

Bandura, A., Grusec, J. E. and Menlove, F. L. (1967). Vicarious extinction of avoidance behaviour. *J. Pers. Soc. Psychol.* **5**, 16–23.

Barker, P. and Frazer, I. A. (1968). A controlled trial of haloperidol in children. *Br. J. Psychiat.* **114**, 855–857.

Bartak, L., Rutter, M. and Cox, A. (1975). A comparative study of infantile autism and specific developmental receptive language disorder 1: the children. *Br. J. Psychiat.* **126**, 127–145.

Basser, L. S. (1962). Hemiplegia of early onset and the faculty of speech with special reference to the effects of hemispherectomy. *Brain* **85**, 427–460.

Becker, W. C. (1964). Consequences of different kinds of parental discipline. *In* 'Review of Child Development Research' (Eds M. L. Hoffman and L. W. Hoffman), Vol. 1. Russell Sage Foundation, New York.

Berecz, J. M. (1968). Phobias of childhood: etiology and treatment. *Psychol. Bull.* **70**, 694–720.

Bowlby, J. (1969). 'Attachment and Loss', Vol. 1: 'Attachment'. Hogarth Press, London.

Bruch, H. (1974a). 'Eating Disorders'. Routledge and Kegan Paul, London.

Bruch, H. (1974b). Perils of behaviour modification in treatment of anorexia nervosa. *J. Am. Med. Ass.* **230**, 1419–1422.

Cantwell, D. (1975). 'The Hyperactive Child: Diagnosis, Management and Current Research'. Spectrum Publications, New York.

Cantwell, D. (1976). Genetic factors in the hyperkinetic syndrome. *J. Am. Acad. Child Psychiat.* **15**, 214–223.

Cantwell, D. (1977). Hyperkinetic syndrome. *In* 'Child Psychiatry: Modern Approaches' (Eds M. Rutter and L. Hersov). Blackwell, Oxford.

Caplan, H. L. (1970). Hysterical 'conversion' symptoms in childhood. M. Phil. Dissertation, University of London.

Clarke, A. M. and Clarke, A. D. B. (Eds) (1976). 'Early Experience: Myth and Evidence'. Open Books, London.

Connell, P. H., Corbett, J. A., Horne, D. J. and Mathews, A. M. (1967). Drug treatment of adolescent tiquers: a double blind study of diazepam and haloperidol. *Br. J. Psychiat.* **113**, 375–381.

Conners, C. (1972). Pharmacotherapy of psychopathology in children. *In* 'Psychopathological Disorders of Childhood' (Eds H. C. Quay and J. S. Werry). Wiley, New York.

Coolidge, J. C., Hahn, P. B. and Peck, A. L. (1957). School phobia: neurotic crisis or way of life? *Am. J. Orthopsychiat.* **27**, 296–306.

Corbett, J. A. (1977). Tics and Tourette's Syndrome. *In* 'Child Psychiatry: Modern Approaches' (Eds M. Rutter and L. Hersov). Blackwell, Oxford.

Corbett, J. A., Mathews, A. M., Connell, P. H. and Shapiro, D. A. (1969). Tics and Gilles de la Tourette's Syndrome: a follow-up study and critical review. *Br. J. Psychiat.* **115**, 1229–1241.

Corbett, J. A., Harris, R., Taylor, E. and Trimble, M. (1977). Progressive disintegrative psychosis of childhood. *J. Child Psychol. Psychiat.* **18**, 211–219.

Cowie, J., Cowie, V. and Slater, E. (1968). 'Delinquency in Girls'. Heinemann, London.

Cox, A., Rutter, M., Newman, S. and Bartak, L. (1975). A comparative study of infantile autism and specific developmental receptive language disorder II: parental characteristics. *Br. J. Psychiat.* **126**, 146–159.

Crisp, A. H. (1967). Anorexia nervosa. *Br. J. Hosp. Med.* May, 713–718.

Crisp, A. H., Palmer, R. L. and Kalucy, R. S. (1976). How common is anorexia nervosa? A prevalence study. *Br. J. Psychiat.* **128**, 549–554.

Critchley, M. (1964). 'Developmental Dyslexia'. Heinemann, London.

Dahl, V. (1971). A follow-up study of child psychiatric clientele with special regard to manic-depressive psychosis. *In* 'Depressive States in Childhood and

Adolescence' (Ed. A. L. Annell). Proc. 4th UEP Congr. Stockholm 1971. Alm-quist and Wiksell, Stockholm.

Douglas, J. W. B. (1973). Early disturbing events and later enuresis. *In* 'Bladder Control and Enuresis' (Eds I. Kolvin, R. MacKeith and S. R. Meadow). Clinics in Dev. Med., Nos. 48/49. SIMP, Heinemann, London.

Douglas, J. W. B. (1975). Early hospital admissions and later disturbances of behaviour and learning. *Dev. Med. Child Neurol.* **17**, 456–480.

Dubowitz, V. and Hersov, L. (1976). Management of children with non-organic (hysterical) disorders of motor function. *Dev. Med. Child Neurol.* **18**, 358–368.

Eisenberg, L. (1958). School phobia: a study in the communication of anxiety. *Am. J. Psychiat.* **114**, 712–718.

Eisenberg, L., Conners, K. and Sharpe, L. (1965). A controlled study of the differential application of outpatient psychiatric treatment for children. *Jap. J. Child Psychiat.* **6**, 125–132.

Field, E. (1967). 'A Validation of Hewitt and Jenkins' Hypothesis'. Home Office Research Unit Report No. 10. HMSO, London.

Folstein, S. and Rutter, M. (1977). Infantile autism: a genetic study of 21 twin pairs. *J. Child Psychol. Psychiat.* **18**, 297–321.

Freud, A. (1966). 'Normality and Pathology in Childhood'. Hogarth Press, London.

Frommer, E. (1967). Treatment of childhood depression with antidepressant drugs. *Br. Med. J.* **i**, 729–732.

Frommer, E. (1968). Depressive illness in childhood. *In* 'Recent Advances in Affective Disorders' (Eds A. Coppen and A. Walk). *Br. J. Psychiat.* Spec. Publ., No. 2.

Gittelman-Klein, R. and Klein, D. F. (1971). Controlled imipramine treatment of school phobia. *Arch. Gen. Psychiat.* **25**, 204–207.

Graham, P. J. (1973). *In* 'Bladder Control and Enuresis' (Eds I. Kolvin, R. Mac-Keith and S. R. Meadow). Clinics in Dev. Med., Nos. 48/49. SIMP, Heinemann, London.

Graham, P. J. (1974). Depression in pre-pubertal children. *Dev. Med. Child Neurol.* **16**, 340–349.

Graham, P. J. and Rutter, M. (1973). Psychiatric disorder in the young adolescent: a follow-up study. *Proc. Roy. Soc. Med.* **66**, 1226–1229.

Gruenberg, F. and Pond, D. A. (1957). Conduct disorders in epileptic children. *J. Neurol. Neurosurg. Psychiat.* **20**, 65–68.

Hampe, E., Noble, H., Miller, L. C. and Barrett, C. L. (1973). Phobic children one and two years post treatment. *J. Abnorm. Psychol.* **82**, 446–453.

Harrington, J. A. and Letemendia, F. J. (1958). Persistent psychiatric disorders after head injuries in children. *J. Ment. Sci.* **104**, 1205–1218.

Hauser, S. L., Delong, G. R. and Rosman, N. P. (1975). Pneumographic findings in the infantile autism syndrome: a correlation with temporal lobe disease. *Brain* **98**, 667–688.

Henderson, A. S., Krupinski, J. and Stoller, A. (1971). Epidemiological aspects of adolescent psychiatry. *In* 'Modern Perspectives in Adolescent Psychiatry' (Ed. J. G. Howells). Oliver and Boyd, Edinburgh.

Herbert, M. (1964). The concept and testing of brain damage in children: a review. *J. Child Psychol. Psychiat.* **5**, 197–216.

Hermelin, B. and O'Conner, N. (1970). 'Psychological Experiments with Autistic Children'. Pergamon, Oxford.

Hersov, L. A. (1960a) Persistent non-attendance at school. *J. Child Psychol. Psychiat.* **1**, 130–136.

Hersov, L. A. (1960b). Refusal to go to school. *J. Child Psychol. Psychiat.* **1**, 137–145.

Hersov, L. A. (1977). School refusal. *In* 'Child Psychiatry: Modern Approaches' (Eds M. Rutter and L. A. Hersov). Blackwell, Oxford.

Hill, O. W. (1972). Child bereavement and adult psychiatric disturbance. *J. Psychosom. Res.* **16**, 357–360.

Howlin, P. A., Marchant, R., Rutter, M., Berger, M., Hersov, L. and Yule, W. (1973). A home-based approach to the treatment of autistic children. *J. Autism Child. Schiz.* **3**, 308–336.

Jenkins, R. L. (1968). The varieties of children's behavioural problems and family dynamics. *Am. J. Psychiat.* **124**, 1440–1445.

Johnson, A. M., Falstein, E. I., Szurek, S. A. and Svendsen, M. (1941). School phobia. *Am. J. Orthopsychiat.* **11**, 702–711.

Kanner, L. (1943). Autistic disturbances of affective contact. *Nerv. Child* **2**, 217–250.

Kellerman, J. (1977). Anorexia nervosa, the efficacy of behaviour therapy. *J. Behav. Ther. Exp. Psychiat.* **8**, 387–390.

Kendell, R. E., Hall, D. J., Hailey, A. and Babigian, H. M. (1973). The epidemiology of anorexia nervosa. *Psychol. Med.* **3**, 200–203.

Kennedy, W. A. (1965). School phobia: rapid treatment of fifty cases. *J. Abnorm. Psychol.* **70**, 285–289.

Klein, M. (1932). 'The Psychoanalysis of Children'. Hogarth Press, London.

Knobloch, H. and Pasamanick, B. (1966). Prospective studies on the epidemiology of reproductive casualty: methods, findings and some complications. *Merrill-Palmer Q.* **12**, 27–43.

Kohut, H. (1972). Thoughts on narcissism and narcissistic rage. *Psychoanalyt. Study Child* **27**, 360–400.

Kolvin, I. (1971). Psychoses in childhood—a comparative study. *In* 'Infantile Autism: Concepts, Characteristics and Treatment' (Ed. M. Rutter). Churchill-Livingstone, London.

Kolvin, I., MacKeith, R. and Meadow, S. R. (Eds.) (1973). 'Bladder Control and Enuresis'. Clinics in Dev. Med., Nos. 48/49. SIMP/Heinemann, London.

Lapouse, R. and Monk, M. A. (1958). An epidemiological study of behaviour characteristics in children. *Am. J. Publ. Hlth* **48**, 1134–1144.

Leslie, S. A. (1974). Psychiatric disorder in the young adolescents of an industrial town. *Br. J. Psychiat.* **125**, 113–124.

Leventhal, R. and Sills, M. (1964). Self-image in school phobia. *Am. J. Orthopsychiat.* **34**, 685–695.

Lockyer, L. and Rutter, M. (1969). A five to fifteen year follow-up study of infantile psychosis. III: psychological aspects. *Br. J. Psychiat.* **115**, 865–882.

Lotter, V. (1966). Epidemiology of autistic conditions in young children. 1: prevalence. *Social Psychiat.* **1**, 124–137.

Lucas, A. R. and Pasley, F. C. (1969). Psychoactive drugs in the treatment of emotionally disturbed children: haloperidol and diazepam. *Compreh. Psychiat.* **10**, 376–386.

McAuley, R. and McAuley, P. (1977). 'Child Behaviour Problems: An Empirical Approach to Management'. Macmillan, London.

Macfarlane, J. W., Allen, L. and Honzik, M. P. (1954). A developmental study of the behavior problems of normal children between twenty one months and fourteen years. *In* 'University of California Publications in Child Development', Vol. 2. University of California Press, Berkeley.

Marchant, R., Howlin, P., Yule, W. and Rutter, M. (1974). Graded change in the treatment of the behaviour of autistic children. *J. Child Psychol. Psychiat.* **15**, 221–227.

Masterson, J. F. (1967). 'The Psychiatric Dilemma of Adolescence'. Churchill, London.

Mays, J. B. (1954). 'Growing Up in the City'. Liverpool University Press, Liverpool.

Miller, L. C., Barrett, C. L. and Hampe, E. (1974). Phobias of childhood in a prescientific era. *In* 'Child Personality and Psychopathology: Current Topics' (Ed. A. Davids), Vol. 1. Wiley, London.

Minde, K., Lewin, D., Weiss, G., Lavigueur, H., Douglas, V. and Sykes, E. (1971). The hyperactive child in elementary school: a 5-year controlled follow-up. *Except. Child* **38**, 215–221.

Moore, T. (1966). Difficulties of the ordinary child in adjusting to primary school. *J. Child Psychol. Psychiat.* **7**, 17–38.

Morgan, H. G. and Russell, G. F. M. (1975). Value of family background and clinical features as predictors of long-term outcome in anorexia nervosa: four-year follow-up study of 41 patients. *Psychol. Med.* **5**, 355–371.

Offer, D. (1969). 'The Psychological World of the Teenager'. Basic Books, London.

Offord, D. R. and Cross, L. A. (1969). Behavioral antecedents of adult schizophrenia. *Arch. Gen. Psychiat.* **21**, 267–283.

Ounsted, C. (1955). The hyperkinetic syndrome in epileptic children. *Lancet* **ii**, 303–311.

Patterson, G. R. (1971). 'Families: Applications of Social Learning to Family Life'. Research Press, Champaign, Illinois.

Pearce, J. (1974). Childhood depression. M. Phil. Thesis, University of London.

Pittman, F. S., Donald, L. G. and Deyoung, C. D. (1968). Work and school phobia: a family approach to treatment. *Am. J. Psychiat.* **124**, 1535–1541.

Pritchard, M. and Graham, P. (1966). An investigation of a group of patients who have attended both the child and adult departments of the same psychiatric hospital. *Br. J. Psychiat.* **112**, 603–612.

Reisman, J. M. (1973). 'Principles of Psychotherapy with Children'. Wiley, New York.

Richman, N., Stevenson, J. and Graham, P. (1975). Prevalence of behaviour problems in 3-year-old children: an epidemiological study in a London borough. *J. Child Psychol. Psychiat.* **16**, 277–287.

Robins, L. (1966). 'Deviant Children Grown Up'. Williams and Wilkins, Baltimore.

Russell, G. F. M. (1977). Editorial: the present status of anorexia nervosa. *Psychol. Med.* **7**, 363–367.

Rutter, M. L. (1965). Classification and categorisation in child psychiatry. *J. Child Psychol. Psychiat.* **6**, 71–83.

Rutter, M. L. (1966). 'Children of Sick Parents: An Environmental and Psychiatric Study'. Maudsley Monograph No. 16. Oxford University Press, Oxford.

Rutter, M. L. (1970). Autistic children: infancy to adulthood. *Semin. Psychiat.* **2**, 435–450.

Rutter, M. L. (1972). 'Maternal Deprivation Reassessed'. Penguin, Harmondsworth.

Rutter, M. L. (1974). The development of infantile autism. *Psychol. Med.* **4**, 147–163.

Rutter, M. L. (1977a). Brain damage syndromes in childhood: concepts and findings. *J. Child Psychol. Psychiat.* **18**, 1–21.

Rutter, M. L. (1977b). Classification. *In* 'Child Psychiatry: Modern Approaches' (Eds M. L. Rutter and L. Hersov). Blackwell, Oxford.

Rutter, M. L. and Bartak, L. (1973). Special education treatment of autistic children: a comparative study, II: follow-up findings and implications for services. *J. Child Psychol. Psychiat.* **14**, 241–270.

Rutter, M. L. and Yule, W. (1975). The concept of specific reading retardation. *J. Child Psychol. Psychiat.* **16**, 181–197.

Rutter, M. L., Lebovici, S., Eisenberg, L., Sneznevskij, A. V., Sadoun, R., Brooke, E. and Lin, T. Y. (1969). A tri-axial classification of mental disorders in childhood. *J. Child Psychol. Psychiat.* **10**, 41–61.

Rutter, M. L., Graham, P. J. and Yule, W. (1970a). 'A Neuropsychiatric Study in Childhood'. Clinics in Developmental Medicine, Nos. 35/36. SIMP, Heinemann, London.

Rutter, M. L., Tizard, J. and Whitmore, K. (Eds.) (1970b). 'Education, Health and Behaviour'. Longman, London.

Rutter, M. L., Shaffer, D. and Shepherd, M. (1975a). 'A Multiaxial Classification of Child Psychiatric Disorders'. WHO, Geneva.

Rutter, M. L., Yule, B., Quinton, D., Rowlands, O., Yule, W. and Berger, M. (1975b). Attainment and adjustment in two geographical areas: III some factors accounting for area differences. *Br. J. Psychiat.* **126**, 520–533.

Rutter, M. L., Graham, P., Chadwick, O. and Yule, W. (1976). Adolescent turmoil: fact or fiction? *J. Child Psychol. Psychiat.* **17**, 35–56.

Sandberg, S. T., Rutter, M. and Taylor, E. (1978). Hyperkinetic disorder in psychiatric clinic attenders. *Der. Med. Child Neurol.* **20**, 279–299.

Sandler, J., Dare, C. and Holder, A. (1973). 'The Patient and the Analyst'. Allen and Unwin, London.

Satterfield, J., Cantwell, D. and Satterfield, B. (1974). Pathophysiology of the hyperactive child syndrome. *Arch. Gen. Psychiat.* **31**, 839–844.

Schaffer, H. R. and Emerson, P. E. (1964). The development of social attachments in infancy. *Monogr. Soc. Res. Child Dev.* **29**, 1–77.

Schopler, E. and Reichler, R. J. (1971). Developmental therapy by parents with their own autistic child. *In* 'Infantile Autism: Concepts, Characteristics and Treatment' (Ed. M. Rutter). Churchill-Livingstone, London.

Seidel, U. P., Chadwick, O. and Rutter, M. (1975). Psychological disorders in crippled children: a comparative study of children with and without brain damage. *Dev. Med. Child Neurol.* **17**, 563–573.

Shaffer, D. (1973a). *In* 'Bladder Control and Enuresis' (Eds I. Kolvin, R. MacKeith and S. R. Meadow). Clinics in Dev. Med., Nos. 68/69. SIMP, Heinemann, London.

Shaffer, D. (1973b). Psychiatric aspects of brain injury in childhood: a review. *Dev. Med. Child Neurol.* **15**, 211–220.

Shaffer, D. (1974). Suicide in childhood and early adolescence. *J. Child Psychol. Psychiat.* **15**, 275–291.

Shaffer, D. (1977a). Enuresis. *In* 'Child Psychiatry: Modern Approaches' (Eds M. Rutter and L. Hersov). Blackwell, Oxford.

Shaffer, D. (1977b). Brain injury. *In* 'Child Psychiatry: Modern Approaches' (Eds M. Rutter and L. Hersov). Blackwell, Oxford.

Shaffer, D., Costello, A. J. and Hill, I. D. (1968). Control of enuresis with imipramine. *Archs Dis. Child.* **43**, 665–671.

Shaffer, D., McNamara, N. and Pincus, J. H. (1974). Controlled observations on patterns of activity, attention and impulsivity in brain damaged and psychiatrically disturbed boys. *Psychol. Med.* **4**, 4–18.

Shaffer, D., Chadwick, O. and Rutter, M. (1975). Psychiatric outcome of localised head injury in children. In 'Outcome of Severe Damage to the Central Nervous System' (Eds R. Porter and D. W. Fitzsimons). CIBA Foundation Symposium No. 34. Elsevier, Excerpta Medica, North-Holland, Amsterdam.

Shapiro, A. K., Shapiro, E., Wayne, H. and Clarkin, J. (1973). Organic factors in Gilles de la Tourette's Syndrome. Br. J. Psychiat. 122, 659–664.

Shepherd, M., Oppenheim, B. and Mitchell, S. (1971). 'Childhood Behaviour and Mental Health'. University of London Press, London.

Silverstone, J. T. and Russell, G. F. M. (1967). Gastric 'hunger' contractions in anorexia nervosa. Br. J. Psychiat. 113, 257–263.

Skynner, A. C. R. (1974). School phobia: a reappraisal. Br. J. Med. Psychol. 47, 1–16.

Slade, P. D. and Russell, G. F. M. (1973). Awareness of body dimensions in anorexia nervosa: cross-sectional and longitudinal studies. Psychol. Med. 3, 188–199.

Slade, R. and Welbourne, J. (1976). Anorexia nervosa: a fresh look. J. Mat. Child Health 1, 31–37.

Slater, E. (1965). Diagnosis of hysteria. Br. Med. J. 1, 1395–1399.

Smith, S. L. (1970). School refusal with anxiety: a review of sixty-three cases. Can. Psychiat. Ass. J. 15, 257–264.

Starfield, S. B. (1967) Functional bladder capacity in enuretic and non-enuretic children. J. Pediat. 70, 777–781.

Stengel, E. (1959). Classification of mental disorders. Bull. Wld Hlth Org. 21, 601–663.

Stores, G. (1975). Behavioural effects of anti-epileptic drugs. Dev. Med. Child Neurol. 17, 647–658.

Stott, D. H. and Wilson, D. M. (1977). The adult criminal as juvenile. Br. J. Crim. 17, 47–57.

Strauss, A. A. and Lehtinen, L. E. (1947). 'Psychopathology and Education of the Brain Injured Child'. Grune and Stratton, New York.

Thomas, A., Chess, S. and Birch, H. G. (1968). 'Temperament and Behavior Disorders in Children'. University Press, New York.

Tolstrup, K. (1975). The treatment of anorexia nervosa in childhood and adolescence. J. Child Psychol. Psychiat. 16, 75–78.

Tyrer, P. and Tyrer, S. (1974). School refusal, truancy and neurotic illness. Psychol. Med. 4, 416–421.

Waldrop, M., Pederson, F. A. and Bell, R. Q. (1968). Minor physical anomalies and behavior in pre-school children. Child Dev. 39, 391–400.

Weinberg, W. A., Rutman, J., Sullivan, L., Penick, E. C. and Dietz, S. G. (1973). Depression in children referred to an educational diagnostic centre: diagnosis and treatment. J. Pediat. 83, 1065–1072.

Wender, P. (1972). The minimal brain dysfunction syndrome in children. J. Nerv. Ment. Dis. 155, 55–71.

Werry, J. S., Weiss, G., Douglas, V. and Martin, J. (1966). Studies on the hyperactive child. III, the effect of chlorpromazine upon behavior and learning ability. J. Am. Acad. Child Psychiat. 5, 292–312.

Werry, J., Minde, K., Guzman, A., Weiss, G., Dogan, K. and Hoy, E. (1972). Studies on the hyperactive child. VII, neurological status compared with neurotic and normal children. Am. J. Orthopsychiat. 42, 441–450.

Wing, L. (1969). The handicaps of autistic children—a comparative study. J. Child Psychol. Psychiat. 10, 1–40.

Wing, L. (1970). The syndrome of early childhood autism. *Br. J. Hosp. Med.* **4**, 381–392.

Wolkind, S. N. (1974). The components of 'affectionless psychopathy' in institutionalized children. *J. Child Psychol. Psychiat.* **15**, 215–220.

Woodmansey, A. C. (1967). Emotion and the motions: an inquiry into the causes and prevention of functional disorders of defecation. *Br. J. Med. Psychol.* **40**, 207–223.

Yates, A. (1958). The application of learning theory to the treatment of tics. *J. Abnorm. Soc. Psychol.* **56**, 175–182.

Young, G. C. and Morgan, R. T. T. (1972). Overlearning in the conditioning treatment of enuresis. *Behav. Res. Ther.* **10**, 147–151.

Yule, W., Sacks, B. and Hersov, L. (1974). Successful flooding treatment of a noise phobia in an eleven-year-old. *J. Behav. Ther. Exp. Psychiat.* **5**, 209–211.

6 Mental retardation

Eric Taylor

The major goals for those dealing with mental subnormality are to prevent the conditions which cause it and to improve the lot of those who are afflicted by it. For many years it appeared that these aims were dishearteningly remote and perhaps even unattainable. In the early part of this century an extreme genetic theory held sway and pessimism was natural. Indeed, the spectre of degeneracy of the intellect of the nation haunted the planners and may well have helped to create the belief that services should be custodial and segregated. Theories, however, have changed. The causes of retardation are becoming clearer and one can be more optimistic about the possible impact of prevention. The President's Committee on Mental Retardation (1972) saw it as feasible to reduce the occurrence of mental retardation by half by the end of this century. Further, the development of methods of psychological treatment—and the focus on retardation as a special problem in learning—make the management of the subnormal a more exciting prospect. It has also become clearer that the dependence of many retarded people can be due to treatable complications, rather than to the mere fact of retardation.

Yet in spite of theoretical grounds for optimism, in practice the care given improves only painfully slowly. Recruitment into the medical speciality of mental handicap is very low in the UK but other disciplines have not yet taken over its function. Special education, nursing, clinical psychology and social work are all very short of trained staff.

Concepts of retardation

The idea of mental retardation has developed as an administrative (not a scientific) concept. We cannot specify all the qualities that are 'mental'.

General intellectual retardation is a necessary part of mental subnormality, but not a sufficient condition. The administrator requires categories of those whose subnormality makes them incapable of independent life or guarding themselves from exploitation (which defines 'severe subnormality' in the Mental Health Act of 1959), and of those whose subnormality requires special care or treatment (which is the essence of the definition of 'subnormality' in that Act). The criterion here is ultimately one of social competence. Now society needs such categories, because society has the duties of sheltering, protecting, caring and treating. But medical science is likely to be confused by them. For instance, it is clear that a proportion of patients in mental subnormality hospitals are of normal intelligence (Castell and Mittler, 1965; Mittler and Woodward, 1966), and that the same is true of some children in schools for the educationally subnormal. The question of what leads to social incompetence and psychiatric symptoms in the retarded becomes a very confused one if the incompetence and the symptoms are part of the definition of retardation.

Intellectual retardation is a more scientific concept. It is true that there is no one measure which will correlate perfectly with performance in every situation that demands cognitive skills. However, the IQ in competent hands can provide an objective and valid measure of current intellectual status (Clarke and Clarke, 1974a). Intelligence in this sense is continuously distributed in the population, and a category of intellectual retardation must have a rather arbitrarily established boundary. It is convenient to regard it as equivalent to an IQ of at least two standard deviations (s.d.) below the mean (i.e. less than 70 on a test constructed to have a mean of 100 and s.d. of 15); and consequently it includes some 2·5% of the population. The upper level of this range (IQ 50 to 70) will certainly contain some who are socially and educationally competent. Indeed, the large majority of the intellectually mildly retarded will never be identified as such. There are three overlapping groups: the educationally subnormal, the socially incompetent, and those of IQ less than 70. A useful administrative definition of the mentally retarded would be those individuals who combine a low IQ with either educational or social failure. By contrast, individuals with an IQ of less than 50 are usually 'severely mentally subnormal'. In this lower range the three criteria of social incompetence, educational backwardness and intellectual retardation are usually all present together.

Considerations of aetiology (below) also make it useful to distinguish between the group with IQs below 50 (roughly equivalent to the 'severely subnormal' and 'idiots and imbeciles' of other classifications) and that with IQs of 50–70 (equivalent to 'mildly subnormal' and 'feeble-minded'). The prognosis of the two groups is also different. The great majority of the mildly subnormal make a good social adjustment, becoming financially and personally independent. They do have a somewhat greater incidence of unemployment, breaches of the law, and marital instability than controls—but even this difference tends to disappear as they get older (Baller *et al.*, 1966). By contrast, only 10 to 20% of the severely subnormal become economically independent (Kushlik and Blunden, 1974). The fact that most of the mildly subnormal disappear in adult life from the sight of those giving care to the handicapped emphasizes that the condition is not 'incurable'. The IQ is not an unvarying property of a person, and it does not predict social adjustment very well.

Causes and prevalence

Intellectual retardation is sometimes the result of specific pathological processes (see Table I) which damage the developing brain. More commonly, however, no disease is responsible and the causes are to be found in the interplay of genetic and environmental factors, which are of the same kind as those operating in the normal population. Naturally these interacting factors will usually lead only to a mild impairment of intellectual function.

Specific pathological processes are much more likely to be found in the severely retarded. Nearly all cases of severe subnormality have gross cerebral pathology at post-mortem (Crome, 1960). With the increasing sophistication of diagnostic aids such as biochemical and cytogenetic analysis, it is possible to identify pathological causes in individuals who would previously have been recognized only as falling within the 'undifferentiated' group. The proportion of the severely retarded whose cause is known varies between studies. In Berg's (1963) well-studied series from the Fountains Hospital, one-third were of known cause; in a community survey reported by Corbett *et al.* (1975) 85% had a cause assigned.

Not even the higher figure should be taken to imply that we now understand the causes of severe subnormality. Even when a biological fault has been established, the aetiology and pathogenesis may remain obscure. How, for example, do chromosomal aberrations cause mental defect? We do not know. What is the cause of such abnormalities as the presence of an extra chromosome of the G group in Down's syndrome? Opinions differ. Certainly there is knowledge about associated factors such as the increase in incidence with increased maternal age (which Penrose (1972) shows to vary from less than 0·1% at a maternal age of less than 35 years to 2·5% at a maternal age of more than 45 years). Certainly there is knowledge about variations in the chromosomal constitution which can occur in Down's syndrome, such as that seen in the small minority of cases who have the normal number of chromosomes (46) in their cells but in whom a large part of a G chromosome has become translocated on to another chromosome (D or G). This knowledge is valuable, and enables useful genetic counselling to be given to older mothers and to mothers who are carriers of an abnormal translocated chromosome. But it is not yet a fundamental biological understanding of aetiology, and accordingly prevention is as yet confined to the early detection and abortion of affected foetuses.

The uncovering of an ever increasing number of pathological conditions has been of great importance; it is only on this foundation that rational schemes of prevention can be established. The details of these conditions are of high intrinsic interest and stimulate consideration of important biological issues (Penrose, 1972).

Table I   *Some pathological conditions causing mental retardation*

(A) *Harmful genes*
      (i)   autosomal dominant, e.g. tuberous sclerosis
     (ii)   autosomal recessive, e.g. phenylketonuria, galactosaemia
    (iii)   sex linked, e.g. Hunter's syndrome

(B) *Aberrant chromosomes*
      (i)   autosomal, e.g. Down's syndrome (tri-G or G-D translocation)
     (ii)   sex chromosomal, e.g. triple-X

(C) *Prenatal environmental causes*
      (i)   infection, e.g. rubella, syphilis
     (ii)   exposure to X-rays
    (iii)   rhesus incompatibility
    (iv)   maternal alcoholism
     (v)   maternal diseases complicating pregnancy, e.g. toxaemia, antepartum haemorrhage
    (vi)   some drugs, e.g. thiouracil
   (vii)   some poisons, e.g. mercury
  (viii)   malnutrition, e.g. cretinism when caused by deficiency of iodine

---

(D) *Birth injury*
      (i)   premature birth
     (ii)   mechanical injury during labour
    (iii)   hypoxia

(E) *Injury during childhood* (especially early infancy)
      (i)   status epilepticus; hypsarrhythmia
     (ii)   metabolic, e.g. hypoglycaemia, hyperbilirubinaemia
    (iii)   infective, e.g. encephalitis, meningitis
    (iv)   toxic, e.g. lead poisoning
     (v)   traumatic, e.g. head injury
    (vi)   gross malnutrition

This is not the place for a full discussion of medical details of these conditions. Some are mentioned in Table II. The student for postgraduate examinations will find succinct accounts in Heaton-Ward (1975) or Dutton (1975); and fuller details in Crome and Stern (1972). Stanbury *et al.* (1971) give a classic account of metabolic errors. An atlas of syndromes is presented by Gellis *et al.* (1971).

The numerical importance of these causes can be judged from a survey reported by Corbett *et al.* (1975) in which all the severely mentally retarded children in a geographically defined area of South London were identified and assessed. Down's syndrome was the commonest condition, accounting for 26% of the 140. All the inherited biochemical errors together accounted for only 4%. There was evidence for other inherited conditions or for associated congenital malformations in 19%. Infections were judged to account for 14% and perinatal injury for 18%. Only 15% were of unknown cause.

It must be stressed that these pathological conditions are frequent only in the severely retarded. The mildly retarded form a much larger group, and one which is more difficult precisely to define. Thus, Kushlik and Blunden (1974) find that by the age of 19 nearly all the severely retarded had been identified and notified to the old Mental Health Departments of local authorities; the prevalence in this age group 15 to 19 was 3·7 per 1000. By contrast, most of those with IQs of 50 to 70 are never identified as such; Kushlik (1961) found the highest prevalence rate (which was also in the 15–19 age group) to be 8·7 per 1000; but theoretical considerations indicate that approximately 20 per 1000 of the population should have IQs in this range. One therefore lacks studies of the mildly subnormal that are firmly based on representative populations. Conclusions about the interaction of genetic and environmental factors are largely based on studies of the normally intelligent.

It is clear that some mildly retarded people will be found to suffer from organic pathology of the kind outlined above. Some of these conditions (such as phenylketonuria) can result in mental states which vary from gross idiocy to levels within the range of normality. Others (such as the triple-X chromosome constitution) are more typically associated with mild than with severe retardation. It is likely that only a minority of mild cases suffer from these forms of pathology.

It is much less clear what factors are causative in the remainder. Nearly all workers in the area would accept that there is an interaction between genetic constitution and environment. But within this generalization there is room for acrid debate between those (such as Jensen, 1973, and Eysenck, 1971) who assert the primacy of genetic make-up and consider 80% of the variance in intellect to be genetic in origin; and those (such as Hunt, 1961) who consider intellectual level to be primarily a reflection of

Table II *Five syndromes causing retardation*

Condition	Prevalence	Aetiology	Clinical syndrome	Associated conditions	Risk of recurrence after one affected child	Other features
Down's syndrome	approx. 1 in 650 live births	*Trisomy-G*; associated with increased maternal age; maternal infective hepatitis (?) conception late in menstrual cycle (?) X-rays to mother (?) *Mosaicism* occurs; maternal mosaicism causes some cases *Translocation* form genetically conditioned	Oblique palpebral fissures, epicanthic folds, Brushfield spots on iris, short hands, wrist tri-radius displaced distally, curved little finger, single transverse palmar crease, small mouth, flat nose, high arched palate, lax joints hypotonia	Congenital heart disease. Intestinal abnormalities, e.g. duodenal atresia, Hirschsprung's disease, Leukemia Low blood serotonin, low serum calcium, increased gamma-globulin. Other chromosome anomalies	*Trisomy*; approx. 1 in 100 *Translocation*: carried by mother: approx. 1 in 10	Affected foetus detectable by amniocentesis and examination of cultured cells Epilepsy is uncommon
Phenyl-ketonuria	approx. 1 in 20,000 live births	Autosomal recessive gene causing lack of hepatic phenylalanine hydroxylase	Dilution of pigment (fair hair, blue eyes). Retardation of growth.	Epilepsy, Microcephaly, Eczema, Hyperactive behaviour	approx. 1 in 4	Treatable by diet excluding phenylalanine from infancy
Homo-cystinuria	approx. 1 in 100,000 live births	Autosomal recessive gene causing lack of cystathionine synthetase	Ectopia lentis Flushed cheeks, enlarged joints, Marfans-type skeletal abnormalities	Epilepsy, Thromboembolic episodes	approx. 1 in 4	Can cause late onset retardation. Sometimes treatable by pyridoxine/restriction of methionine
Tuberous sclerosis	approx. 1 in 100,000 live births	Autosomal dominant gene	Epilepsy Adenoma sebaceum white skin patches, shagreen skin, retinal phakomata, subungual fibromata.	Multiple tumours in heart, stomach, spleen, lungs. Autism.	If parent heterozygote, 1 in 2; If parents unaffected very low risk	
Rubella embryopathy	approx. 15% of offspring of mothers infected in first trimester	Viral infection of mother causing damage to foetus	Cataract, microphth-almia, deafness, microcephaly, con-genital heart disease; affected newborn sheds virus	Cerebral palsy, Autism	very low risk	Irregular epidemics; large-scale epidemic in 1964.

environmental circumstance. No attempt need be made here to give a numerical estimate of 'heritability' (the proportion of the variance in intellect accounted for genetically). Any such estimate is useful only for the precise group for whom it was derived. Where the environment for two people is very similar (as it usually is for twins reared together and for children in the same institutional home), then the difference between them is likely to be due largely to heredity. Where the heredity of two people is very similar (as it is for monozygotic twins) then the difference between them will be due largely to environment. In the same way heritability varies with the homogeneity of the group in which it is estimated; it is not a fixed property of intelligence.

There is firm evidence for an important genetic contribution to the determination of IQ. Erlenmeyer-Kimling and Jarvik (1963) summarize the results of more than 50 studies which correlate the IQs of individuals and their relatives, and show that the correlations increase as the genetic relationship becomes closer. The median correlation of IQ for parent and child is 0·50; for foster-parent and child it is low (0·20). The correlation for monozygotic twins reared together is quoted at 0·87; and it is still high (0·75) for monozygotic twins reared apart. For siblings reared together the figure is 0·49, for siblings reared apart 0·40, and for unrelated children reared together 0·23. Furthermore, unrelated children who live for long periods in the rather uniform environment of a residential institution nevertheless preserve a wide range of individual differences—and this, too, argues for a powerful effect of innate factors. These findings, however, do not argue for the absence of an environmental effect. An example is a well-known study by Skodak and Skeels (1949) which examined 100 children with a poor social background who had been adopted in infancy into superior homes. At the age of 13 there was a substantial correlation (0·44) between the IQs of the child and the biological mother, which points to the influence of genetic make-up on intellectual development. But there was also a substantial difference of more than 20 points between the mean IQ (117) of the 13-year-olds and that of their biological mothers. This kind of finding points to the theoretical view that environment, too, is a potent influence on intellectual development and to the practical suggestion that changing a child's environment can increase his IQ. A study by Skeels (1966) supports these views. This study followed 13 children (average age 19 months) from an under-stimulating orphanage who were placed in a state school for the mentally deficient, where they were the only young children and therefore received much attention. They were compared with 12 children remaining in the orphanage. Those in the state school increased their IQ from a mean of 64 to a mean of 92; those remaining in the orphanage declined in IQ from a mean of 87 to a mean of 60. All but two of the experimental group were adopted;

the controls were not. Follow-up 20 years later showed very marked differences between the groups in education and in occupation; the experimental group—whose whole childhood had been changed—were functioning at a much higher level.

This kind of institution represents a severely impoverished environment. It seems probable that less extreme variations, as occur between the different social classes, can also be involved in causing mental handicap. It has long been known that in industrial societies parents of severely retarded individuals are distributed evenly among all the social classes; whilst by contrast the parents of the mildly retarded are predominantly from the lower social classes. Indeed, mildly retarded subjects who are otherwise clinically normal (i.e. who do not suffer from one of the pathological conditions considered above, and do not have neurological or sensory abnormalities) are almost always from lower working class families (Birch *et al.*, 1970). It is hard to account for the strength of this association without invoking environmental causes.

These environmental causes might be psychological or physical. There is an increased frequency among the mentally retarded of large families, poor housing, overcrowding and disrupted schooling (Birch *et al.*, 1970), arguing that psychological and social aspects are important; but the role of physical factors is not agreed. For instance, Knobloch and Pasamanick (1962) argue that the mildly subnormal may have 'minimal brain damage' due to perinatal injury even in the absence of neurological signs. This could account for social class differences since the lowest classes get less antenatal care, more obstetric complications, and more children of low birth weight. However, McDonald (1964) reviews the question of low birth weight and concludes that it is less important as a cause than low social class. Gottfried (1973) finds at most a small effect of neonatal asphyxia on later IQ. Exposure to lead is another feature of the physical environment that is sometimes said to be a major cause of mild mental retardation. It is generally accepted that overt lead poisoning is a rare event, but that it can cause an encephalopathy resulting in mental retardation. There is much more controversy about whether intellect and behaviour can be altered by subclinical intoxication with lead. Most studies (Editorial, 1977) are compatible with the view that minor elevations of blood lead have, at worst, only slight effects on the IQ.

It is still difficult to disentangle these various factors which tend to occur together in the poor. It seems that mild intellectual retardation in otherwise normal individuals is often due to the psychological environment of a lower working class sub-culture with low aspirations. This retardation usually presents when people cannot meet the demands of the educational system. Psychologically harmful aspects of the environment are difficult to define with precision. Lack of stimulation at home and unsuitable education in school are commonly blamed; but what sort of stimulation is necessary for full development? One attempt to be more precise is the notion that the kind of language used at home conditions intellectual development. Luria (1961) has been a strong exponent of the view that speech is intimately related to thinking and determines the development of abstract reasoning and of specificity in all aspects of behaviour. Middle class language may be more elaborate than working class (Bernstein, 1960); lower class mothers may talk to their children less and with less complexity and tend less to explain the need for rules (Hess and Shipman, 1965). Even if language differences are just a part of cognitive differences, it is by the testing of such hypotheses that one can get the information to plan a programme of intervention.

Psychological function and brain structure are of course interdependent. Wiesel and Hubel (1965) have shown that deprivation of vision during a critical period in kittens leads to a loss of neurones in the optic radiation and occipital cortex.

Nature of the primary handicaps

The intellectually retarded have (by definition) serious problems in learning, in the use of concepts and in problem-solving. If these difficulties were due to impairment of a specific psychological function, they would become more comprehensible. Remediation could become more rational and strategies of education would follow. The methods of experimental psychology have been used very extensively to examine the intellectually retarded and to compare them with normal people matched for chronological age or for mental age. No specific disability has reliably been found; the overall picture is one of general impairment of intellectual abilities; and of course this fits with the usual pathological picture of diffuse and widespread brain damage among the severely subnormal.

Short-term memory appears to be inferior in the intellectually retarded, the acquisition of new material being impaired (Scott and Scott, 1968). On the other hand, long-term retention of material—once it has been learned—seems to be as good as in normals (Haywood and Heal, 1968). Zeaman and House (1963) have analysed discrimination learning in the retarded: the major impairment is in attention to the relevant dimension of experience; once the process of learning starts it may proceed as effectively as in normals. Operant conditioning takes place even in the profoundly subnormal, and the possibility of using this to inculcate skills of self-care, communication, social interaction and occupation has repeatedly been demonstrated. There is impairment of verbal ability, of ability to use other symbols, and of forming abstract concepts.

The coding of sensory input is a basic psychological process whose impairment in the intellectually subnormal is emphasized by O'Connor and Hermelin (1974). Several measures of the EEG are related to IQ levels (Ellingson, 1972). Quantitative analysis of the reaction of the EEG to stimuli also suggests an impaired responsiveness in the intellectually retarded. Callaway (1973) reviews the associations between IQ and the averaged response evoked by stimuli and concludes that lower IQ entails a slower and more variable response. This may reflect an impairment of attention or of the processing of stimuli.

In general, the differences between the subnormal and the normal are probably of the same kind as the differences between normals and the intellectually gifted (Clarke and Clarke, 1974b). This, if confirmed, argues that the subnormal are not a race apart. Their difficulties are better conceptualized as a 'retardation' of development than as a pathological 'defect'.

Some of the subnormal may show specific intellectual or perceptual defects superimposed on a background of more general handicap. It is important to detect these in the individual case. Comparison of the organically damaged with subnormal people in whom no organic damage is demonstrated suggests that they are similar in their patterns of psychological performance (Zeaman, 1965).

Secondary handicaps

It is common for the intellectually retarded to display other handicaps. Indeed, it is often these complicating features which make the difference between success and failure in reaching independence or in fulfilling potential. Immobility, severe incontinence, severe behaviour disorder and uncontrolled epilepsy are powerful causes of incapacity, and are all more common in the severely retarded. Kushlik and Cox (1968) measured the range of handicaps on a large scale in Wessex. As a population of the retarded ages, the amount of incapacity falls (and by age 15–19 71% of the severely mentally subnormal were ambulant, continent and free of severe behaviour disorder); yet the proportion in residential care rises.

1 Psychiatric disorder

This deserves special consideration by the student of psychiatry, but we lack the information on which to base a sound understanding of psychiatric problems in the intellectually retarded. Certainly patients in subnormality hospitals present a high rate of disordered behaviour, but some of this may be caused by the institutional environment, and some may be over-represented as it has been the precipitating cause of hospital admission. However, several lines of evidence suggest that the intellectually retarded have a higher prevalence of psychiatric illness as well as of disordered behaviour.

Schizophrenia

The diagnosis may be difficult, and the clinical picture is altered by the presence of retardation. In particular there is a marked poverty of thought. Childish and silly behaviour is typical, but it needs distinguishing from the social immaturity that is an expected part of retardation; and this may lead to over-diagnosis of schizophrenia. Again, over-diagnosis may result from not appreciating the frequency in childhood (and accordingly in the retarded) of archaic patterns of thought and of blurring of the distinction between fantasy and reality. Massive hallucinations of a rather primitive and monotonous character are also typical. The impoverished presentation has been dignified by the term 'Pfropfschizophrenie' but it seems clear that this is not a separate entity. Uncertainty about the diagnosis may also result from prominent motor symptoms. Isolated stereotypies and mannerisms are not uncommon in the retarded and do not run the course of fluctuating deterioration that would be expected if they were regarded as catatonic. Hallgren and Sjögren (1959) studied a large Swedish rural population and found that schizophrenics had a high prevalence of 'low-grade mental deficiency'—around 10%.

Manic-depressive psychosis

Manic-depressive psychosis is usually regarded as being less common in the intellectually retarded, and this may well be so. Nevertheless it does occur and it is important to recognize and treat it. Increases in agitation or hyperkinesis, increased withdrawal and obsessional behaviour may all be the presentation rather than overt distress.

Neurotic symptoms

Neurotic symptoms and hysterical conversion symptoms are more common in the retarded, at any rate in the mildly affected (Penrose, 1972). The retarded are likely to react more severely than normals to minor changes in their environment. Improving environmental circumstance may be much more helpful than prescribing psychotropic drugs.

Childhood disorders

Childhood disorders have been carefully examined in an epidemiological study of children in the Isle of Wight (Rutter *et al.*, 1970b). Eight to

162   E. Taylor

ten-year-old children with intellectual retardation were identified and compared with a control group of the same chronological age but of normal IQ. Psychiatric disability was much more common in the retarded, being diagnosed in more than a fifth. It is present in an even higher proportion of the severely retarded—40 to 50%. All epidemiological surveys agree that deviant behaviour is more common in the lower range of IQ. The association, though strong, is not specific. There is no one pattern of abnormal behaviour that is characteristic of all the retarded. Intellectually subnormal children suffer a higher incidence of antisocial conduct problems, neuroses and emotional disorders, and these common problems account for the bulk of psychiatric disorder in the retarded, as in the normal. Indeed, for the mildly subnormal, these problems occur in very much the same proportions as in the normal. However, some conditions which are rare in the general population are disproportionately frequent in the severely retarded. Autism and hyperkinetic syndrome are major diagnoses among the severely subnormal; and individual items of behaviour such as stereotyped movements, pica and self-mutilation are relatively more important.

Pathogenesis of psychiatric disorders

Rather little evidence has been gathered on the reasons for this high rate of psychiatric disorder; it is reviewed by Rutter (1971) for the disorders of childhood. Some possible reasons need to be considered because of their implications for a programme of prevention and management.

Firstly, psychiatric disorder might be genetically linked to intellectual retardation. However, it seems unlikely that this is in fact so. Even for an illness such as schizophrenia whose genetic basis has often been examined, there are no convincing grounds for the view that there is a high incidence of retardation in the families of schizophrenics. Hallgren and Sjögren (1959), for example, found that the siblings of schizophrenics had only the same incidence of mental deficiency as the rest of the population; and that the siblings of the defective had no raised incidence of schizophrenia. Kallman et al.'s (1941) twin study showed no association between schizophrenia and mental defect.

Secondly, psychiatric disorder might cause intellectual retardation. This cannot usually be the case in children, for longitudinal studies such as that of Douglas et al. (1968) indicate that a low IQ precedes overt psychiatric disturbance. Nevertheless, schizophrenia in adults can lower scores on IQ tests (Payne, 1973).

Next, brain damage may cause both a psychiatric problem and subnormality. This seems to be a real and important cause, particularly for those with severe subnormality. At any level of intelligence neuro-epileptic conditions can cause abnormality; they give rise to a five-fold increase in the psychiatric disorders of childhood over normal children, and a three-fold increase over children with chronic physical illness not involving the brain (Rutter *et al.*, 1970a). Psychological symptoms were more frequent in children with brain damage than with other chronic conditions producing visible and restricting physical handicap (Seidel *et al.*, 1975). Further, the site and the nature of cerebral pathology can influence the kind of symptoms produced and the rate of symptoms (Davison and Bagley, 1969). For example, the hyperkinetic syndrome is more likely to be seen when epilepsy is also present; and seems to be associated particularly with temporal lobe epilepsy (Ounsted, 1955). People with Down's syndrome are by no means free of psychiatric problems, but they do have lower rates of aggressive hyperactive and antisocial behaviour than other retardates (Moore *et al.*, 1968). Phenyl-ketonurics, by contrast, have been shown by Johnson (1969) to be more aggressive and more destructive than their fellows in the same institu-tion. In older phenylketonurics, with irreversible brain damage, a low phenylalanine diet may still produce an improvement in their behaviour problems (Bruhl *et al.*, 1964). The Lesch-Nyhan syndrome (which is a recessively inherited error of uric acid metabolism) is specifically associ-ated with a kind of self-mutilation involving chewing of the lips; this behaviour can be reduced by physical treatment with L-/5-hydroxy-tryptophan (Mizumo and Yugari, 1974). These findings all indicate the capacity of brain injury to determine behaviour.

Brain injury is not the whole story. The intellectually retarded who have no evidence of neurological damage still have a high incidence of psychiatric symptoms. A fourth factor that could be important, therefore, is that psychiatric disorder may be a consequence of other psychological abnormalities which are associated with intellectual retardation. A deviant temperament may be associated with retardation and may con-tribute to later behaviour disorder (Rutter *et al.*, 1964). Impairment of attention may start adverse interaction between a retarded child and his parents. The failure to acquire social skills might also impair personal relationships and so predispose to mental ill health. Educational failure (consequent upon retardation itself, upon language delay or upon the above associated features) can have profound effects on the individual's view of himself and on his reception by peers and teachers: repeated failure may be compensated for by delinquency.

Psychiatric disorder may also be a consequence of the reaction of others to a handicapped individual. Some possible reasons for adverse reactions have been touched on above. However, the arrival of a retarded child can of itself have profound consequences upon his family. Excessive protectiveness is sometimes encountered clinically. This may be rooted in compassion, but can represent an over-reaction to natural feelings of guilt and inadequacy. Overt rejection may be communicated to a child who is regarded as abnormal or frightening. Inappropriate expectations of the child—whether they are too high for him to meet or suffocatingly low—can engender emotional problems. In spite of these possibilities, one must not forget that most families cope well.

Factors such as parental ill health, marital discord and inadequate discipline are associated with disordered behaviour in children of normal intelligence, and will have the same effect on retarded children. However, they are not necessarily more common in the families of the retarded than in other families. It is true, as already noted, that poverty and large families are frequently encountered among the mildly retarded; but these are not the chief factors which lead to disturbed behaviour.

A further potential cause of emotional disturbance is the retarded individual's distorted view of himself. The results of failure have already been stressed. Edgerton (1967) has graphically described how an individual's life may be dominated by the effort to escape the stigma of deficiency and to 'pass as normal'. This urge may have stemmed from the fact that all his subjects had spent years in a State institution.

Finally, psychiatric disorder may be a consequence of the care given. The depriving environment of the bad institution has been referred to; when present it may be the dominant fact in the development of symptoms. Anticonvulsant, hypnotic and psychotropic drugs may all worsen or create behaviour problems.

In summary, brain dysfunction—or the mere presence of intellectual retardation—interacts with other psychological abnormalities and the reactions of other people to cause a high rate of most psychiatric disorders. The task of disentangling these factors is a considerable challenge to both clinician and researcher. It is likely that some of the causes are preventable.

2 Epilepsy

Fits are common among the mentally retarded. In the survey reported by Corbett *et al*. (1975), 19% of children with an IQ under 50 or with a specific syndrome of retardation had suffered seizures during the previous year. A figure of around 25% is often given for the prevalence of epilepsy in institutionalized adult subnormals (Tredgold and Soddy, 1970).

Usually the fits and the retardation are both consequences of damage to the brain. Perinatal and neonatal injury is especially important, and some inborn errors of metabolism (e.g. pyridoxine dependence, phenyl-ketonuria, galactosaemia) are associated with epilepsy.

Sometimes epileptic convulsions are the direct cause of the mental retardation. Hypoxia during prolonged and repeated convulsions (as in status epilepticus) may cause damage to the developing brain. Infantile spasms may be associated with the EEG changes of 'hypsarrhythmia': this pattern is very often followed by gross developmental delay. Sometimes this is because of an underlying cause such as tuberous sclerosis; but whatever the cause the prognosis for intellectual development is grave. In the 'Lennox syndrome' progressive mental deterioration is associated with myoclonic or akinetic epilepsy.

Both epilepsy and retardation are common conditions and sometimes their association will be due to chance. Whatever the relationship, the presence of epilepsy can profoundly alter the individual's life. Frequent fits can disrupt the ability to concentrate and to learn; and sometimes these fits will produce little motor change and so will go undetected by teacher or parent. Episodic behaviour disturbance occasionally proves to be a post-ictal automatism. The supervision and protection needed by the uncontrolled epileptic may limit his capacity for independent life. Epilepsy powerfully evokes fear and prejudice in other people.

The treatment of epilepsy follows the same principles as in the intellectually normal. Particular care is necessary in the monitoring of anticonvulsant drug therapy. Behavioural and cognitive side-effects are not rare, and poisonously high blood levels of drugs may be reached without the warning of the neurological signs (such as nystagmus and ataxia) which are usual in the non-retarded (Reynolds and Travers, 1974).

Services for the retarded

In an ideal service there will be ready access to assessment, education, appropriate residential placement, guidance for the family, and treatment. As yet we are very far from achieving this, and many of the mentally retarded are managed by their parents with no professional help (Carr, 1975; Corbett and Wing, 1972). Many different professions are inevitably involved; they need to work as a team and to be adequately coordinated.

Assessment

The *medical causes* of retardation should always be sought, even though assessment has only begun when a diagnosis is made. The detailed

Table III   *Some psychological measures of development*

Test	Age range	Examiner	Features
IQ Tests			
Wechsler Intelligence Scale for Children (WISC)	6½ to 15 yrs.	Trained psychologist	Profile of abilities from subtests of verbal and non-verbal items. Un-suitable for those with mental age < 6 yrs; pre-school scale (WIPPSI) available for 4 to 6½ yrs.
Stanford Binet Intelligence Scale	2½ to 18 yrs.	Trained psychologist	Tests weight verbal ability highly, which may increase cultural bias.
Merril-Palmer	1½ to 6 yrs.	Trained psychologist	Performance and picture tests; useful for lower range of mental ages than WISC.
Developmental Assessments			
Denver Development Scale	Infancy to 6 yrs.	No special training required	Separate assessment of gross and fine motor, language and social development with simple tests. Least useful for youngest children.
Griffiths Mental Development Scale	Infancy to 8 yrs.	Psychologist or doctor after formal training course	Probably more accurate than Denver. Tests of locomotor, social, language, eye-hand, performance and practical reasoning abilities with standardized equipment.
Social Development			
Vineland Social Maturity Scale	Infancy to maturity	Usually psychologist	Wide range of skills tested; items can be passed by report of informant as well as by examination, therefore useful for uncooperative children. Social age correlates with mental age.
Gunzburg Progress Assessment Charts	Infancy to maturity	Personnel involved in care of the individual; no special training needed	Not standardized; clear visual display of abilities in self-help, communication, socialization and occupation. Useful for following progress and as a profile.

history, family history, general examination, and detailed neurological examination will be supplemented with as full a pathological screen as is in the patient's interests. Some of the more fruitful pathological tests are: full blood count and film; blood and urine aminoacid chromatography; serum calcium, blood lead, acid/base studies, fasting blood sugar; thyroid function tests; serological tests for syphilis; urinalysis; skull X-ray, electroencephalography; and perhaps chromosomal analysis.

Developmental assessment is now widely practised as a screening test, usually carried out clinically by a trained examiner. The aim is to focus attention early on children in need of help. In the assessment of suspected retardation, however, reproducible and standardized tests are required. The IQ, properly measured, is the best index of general intellectual development. But it is an unreliable guide in the earliest years of life. Moreover, standardization has usually been carried out on populations of normal children, and so accuracy is reduced at the extremes of the distribution. A single, general test is usually not enough; a large number of tests of specific functions is available. A few tests are briefly described in Table III.

The weaknesses and strengths of a retarded person need to be comprehensively assessed. This is best done by a multidisciplinary team who discuss their findings together. The specialized teacher, psychiatrist, psychologist, social worker, paediatrician, physiotherapist, occupational therapist, nurse, and speech therapist all have a place in such a team. Some of these roles overlap, fortunately, and it will be a lucky team that can assemble all these members. Even then, they will need to call on a large number of specialized disciplines, including paediatric neurologist, orthopaedic surgeon, audiologist, geneticist and dentist.

Testing sensory capacity is important: minor impairments of hearing and vision can have a disproportionate effect. Objective measures, such as evoked response audiometry, will sometimes be necessary. Full assessment will include judgements about family abilities and interactions and the social situation. Complicating factors (see above) and physical ill health have to be considered.

There needs to be good liaison between those assessing and those treating: communication must be two-way, or assessment will be aridly theoretical and management will be ignorant. Plans for management need to be flexible; regular reassessment should be the rule. For most families the health visitor and the general practitioner will be the agents most closely involved.

Education

The distinction between education and treatment is artificial: most treatment aims to assist the development of new skills, and all good treatment takes account of the whole individual's development. Since 1971 the responsibility for the education of all children in the UK has been laid on the local education authorities. There are special schools for the 'educationally subnormal'; provision of schools for the 'severely subnormal' is increasing. It remains a matter for debate whether the good that is done by increased acceptance in a special school is outweighed by the segregation and labelling. The most severely handicapped children—often those with major physical handicap as well—are commonly placed in a 'Special Care Class' within a school for the severely subnormal.

The methods, and indeed the goals, of special education are also matters under debate. Usually there is emphasis on structure in the classroom and on cultivating self-expression. Many skills (such as those of social and locomotor development) which those of normal intellect can acquire informally require specific inculcation in the handicapped. Increasingly people are using the powerful techniques of behaviour modification (see Gardner, 1971 and Chapter 21). These methods can be taught to teachers and to parents (Gardner, 1972).

On leaving school many will transfer to an adult training centre. Education needs to be prolonged beyond the age of 16, and the teaching of social skills and leisure activities ought to be taken as seriously as vocational training. Employment in sheltered workshops and, for some, in the community can follow—but the outlook for the severely retarded remains gloomy. The provision of day educational facilities for adults falls greatly short of the need (Department of Health and Social Services, 1971). The size of day centres will be limited by their accessibility. Tizard (1974) sets out estimates for the facilities required for a total urban population of 100,000 and considers that about 140 places in sheltered workshops will be necessary.

Residential placement

For the mentally retarded, as for anyone else, it is best to grow up in a family. Most do so. With increasing age a place outside the natural family may become increasingly necessary, particularly for the most severely handicapped. Foster homes can seldom be found, and ordinary children's homes are usually reluctant to admit a retarded child.

In the past hospitals provided almost the only special care. Large hospitals, often isolated, were treated as dumping grounds. Financial neglect, under-staffing, overcrowding of patients, and the habit of institutional patterns of care conspired to create an antitherapeutic environment, and ultimately a series of scandals. Since the Mental Health Act of 1959, it has been official policy that purely residential provision for the handicapped should be made in the local community and not the hospitals. Unfortunately, the local authorities have not provided anything like enough homes and hostels. The Department of Health and Social Security's own document on 'Better Services for the Mentally Handicapped' (DHSS, 1971) estimated a need for 70 such places for a total population of 100,000. The actual figure provided was more like 12/100,000. It seems that—at least for this generation—many will remain in hospital whose need is only for a supervised place to live. From 1959 to 1973 the number of NHS hospital beds for the mentally subnormal actually rose.

It is not easy to predict the requirement for residential places. The prevalence alone of subnormality is not an adequate guide. Where good community services are available to support families, the demand for residential places may fall. On the other hand, a family reluctant to see a handicapped member in a remote and unattractive institution may press for a place in an improved service offering small local units. Kushlik and Blunden (1974) estimate the needs on the basis of epidemiological surveys, such as that in Wessex described by Kushlik and Cox (1968). In a population of 100,000 they expect about 100 severely subnormal children younger than 16 years. Of these, 69 will be at home, 19 in hospital, and 12 will need residential care in the community. In the same population they expect 375 adult retardates, 180 of them employable. Of the remaining 195, 55 will be at home, 65 in hospital and 75 in residential hostels.

It follows from the consideration of social causes of handicap that residential homes (whether in large hospitals, small community hospitals, or local authority hostels) should aim at small, family-type units that can give stimulation, affection and stability. A unit such as this was compared by Tizard (1964) with a large, poorly staffed hospital: the success of the smaller and better unit was reflected in a rise of the IQ of its residents, whilst the IQ of those in hospital for the same period fell. Tizard (1974) finds that the reasons for the superiority of some units were not their small size alone, nor their staffing ratios. Their social organization and their staff training were the key features. The hostel units were child-oriented, with sharing of responsibility and with staff interacting with children a lot; the hospital units were institution-oriented and hierarchical.

Making residential places available for short periods of a few days or weeks may give the rest and support to parents that will enable them to continue with their burden of care. A period of time spent in a supervised hostel after leaving school may well help the less severely handicapped adolescent to increased independence at home or in lodgings. The value of a family-type unit for adolescents has been described by Baranyay (1971).

One may hope that hospital care will be reserved for the most severely handicapped, who present a medical and nursing challenge. Special units increasingly focus on problems such as psychosis, epilepsy, sensory handicap and rehabilitation.

Guidance for parents

From the initial discovery of retardation, parents have a pressing need for factual information and for the reassurance of knowing that the condition is understood and manageable. It is kind for an emphasis to be laid on what they can do to help development by responsive play, by talking and by training. The view that 'nothing can be done' is sometimes reinforced by medical advice and can make life more difficult. Where inherited conditions are involved, genetic counselling should be available. As the child grows, the increasing burden of care will need practical help. Advice on managing problems of behaviour is one kind of help. The organization of babysitters and short-term admissions to care will serve not only as a relief but as a prelude to the natural separation of the handicapped adult from his ageing parent. The social worker may arrange for the incontinence laundry services, the constant attendance allowance, the mobility allowance, the provision of apparatus and aids and for grants from charities.

Some parents will be helped by listening and counselling—for example, to work through a process of mourning for the ideal child they have lost. Another profitable area for counselling is in helping some parents to a suitable acceptance of their child's developmental level. Some parents become isolated as they encounter the prejudice which our society shows to its handicapped members. Contact with other parents of the retarded can be very helpful.

Treatment

(i) Medical

Specific medical remedies for a causative condition are rare: but where they exist, as in phenylketonuria and cretinism, treatment needs to be prompt and of high quality. Treatment of associated physical illness can improve the quality of life.

It seems likely that the future will bring the possibility of the direct replacement of missing enzymes. Exogenous enzymes must, of course, be protected from the immune systems of the body. One possibility is the transplantation of bone marrow or liver (Groth, 1972). In theory, endogenous enzyme synthesis could be stimulated by 'genetic engineering'. Merril *et al.* (1971) infected a culture of fibroblasts from a galactosaemic patient with a bacteriophage that contained the gene for the missing Galactose-1-phosphate uridyl transferase; they found that the culture acquired the ability to make this transferase.

(ii) *Psychiatric*

Even when psychiatric disorder has a biological cause, it does not follow that *organic treatment* will be the most effective. It has been argued that the organically damaged are often highly susceptible to environmental change, and manipulation of that environment may be much more effective than any drug. Sprague and Werry (1971) have thoroughly reviewed psychopharmacological studies. They conclude that there are very few methodologically sound trials, and fewer still which show a positive effect of drugs; that we know practically nothing about the effects of drugs on development; and that in spite of this the prescription of psychotropic drugs for retarded people in hospital is very widespread, often using high doses of phenothiazines for long periods. Certainly these drugs have their uses: phenothiazines can control agitated, aggressive and destructive behaviour, stimulants sometimes benefit the hyperkinetic, the tricyclic antidepressants help the depressed, and the anti-androgen cyproterone acetate is used to reduce sex drive in those misbehaving sexually. But all these treatments should be given subject to careful review and in the spirit of a clinical trial. *Psychotherapy* (see Chapter 22) has also lacked adequate evaluations. Some evidence for an effect of group therapy has been presented by Mehlman (1953) and Zisfein and Rosen (1973). It must, of course, be pitched at a level appropriate to the individual's mental age; verbal interventions are of little use for the very severely handicapped. The methods of *behaviour modification* (Gardner, 1971) have become major tools. They can be used for the very young and the very handicapped. A great deal has now been published on techniques suitable for individual problems. They do not depend on formal psychiatric diagnosis but are suggested by a detailed functional analysis of the individual's behaviour.

Successful behaviour therapy concentrates on modifying clearly specified, recordable behaviours. Another important principle is that a

desired behaviour should be followed very rapidly by a reward. A programme suggested by Azrin and Foxx (1971) for toilet training involves
instant rewards for using the toilet and also for being dry at regular
checks. An ideal reward can be given swiftly and repeatedly—praise and
affection are often used. Access to toys and to tokens for privileges suit
many people. Sometimes tit-bits of food are the only effective reinforcers.

New behaviours can be instilled by instruction, but often it is more
helpful for the therapist to model the behaviour or to prompt the patient
physically through it. As learning proceeds, the prompts can be gradually
faded out. Complex skills such as dressing and playing games can be
taught in this way, by analysing the activity into small, separate pieces of
behaviour which can then be learned separately (usually starting with the
last link in the chain).

Teaching a person to be constructively occupied and to communicate is
usually the best way of diminishing undesirable behaviour such as
aggression or stereotypies. Sometimes, however, it is necessary to intervene to reduce the frequency of some activity: repetitive self-injury is an
extreme example. Several techniques are available; the choice will
depend on what factors maintain the self-damage. For example, it may be
rewarded by the attention and concern it evokes; and in this case it may be
extinguished by a studied ignoring of the behaviour. Failing this, a brief
period of 'time out' from positive reinforcement may be effective, e.g. by
placing a patient for three minutes in a featureless room when he starts to
injure himself (with protection against injury). Periods of time when the
behaviour is not produced can be rewarded, as above. Mild punishment—such as loss of tokens—may be made to follow directly on
attempts at self-injury. As a last resort in life-threatening and very serious
cases, it may be justifiable to use a painful punishment such as electric
shock.

Prevention

New possibilities of preventing handicap have appeared with our
improved understanding of causes.

Preconceptual causes are attacked in several ways. Where a genetic condition is known to be present in a family (as after the birth of an affected
child) then genetic advice may lead to carriers deciding against conceiving
future children.

It may also be possible to detect an affected foetus before birth. The
most important method is by amniocentesis, with subsequent abortion of
an affected foetus. Foetal cells can be examined for chromosome composi-

tion (and, given time, for enzyme assay in cultured cells). The cell-free liquor amnii is available for biochemical analysis. The commonest analyses done are for the presence of the extra chromosome of Down's syndrome and for the presence of alpha-foetoprotein in open neural tube defects. Amniocentesis is usually offered to women with an affected child, a positive family history, or who are over the age of 35. The procedure carries a small but definite risk. The risks of unplanned abortion, placental injury and uterine haemorrhage may well be unacceptable in a long-awaited or precious pregnancy; uterine infection, injury to the foetus, and isoimmunization of the mother must also be reckoned with. X-ray examination, ultrasound, and foetoscopy may also show foetal abnormality.

A few genetic causes (e.g. phenylketonuria and galactosaemia) if detected very early in life, can be managed by excluding specific metabolites from the diet and so preventing damage to the brain. The screening of blood samples from all neonates for phenylketonuria is now routine in developed countries; tests for histidinaemia, homocystinuria, hyperprolinaemia, galactosaemia, maple syrup urine disease and some other conditions are commonly done on the same blood sample.

Prenatal environmental causes. Kernicterus due to rhesus incompatibility should be in part preventable. This can be done, firstly, by preventing Rhesus negative mothers from being sensitized by Rhesus positive foetal blood in childbirth by giving anti-D antibody (Clarke, 1967); and secondly by detecting affected foetuses with amniocentesis and treating them where necessary (with exchange transfusion).

Infections during pregnancy have become more controllable. Congenital syphilis is now rare; the treatment of maternal syphilis with penicillin remains effective. Immunization against rubella gives long-lasting resistance to the disease, and is offered routinely to schoolgirls of 11–14 years. (Pregnant women should not be immunized.) Maternal infection with toxoplasma can be detected by repeated serological testing: in Paris 47 of 15,000 pregnant women were found to convert from seronegative to seropositive: treatment of these women lowers the incidence of infected children but can clearly make little impact on the total number of mentally retarded (Desmonts et al., 1965). However, the improvement of antenatal services in general can be expected to have some effect; especially if services can successfully be delivered to the poor and careless girl, perhaps herself of low intelligence, who is at increased risk of producing a handicapped child.

Perinatal casualty. The improvement in the care of the neonate has had some effect in diminishing retardation, especially that due to metabolic causes. It is inevitable, however, that a few children of very low birth weight will survive and be handicapped who would have died without the intervention of modern medicine.

Paediatric care outside the neonatal period is likely to prevent only a relatively small number of cases of handicap—but is all the more important since the damage of a normal child is particularly hard on his family. Public health measures for the prevention of accidents and the reduction of serious pollutants deserve the support of those concerned with retardation. The role of malnutrition in developing countries needs more research.

Psychosocial causes. If effective measures for counteracting the impoverishment of the psychological environment were available, they would represent the largest contribution to the prevention of mild retardation. The Headstart programme in the United States aimed to enrich the environment of pre-school children. Klaus and Gray (1968) described a similar programme which did make some immediate difference to children's cognitive attainment as measured by IQ. Nevertheless, in many areas the Headstart programme was a failure; and in no area was there dramatic success. This absence of effect has been taken as evidence of the overwhelming importance of genetic inheritance, but another explanation is likely: the educational intervention was too little, and too late, and too hastily planned. A massive effort has been made in Milwaukee by Heber and his associates (Heber and Garber, 1975). They identified mothers with an IQ of less than 75 in slum areas, and offered an educational package. The children's teaching began at the age of three months and continued in small groups until school age. The emphasis was on teaching cognitive and language skills in a structured way, seven hours a day, five days a week. At the same time the mothers were trained in home economy, child care, hygiene and job skills. At the age of five, the children given this programme had a slightly above average IQ, which was nearly 30 points higher than the control children who did not receive it. It may well be that these gains will gradually fade if the children receive only routine schooling, but the clear implication is that a large investment of resources has a major effect.

The conclusion is similar to that which can be drawn from studying many parts of the complex field of mental retardation. Current knowledge shows many ways in which we can help the retarded and their families. Admittedly, large areas of ignorance remain—perhaps none larger than the psychiatric disorders of the mentally handicapped. But the most pressing need is to use the knowledge we already have. A high standard of care can be achieved now; the difficulty is to deliver it to a group of people who have for long been starved of professional and material resources.

References

Azrin, N. H. and Foxx, R. M. (1971). A rapid method of toilet training the institutionalised retarded. *J. Appl. Behav. Anal.* **4**, 89–96.

Baller, W. R., Charles, D. C. and Miller, E. L. (1966) 'Mid-Life Attainment of the Mentally Retarded: A Longitudinal Study'. University of Nebraska, Lincoln.

Baranyay, E. P. (1971). 'The Mentally Handicapped Adolescent'. Pergamon, Oxford.

Berg, J. M. (1963). Causal factors in severe mental retardation. *In* 'Proceedings of the Second International Congress on Mental Retardation', Vienna, 1961 (Ed. O. Stur), Part I. S. Karger, Basel and New York.

Bernstein, B. (1960). Language and social class. *Br. J. Sociol.* **11**, 271.

Birch, H. G., Richardson, S. A., Baird, D., Horobin, G. and Illsley, R. (1970). 'Mental Subnormality in the Community: A Clinical and Epidemiologic Study'. Williams and Wilkins, Baltimore.

Bruhl, H., Arnesen, J. and Bruhl, M. (1964). Effect of a low phenylalanine diet on older phenylketonuric patients. *Am. J. Ment. Def.* **69**, 225–235.

Callaway, E. (1973). Correlations between average evoked potentials and measures of intelligence. *Arch. Gen. Psychiat.* **29**, 553.

Carr, J. (1975). 'Young Children with Down's Syndrome'. Butterworth, London.

Castell, J. H. F. and Mittler, P. J. (1965). Intelligence of patients in subnormality hospitals: a survey of admissions in 1961. *Br. J. Psychiat.* **111**, 219–225.

Clarke, A. M. and Clarke, A. D. B. (1974a). The changing concept of intelligence. *In* 'Mental Deficiency: The Changing Outlook' (Eds A. M. Clarke and A. D. B. Clarke) (3rd edn). Methuen, London.

Clarke, A. M. and Clarke, A. D. B. (1974b). Experimental studies: an overview. *In* 'Mental Deficiency: The Changing Outlook' (Eds A. M. Clarke and A. D. B. Clarke) (3rd edn). Methuen, London.

Clarke, C. A. (1967). Prevention of Rh-haemolytic disease. *Br. Med. J.* **4**, 484–485.

Corbett, J. A. and Wing, L. (1972). A plan for a comprehensive service for the mentally retarded. *In* 'Evaluating a Community Psychiatric Service: The Camberwell Register 1964–1971' (Eds J. K. Wing and A. M. Hailey). Oxford University Press, Oxford.

Corbett, J. A., Harris, R. and Robinson, R. (1975). Epilepsy. *In* 'Mental Retardation and Developmental Disabilities: an annual review' (Ed. J. Wortis), Vol. 7. Brunner/Mazel, New York.

Crome, L. (1960). The brain and mental retardation. *Br. Med. J.* **1**, 897–904.

Crome, L. and Stern, J. (1972). 'Pathology of Mental Retardation' (2nd edn). Churchill Livingstone, Edinburgh and London.

Davison, K. and Bagley, C. R. (1969). Schizophrenia-like psychoses associated with organic disorders of the central nervous system: a review of the literature. *In* 'Current Problems in Neuropsychiatry' (Ed. R. Herrington). Headley Bros. and RMPA, Ashford.

Department of Health and Social Services (1971). 'Better Services for the Mentally Handicapped'. HMSO, London.
Desmonts, G., Couvreur, J. and Ben-Raschid, M.-S. (1965). Le Toxoplasme, La Mère et L'Enfant. Arch. Fr. Pediat. 22, 1183.
Douglas, J. W. B., Ross, J. M. and Simpson, J. R. (1968). 'All Our Future'. Davies, London.
Dutton, G. (1975). 'Mental Handicap'. Butterworths, London.
Edgerton, R. B. (1967). 'The Cloak of Competence: Stigma in the Lives of the Mentally Retarded'. University of California, Berkeley.
Editorial (1977). Child health and environmental lead. Br. Med. J. 1, 255–256.
Ellingson, R. J. (1972). Neurophysiology. In 'Mental Retardation: An Annual Review' (Ed. J. Wortis), Vol. 4. Grune and Stratton, New York.
Erlenmeyer-Kimling, L. and Jarvik, L. (1963). Genetics and intelligence. Science 142, 1477–1479.
Eysenck, H. J. (1971). 'Race, Intelligence and Education'. Temple Smith, London.
Gardner, J. M. (1972). Teaching behaviour modification skills to non-professionals. J. Appl. Behav. Anal. 5, 517–521.
Gardner, W. I. (1971). 'Behaviour Modification in Mental Retardation'. University of London, London.
Gellis, S. S., Feingold, M. and Rutman, J. Y. (1971). 'Atlas of Mental Retardation Syndromes'. US Dept. of Health Education and Welfare, Washington DC.
Gottfried, A. W. (1973). Intellectual consequences of perinatal anoxia. Psychol. Bull. 80, 231–242.
Groth, G. C. (1972). 'Enzyme Replacement in Genetic Disease'. The National Foundation.
Hallgren, B. and Sjögren, T. (1959). A clinical and genetico-statistical study of schizophrenia and low-grade mental deficiency in a large Swedish rural population. Acta Psychiat. Scand., Suppl. 140, 1.
Haywood, H. C. and Heal, L. W. (1968). Retention of learned visual associations as a function of IQ and learning levels. Am. J. Ment. Def. 72, 828–838.
Heaton-Ward, W. A. (1975). 'Mental Subnormality' (4th edn). Wright, Bristol.
Heber, R. and Garber, H. (1975). Progress Report II: An experiment in the prevention of cultural-familial retardation. In 'Proceedings of the Third Congress of The International Association for the Scientific Study of Mental Deficiency' (Ed. D. A. A. Primrose). Polish Medical Publishers, Warsaw.
Hess, R. D. and Shipman, V. C. (1965). Early experience and the socialisation of cognitive modes in children. Child Develop. 36, 869–886.
Hunt, J. McV. (1961). 'Intelligence and Experience'. Ronald Press, New York.
Jensen, A. R. (1973). 'Educability and Group Differences'. Methuen, London.
Johnson, R. R. (1969). Behavioural characteristics of phenylketonurics and matched controls. Am. J. Ment. Def. 74, 17–19.
Kallmann, F. J., Barrera, S. E., Hoch, P. and Kelly, D. M. (1941). Role of mental deficiency in incidence of schizophrenia. Am. J. Ment. Def. 45, 514–539.
Klaus, R. and Gray, S. (1968). The early training project for disadvantaged children. Monogr. Soc. Res. Child Dev. (Serial No. 120) 33, 4, 1–55.
Knobloch, H. and Pasamanick, B. (1962). Medical progress: mental subnormality. New Engl. J. Med. 266, 1045–1051, 1092–1097, 1155–1161.
Kushlik, A. (1961). Subnormality in Salford. In 'A report on the Mental Health Services of the City of Salford for the year 1960'. (Eds M. W. Susser and A. Kushlik). Salford Health Department.
Kushlik, A. and Blunden, R. (1974). The epidemiology of mental subnormality. In

'Mental Deficiency: The Changing Outlook' (Eds A. M. Clarke and A. D. B. Clarke) (3rd edn). Methuen, London.

Kushlik, A. and Cox, G. (1968). Planning services for the subnormal in Wessex. *In* 'Psychiatric Case Registers'. (Eds J. K. Wing and B. R. Bransby). HMSO, London.

Luria, A. R. (1961). 'The Role of Speech in the Regulation of Normal and Abnormal Behaviour'. Pergamon, Oxford.

McDonald, A. (1964). Intelligence in children of very low birth weight. *Br. J. Prev. Soc. Med.* **18**, 59–73.

Mehlman, B. (1953). Group play therapy with mentally retarded children. *J. Abnorm. Soc. Psychol.* **48**, 53–60.

Merril, C. R., Geier, M. R. and Petricciani, J. C. (1971). Bacterial virus gene expression in human cells. *Nature* **233**, 398–400.

Mittler, P. J. and Woodward, M. (1966). The education of children in hospitals for the subnormal: a survey of admissions. *Dev. Med. Child Neurol.* **8**, 16–25.

Mizumo, T. and Yugari, Y. (1974). Self-mutilation in Lesch-Nyhan syndrome. *Lancet* **1**, 761.

Moore, B. C., Thuline, H. C. and Capes, L. V. (1968). Mongoloid and non-mongoloid retardates: a behavioural comparison. *Am. J. Ment. Def.* **73**, 433–436.

O'Connor, N. and Hermelin, B. (1974). Specific defects and coding strategies. *In* 'Mental Deficiency: The Changing Outlook' (Eds A. M. Clarke and A. D. B. Clarke). Methuen, London.

Ounsted, C. (1955). The hyperkinetic syndrome in epileptic children. *Lancet* **ii**, 303–311.

Payne, R. W. (1973). Cognitive abnormalities. *In* 'Handbook of Abnormal Psychology' (Ed. H. J. Eysenck) (2nd edn). Pitman Medical, Kent.

Penrose, L. S. (1972). 'The Biology of Mental Defect' (4th edn). Sidgwick and Jackson, London.

President's Committee on Mental Retardation (1972). 'Entering on the Era of Human Ecology'. Dept. of Health Education and Welfare, Washington DC.

Reynolds, E. H. and Travers, R. D. (1974). Serum anticonvulsant concentrations in epileptic patients with mental symptoms. *Br. J. Psychiat.* **124**, 440–445.

Rutter, M. (1971). Psychiatry. *In* 'Mental Retardation' (Ed. J. Wortis), Vol. 3. Grune and Stratton, New York.

Rutter, M., Birch, H. C., Thomas, A. and Chess, S. (1964). Temperamental characteristics in infancy and the later development of behavioural disorders. *Br. J. Psychiat.* **110**, 651–661.

Rutter, M., Graham, P. and Yule, W. (1970a). 'A Neuropsychiatric Study in Childhood'. Spastics Int. Med. Publ. and Heinemann, London.

Rutter, M., Tizard, J. and Whitmore, K. (1970b). 'Education, Health and Behaviour'. Longmans, London.

Scott, K. G. and Scott, M. S. (1968). Research and theory in short-term memory. *In* 'International Review of Research in Mental Retardation' (Ed. N. R. Ellis), Vol. 3. Academic Press, New York and London.

Seidel, U. P., Chadwick, O. and Rutter, M. (1975). Psychological disorders in crippled children: a comparative study of children with and without brain damage. *Dev. Med. Child Neurol.* **17**, 563–573.

Skeels, H. (1966). Adult status of children with contrasting life experiences: a follow-up study. *Monogr. Soc. Res. Child. Dev.* **31**, 3.

Skodak, M. and Skeels, H. (1949). A final follow-up study of one hundred adopted children. *J. Genet. Psychol.* **75**, 85–125.

Sprague, R. L. and Werry, J. S. (1971). Methodology of pharmacological studies with the retarded. In 'International Review of Research in Mental Retardation' (Ed. N. R. Ellis), Vol. 5. Academic Press, New York and London.

Stanbury, J. B., Wyngaarden, J. B. and Frederickson, D. S. (1971). 'The Metabolic Basis of Inherited Disease' (3rd edn). McGraw-Hill, New York.

Tizard, J. (1964). 'Community Services for the Mentally Handicapped'. Oxford University Press, Oxford.

Tizard, J. (1974). Services and the evaluation of services. In 'Mental Deficiency: The Changing Outlook' (Eds A. M. Clarke and A. D. B. Clarke) (3rd edn). Methuen, London.

Tredgold, R. F. and Soddy, K. (1970). 'Tredgold's Mental Retardation' (11th edn). Baillière Tindall and Cassell, London.

Wiesel, T. and Hubel, D. (1965). Comparison of the effects of unilateral and bilateral eye closure on cortical unit responses in kittens. J. Neurophysiol. 28, 1029–1040.

Zeaman, D. (1965). Learning processes of the mentally retarded. In 'The Biosocial Basis of Mental Retardation' (Eds S. Osler and R. Cooke). Johns Hopkins, Baltimore.

Zeaman, D. and House, B. J. (1963). The role of attention in retardate discrimination learning. In 'Handbook of Mental Deficiency' (Ed. N. R. Ellis). McGraw-Hill, New York.

Zisfein, L. and Rosen, M. (1973). Personal adjustment training: a group counselling program for institutionalised mentally retarded persons. Ment. Retard. 11, 16–20.

7 Neurosis and personality disorder

Anthony Thorley and *Richard Stern**

Problems of concept and classification

The neuroses

The term neurosis originated in the late eighteenth century and applied to any disease due to a dysfunction of the nervous system, but the meaning changed when Freud and the analytic movement gave the word a completely different aetiological connotation. Far from signifying a neurologically based set of hereditary and degenerative diseases, neurosis became a synonym for psychogenic disorder. Gradually the concept of a psychological, psychogenic or neurotic aetiological factor has grown in importance and now plays a prominent role in the International Classification of Diseases (Katschnig and Shepherd, 1976).

In psychoanalytical theory the neuroses are associated with fixation at various levels of psychological development, e.g. oral or anal level. Classic analytic theory distinguishes between *psychoneuroses*: conversion hysteria, anxiety hysteria (phobia) and obsessional neurosis, and *character neuroses* in which the symptoms are character traits (Rycroft, 1972). This technical psychoanalytic use of neuroses, like the analysts' use of the term psychosis, differs from the narrower syndromal view of the general psychiatrist, and yet essentially informs the more specific neurotic and personality disorder category descriptions found in the International Classification. Another strand of psychoanalytic influence lies in the

* Richard Stern contributed to the section on obsessional states.

traditional stress placed on the importance of insight in distinguishing neurosis from psychosis; whilst insight appears very variable and complex in clinical practice, its importance is still reflected in the current WHO definition of the neuroses as:

> mental disorders without demonstrable organic basis in which the patient may have considerable insight and unimpaired reality testing, in that he usually does not confuse his morbid subjective experiences and fantasies with external reality. Behaviour may be greatly affected, although usually remaining within socially acceptable limits, but personality is not disorganised. The principal manifestations include excessive anxiety, hysterical symptoms, phobias, obsessional and compulsive symptoms, and depression.   (WHO, 1974)

The immensely broad range of 'neurotic' disorders in the International Classification of Diseases has led one Swedish worker (Hagnell, 1970) to define neurosis as 'non-psychotic mental illness in the absence of obvious brain disease'. This wide definition only clarifies what neurosis is not rather than what it is. By contrast Eysenck (1977) stresses the behavioural and maladaptive elements of neurosis and defines it as

> behaviour which is associated with strong emotion, which is maladaptive, and which the person . . . realises is nonsensical, absurd, or irrelevant, but which he is powerless to change.

If there are minor variations in these definitions of neurosis with different stresses laid upon behaviour, personality, maladaptation and insight, major problems of reliability and validity arise with regard to separating neurosis into types. Noyes and Kolb (1958) state:

> The so-called 'types' are not disease entities in genesis, mechanisms or manifestations. Rather should the psychoneuroses be regarded as a series of varying types of reaction brought about by multiple causative factors which vary from case to case. The more carefully the reactions of the neurotic are examined, the more frequently it will be found that there are no sharply defined lines amongst the various types of neuroses.

These remarks are equally relevant when we attempt to separate neurosis from personality disorders, or categorize personality disorders.

Reliability of diagnosis has been tested in various studies (Kreitman, 1961; Ley, 1972) and has usually been found to be substantially lower for neurosis than for organic psychiatric and psychotic illness. Kreitman (1961) found that there was 52% agreement about what constituted a neurosis, but only 28% agreement about what type of neurosis might be present. Greer and Cawley (1966) concluded from their study of the natural history of neurotic illness that 'differentiations between depressive, anxiety and hysterical reactions appear difficult; in many cases admixtures of symptoms were found in all categories'. While the clinician may not feel very inconvenienced by these admixtures of symptoms, the categorical approach to the neuroses has severe limitations for the research worker and Kendell (1976) concludes that in the long term there must be a move towards a dimensional representation of these phenomena.

Personality disorders

If the neuroses present nosological problems but at least are generally recognized as illnesses, the personality disorders may not strictly merit consideration as diseases or illnesses at all. Lewis (1955) raised the whole question of what constitutes a mental illness in his analysis of health as a social concept. Anticipating the psychiatrization of everyday life, Lewis points out the dangerous implications of judging the existence of mental illness by the presence of social factors. He states: 'it is misconceived to equate ill health with social deviation or maladjustment'. Lewis develops this theme by stating that mental illness can be inferred only from deviant, maladaptive or non-conformist behaviour, when like physical illness, there is present some disorder of part-function of the whole. This may rarely be physical, e.g. brain damage, or more commonly psychological, e.g. a disturbance in perception, memory, mood etc. Lewis is quite clear that 'if nonconformity can be detected only in total behaviour, whilst all the particular psychological functions seem unimpaired, health will be presumed not illness'.

Clare (1976) has pointed out that whilst many people with so-called personality disorders probably have no part-function disorder, or at least none detectable by present techniques, and hence are not essentially ill, they are nevertheless treated by psychiatrists *as if* they were. Certainly, some psychiatrists return such people to the legal or social services having detected 'no overt psychiatric illness' whilst others assume that a disease is present but with as yet an unidentified biological basis, and offer treatment; others may be doubtful about whether disease is present but respond recognizing that their skills are as valid as anyone elses to cope with the problem. Psychiatry has probably offered itself too enthusiastically, or been pressured too easily by society into providing a medical response to personality disorder, and now it has the problem squarely on its lap. Hence although psychiatrists today may be rightly uneasy about the majority of cases, illness is usually legitimized as this facilitates an assisting response. Thus personality disorders have become psychiatric illnesses.

It is perhaps in this dubiously medical area of personality disorder that the social scientist has the strongest case to make for the sociological model of mental illness as a rationalization of unacceptable deviance. Indeed, had social scientists concentrated on the vagaries of disturbed personality rather than on schizophrenia, labelling theory and sociological explanations might have been more readily accepted by orthodox psychiatrists. Thus while we may agree with Kendell (1976) that 'it is simply mischievous to suggest that schizophrenia is nothing more than the product of social and intrafamilial pressures', it is perhaps not so mischievous to consider personality disorder in this way. One of the central sociological assertions is that the deviant individual and his actions, once having been judged abnormal and hence ill, are no longer socially disturbing and need not be taken seriously as a challenge to current standards and beliefs (Pearson, 1975). Once the behaviour is construed as illness, there is no requirement placed upon society to conceptualize it in other ways. Medicine, it is argued, becomes one of society's agents in quiescing challenges to the social order, and whilst such processes may not be immediately apparent to the busy psychiatrist in his out-patients, he recognizes this 'misuse' of psychiatry in other countries (Baruch and Treacher, 1978; Wing, 1978).

If we accept that for practical purposes personality disorders are mental illnesses, we may now ask how effectively can they be defined and typed, and is it possible to separate them satisfactorily from neuroses? Schneider's rich description of psychopathic personalities has been particularly influential on British psychiatry (Schneider, 1950). Schneider used the term psychopathic personality in the classical German sense, encompassing what we now commonly regard as neurosis and personality disorder, and established an important and enduring principle. He stated that psychopathic personalities are those abnormal personalities who suffer from their abnormality or cause society to suffer. Abnormal personalities who are not psychopathic personalities are seen as eccentrics, tolerated, non-problematic, and in the case of great men, highly valued by society. Psychopathic personalities who personally suffer broadly correspond to our narrow view of neurosis, and those who cause society to suffer are 'sociopathic' personality disorders.

Schneider's distinction between personal and social suffering influenced an experimental typology of personality disorder used by Walton and his colleagues to test reliability and validity of the types (see Table I) (Walton et al., 1970). Six male psychiatrists were asked to assign 40 patients to one of 11 categories. Results showed that although four broad types of personality disorder emerged, precise descriptive labels were not reliably applied, and there was a strong tendency to categorize men as aggressive psychopaths and women as hysterical personalities. Later studies (Walton and Presly, 1973; Presly and Walton, 1973) further investigated the above typology and found a minor improvement in

Table I *Experimental classification of abnormal personality (from Walton* et al.*, 1970)*

1 *Mild:* Character disorder (usually complained of by the patient himself):
  (a) dependent type
  (b) detached type
  (c) assertive type

2 *Moderate:* Personality disorder (usually identified clinically):
  (a) obsessional type
  (b) hysterical type
  (c) schizoid type
  (d) paranoid type
  (e) cyclothymic type

3 *Severe:* Sociopathy (usually identified socially):
  (a) aggressive type
  (b) inadequate type

reliability, but agreement between psychiatrists failed to reach 50% for both type and severity. However, the reliability of ratings for the same patients on 46 personality traits, measured on four-point scales, was much higher, and led the authors to suggest abandoning a categorical approach to personality disorders in favour of a dimensional approach.

The woeful lack of reliability in these results may lead some to renew their doubts about the value of personality disorder at all, but Shepherd and Sartorius (1974) state that despite these confusions 'the concept of personality disorder remains indispensable to psychiatric practice'—an opinion which no doubt confirms any suspicions among social scientists! These authors draw attention to the latest WHO definition which states that personality disorder includes

> deeply ingrained maladaptive patterns of behaviour generally recognisable by the time of adolescence or earlier and continuing throughout most of adult life, although often becoming less obvious in middle or old age. The personality is abnormal either in the balance of its components, their quality and expression or in its total aspect. Because of this deviation or psychopathy the patient suffers or others have to suffer and there is an adverse effect upon the individual or on society. (WHO, 1971)

Clearly the problems of defining more explicit categories of personality disorder which can satisfy international requirements can only be solved by further research. Shepherd and Sartorius (1974) advocate two lines of approach. First to identify sharper and more precise definitions which would command more general acceptance. Second to investigate the feasibility of a multiaxial or dimensional classification such as that introduced for the psychiatric disorders of childhood (see Chapter 5).

The choice between categories and dimensions is further confused by the observation that some neurotic symptoms are apparently discontinuous, are not found distributed in the normal population, and therefore lend themselves to category representation, whereas the abnormal or accentuated traits of personality disorder are continuous, distributed as traits throughout the normal population, and so lend themselves to dimensional representation. In addition there is the inescapable clinical observation that some patients with neurosis have personality disorder, and some do not, and some patients with personality disorder have neurotic symptoms, and again some do not.

Foulds' universe of personal distress

One person who attempted to tackle this complexity was the late G. A. Foulds. Over the last twenty years, Foulds described and provided evidence for a hierarchy of diagnosis, such that patients characteristically not only display the manifestations of their disorder, but also those of disorders at all lower levels on the hierarchy. Foulds (1965) proposes that patients with non-integrated psychosis (schizophrenia) will also have integrated psychosis (melancholia or paranoia), also have personal illness (neurosis) and also have personality disorder. In his original scheme Foulds proposed that all those with personal illness, i.e. neuroses, were personality disordered, and those who were personality disordered but had no personal illness, i.e. no neurotic symptoms, were psychopaths. Since first making these proposals, there have been many developments in the investigation of symptoms and of personality, and Foulds (1976) has responded to the potentially wide range of combinations of personality dysfunction, psychiatric symptoms and social disturbance, by proposing two basic classes: personal symptomatology and maladaptive personality deviance. He also makes use of the Schneiderian distinction between suffering to self and to society, but introduces a concept of unmanageability or not coping, which pays credence to symptoms and behaviours which although the cause of personal or social suffering are nevertheless tolerated, coped with, and so do not emerge as illness, crime or social casework.

Personal symptomatology concerns the presence of psychiatric symptoms from minor mood change, through neurosis to psychosis. There are those who are personally ill (X), whose symptoms are distressing either to society or to the individual and are unmanageable by the individual or by society. The personally disturbed (y) have distressing symptoms that are tolerated by the individual or by society. There are those who are symptom free and who are personally healthy ($\bar{Y}$).

Maladaptive personality deviants are 'people who deviate extremely from the general run of the population on personality characteristics which appear likely to have an adverse bearing on the capacity to enter into mutual relationships' (Foulds, 1976). This is not an implicitly medical definition. Personality disorders (A) are those whose personality attributes and effects are distressing to the individual or to society, and are unmanageable by the individual or by society. Discordant personalities (b) are those whose personality attributes and effects are distressing either to the individual or to society, but are tolerated by the individual and by society. Normal personalities (B̄) are those whose personality attributes and effects are not distressing to either the individual or to society.

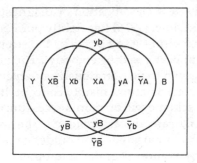

Fig 1 Foulds' universe of personal distress: personal symptomatology and maladjustive personality deviance. Taken from 'The Hierarchical Nature of Personal Illness' (Foulds, 1976, p. 50), Academic Press.

As can be seen in the Venn diagram in Fig. 1 the six groups in these two basic classes can be combined in nine different ways which allows a good deal of flexibility. For example, a personally ill normal personality (X:B̄) could be a man of normal personality who has a series of traumatic experiences and develops an acute anxiety state. This is not tolerated, he presents for treatment, and the anxiety is alleviated so as to become tolerable. Now the man is clinically well, and can be classified as personally disturbed normal personality (y:B̄). The reader can experiment with various other combinations for himself, but as can be seen these do not have to imply mental illness, but take into account normal functioning, tolerable functioning, and dysfunction which may require a non-medical (i.e. social work or legal) response. An added value of this scheme is that the categories link in with the hierarchy of other psychiatric illnesses through the medium of personal illness, and hence psychotic states and neurotic disorders can be considered alongside pre-existing or concomit-ant personality dysfunction.

Foulds' classification of personality function and symptomatology linked to his hierarchy for other disorders makes an important contribu-tion because it provides another alternative to unreliable categories, and dimensions which are at present alien to the average clinician. Foulds' scheme is pragmatic and integrationist, and is more likely to appeal to those concerned with clinical practice than those who favour a refined categorical classification in the belief that when the precise types can be eventually defined we may discover a relatively simple causality. Defin-ing personality disorder in more precise unitary categories is likely to prove very elusive, and it is arguable that reductionist thinking is least appropriate to the classification of personality disorders and neuroses. A final problem for any new classification or diagnostic scheme is that of prognostic validity. Kendell (1976) has rightly pointed out that 'in the last resort all diagnostic concepts stand or fall by the strength of the prognos-tic and therapeutic implications they embody'. The neuroses and person-ality disorders are known to be notoriously variable in their longitudinal course and virtually deny a natural history concept. It is impossible at this stage to know which scheme will be more successful: the refined, possibly operationally defined, categorical approach; the integrated categories linked to a hierarchy advocated by Foulds; or a multi-dimensional approach favoured by Walton, Kendell and others.

Biological and social aspects of personality development

In order to place personality dysfunction and neurotic symptomatology in context it is important to understand the broad range of social and biological factors which play a part in the development of normal person-ality. This massive subject is more properly the concern of developmental psychology but in this short account attention will be drawn to some of the key processes.

First, the development of normal personality rests on a genetically endowed biological and behavioural substrate, but this genetic base is very difficult to isolate experimentally. Shields (1976) indicates that twin studies have shown clearly that specific factors like intelligence, and personality traits as tested on the Eysenck Personality Inventory, are more likely to be concordant in MZ rather than DZ twins. There is also a body of evidence which suggests that various temperamental attributes are identifiable within weeks of birth and remain relatively stable in each child during the first three years (Thomas et al., 1963). These early behavioural characteristics, apparently constitutional, influence the later development of childhood behavioural disorders (Rutter *et al.*, 1964). For many years there was a belief that body build was linked to basic personality and to predisposition to certain mental illnesses. Classically, cyclothymic personalities were associated with a pyknic body-build, whereas schizoid personalities, predisposed to schizophrenia, were associated with an asthenic build. However attractive these associations may be to the clinician, they have not stood up to rigorous experimental examination (Fowlie, 1962).

Constitutional factors contributing to personality development may be identified as separate from genetic factors, e.g. inter-uterine development and insult. Animal experiments indicate that unnatural hormonal influences in the neonatal period can affect subsequent sexual characteristics and it is possible that these mechanisms affect human gender identity and sexual development. There is also evidence that drugs taken during pregnancy may not simply affect physical growth, but also more subtle development of the central nervous system which carries implications of behavioural dysfunction (Nelson and Forfar, 1971).

Whereas there is no doubt that substantial brain damage in early life causes deficits in personality development, Pasamanick and Knobloch (1961) have suggested that prematurity and perinatal complications may lead to minor brain damage not detectable by neurological signs but evidenced by personality dysfunction. Such a 'continuum of reproductive casualty' is difficult to establish but studies suggest that children born with low birth weight (Drillien, 1969), or perinatal hypoxia (Corah *et al.*, 1965) are likely to show reduced social maturity and intellectual ability, and experience problems of personality adjustment in the first decade. As severe undernourishment within the first year is associated with reduced brain weight and fewer brain cells, Oswald and Wolff (1973) have speculated that chronic malnutrition might affect the development of intellectual and social skills.

The biological and constitutional factors described above cannot be viewed in a causal vacuum as personality develops in a constant interactive process between biological potential, environmental circumstance and social opportunity. Thus attachment behaviour is the basis for the infant's earliest social interaction, but effective bonding and associated personality development depend on an intact and viable biological base; developmental impairment may result when there is interference between the biological system and environmental stimuli. Thus blind children develop specific attachments more slowly than the sighted, but their attachments are more intense and last longer. The development of social behaviour in children has been reviewed by Schaffer (1971) and an important re-examination of interference in bond formation has been made by Rutter (1972a).

Between two and five years the child develops especially in the areas of self-control, social and sexual identity. At school the intimate dependence on parents and family lessens and in early adolescence the child increasingly experiments with personal responsibility and independence. This emotional and social development is paralleled by a complex cognitive development (Piaget and Inhelder, 1970). Adolescence itself is a period of rapidly changing biological function and potential, and normally great ambivalence is experienced separating from childhood and embracing adulthood. Personality development here reaches a critical phase as self-esteem, attitudes and future patterns of behaviour are continuously tested and explored in social, sexual and vocational outlets. In this maturational process from infant to young adult consistent parental, family and peer encouragement, support, and not a little love, are at a premium. Inadequate or culturally atypical child rearing practices, parental illness, marital disharmony and family disturbance are all associated with personality disorder.

In this maturational process the role of learning cannot be overestimated. Much of what we identify as personality disorder can be described in terms of inappropriate thresholds to incoming stimuli. Thus we identify as maladaptive low thresholds to frustration or tolerance, leading to impulsive behaviour or loss of temper, and a high threshold in relation to emotional insensitivity leading to overdefendedness and emotional coldness. Personality is in part created by myriads of constitutionally determined threshold levels being altered, by social learning in the family, with peers and at school. Thus the child with little innate tendency to loss of temper but brought up in a family setting where tempers are regularly lost and are socially effective and valued, will model this behaviour, lower his threshold and develop a more ready temper. Impulsive behaviour will be found in children where impulsive behaviour already flourishes in the family or sub-culture. Most social skills (and lack of them) are generated in this subtle high order learning situation, and it is the implicit plasticity in the human organism that holds out the greatest promise for later therapeutic endeavour.

It is generally considered that gradually the plasticity diminishes and the personality becomes set in early middle age. Whilst there is no doubt about this socially and culturally (witness how youthful flexibility and radicalism give way to conservatism) and that there are a whole mass of biological factors associated with ageing, it may be unwarranted to assume a predominant underlying biological process of personality concretization. It may be more true to say that personality development as observed, or personal growth as experienced, is a continuous but fluctuating process which only ceases when dementia or death intervenes.

Contributions to an understanding of neurosis

Epidemiological aspects

Studies of the prevalence and distribution of neurosis in society and in selected groups, e.g. hospital in-patients, are rarely satisfactory because of the vagueness of the category. Thus in the studies discussed below neurosis usually includes minor depression (depressive neurosis) as the major contributing diagnosis. Detailed studies of whole communities are rare but Hagnell (1970) has estimated from his community survey that the life-time expectancy rate for neurosis in Sweden is 13%, and that the average duration of an illness for men, 5–9 months, is a little less than for women. Cross-cultural studies have revealed widely differing prevalences of neurotic illness and various culture-bound neurotic syndromes and anomalies, e.g. Koro (see Chapter 15). For instance in the Leightons' study of mental disturbance in defined rural Canadian populations as compared with a Nigerian tribe, the Yoruba, it was found that women had more neurotic symptoms than men in Canada, whereas the opposite held in Nigeria (D. C. Leighton *et al.*, 1963; A. H. Leighton *et al.*, 1963).

In a large survey of general practice consultations in London, Shepherd and his colleagues (1966) estimated that the patient consulting rate per 1000 at risk for neurosis was 89 (117 per 1000 for women and 56 per 1000 for men). There is no adequate explanation for this marked sex difference, but it is difficult to avoid the speculation that neurotic symptomatology is one way women can communicate underlying needs in a male dominated and doctored society (Kendell, 1974).

Cooper and Sylph (1973) found that new cases of neurotic illness identified in a London general practice setting had experienced significantly more life events during the three months before the onset of their illness than matched controls. Hare and Shaw (1965) surveyed a new suburban housing estate, and an older and more densely populated inner urban area, and found no difference in the neurosis rate. Such broad based epidemiological studies face problems of 'treated' and 'true' prevalence in society and to what extent there is an iceberg of untreated disturbance. A major contribution, arising from findings in a 'normal' group of women in South London, has been the identification of important class related and protective social factors which affect the prevalence of depressive illness (Harris *et al.*, 1976) (see Chapter 12).

It is well known that a majority of neurotic illnesses remit and that spontaneous remission may be common. Harvey-Smith and Cooper (1970) found that 75% of neuroses in a general practice setting remit within three years. Greer and Cawley (1966) followed up 181 hospitalized neurotic patients and found that four to six years after discharge 53% were symptom-free and satisfactorily socially adjusted. Cases of obsessive compulsive neurosis and hypochondriacal states had the worst prognosis. In another follow-up of hospitalized neurotic patients Sims (1975) found that factors predictive of a poor outcome 12 years after admission, included abnormal personality, long duration of the pre-admission illness, onset before 20 and an early or late marriage.

Genetic aspects

The genetic contribution to neurotic illness may be symptom or disorder specific or may take the form of a more general vulnerability. At present there is no disorder which merits a predominantly genetic explanation, but the accumulating evidence is impressive. Shields (1976) reports 47% concordance for neurotic illness in MZ twin pairs compared with 24% concordance in DZ pairs. Similarly, Schepank (1973) in reviewing 13 international studies carried out over the last forty years found a 59% concordance in 184 MZ twin pairs as against 28% concordance in 163 DZ pairs. What evidence there is suggests that anxiety neurosis is more genetically influenced than hysterical and depressive illnesses (Miner, 1973; Shields, 1976).

Animal studies and experimental neurosis

Increasing knowledge relevant to neurosis is being collected from animal behaviour in the wild and in the laboratory, particularly with regard to specific cues causing fear and flight and behaviourally conditioned responses. Kumar (1976) in reviewing this area has cautioned those who would enthusiastically extrapolate from crude 'experimental neuroses' in animals to the human condition, but asserts that animal studies, especially when supported by concurrent physiological data, will eventually help to elucidate aspects of human psychopathology. In particular animal conditioned avoidance responses can serve as a paradigm for phobic illnesses, and the specificity of some of the cues and the facility with which the response is sometimes learned has led Marks (1973) to speculate whether there are not certain stimuli which are pre-potent elicitors of fear in animals, and facilitators of phobic responses in man.

Experimental neurosis in humans, other than experiments on volunteers with fears, is at an early stage, but would seem to offer much promise for the investigation of obsessive compulsive and dissociative (hysterical) phenomena (Marks, 1973, 1976).

Childhood emotional disorders and adult neurosis

Traditionally it has always been considered that there is a strong continuity between childhood and adult neurosis, but Rutter (1972b) in reviewing this area suggests that this view may be partly mistaken. More recently, Cox (1976) has critically appraised the evidence for continuity. In a now classic thirty year follow-up study of over 500 child psychiatric clinic attenders Robins (1966) showed that neurosis in adult life was no more common in former clinic attenders than in a control group, but that children referred with non-conduct problems had a higher rate of adult psychiatric disorder in general, compared with the controls. However, as has been confirmed in many other studies, the risk of future adult psychiatric illness, including neurosis, was much higher in children referred for antisocial behaviour and conduct disorders. By contrast, Pritchard and Graham's (1966) study of individuals who had attended both childrens and adult departments at the Maudsley Hospital found that children with neurotic disorders more often had neurosis in later life compared with other disorders, and childhood neurosis was the most common antecedent for adult neurosis. This combination of a good prognosis for childhood neurosis with some evidence of continuity led Rutter (1972b) to conclude that 'most neurotic children become normal adults and most neurotic adults develop their neurosis in adult life'. Some idea of the degree of continuity has been provided by Melsopp (1973) in an Australian study. Children attending a department of child psychiatry with neurosis were 4–5 times as likely to attend as neurotic adults as the general population, but the proportion of child attenders who became neurotic adult clinic attenders was only 3–4%. Similarly only 8% of all adult neurotic clinic attenders had attended as children. Clearly, emotional disorder in childhood carries an increased risk of adult neurosis but this continuity applies to very few individuals (Cox, 1976).

Neurosis and the family

Although popular opinion would impute family disturbance and marital discord as being major factors in the production of mental illness (see Chapter 11) very little specific evidence has been brought to bear on the problem of neurosis and the family, but some important work has been done on neurosis and marriage. Kreitman and his colleagues (1970, 1971) have carried out a series of studies into the effect of neurosis on a patient's marriage and marital partner, and have tested the hypothesis that any concordance of psychiatric disorder in the couple occurred principally by assortative mating. Using detailed conjoint interviews and psychometric tests, they examined 60 normal couples matched with 60 male out-patients treated for neurosis or personality disorder, together with their wives. Patients' wives scored significantly higher than control wives for incapacitating ill health, neurotic problems, number of previous psychiatric illnesses, and their disabilities appeared to increase as the marriage progressed. Interspouse correlations on various measures were lower in patients than in controls, and overall these findings suggested that the couples did not come together by assortative mating, but rather that increasing disturbance in patients' spouses was due to a pathogenic marital interaction. A further study examined the nature of this interaction and identified conflict over role function especially with regard to leisure and child-rearing to be of importance (Ovenstone, 1973).

Sociological aspects

Sociological contributions to an understanding of neurosis parallel contributions to mental illness in general, and centre on three related areas: labelling theory, concepts of deviance and deviancy amplification, and concepts of the sick role and illness behaviour. More specifically, neurosis (and personality disorder) may be better understood by application of the concept of abnormal illness behaviour.

First it is clear that unacceptable behaviour or symptoms or complaints can be interpreted in various ways by the individual and variously construed by relatives, friends and society in general. This 'primary deviance', which Lemert (1967) has argued may only have marginal implications for the stability of the individual and society, can be seen as 'bad behaviour', 'maladjustment', 'mental illness' or simply as a social nuisance. To choose a construct of 'mental illness', or more specifically a diagnosis of some kind of neurosis, is to attach a label to the person which carries profound implications of its own. These implications include assumptions about altered responsibility of the individual for his actions or behaviour, reactions of other people which may be stigmatic, and an invitation to take up the sick role and show appropriate illness behaviour. When such a labelled person reacts to these implications and begins to employ his deviant behaviour, or a role (e.g. the sick role) based upon it as an adjustment to the overt and covert problems created by society's reaction to him, he may enhance his apparent psychopathology or behaviour and assume 'secondary deviance' (Wing, 1978).

Secondary deviance is usually considered more extreme or severe than primary deviance, and for the patient free in society (or even in a mental hospital), the process of deviancy amplification may become important. Deviancy amplification can take many forms and the example described in Chapter 9 with regard to drug addicts is just as relevant for others with unacceptable behaviours, e.g. sexual variations or antisocial behaviour, who are likely to form sub-cultures and pursue deviant illness careers.

Labelling in mental illness can be seen as the way in which the deviant is confronted by society's agent, the doctor, and judged ill in the process of psychiatric diagnosis (Clare, 1976). Although this diagnostic process claims to be objective and dispassionate, inevitably, and particularly with regard to neurosis and personality disorder, it carries evaluative and judgemental constructs (Orford, 1976). How else do doctors respond when faced with symptoms and behaviour which appear to manipulate or compromise their authority and position (e.g. suicidal or histrionic acting out behaviour) or else are morally or socially repugnant (e.g. sexual problems or vagrancy)? Orford (1976) argues that inevitably these evalua-tive constructs affect the objective assessment of psychopathology and colour not only the final diagnostic label but the likely clinical manage-ment. Thus being diagnosed hysterical personality, psychopath, or more loosely 'neurotic' and having this entered in the clinical notes, carries unenviable long-term implications.

It is important to appreciate how much the diagnostic process, or psychiatric interview, is a negotiation about appropriate constructs be-tween doctor and putative patient (Scheff, 1968). The psychiatrist recog-nizes illness, albeit neurotic illness, but the patient may construct his behaviour or explain his disability in other ways. For effective psychiatric treatment acceptance of the doctor's contribution is crucial (and inciden-tally often very relieving for the patient: 'Now I know what it is. I feel so much better!') and essential for initiation of an appropriate sick role. Equally crucial is the much more diffuse negotiation which may occur with relatives of the patient. Baruch and Treacher (1978) have provided rich anecdotal evidence of the process by which relatives of in-patients in a leading British psychiatric unit have their non-psychiatric constructs and explanations medicalized.

Parsons (1951) regards the patient in his sick role as obligated to want to get well, and to co-operate with others for the purpose of achieving health as soon as possible. Mechanic (1962) has called attention to illness behaviour and its variety in different settings. For instance, given the same disability, patients who are lonely or isolated seek medical aid significantly more often than other patients. Thus appropriate illness behaviour (for the disability) may dissolve into arguably inappropriate illness behaviour (for the disability and in addition the loneliness). This idea has been elaborated and developed by Pilowsky (1969, 1978) as the concept of abnormal illness behaviour.

Pilowsky argues that many psychiatric illnesses and processes vari-ously labelled hysteria, hypochondriasis, functional overlay, pathogenic pain, compensation neurosis and malingering do not present clear objective underlying pathologies to the doctor which entitle the patient into the sick role that he expects. Many of these patients do not fulfil the Parsonian sick role because they manifestly do not appear to want health, but have other or more powerful gains and advantages in prolonging or generating illness (Kendell, 1974). Pilowsky considers that those patients who are uninfluenced by medical explanations of the problem and the way it should be managed, should be considered as manifesting abnormal illness behaviour. In these cases the diagnostic negotiation is unsatisfactory or unresolved and a gap remains between physician and patient. The patient feels he is ill, but not in the way the doctor sees it or explains it. Thus the paralysed leg following an industrial accident remains paralysed not because of prolonged neurological damage, but because of the financial gain of compensation.

The significance of this concept in clinical work is that it calls upon the psychiatrist or physician to look beyond the behaviour or symptoms, and any underlying pathology, to examine the psychological gains and advantages which the patient accrues from their prolongation, and so be able to approach these dynamics in a more appropriate way (Pilowsky, 1978).

Obsessional states

Obsessive-compulsive neurosis

The first published report was probably Esquirol in 1838, but it was not until 1877 that Westphal gave the first comprehensive definition. Today most authorities stand by Schneider's (1959) definition:

> Compulsion may be said to occur when an individual is haunted by conscious contents although at the same time he judges them as senseless or at any rate senselessly insistent.

Lewis (1936) claimed that there are two essential components of obsessional ruminations and rituals, the first being compulsion and the second resistance to the obsession which is experienced as part of the patient's free will. Textbooks (e.g. Mayer-Gross et al., 1969; Beech, 1974) and research papers until now have continued to reiterate Lewis's definition. A recent study (Stern and Cobb, 1978) in keeping with Walker (1973) suggests, however, that resistance is not an essential component. There was evidence that where resistance to a ritual occurs it is to the repetition of an activity. In other words, a patient with obsessional hand-washing does not resist the hand-washing *per se* but resists repeating this activity several times.

Common obsessional themes

Obsessional ruminations and their resistance, however variable, often give rise to uncomfortable tension and anxiety. When obsessional thoughts are strongly associated with danger to others, e.g. family in a car crash, secondary thought rituals or repetitive actions, e.g. thinking or counting aloud up to a specific number, are developed as a kind of magical activity to neutralize the danger and reduce the anxiety. The content of these unpleasant thoughts and actions is partly determined by cultural, social and personal experience (Black, 1974). Common themes include ritual hand-washing to cope with harmful contamination, crippling indecisiveness, elaborate checking and compulsions to shout out obscene or blasphemous thoughts. In spite of and after years of successful resistance to carrying out an unpleasant or harmful ritual, the individual may still greatly fear that he may give way to his impulses. At another time and quite without explanation the obsessional may deliberately carry out the previously resisted compulsive act and, for example, engage in purposeful contamination (Beech and Perigault, 1974). Thus even successfully practising resistance over a period of time does not appear to necessarily make it easier to manage. An individual can be totally preoccupied with cleanliness and tidiness and yet live in the midst of indecision and chaos, or divide his house into a part which is obsessively clean to the point of medical sterility, and another part which is filthy and squalid. Finally, an obsessive-compulsive may keep his experience secret for years and somehow struggle to manage an apparently normal life.

Aetiology

Prevalence and genetic studies. The problems of the genetic aspects of aetiology are connected with the rarity of obsessive-compulsive neurosis. The prevalence in the general population was assessed at 0·05% by Rudin (1953), and Shields (1962) calculated that one in 200 adults is an identical twin. The expected incidence of an index identical twin with obsessional neurosis is therefore between 1:300,000 and 1:400,000. Of these cases 0·05% (approximately 1:700 million) could be expected to be a co-twin with obsessional neurosis if concordance were random. In fact the number of reported cases in the literature exceeds that which would be expected, but often there are doubts as to diagnosis and criteria for zygosity.

Rudin (1953) reported on 10 pairs of monozygotic twins with six being concordant. Lewis (1936) cited two concordant pairs, and Ihda (1965) reported 10 out of 20 identical pairs were concordant for neurosis. Inouye (1965) included 10 monozygotic pairs of which eight were concordant, and four dizygotic pairs of which one was concordant for obsessional neurosis. The MRC Psychiatric Genetics Unit at the Maudsley Hospital reported six cases of obsessional neurosis in identical twins, three of which were probably concordant. Marks *et al.* (1969) report the treatment of an identical twin with obsessive-compulsive neurosis whose twin brother had a similar neurosis which began at age 10 years almost simultaneously.

Psychological models. The apparent relationship in obsessional phenomena between a thought, e.g. a rumination, and an act, e.g. a ritual, has received most attention from psychologists. Rachman (1971) speculates that ruminations are examples of noxious stimuli that arise often in the context of altered mood states. Obsessionals become particularly sensitized to such stimuli and are unable to speedily habituate, and Rachman suggests that the sensitization may lead to a further deterioration in mood. Attempts to escape the unpleasant ruminations, by neutralizing thoughts or repetitive behaviours, will only temporarily reduce anxiety, and the relief will positively reinforce the occurrence and expression of both rumination and ritual. Beech and Perigault (1974) are critical of a simple 'anxiety reduction' hypothesis and are more concerned with the nature of the pathological mood or emotional state which they believe is implicit to the origin of obsessional phenomena. Beech (1978) considers that there is a defect of the arousal system so that minor alterations to incoming stimulation precipitate major defensive reactions to cues experienced as distressing or dangerous to which the individual must respond. The reaction is seen as a preventive or placatory activity which serves as a failing defence in the control of unpleasant internal states. The important implications of these psychological models relate to clinical treatment: the abnormal mood state may be stabilized with drugs; the abnormal thoughts and actions may be attenuated with behavioural treatments (Beech, 1978).

Premorbid personality. The relationship between premorbid obsessional traits and symptoms of obsessive compulsive neurosis has received much attention (Black, 1974). Slater (1943) correlated personality traits and type of symptoms in 400 neurotic patients and found the highest correlation (+ 0·76) was between obsessional traits and symptoms. Black (1974) found that amongst obsessive-compulsives there was a high incidence of premorbid so-called non-specific 'immature' personality traits and an average of 71% with premorbid obsessional personalities. But there is no predictable relationship between traits and the onset or course of obsessional symptoms.

Obsessional phenomena and other psychiatric syndromes. There has long been recognized a relationship between obsessional symptoms and depressive illness, and depressive symptoms in obsessive compulsive neurosis. However there is no conclusive evidence that patients with obsessional neurosis are more likely over a ten-year period to have any more depressive illness than patients with anxiety neurosis (Rosenberg, 1968); about 30% of both neurotic groups receive treatment for depression over this period. Gittleson (1966a, b) examined the case notes of 398 in-patients with depressive psychosis; 13% showed definite premorbid obsessional neurotic symptoms, and a quarter of these lost their symptoms during their depressive illness. Similarly a quarter of those patients with no premorbid obsessional symptoms developed them during their depressive illness, and amongst the total number of patients with obsessional symptoms during their depression the incidence of premorbid obsessional personality was twice as great, and premorbid obsessional symptoms, ten times as great, as the depressed patients without obsessional symptoms.

There is an intriguing relationship between obsessional neurosis and psychotic states and it was Lewis (1936) who aptly remarked, 'It must be a very short step, one might suppose, from feeling that one must struggle against thoughts that are not one's own, to believing that they are forced upon one by an external agency'. In psychotic depression Gittleson (1966a) found that 5% of his series made the transition from an obsession to a delusion. Rosen (1957) reviewed 848 schizophrenic in-patients at the Maudsley Hospital and found that 3·5% exhibited obsessional symptoms before or at the onset of their psychosis, and none developed obsessional symptoms during their psychosis. Rosen (1957) also found that the more elaborate and long-lived the pre-psychotic obsessional symptoms the more benign was the psychosis itself. There is no convincing evidence that obsessional neurotics are strongly predisposed to develop schizophrenia as such, but a small number may develop a mixed psychosis (Black, 1974).

Obsessional symptoms may appear as a result of various organic brain lesions or brain injury. Compulsive symptoms are classically associated with encephalitis lethargica and post-encephalitic states. Goldstein (1942) has reported that brain injured patients with personality defects also have an extreme 'organic orderliness' which borders on compulsive behaviour. Hillbom (1960) has described the occurrence of severe obsessive compulsive neurosis in patients suffering from brain injuries with epilepsy following gunshot wounds of the head. There is no cerebral localization for these phenomena.

Natural history

Goodwin *et al.* (1969) has reviewed 13 follow-up studies of obsessive-compulsives and noted that the condition is one of the rarest psychiatric illnesses, representing no more than 1% of the psychiatric in-patient or out-patient populations and no more than 4% of the 'neurotic group'. In 6·5% the onset was before the age of 25 years and less than 15% developed after 35 years.

The natural history of the condition has been a matter for some dispute. Pollitt (1957) traced 101 patients for a period of from three months to 15 years. Of the 82 patients followed for a year or more 67% had become either free of symptoms or able to lead a normal life. From this he concluded that obsessional illness has a better prognosis than is usually thought. However in the long term follow-up study conducted by Kringlen (1965) 75% of the sample were unchanged at follow up 13 to 20 years later. A 'severe clinical picture' at first admission predicted a less favourable prognosis in the study. One cannot but agree with Goodwin *et al.* (1969) that there seems to be great variability in the course of the illness. Goodwin also suggests that about 70% of 'mild' cases improve after one to five years, but in cases where admission to hospital is necessary only about 33% improved. All these studies have not taken into account therapeutic advances using the newer behavioural approach which radically affect the outcome.

Treatment

Psychoanalytic. Many consider that Freud originated the term 'obsessional neurosis' in 1895 and his views were so influential that psychoanalytic therapy for obsessional neurosis dominated the field for seventy years. Freud presented his classic account 'Notes upon a Case of Obsessional Neurosis' (known as the Rat Man) to the first Psychoanalytic Congress in 1908 (Freud, 1909). Freud's explanations of his patient's symptoms and behaviour, relying on highly symbolic word associations and the concept of regression to anal eroticism, still occupied psychoanalysts at the twenty-fourth International Psychoanalytic Congress in 1965. Some psychiatrists today would still recommend formal psychotherapy as a first line of treatment, but most would agree with Cawley's (1974) summary that:

> there is no evidence to support or refute the proposition that formal psychotherapy helps patients with obsessional disorders. The hypothesis has not been examined by methods which could produce valid evidence.

Psychological. Marks *et al.* (1975) have described their treatment of a typical obsessional:

> One patient worried that her vagina would be harmed by contact with glass or contaminating substances. To avoid such harm she checked for glass on chairs and toilet seats before she sat down, would not wear flared dresses because they were more likely to pick up bits of glass, kept her panties in a special part of her drawer away from any possibility of dirt or contamination and would not run for fear of knocking something over and breaking glass. After two weeks of treatment she said that her greatest problem would be to wear an internal tampon.
>
> She was encouraged during treatment to carry out the therapist's instructions no matter how much anxiety she felt and was assured that difficult tasks would become easier with repetition. During the first few weeks of treatment she was asked, and managed, to sit on breadcrumbs repeatedly and to touch glass and then touch the clean panties in her drawer and later wear them without checking. She was encouraged by a nurse to sit on the toilet seat without undue checking, and with difficulty managed to sit on the floor, surrounded by pieces of broken glass and with broken glass on her lap. Each day a glass bottle was broken in her presence. She was helped and encouraged by a nurse to insert an internal tampon, to keep it in place and to change it daily.
>
> Treatment evoked much anxiety and some depression. She needed a lot of encouragement and attention to persuade her to continue with the programme. However, within two months of treatment (39 sessions) her main obsessions and rituals had disappeared, and at two-year follow up there were no signs of any of them returning.

The behavioural approach just described (exposure *in vivo*), is very similar to the treatment Janet described in 1903. This leads us to ask: Why did it take seventy years for Janet's ideas to catch on? Indeed, the first impressive report of successful treatment using a behavioural approach was in 1971, when Levy and Meyer reported an uncontrolled study in which patients' rituals were totally restricted. This involved continual supervision during the waking hours by nurses who were instructed to prevent the patient carrying out any rituals. This supervision was carried out for between one and four weeks during which the patient was gradually exposed to situations which evoked rituals and again prevented from carrying these out. The relative importance of modelling and flooding was examined in a study of 10 patients by Rachman *et al.* (1971). All patients were treated in hospital, and in the first three weeks had 15 sessions of control treatment (relaxation). Over the second three weeks patients were assigned at random to 15 sessions either of modelling or of flooding. All measures showed improvement after flooding and modelling, both of which were significantly superior to the relaxation control treatment. Flooding and modelling did not differ significantly from each other. The authors suggest that this could be because both treatments act through a common factor which might also be present in Levy and Meyer's (1971) technique. What all three techniques have in common is exposure to the situations which cause discomfort, along with tacit prevention of rituals in each case.

Following reports of short-term improvement after behavioural treatment, Marks *et al*. (1975) reported the results over two years follow-up of 20 patients who were treated by real life (*in vivo*) exposure (alone or with modelling) in a partially controlled design. The patient's relations and friends were advised to refuse requests for reassurance about possible effects of *not* carrying out the ritual, and were told to reply to the patient 'I am afraid I cannot answer that sort of question'. It should be stressed that patients were asked to give permission for relatives to co-operate in this way. Skill is often needed to teach helpful behaviour to relatives without them becoming coercive or bullying.

The results of that study showed there was no significant improvement after three weeks of relaxation, but improvement occurred within the first three weeks of treatment by real life exposure. This was significantly greater than after relaxation, and the gain continued until six months follow-up.

Treatment by real life exposure with self-imposed response prevention effectively reduced rituals in two-thirds of the chronic obsessional patients. Treatment was short and did not involve continual supervision. All eight patients who were much improved after three weeks' exposure treatment remained so at two-year follow-up, as did all 12 patients who were much improved at six months follow-up. This treatment has proved so effective that patients with some types of compulsive rituals represent some of the most treatable disorders, and the 'natural history' or outcome for these patients has radically improved.

It should be emphasized, however, that we have not yet developed proven remedies for the minority of obsessional patients who have obsessional *ruminations* as their main problem. Obsessional ruminations are repetitive, intrusive and unacceptable thoughts which may be distasteful, shameful, worrying or abhorrent. Thought-stopping treatment for obsessive ruminations was described by Wolpe and Lazarus (1966) and recently there have been several reports of successful treatment involving single cases (Stern 1970; Kumar *et al*., 1971; Yamagami, 1971). When thought-stopping is given the patient is usually first relaxed and then asked to ruminate. The therapist then shouts 'STOP' while making a sudden noise at the same time. At this point the patient is told that he should cease thinking his ruminative thought at the moment he hears the noise. After a pause this procedure is repeated several times until the patient learns control over the thought. The value of this technique remains to be demonstrated by a controlled trial.

Drug treatment. Chemotherapy of obsessional neurosis has been reviewed by Sternberg (1974) and whilst obsessional symptoms often remit when present in depressed patients treated with conventional antidepressants, only the tricyclic clomipramine is reported as specifically alleviating obsessional symptoms when depression is absent (Capstick, 1975). However, there is need to assess the efficacy of this drug on obsessional-compulsive patients uncomplicated by depression in a satisfactorily controlled clinical trial.

Physical treatments. Physical treatment methods used for obsessive compulsive neurosis include ECT and leucotomy (Sternberg, 1974). Of course obsessional symptoms are common in depression and it is in these cases where ECT may be beneficial. Limited benefit appears to accrue with modified leucotomy to a number of the most severely disordered obsessional patients (Tan *et al.*, 1971). Sykes and Tredgold (1964) found that improvement was associated with a decrease in tension and although obsessional symptoms persisted in many patients they were less disabling. These and other studies of leucotomy were carried out before the advent of behaviour therapy, and today leucotomy operations are usually only carried out after failure of behaviour therapy.

Obsessional personality

Minor obsessional traits are often present within the range of normal personality and it is clear that clusters of traits like 'clean and tidy', 'perfectionism' and 'thoroughness and checking behaviour' have particular advantages both in the domestic setting and in many walks of life. Such traits are clearly valuable in diagnostic medicine and arguably essential in accountancy.

Problematic obsessional personalities in the absence of depressive illness or obsessive-compulsive neurosis rarely constitute psychiatric disorders in their own right although such people may be difficult to live and work with. Traits which usually characterize obsessional personality are excessive cleanliness, orderliness, pedantry, conscientiousness, uncertainty, inconclusive ways of thinking and acting and perhaps a fondness for collecting things.

In general obsessional personalities prefer their world to be orderly and to that extent predictable and secure. Disorder leads to insecurity and anxiety and is usually met by increased obsessional and ordering activity. It is only when these natural defensive activities break down that the obsessional personality will present for help, or develop more significant symptomatology. Thus as well as depression and obsessional neurosis, obsessional personality is associated with anxiety states, anorexia nervosa, migraine and duodenal ulcer (Black, 1974).

Gilles de la Tourette's syndrome

The rare Gilles de la Tourette's syndrome commonly has some elements of obsessional symptomatology and thus for convenience will be considered at this point. First described in 1885 by Charcot's pupil Gilles de la Tourette, today the syndrome is generally recognized by the following features: (1) onset in childhood (below the age of 16); (2) multiple motor tics; (3) unprovoked loud utterances which may progress to the forced shouting of obscenities (coprolalia) (Fernando, 1976). Although the disorder usually starts in childhood with symptoms progressing from minor muscular twitches to coprolalia or more violent movement, there is often a variable latent interval, followed by a fluctuating course in adulthood. The syndrome may spontaneously remit at any time, particularly as the personality matures, but untreated, the symptoms may be life-long and profoundly disabling.

Aetiology of the syndrome remains uncertain (Fernando, 1976). Tics occurring in children can be understood in terms of organic, developmental, emotional and mixed models (Corbett *et al.*, 1969). In adults there is often a history of emotional disturbance and familial psychiatric illness, suggesting developmental and psychopathological factors. Sweet and his colleagues (1973) analysed 22 adult cases and found that a majority had enough minor physical signs and EEG abnormalities to strongly suggest a non-specific neurological basis to the disorder.

Treatment and management of the syndrome has become more effective in recent years. Fernando (1976) has outlined three main areas of clinical endeavour. First, the use of Haloperidol (or other butyrophenone) to suppress the tics. Second, the use of massed practice techniques as an alternative or in conjunction with medication. Third, the promotion of personality maturation with an emphasis on discouraging dependence and encouraging personal responsibility.

Anxiety states

Anxiety is a normal and universal emotion essential for the effective functioning of human behaviour and sensibility. It is usually experienced as unpleasant and it has the subjective quality of ineffable foreboding. Generally it is unrelated to any recognizable threat, or the threat is disproportionate to the emotion it evokes, and commonly there is subjective bodily discomfort (Lewis, 1967). Lader (1975a) distinguishes between 'state anxiety' and 'trait anxiety'. State anxiety refers to anxiety felt at a moment in time: 'I feel anxious now', whereas trait or personality anxiety is a habitual tendency to be anxious in a wide variety of circumstances: 'I often feel anxious'. The appearance of anxiety symptoms surmounting a critical threshold of tolerance to anxiety is seen as the result of an interaction between situational and cumulative life stresses and an individual's level of trait anxiety.

Pathological or morbid anxiety can only be defined in relative terms, but is generally recognized as when a person complains of anxiety which is more frequent, more severe or more persistent than he is used to or can tolerate. In consequence he may seek medical help. In contrast, normal, but painful or uncomfortable anxiety may be experienced after separation, or bereavement, in acute but realistic stress (e.g. examinations, going to the dentist) but usually this will be tolerated without resort to medical help. It follows that there can be no minimal level or type of anxiety which is essentially pathological (Lader and Marks, 1971).

Anxiety symptoms commonly reported in the clinical setting are usually distinguished as psychological or central, and somatic or peripheral. Psychological symptoms include weakness, dizziness, malaise, insecurity and irritability, and more cognitively, dread, and most threatening, an imminent loss of control: panic. Somatic symptoms are legion but commonly include palpitations, dyspnoea, chest pain, paraesthesia, headache, tremor, fatigue, sweating, flushes, dry mouth and frequency. There are wide individual and culturally related variations of normal and morbid anxiety (Lader and Marks, 1971).

The psychophysiology of anxiety

This subject has received much attention in recent years and has been extensively reviewed by Lader and Marks (1971) and Lader (1975a, b; 1976). In essence, psychophysiology utilizes standard physiological techniques of measurement, e.g. pulse rate, salivation and sweating, electromyographic (EMG) recordings and peripheral blood flow, under conditions which ensure that the psychological correlates of the measure can also be detected. It is important to appreciate that as the emotion of anxiety is a complex phenomenon and largely a subjective experience, it follows that there is no direct or single physiological measure of it. At best what can be measured are physiological changes related most directly to somatic elements, and less directly to the subjective experience, of anxiety.

Arousal is a concept which furnishes the means for interpreting results of psychophysiological studies. Lader (1975a) defines arousal as an individual's level of behavioural activity ranging from relaxed sleep to emotional excitement. It underlies all affective states and is particularly high in emotions such as anger, panic and revulsion. Psychophysiology is only able to measure general levels of arousal rather than a specific emotion, but enables a clearer interpretation of the relationship between psychophysiological changes and emotion. In contrast to this measure of general arousal, specific arousal refers to physiological changes specific to certain emotions, for example penile erection occurring with sexual excitement.

A number of basic psychophysiological measures have consistently differentiated between anxious patients and normal controls. Anxious patients show raised mean forearm extensor EMG levels, pulse rates, skin conductance and increased forearm blood flow (Lader, 1975a). The amount of alpha activity in the EEG decreases with increasing anxiety and there are differences in dominant alpha frequencies between anxious subjects and controls (Lader, 1975a). Lader and Wing (1966) demonstrated that spontaneous skin fluctuations in skin conductance are significantly more frequent in anxious patients than controls, and have suggested that this finding reflects a greater spontaneous activity at some level of central nervous system function. Another approach to distinguish between anxious patients and normal subjects has been to measure changes associated with the onset of sleep. For example anxious patients show increased peripheral vasodilatation and greater drops in pulse rate with the onset of sleep than do controls (Ackner, 1956). Finally, a number of experiments have shown how psychophysiological measures can be quite specifically related to symptoms. Sainsbury and Gibson (1954) demonstrated that patients with aches and pains in the limbs had high forearm EMGs and contrasted with patients with headaches who had high frontalis EMG levels.

Anxious patients also show clear evidence of impaired homeostatic processes in relation to external stimuli. Normal subjects soon lose a response of pupillary dilatation after a pain stimulus has been discontinued, in contrast to anxious patients whose pupils remain dilated for some time, i.e. they showed impaired adaptation. Similarly, anxious patients also habituate more slowly to a discrete repeated stimulus than to normal subjects (Lader, 1975a).

Superimposed on all these basic parameters of anxiety is a most important cognitive component. In a series of experiments Schachter (1966) has explored the relationship between cognitive factors and states of arousal. It appears that an emotion like anger or euphoria is induced by the interaction of at least two states: high general physiological arousal and an appropriate sensory input. The quality and expression of the emotion is not inevitable but can be greatly modified by cognitive factors, e.g. anger felt, but barely shown, because of an understanding of the disadvantageous consequences of showing it.

All this evidence shows how psychophysiological techniques have primarily been used in research into anxiety states, but there is also a valuable clinical application for selected cases, e.g. EMG levels in systematic desensitization of phobic disorders (Lader, 1975a).

A general model of anxiety

Lader (1975b) has proposed a general model of anxiety which seeks to draw together the basic findings discussed above (see Fig. 2). A continuous interaction of past experience and genetic endowment produce basic internal drives. At any time internal and external stimuli are monitored and evaluated for possible degrees of threat. If a danger is perceived, a

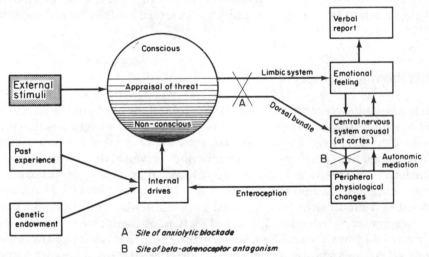

A *Site of anxiolytic blockade*

B *Site of beta-adrenoceptor antagonism*

Fig. 2 A general model of anxiety. Taken from Lader (1975b) *Medicine Series* **2**, No. 10. p. 432.

central nervous system arousal ensues which remains coordinated and integrated at all but extreme levels. The resultant affect which is experienced depends on the conscious level at which the threat is perceived. If the threat is conscious it is experienced as fear of an event, object etc. If it is subconscious, it is experienced as anxiety, and the basis of the emotion is not immediately apparent either to the subject or to an observer. The CNS arousal produces peripheral physiological changes which may be perceived as unpleasant and thus secondarily reinforce the anxiety.

Psychological aspects

Psychologists concerned with learning theory identify anxiety as an example of a secondary drive, and also as a source of secondary reinforcement. The primary drive is pain, and neutral stimuli associated with pain give rise to conditioned fear responses: the psychologist's conception of anxiety. As a continuous state anxiety has the properties of a drive in that anxiety reduction, being more comfortable, is a reinforcer and hence can serve to cause learning (Eysenck, 1969). However, as a drive, anxiety has important effects on performance. Very high or very low levels of anxiety may cause inefficiencies in performance and so affect learning. Most people studying for exams are aware of an optimal level of anxiety which aids their motivation and learning ability. Psychologists have more difficulty in explaining how minimum cues with minor fear responses (i.e. anxiety) may apparently summate into overwhelming clinical anxiety, but Eysenck believes that the failure to extinguish the conditioned fear response is related to the unusual feature of anxiety being a conditioned response and simultaneously a drive state (Eysenck, 1976).

Psychoanalytic aspects

It is generally accepted that Freud (1894) coined the term anxiety neurosis (Angstneurose) and originally proposed that morbid anxiety was due to a failure to discharge somatic sexual arousal. In a later revision Freud abandoned this specific sexual dynamic and arrived at the conclusion that anxiety is the reaction to the danger of loss of an object, or the pain of mourning as a reaction to the actual loss of the object. Bowlby (1969) has discussed Freud's contribution and drawn attention to the distinction between escape behaviour governed by fear, and attachment behaviour governed by anxiety and loss. Bowlby proposes that whilst all anxiety is related to separation experiences, major child–parent separations and disruption of affectional bonds may lead to pathological anxiety states in adulthood.

Clinical anxiety

Anxiety is a common symptom in the clinical setting and an important component of many psychiatric and organic disorders. Although it has been remarked that 'there is never depression without anxiety and probably never anxiety without depression', close examination of the nature and course of the illness together with an assessment of early life and personality features usually allows a distinction to be made between anxiety states and depressive illnesses (Roth *et al.*, 1972) (See Chapter 12 for a further discussion of affective disorders and anxiety). Schizophrenic illnesses commonly have anxiety as a prominent feature and anxiety is also variably present in other neurotic illnesses; in particular in phobic disorders, obsessional states and hysterical syndromes. On occasion syndromes of alcohol or drug dependence arise in relation to high resting anxiety or phobic symptoms.

Organically derived symptoms of chronic anxiety may be due to a constitutionally high level of beta adrenergic sensitivity, the so-called hyperdynamic beta-adrenergic state (Lader and Wing, 1971). Various symptoms of acute anxiety can be present in thyrotoxicosis, paroxysmal tachycardia, hypoglycaemia, phaeochromocytoma and toxic confusional states. Anxiety lasting a few seconds may be associated with the aura of temporal lobe epilepsy. In general, anxiety symptoms presenting *de novo* in middle-aged patients should raise the suspicion of an underlying organic disorder.

Anxiety neurosis

The patient with anxiety neurosis presents with a cluster of symptoms centred on anxiety, the source of which is usually not, or only partially, comprehended. In its characteristic form it may present as an attack of anxiety, or panic attack: an acute onset of symptoms which may last for minutes, hours or days, or occasionally become chronic. Common symptoms include apprehension, inattention, difficulty in concentration, fears of losing control or being rooted to the spot, fears of impending disaster or disease, irritability, depersonalization, derealization, dizziness, faintness, sweating, tremor, chest pain, palpitations and respiratory distress (Lader and Marks, 1971). As anxiety is a dimensional trait, mild cases of anxiety neurosis may be described as persons handicapped by anxious personality, but a specific anxious personality disorder is not recognized clinically. Prominent symptoms of anxiety can clearly interfere with effective social and everyday functioning, and when they are present a differential diagnosis of organic conditions must be considered.

Prevalence

Anxiety neurosis constitutes the commonest form of neurotic illness in developed countries, and in the UK, USA and Sweden prevalence has been estimated at 2·0–4·7% in a normal population and 10–14% of cardiology patients (Marks, 1973). One London general practice found that anxiety states constitute 27% of all psychiatric consultation (Kedward and Cooper, 1966), and for several years 8% of Maudsley Hospital out-patients have had anxiety neurosis (Marks, 1973). Anxiety states are predominantly found in young adults, sex distribution of hospital patients being equal, whereas in general practice two-thirds of the patients are women.

Genetic aspects

Many of the psychophysiological responses and measures associated with anxiety are more concordant in MZ than DZ twins, suggesting a substantial genetic influence. Family studies have found that 15% of parents and siblings of anxiety neurotics were similarly affected as com-pared with up to 5% of relatives of control groups (Marks, 1973). One British twin study found that 50% of MZ twins of anxiety neurotics had the same diagnosis and 65% had marked anxiety traits. In marked con-trast, in DZ twins concordance of anxiety neurosis was only 4% and marked anxiety traits were present in only 13% (Slater and Shields, 1969). The effects of family environment have not been excluded from these large studies, but Shields (1962) has described three pairs of MZ twins reared apart, all of whom showed marked anxiety traits in later life.

Course and prognosis

Although little is known about the outcome of mild anxiety reactions in general practice, it is probable that the majority remit within a few months. Kedward and Cooper (1966) found that in a general practice population of chronic anxiety neurosis, only 18% had recovered or improved at a three-year follow-up. Greer (1969) has reviewed systematic follow up studies of anxiety states in hospital patients. After a period of up to 20 years 41–50% of cases were recovered and much improved, and none of the studies found a high or excessive incidence of other serious physical or psychiatric illnesses at follow-up. Kerr and his colleagues (1974) have found that male patients are more likely to improve than females and that premorbid stability has an important influence on even-tual recovery.

Treatment

General. Many acute anxiety states which form understandable reactions to stress in relatively stable individuals respond to reassurance and explanation of the basis of the condition. In cases of chronic social disturbance and stress, e.g. unemployment or debt, support by counselling and social work assistance may be of value. These approaches may be used in conjunction or in combination with the techniques described below.

Behaviour therapy. In spite of the clear psychological elements in its onset and prolongation chronic anxiety neurosis is not particularly susceptible to behavioural treatments. Limited success has been gained using techniques of flooding coupled with coping and anxiety management training (Marks, 1974) (see Chapter 21). Bonn (1971) has artificially induced high levels of anxiety in patients with anxiety states using intravenous lactate infusions, a technique of chemical flooding, on the assumption that anxiety will extinguish after several trials, but as yet this experimental technique remains unproved.

Drug therapy. Drug therapy plays an important part in the treatment of anxiety neurosis, and following a careful assessment of the predominant symptomatology, e.g. central or peripheral, it may be necessary to try several drugs before the most effective anxiolytic or combination is discovered. Benzodiazepines are now the tranquillizing anxiolytics of choice and have replaced barbiturates, largely because of their increased safety in cases of self poisoning and more limited risk of producing a serious dependence problem. Great care must be taken to minimize side-effects and where there is a risk of suicidal behaviour small doses should be prescribed regularly. Long-term prescribing of anxiolytics is all too common, and every attempt should be made to minimize tolerance by moving from one drug to another. For those who are tolerant to benzodiazepines, benzoctamine, a drug which possesses both anxiolytic and muscle relaxant properties, is a useful alternative.

When peripheral symptoms of anxiety predominate beta-adrenergic blocking drugs may be considered, singly or in combination with central anxiolytics. However, as these drugs are associated with harmful side-effects, they should be prescribed only after a full assessment, and then with great caution.

Psychosurgery. Although psychosurgical techniques have been widely reported as being of value for cases of chronic intractable anxiety that have not responded to other treatments, there is still only limited evidence as to their effectiveness when refined stereotactic procedures are used (see Chapter 20). One British study has shown that 16 months after a stereotactic limbic leucotomy, 66% of patients were improved (Mitchell-Heggs *et al.*, 1976). This is similar to 63% of patients improved at least two and a half years after a stereotactic subcaudate tractotomy (Göktepe *et al.*, 1975). However both studies base their results on small samples of patients with a primary diagnosis of anxiety and the proportion improved is only marginally superior to 55% who improve after free hand leucotomy.

Phobic disorders

Fear and fears, whether general or specific, are an essential and universal component of human experience. Mechanisms of their onset, and their role in animal and human survival have been studied by many disciplines, and a detailed review has been provided by Marks (1969). Many normal fears (e.g. fear of road accidents) lead to appropriate and life-saving avoidance, whereas some fairly minor fears (e.g. fear of spiders or heights) do not lead to total avoidance of objects and situations, but are still considered within the cultural norm. However, when any fear becomes sufficiently intense to handicap the individual in his daily life, then it can be considered as a phobia. Phobos, the Greek word for fear, was also the name of a god who struck panic in one's enemies.

More specifically, a phobia is a morbid fear which is disproportionate to the stimulus, is involuntary, cannot be explained away, and leads to avoidance of the feared object or situation (Marks, 1969). Hence panic attacks commonly occur when the individual is in contact with the phobic object, and anxiety in certain specific situations may be considered as phobic anxiety.

A distinction is made between phobic symptoms and phobic disorder. Phobic symptoms often occur as part of depressive illness, obsessional neurosis, diffuse anxiety states, alcohol and drug dependence, personality disorder and schizophrenia. In these conditions the severity of the phobic symptoms is largely related to the overall treatment and management of the primary illness in which the phobia arises. Thus phobic symptoms wax and wane with mood alterations in depressive illness. When the phobia is itself the predominant feature and major cause of distress, then the illness is a phobic disorder. Phobic disorders are broadly categorized in terms of their fear stimulus, and range from the common agoraphobia (fear of open places) to the rare and bizarre thassophobia (fear of sitting idle). A full list of prefixes for the curious, and the crossword puzzle devotee, is presented by Marks (1969).

Epidemiological aspects

Several studies in the UK and USA have found that phobic symptoms are found in as many as 20% of all psychiatric patients, and phobic disorders comprise about 3% of all psychiatric out-patients (Marks, 1973). However this psychiatric prevalence appears to represent the tip of a phobic iceberg as a community survey carried out in Vermont by Agras and his co-workers (1969) estimated that the total prevalence of all phobias was 77 per 1000 of the normal adult population. It is noteworthy that severely disabling phobias only accounted for 2·2 per 1000 and fewer than 1 in 1000 was currently receiving treatment. The majority of untreated phobias were of injury, illness and death, whereas agoraphobia, presumably because of its particularly disabling nature, accounted for 50% of the treated cases (Agras *et al.*, 1969).

Specific phobias tend to be related to age. Childhood phobias are equal in sex incidence (see Chapter 5) as are adult miscellaneous specific phobias, but agoraphobia and animal phobias are markedly more common in women. Marks (1973) has speculated that this sex difference may be due to men being biologically stronger, culturally expected to be more fearless, and possibly less willing to admit fear than women.

Phylogenetic influences

There seems little doubt that both animals and humans are phylogenetically predisposed to learn certain stimulus–response links rather than others, even though all classes of stimuli may be encountered with equal frequency. Marks (1969, 1973) has reviewed evidence of certain stimuli being prepotent in triggering phobias. He speculates, for instance, that normal instinctual depth avoidance in infants may become elaborated by subsequent specific experiences into a persistent phobia of heights. Similarly, traces of innate elements of cue specific behavioural responses are seen in patients with animal·phobias; like animals themselves, they find sudden sharp movements, or snakelike writhing movements, particularly threatening (Marks, 1969).

Genetic, personality, family and cultural influences

In contrast to anxiety neurosis there is no strong evidence that genetic influences play a significant part in the development of specific phobias in particular patients. Concordance of MZ twins may be extremely rare and as yet none are reported in the literature (Marks, 1973). A majority of phobics seen in hospital out-patients have normal personalities before the onset of their illness, but there is some association between agoraphobia and a childhood history of separation anxiety (Marks, 1969). Fears, however, tend to run in families, and a minority of phobic patients have a relative with the same phobia; probably the effect of learned behaviour and modelling rather than of inheritance. Inevitably, there are broad cultural differences with regard to specific phobias, and historical changes and technological innovation have produced new object and situational phobias. However certain basic phobias, e.g. heights, open spaces, animals, illness, insanity and death, have persisted over the centuries and appear to be common to all cultures (Marks, 1969).

Psychophysiological aspects

Psychophsiological studies have not revealed specific measures highly associated with particular phobias, but they do show important differences between common phobic categories. Lader (1967) measured galvanic skin response habituation and spontaneous skin conductance fluctuation on the following groups: (1) anxiety with depression; (2) anxiety states; (3) agoraphobics; (4) social phobics; (5) miscellaneous specific phobics; (6) normal subjects, and found that habituation was slowest, and fluctuation rates were highest, in group 1 and graded down through the other groups to normal levels in groups 5 and 6. Evidence from a subgroup showed that subjects with slow habituation and high spontaneous fluctuation rates were associated with a poor response to systematic desensitization (Lader et al., 1967).

Psychological mechanisms

It is well known that the onset of some phobias is associated with a traumatic event and that the phobic object relates to that event, e.g. height phobia after falling downstairs, or a car phobia after a driving accident. Often there is a lag of several days between the trauma and the onset of the phobia and the psychological mechanisms of the time lag are not understood (Marks, 1969). In specific phobias associated with trauma, classical learning theory proposes that the future phobic stimulus (CS) is paired together with or slightly before a noxious stimulus (UCS). Conditioning occurs through their temporal contiguity, and the strength of the phobia relates to the frequency of the pairing and the strength of the noxious stimulus. Once fear causes avoidance of the phobic situation, the phobia is maintained by drive reduction and is difficult to extinguish—a form of operant conditioning (Marks, 1969). However it is very clear that many phobias are not associated with obvious trauma, or easily remembered noxious stimuli, and appear to originate spontaneously at times of mood change or emotional turmoil. In these cases learning theory provides no adequate explanation of the onset.

Two other psychological mechanisms play an important part in maintaining and elaborating phobic behaviour. Specific phobic behaviour may be *modelled* from other phobias in the family: a mechanism often seen in agoraphobia. It may also be extended through the mechanism of *sensory association* (stimulus generalization), so that phobias to single objects or situations can become phobias to many objects and varied situations associated with the original stimulus in time or place.

Psychoanalytic aspects

Psychoanalysts have long recognized that phobias generalize not only by simple sensory association, but also through symbolic cues of particular significance to the patient. Thus Freud and other psychoanalytic writers regarded phobias as symbols for other more fundamental and hidden fears. Initially, Freud considered phobias as part of anxiety neurosis, but later he separated them out as examples of 'anxiety hysteria'. Always aware of the importance of emotional factors in the onset of phobias, psychoanalysts proposed that the basic mechanism was neurotic repression arising out of mental conflict. Thus free floating anxiety associated with some basic psychodynamic problem (e.g. unexpressed fear of father's anger), would become concentrated upon an easily avoidable symbolic object (e.g. a horse), to emerge as a horse phobia (Marks, 1969). Later psychoanalytic writers have stressed that all phobias mask the real unconscious source of the anxiety. However, Marks (1969) has argued that symbolic material in phobic patients may in fact be a secondary effect of the phobia, and that abreaction of such significant material (with or without phobic improvement) does not necessarily prove the significance of the material in the genesis of the phobia.

Clinical syndromes

Agoraphobia. This is the commonest and most handicapping phobic syndrome seen by psychiatrists and makes up 60% of phobic patients seen at the Maudsley Hospital (Marks, 1969). In its narrowest sense agoraphobia (Greek root *agora*: market place, place of assembly) means fear of open spaces, but many patients also have fears of shopping, crowds, travelling and enclosed spaces. Over two-thirds of agoraphobics are women and most develop their symptoms between 15 and 35. The established syndrome has a fluctuating course related to internal and external events and may persist for many years. A majority of patients come from stable families, have passive, anxious and rather dependent premorbid personalities, and with regard to education, occupational status, income and religion are like the general population (Marks, 1969).

Many agoraphobic illnesses clearly start after a major change in the patient's life situation (e.g. serious family illness, bereavement, marriage) which usually threatens individual security, but the speed of onset may be a matter of hours following a severe panic attack, or a matter of months following a prodromal stage of vague intermittent anxiety. A minority of patients will develop agoraphobia following some major organic episode, e.g. brain tumour, surgical operation, encephalitis, or hypothyroidism (Marks, 1969).

Clinically, the patient presents with intense fear of leaving home or a secure place. In addition many patients develop phobias generalized to objects and situations associated with the outside world: shopping, modes of transport etc. Many patients are virtually or completely house-bound and therefore severely socially handicapped. Other non-phobic symptoms are very common and include general anxiety, panic attacks, depression, obsessions, and depersonalization. Harper and Roth (1962) found that depersonalization and derealization occurred in 37% of a series of agoraphobics. Previously, Roth (1959) had described a phobic-anxiety-depersonalization syndrome in which 80% of patients had phobic symptoms, and many of whom closely resembled agoraphobics with prominent depersonalization. Thus although agoraphobia is without doubt a coherent clinical syndrome, in its more diffuse forms it may overlap and merge imperceptibly with anxiety states, affective disorders and even obsessional neurosis.

Social phobias. Social phobias are probably the next most common syndrome seen in psychiatric practice and account for 8% of Maudsley Hospital phobic patients. Little systematic work has been done on this group, but it is known that 60% are women, and the illness usually starts shortly after puberty and peaks in the late teens (Marks, 1969). A third of social phobias come from broken homes, and about half are noticeably timid and fearful in childhood. The disorder usually presents as an intense fear of eating, drinking, speaking, writing, blushing, shaking, fainting or vomiting in the presence of other people, particularly strangers. Situational fears may be quite specific, like a crowded restaurant or shop, or more general: a fear of all social contact leading to the life of a recluse. Most social phobics are free of other symptoms, although depression and anxiety occur occasionally and many have a poor level of general social skills. Some social phobics deal with their handicap by recourse to alcohol or drug-taking and may develop dependency problems.

Animal phobias. These phobias present rarely and only account for 3% of Maudsley Hospital phobic patients. They almost wholly occur in women and usually the onset is before the age of seven and is often lost in the mists of childhood (Marks and Gelder, 1966). Patients tend to come from stable phobia free families, but like social phobics, a high proportion were manifestly shy and timid as children. A marked feature is the relative absence of other psychiatric symptoms, and the specificity of the phobia to the particular animal with very little stimulus generalization. Without treatment the illness has a steady course for many years.

Miscellaneous specific phobias. Whilst individual specific phobias are rarer than animal phobias, collectively this group comprises 14% of Maudsley Hospital phobics. A vast range of fears have been reported in the literature: heights, wind, darkness, thunderstorms, dolls, voices in another room, running water and even textures of cloth. Some patients may have a specific travelling phobia, e.g. travelling by plane or underground train, but otherwise find that they can travel without fear in an unrestricted fashion. The onset of these phobias is variable, the sex incidence is about equal, and the course is usually continuous (Marks, 1969)

Illness phobias. These phobias may be distinguished from the preceding clinical types in that they are phobias to internal rather than external stimuli (Marks, 1969). They comprise 15% of Maudsley Hospital phobic patients. Usually they present as intense fears of illness, centred round specific disorders such as cancer, heart disease, venereal disease, or, as intense fears of death and dying. The endless ruminations about the possibility of suffering from any of these diseases may resemble an obsessional illness, except that there is never any subjective feeling of resistance (Marks, 1969). Occasionally patients have concomitant depressive illness and the illness phobias fade as the depression improves. Other patients have fears of illness which persist independently of non-phobic symptoms, and it may be more correct to consider these as extreme forms of hypochondriasis (see p. 228). Illness phobias occur in both sexes, and the particular illness feared depends on current fashion, media influences, and cultural background.

Treatment

The treatment and management of phobic disorders has been extensively reviewed by Marks (1969, 1974). A variety of approaches is employed, and the ess ential principles are similar to those outlined for anxiety neurosis. One specific treatment adjunct may be to put agoraphobics in contact with the self-help Open Door organization as many patients benefit from this support.

Behaviour therapy. Behavioural techniques have produced the most effective therapy for phobic disorders over the last few years. In essence these involve exposing the phobic stimulus to the patient until he habituates to it and extinguishes his avoidance response. Principal behavioural techniques are desensitization, flooding and modelling and are described in detail in Chapter 21.

It appears that desensitization in fantasy is effective and superior to contrasting procedures especially for very specific phobias but less effective for patients with much free floating anxiety e.g. agoraphobics (Marks, 1974). However, flooding techniques, especially exposure *in vivo*, are effective for phobias where free floating anxiety is prominent. There is some evidence that a combination of flooding, associated modelling, and moderate doses of diazepam given four hours before sessions is particularly effective. Phobic patients with marked social skills deficits may improve with structured social skills training (Falloon *et al.*, 1977).

Drug therapy. In general benzodiazepine anxiolytics are most effective when, as described above, they are used in a specific manner in combination with behavioural techniques. There is some evidence that beta-adrenergic blocker drugs used in a similar manner enhance the effects of exposure *in vivo* (Marks, 1974). Antidepressant medication can clearly be of use in helping phobics with marked depressive features. More specifically, imipramine has been shown to reduce the frequency of panic attacks in agoraphobia (Klein, 1964). Tyrer and his colleagues (1973) have convincingly shown that phenelzine given for at least two months was significantly superior to placebo in relieving agoraphobia, the chemotherapeutic effect being apparently comparable with desensitization in fantasy.

Hysterical syndromes

The status of hysteria as a disease has been as unclear and elusive as its cause; yet in spite of constant assault, and being regarded as the most mythical of mental illnesses (Szasz 1961), hysteria 'tends to outlive its obiturists' (Lewis, 1975). It is doubtful whether there is a unitary disease of hysteria, but there does appear to be a disparate group of syndomes best collected together under its flag. Several authors have emphasized the multiple meanings attached to the word hysteria (Cleghorn, 1969; Chodoff, 1974). Kendell (1974) described (1) conversion hysteria; (2) dissociative states; (3) hysterical personality; (4) St Louis Hysteria (Briquet's Syndrome); (5) epidemic hysteria; (6) anxiety hysteria (see p. 213); (7) hysteria: a pejorative term reflecting an unsatisfactory doctor–patient relationship.

Do these syndromes and labels have anything in common? The nearest common factor appears to be the mental mechanism of dissociation.

Dissociation is used to cope with unacceptable reality and conflict, and involves a splitting of consciousness so that certain aspects of thought or behaviour are not regarded as such by the patient. A capacity to dissociate is a property of all individuals, but a propensity to dissociate may be the hallmark of hysteria. Closely allied to this phenomenon is the apparent gain to the patient that hysterical symptoms provide. Finally, within the range of hysterical syndromes are included some of the most bizarre mental states and somatic symptoms seen in medicine, providing insights into some most fundamental personal, psychological and social phenomena.

Historical development

Hysteria was first clearly described by Hippocrates, and Plato presented a classic account of the role of the uterus. Although the uterine theory of hysteria as a woman's disease lingered on until the end of the nineteenth century (Veith, 1965; Thorley, 1974), it was Thomas Sydenham in 1681 who first proposed that hysteria was a disease of the mind.

In the nineteenth century Robert Brudenell Carter described primary and secondary gain, stimulus generalization, appreciated the role of learning in symptom prolongation and in many ways anticipated Pilowsky's 'abnormal illness behaviour'. Carter's clear-headed use of social isolation and negative reinforcement to encourage the extinction of symptoms, combined with positive rewards for appropriate behaviour, matches our contemporary behavioural programmes.

Sadly, Carter's insights were outside the mainstream of nineteenth century thought, and were clearly absent during the final two decades in what has been described as the 'golden age of hysteria'. At that time, women in particular, were strongly bound by cultural expectations of sexual, emotional and social control. A common outlet and expression of a middle class woman's repressed needs and passions was illness: hysterical fits, faints, the vapours, trance states, somnambulisms, spectacular paralyses and bizarre multiple personalities. This was a society which placed the powerful charismatic doctor in high esteem, especially when like Charcot (so unaware of Carter's insights), he accomplished neurological miracles in public demonstrations. There was a popular and insatiable curiosity for literary accounts of suggestibility and multiple personality epitomized and immortalized in characters like du Maurier's Svengali and Stevenson's Dr Jekyll and Mr Hyde.

Janet, Charcot's pupil, emphasized suggestibility and dissociative features of hysteria, and gradually dissociation emerged as a crucial factor. Freud was deeply impressed by Charcot's demonstrations, and with

Breuer formulated (1893) the 'hysterical conversion' as the mechanism by which repressed emotional affect was converted into a somatic symptom. This first primitive psychodynamic, and its association with repressed sexual material, provided Freud with the basis upon which he was to develop his subsequent psychoanalytic theories. With the contributions of Janet and Freud, hysteria was now firmly within the province of psychiatry, although its multiple somatic manifestations ensured that it continued to be commonly seen in the rest of medicine.

Prevalence and epidemiology

It is not surprising that there is little epidemiological work of substance. Hysterical neurosis (conversion reactions and dissociative states) accounted for 6% of annual admissions to the Bethlem Royal and Maudsley Hospitals from the mid-nineteenth century up to the 1950s, but since then the annual rate has dropped to 3% (Hare, 1965). Stefansson and his colleagues (1976) examined psychiatric case registers in Munroe County, New York State, and Iceland, and estimated that the annual incidence of hysterical neurosis (conversion type) was 22 per 100,000 in Munroe County and 11 per 100,000 in Iceland. Conversion reactions accounted for 4·5% of all psychiatric consultations, and were most common in women, non whites, and in lower socio-economic groups. Although more common in women, hysterical neuroses are also found in men, and conversion reactions and dissociative states are particularly common amongst soldiers under stress. The prevalence of hysterical phenomena varies widely from culture to culture, and is often associated with religious and cult healing ceremonies (Ellenberger, 1970).

Genetic, personality, familial and social aspects

Slater (1961) examined 12 MZ and 12 DZ twin partners of 24 probands diagnosed with hysteria, but found no twin pairs concordant from either group. Eysenck has long asserted that in a neurotic illness, extraverts tend to develop hysterical symptoms, and there is evidence that 'hysterics' have high extraversion scores on the Eysenck Personality Inventory (Eysenck, 1958). However, Ingham and Robinson (1964) have criticized Eysenck's unclear use of hysteria, i.e. not distinguishing between hysterical/histrionic personality characteristics and conversion reactions, and have shown that whilst hysterical personalities scored higher E scores than normals, conversion hysterics were slightly more introverted than, but essentially very similar to, the normal sample.

The association between hysterical neurosis and hysterical personality is by no means as strong as traditional clinical opinion would suggest. Only 12–21% of hysterical neurotics have premorbid hysterical personalities, 16–55% have essentially normal premorbid personalities and a small group (especially men) have passive dependent premorbid personalities (Reed, 1975a). Although earlier reports indicated high incidence rates for hysterical reactions and personality disorders amongst first degree relatives of patients with hysterical symptoms, more recent studies report incidence rates of about 5%, lowest in fathers and highest in mothers and daughters (Reed, 1975a). This level of family loading is more likely to be explained by social learning rather than by a hereditary factor.

Psychophysiological aspects

Traditional clinical observation suggests that patients with hysterical conversion reactions show 'la belle indifference' or 'la belle complaisance': a marked lack of concern or anxiety about their symptoms. Lader and Sartorius (1968) investigated ten subjects with chronic conversion reactions and compared them with phobic and anxiety states, and normal subjects. The hysterics rated themselves as significantly more anxious than the anxiety states, and were more anxious than as rated by the investigators. These discrepancies between observed and experienced anxiety were supported by psychophysiological measures which confirmed that chronic hysterical symptoms are associated with high levels of anxiety. The relationship between hysterical symptoms and anxiety is further complicated by Lader's finding that symptom improvement led to increased or reduced anxiety levels in different individuals (Lader, 1974). Meares and Harvath (1972) distinguish between those with acute conversion symptoms and normal backgrounds, and those with chronic symptoms and backgrounds of personal failure and high morbidity. The acute group had essentially normal psychophysiological function (possibly to be seen as 'la belle indifference') whereas the chronic group showed many indices of anxiety. Lader (1974) has suggested that there appears to be a group of polysymptomatic neurotic patients with high anxiety levels who eventually develop conversion symptoms under stress, such that the symptoms provide enough secondary gain to prolong the illness, but insufficient to lower the anxiety level. By contrast, individuals with histrionic or more stable personalities may develop acute anxiety in response to stress, and then reduce the anxiety by the formation of a conversion reaction. As the stress is removed the conversion reaction fades without recurrence of the anxiety.

Levy and Mushin (1973) have presented detailed analyses of evoked responses of patients with hysterical anaesthesias and conclude that there are at least two underlying physiological mechanisms: (1) a lowering of peripheral receptor sensitivity, and (2) a central mechanism of inhibition along the afferent pathways. Further research in this area could provide the basis for a neurophysiological understanding of dissociation.

Psychoanalytic aspects

Following Freud's classic early work on hysteria and the establishment of psychoanalysis, most psychoanalytic writers made the distinction between anxiety hysteria (phobic anxiety) and conversion hysteria (Fenichel, 1945). The key assumption made by most contemporary analysts is that the conversion symptom, in contrast to the more vague psychosomatic symptoms, e.g. peptic ulcer, possesses specific psychic content, and may be a precise symbolic representation communicating some otherwise hidden or unexpressed intrapsychic conflict. Thus its essential and distinctive feature is the substitution of a bodily state for a personal problem.

Psychological aspects

Kendell (1974) has called attention to the importance of social learning, implicit in the sick role and abnormal illness behaviour, which is common to all hysterical syndromes. A hysterical symptom may have primary gain (e.g. reduction of anxiety, avoidance of social responsibility) and secondary gain (e.g. care and attention from others) which ensures that it becomes more frequent and persistent. Some theorists propose that hysterical conversion is a non-verbal communication that arises in the context of the doctor–patient relationship (Pilowsky, 1969; Chodoff, 1974). Kendell (1974) believes that it is those who lack an effective conventional verbal communication, or those who are in an inferior or dependent role, e.g. women, children, passive men, who are most likely to utilize hysterical symptoms and behaviour to gain their ends.

Hysteria and organic disease

There is a strong association between hysterical symptoms and organic disease (Slater, 1965; Merskey, 1978), and Lewis (1975) has noted that hysterical patients seen in neurology clinics are more likely to have identifiable organic illness than those seen in psychiatric clinics. Merskey and Buhrich (1975) examined 89 patients with conversion symptoms attending a neurology clinic; 67% had some organic diagnosis, and 48% had some organic cerebral disorder or systemic illness affecting the brain. Merskey (1978) has drawn attention to traditional hysterical symptoms which are increasingly found to have an organic basis: globus hystericus and disorders of swallowing, abnormal movements, choreas, tics, hemifacial spasm, facial dyskinesia and spasmodic torticollis are common examples.

Follow-up studies and the status of hysteria as a disease entity

Slater was in no doubt about the spurious nature of hysteria: 'If in our patients we find the signs of hysteria and no more, then these are signs that we have not yet looked deeply enough' (Slater, 1961). He brought further evidence to bear in a study of 85 young or middle-aged patients (53 women and 32 men) with a diagnosis of hysteria who attended Queen Square neurology hospital (Slater, 1965). After a nine-year follow-up, 12 patients had died and only 19 were symptom free. Most significantly, for 28 patients, a third of the sample, the original diagnosis of hysteria had been replaced by an organic diagnosis, and of the 12 who died, three had diseases that would have accounted for their previous hysterical symptoms. Finally, of the 33 patients with no significant organic disease, 13 had developed significant psychiatric illness. Slater (1965) used this heterogeneous outcome to pour scorn on the disease entity of hysteria: 'The diagnosis of "hysteria" is a diagnosis for ignorance and a fertile source of clinical error'.

For a while in the UK, any diagnosis of hysteria was evidence of bad psychiatric practice. Then Lewis (1975) reported a 7 to 12 year follow-up of 98 Maudsley Hospital psychiatric patients diagnosed with hysteria and found that 54 were completely well and working. Although some developed organic and psychiatric illness, Lewis considered that 'residual illness in those who had not recovered was remarkably close in its main features to the clinical picture presented at the time of the original admission'. Reed (1975b) followed up a further 113 Maudsley Hospital in-patients for a mean of 11·3 years and found that 13% showed only hysterical symptoms, 33% showed hysterical and affective symptoms, 28% showed only affective symptoms and the remainder were of other or uncertain diagnostic groupings. Reed (1975b) concludes that 'the 13% are suffering from a condition that can only be diagnosed as hysteria'. Thus, it appears that the latest assault on hysteria has been rebuffed.

Hysterical neurosis

Conversion reactions and dissociative states

Accepting that dissociation is the underlying mechanism in hysterical neurosis, Merskey (1978) has proposed a basic definition for conversion or dissociative symptoms as follows: (1) they correspond to an idea in the mind of the patient concerning physical or sensory changes or psychological function; (2) they are definable, if somatic, in terms of positive evidence and, if psychological, by techniques of clinical examination; (3) they are related to emotional conflict. He lists five other characteristics which may be associated: primary gain, secondary gain, a symbolic choice of symptom, manipulation of other persons and the environment, and a hysterical personality.

Thomas Sydenham said that hysteria could mimic all other physical diseases. Conversion reactions principally occur as disorders of mobility or perception. Hysterical paralysis may occur anywhere, but the muscles are usually found to show no wasting and normal tone. Passive movement of a paralysed limb may produce contraction in antagonist muscle groups, but there is no absolutely foolproof method of clinical examination which will eliminate hysterical symptoms and it may be necessary to carry out special tests, e.g. an EMG. Similarly, hysterical blindness, tunnel vision, deafness or aphonia may be established only when normal EEG changes are produced when the particular organ is stimulated. Hysterical seizures and epileptic phenomena are more difficult to distinguish on EEG examination, as some epileptics have superimposed hysterical convulsions, and non epileptics with markedly disturbed personalities can show EEG abnormalities of a paroxysmal type (Hill and Watterson, 1942). Hysterical anaesthesias are more easily established as often the affected area bears little relationship to anatomical cutaneous nerve distribution. Symptoms which are less commonly hysterical are vomiting, urine retention, pseudocyesis, blushing, diarrhoea and pain. Pain is particularly difficult to assess (Merskey and Spear, 1967).

Dissociative states include the trance states, somnambulisms and twilight states which so fascinated the nineteenth century neuropsychiatrists, but today, the main areas of clinical significance are disorders of memory, consciousness and intellect.

Hysterical amnesias occasionally consist of forgetting a specific or traumatic episode, but more commonly the patient, in a setting of clear consciousness, complains that he knows nothing of his earlier life. This lost memory contrasts markedly with a completely intact preservation of cognitive function and the ability to use learned information from the past that does not have personal or emotional connotations. These inconsistencies aid the diagnosis but it is important to eliminate the possibilities of organically based amnesias e.g. transient global amnesia. Hysterical amnesias tend to occur in patients with previous history of head injury and loss of consciousness (Kennedy and Neville, 1957). Recovery commonly occurs within a few days, but in some cases the patient may never clearly recall the precipitating events.

Amnesic symptoms may be associated with a fugue state. Here, usually to escape from a disagreeable or threatening situation, e.g. avoiding police arrest, the patient wanders from his usual environment, travels to a new vicinity or town, and may sleep rough for a period of hours or days. The patient may be astonished to find himself some distance from home and be unable to explain how he got there. It is important to distinguish hysterical fugue states from those which occur after head injury, in epilepsy, during depressive illness, and in the context of heavy drinking (alcoholic amnesic episodes). It is sometimes difficult to decide whether a fugue is simulated, an act of malingering, or genuinely beyond the patient's comprehension and control.

Treatment of hysterical symptoms associated with underlying organic or psychiatric illness, e.g. depression, usually presents no problem. The hysterical element will tend to fade as conventional treatment causes the underlying illness to remit. Hysterical neurosis, as a primary state, is a diagnosis to be made with great caution, and regular clinical review and examination of the patient will probably pay dividends in revealing a more appropriate diagnosis. Where hysterical neurosis is established, a very careful analysis must be made of the circumstances of the patient and the onset of the symptoms. Where symptoms have obvious symbolic value, psychotherapeutic techniques can be employed. Generally we cannot better the practice of Carter (1853) in setting up a regime of consistent personal management which sets out 'not only entirely to withdraw the motives for the production of convulsive hysterical action, but also to put in their place the strongest inducements for the preservation of health'.

The Ganser syndrome

Hysterical pseudodementia is a disorder in which a patient tries to give the impression that his intellectual capacity is impaired. The classic symptom is the approximate answer: a patient may answer that 2 + 2 is 5 or that a camel has five legs. Usually, careful testing of cognitive function can distinguish pseudodementia from true dementia. Ganser in 1898 described a clinical state which he considered to be a true hysterical pseudodementia. The Ganser syndrome has four clinical features: (1) the approximate answer; (2) clouding of consciousness; (3) somatic conversion features; (4) hallucinations (Enoch *et al.*, 1967). Although the crucial feature is again the approximate answer which 'passes by' the correct one, the syndrome is difficult to objectively define and may be so rare as 'to occur exclusively in gaols and in old fashioned German psychiatric text books' (Mayer-Gross *et al.*, 1969). Enoch and his colleagues (1967) point out the need to bear in mind the possibility of schizophrenic illness when a Ganser-like state is encountered.

Multiple personality

Multiple personality was common at the turn of the century and more and more bizarre forms seemed to occur in direct response to the increasing fascination of clinicians. Almost all the cases were women, and once it became general knowledge that the role of the doctor's expectations was crucial, multiple personality rapidly became rare (Ellenberger, 1970). Cutler and Reed (1975) suggest that multiple personality is best considered as a variant of a fugue state or partial amnesia in which alternative personalities are adopted. Congdon and his co-workers (1961) have emphasized the importance of role playing and report a case which shows a gradual transition from an imaginary playmate, through conscious role playing, to unconscious alternation between two separate personalities. An extraordinary and detailed report, including evidence of benefit from psychotherapy, has recently been made of 'Sybil', a lady with no less than 16 separate personalities (Schreiber, 1975). Cutler and Reed (1975) conclude that there are three basic determinants of multiple personality: (1) dissociation; (2) suggestion, including secondary gain from medical attention; (3) role playing. There is no relationship between multiple personality and schizophrenia.

Epidemic hysteria

Throughout history hysterical symptoms and behaviour have been reported as spreading, as it were by contagion, in crowds and through society (Sirois, 1974). In his classic work Hecker (1867) reports bizarre examples from mediaeval times: 'I have read . . . that a nun began to mew like a cat; shortly afterwards other nuns also mewed. At last all the nuns mewed together every day at a certain time for several hours together'; and in fifteenth century Germany a nun 'fell to biting all her companions. In the course of a short time all the nuns of the convent began biting each other. The news of the infatuation soon spread; and now it passed from convent to convent . . . even as far as Rome.'

Some light has been thrown on the mechanisms involved by detailed studies of mass fainting or overbreathing in schoolgirls (Moss and McEvedy, 1966; Benaim *et al.*, 1973). The setting is often institutional (e.g. school, convent) and there is commonly a good deal of background tension and emotional apprehension (e.g. examinations, fear of pregnancy, death of a school friend). Benaim *et al.* (1973) have noted that the hysterical behaviour is usually initiated by a powerful and subtly charismatic personality who is admired, feared or copied by other girls: a kind of unconscious pathological leadership. The behaviour spreads to younger and less strong girls, and excludes minorities and outsiders: the very bright, Jewish or black pupils. The background anxiety and emotionality creates a culture medium for dissociation; the institutional setting provides a basis for such symptoms making some kind of protest against the social order. Epidemics tend to be self-limiting, and may be controlled more swiftly by isolation of the initiators or protagonists. A splendid historical account of epidemic hysteria and its consequences has been detailed by Huxley (1952) in 'The Devils of Loudun'.

Briquet's syndrome (St Louis Hysteria)

Charcot and his colleagues were considerably influenced by the description of hysteria presented by the French physician Briquet in 1859. Over the last twenty-five years psychiatrists in St Louis have adopted Briquet's description to best account for a distinct and recognizable syndrome in women, and some have advocated that it replace conventional descriptions of hysteria (Purtell *et al.*, 1951; Perley and Guze, 1962). Women with Briquet's syndrome have longstanding multiple somatic symptoms, manipulate their doctors and generally refuse to accept psychological or psychodynamic explanations. Sexual and gynaecological symptoms are common, and most patients have a history of hospitalization and surgery before the age of 30. Conversion and dissociative symptoms are not an essential part of the clinical picture, and although many women are described as histrionic, no single personality type emerges (Perley and Guze, 1962; Chodoff, 1974). The prevalence is estimated at 1–2% in women (Woodruff *et al.*, 1971) and so far there is an apparent aversion to find the syndrome in men. It is claimed that there is a considerable genetic component as Briquet's syndrome occurs in 20% of first degree relatives of index cases, and is related to increased sociopathy in male relatives (Woerner and Guze, 1968; Cloninger *et al.*, 1975).

There is no doubting the existence of this type of female patient and the energies of the St Louis group in demonstrating its validity as a distinct syndrome (*Lancet*, 1977). Protagonists of the syndrome appear to emphasize its organic-somatic and genetic components and eschew psychological and psychiatric explanations. However, we are bound to ask, is this a new positive diagnosis with a distinct aetiology, course and treatment, is it a diagnosis by exclusion and therefore little better than traditional hysteria, or is it a new and convenient somatically orientated label which male doctors can use to legitimize a particularly common form of abnormal illness behaviour seen in middle class American psychiatric practice? At present there may be no clear answers to these questions, but it is notable that the syndrome shares many of the characteristics of hypochondriacal neuroses and histrionic personalities, and already doubts have been expressed about its validity (Cleghorn, 1969; Chodoff, 1974; *Lancet*, 1977).

Hysterical personality

Thorley (1974) has traced the origins and derivation of the modern concept of hysterical personality and shown how it relates to the changing face of traditional hysteria. Thus it was Griesinger in 1845 who first made a clear distinction between 'hysteria proper' and the 'hysterical disposition' and showed that each could exist independently of the other. Janet stressed that a major feature of the personality of 'hystericals' was their enhanced suggestibility and propensity to dissociate, but a more modern and influential definition of hysterical personality reflects the plasticity of the personality type as it abandons the mildly antiquated concept of suggestibility and incorporates the more modern one of dependence (Chodoff and Lyons, 1958).

Chodoff and Lyons (1958) list the following characteristic traits: (1) egotism, vanity, self-indulgence; (2) exhibitionism, dramatization, histrionic, pseudologia phantastica; (3) irrational, unbridled and capricious emotionality; (4) emotional shallowness, fraudulent affect; (5) lasciviousness, sexualization, coquetry; (6) sexual frigidity, fear of mature sexuality; (7) demanding, dependent. Foulds (1965) remarks, 'number eight should be a Thurber drawing of a predatory female bearing down on a timorous male psychiatrist', and indeed it is undeniable that the above description is a distorted caricature of femininity.

Apart from the enduring needs of male doctors to deal with manipulative lady patients, is there any more fundamental feature of this personality type other than the loose collection of traits described above? Jaspers (1923) presented the first description of hysterical personality which integrated observed behaviours and existential experience. He advocated the need to fall back on one basic trait, that is that 'hysterical personalities crave to appear, both to themselves and others, as more than they are and to experience more than they are capable of'. The personality is therefore like some kind of pathetic actor and all experience is contrived and forced. Jaspers points out that the experience 'is not contrived "consciously"', but reflects the ability of the true hysteric to live wholly in his own drama, be caught up entirely for the moment and succeed in seeming genuine. All other traits can be understandably deduced from this. In the end the hysterical personality loses its central 'core', and consists simply of a number of different exteriors.

American studies have found that the fundamental traits of Chodoff and Lyons tend to cluster together when measured by a factor analysis of patients self-rating their symptoms (Lazare *et al.*, 1966) and that hysterical personalities are often clinically depressed (Lazare and Klerman, 1968). However, a more recent study of in-patient hysterical personalities compared with general psychiatric controls revealed that none of the traditional traits clearly distinguish the hysterical personalities (Slavney and McHugh, 1974), and that the MMPI, whilst able to distinguish between psychotic states and hysterical personality, was unable to distinguish between hysterical personality and depression (Slavney and McHugh, 1975). Also, and in contrast with traditional assumptions, these authors found no evidence of hysterical signs and symptoms in the 32 hysterical personalities studied. We are left therefore with evidence which confirms Walton and Presly's (1973) finding that very little objective reliability or validity can be attached to the diagnosis.

Munchausen syndrome

In 1951 Asher drew attention to a type of patient who repeatedly sought medical or hospital treatment for consciously and unconsciously feigned symptoms. He chose the eponym Munchausen because of the similarities between the wandering and fabrication of these patients and the fantastic adventures and anecdotes attributed to Baron Munchausen (1720–1797). Although many authors have pointed out that the eponym is invalid as medical treatment did not feature in the Baron's adventures, and suggested alternative labels like hospital addiction, peregrinating patients, hospital hoboes etc., the term Munchausen syndrome has survived (Enoch *et al.*, 1967).

The essence of the syndrome is a dramatic presentation of the symptoms and history suggesting an acute organic emergency, leading to concentrated medical care, admission or even surgery. Asher (1951) described three basic varieties: abdominal type, e.g. recurrent laparotomies; haemorrhagic type, e.g. haemoptysis; neurological type, e.g. convincing fits, etc. Reed (1977) states that the first two varieties still account for the majority of presentations, and other presentations now include almost every symptom and syndrome imaginable, and often those of particular rarity and interest to aspiring physicians in the hospital casualty department. Reed (1977) reviews 43 cases described in the literature since 1967 and finds that the mean age is 36, the mean time of Munchausen illness career is nine years and just over half of the cases are men. Many of the patients have had hundreds of admissions in different parts of the country over a number of years and consequently effective follow-up studies are virtually impossible.

The basis of the syndrome is best seen in terms of abnormal illness behaviour, elements of institutional dependency, and the whole constituting a sophisticated form of abnormal illness career. Most patients studied in any depth appear to need to be the centre of attention, need to be passive but controlling, and need a relationship with a parental authority figure (doctor) in which they can cheat and manipulate. Thus conventional social inadequacy is turned into extraordinary adequacy as a patient! Symptoms are usually feigned or fabricated, but there may be an unconscious dynamic utilizing dissociation or conversion (Cramer et al., 1971).

Investigation and treatment only reinforce the likelihood of the patient repeating the behaviour. To turn the patient away or blacklist him only serves to aid the hospital and not the individual. The challenge remains for an appropriate medical response: to identify and isolate the underlying problems and help the patient cope with them.

Hypochondriasis

Hypochondriasis is as venerable as hysteria and so closely are they intertwined that in the late seventeenth century Thomas Sydenham considered them to be a single disease expressing itself as hysteria in women and hypochondriasis in men. Indeed, it is arguable that this inclusive concept, in the light of our insights into sick role and abnormal illness behaviour, merits a reconsideration (Pilowsky, 1969; Kendell, 1974). Originally, however, hypochondriasis was barely distinguishable from melancholy or affective illness, and became particularly associated with England and was known throughout Europe as the 'English Malady'. Although Molière's classic comedy play 'Le Malade Imaginaire' was first performed in 1693 and clearly reflected contemporary public attitudes about illness and physicians, it was not until the early nineteenth century that the term hypochondriasis became primarily associated with a morbid preoccupation with physical health (Kenyon, 1965, 1976).

The use of the term hypochondriasis is hardly less confused than that of hysteria, but whereas hysteria can be examined as a set of broadly identifiable syndromes, hypochondriasis does not easily fall into any natural categories. Thus Kenyon (1965) after a detailed review of the confused aetiology lists eighteen different uses of the term hypochondriasis ranging from a 'synonym for mad or senseless' to 'a form of schizophrenia'! However, one strict (and therefore unsatisfactory) but influential definition of hypochondriasis has been provided by Gillespie (1928):

> a mental preoccupation with a real or suppositious physical or mental disorder; a discrepancy between the degree of preoccupation and the grounds for it so that the former is far in excess of what is justified; and an affective condition best characterised as interest with conviction and consequent concern, and with indifference to the opinion of the environment, including irresponsiveness to persuasion.

Pilowsky (1967) has found support for Gillespie's definition from a factor analysis of symptoms and attitudes reported by hypochondriacal patients which identified three major factors: (1) bodily preoccupation; (2) morbid fear of disease; (3) conviction of the presence of disease with non response to reassurance.

Broadly speaking the basic nosological dispute turns on whether hypochondriasis can be considered as a primary disease entity or syndrome, or whether inevitably it is always symptomatology secondary to some other disorder, e.g. depressive illness. Kenyon (1964) surveyed 512 patients diagnosed as having primary or secondary hypochondriasis seen at the Maudsley Hospital. The vast majority presented with pain and other diffuse or generalized symptoms, and so common was anxiety and depressive illness in both groups of patients that Kenyon concluded that 'hypochondriasis particularly when as rigidly defined as by Gillespie, does not form an entity but is rather part of another syndrome, most commonly an affective one' (Kenyon 1964). In contrast Pilowsky (1970) compared 66 patients with primary hypochondriasis and 81 patients with secondary hypochondriasis and found that they differed on a variety of social and clinical variables which strongly suggested that primary hypochondriasis was a true entity. Further weight is given to the concept of primary hypochondriasis by Bebbington (1976) who has described two cases of chronic monosymptomatic psychogenic eye pain in the absence of significant depressive illness. It seems likely therefore that primary hypochondriasis is a viable entity, but it may be far less common than secondary hypochondriasis. However, in a more recent review Kenyon (1976) continues to distrust the primary form and advocates abandoning the terms 'hypochondriasis' and 'hypochondria' in favour of the more symptomatic 'hypochondriacal states'.

Kendell (1974) considers that the current concept of hypochondriasis is in no better shape than hysteria and that it survives 'because no better concept has been produced to fill in the void left by its disappearance'. Kendell (1974) proposes that hypochondriasis is best seen as learned abnormal illness behaviour and draws heavily on the ideas of Pilowsky (1969, 1978). The main advantage and promise of this approach is that learned abnormal illness behaviour may be therapeutically unlearned. Bebbington (1976) has noted that people respond to the presence of a noxious internal stimulus in a continuum from the stoical to the hypochondriacal. The extent to which people respond to this interoceptive stimulus has been called perceptual reactance (Petrie, 1967), and Bianchi (1973) has claimed that stimulus augmentation and consequent sensitivity may be programmed, i.e. by early learning experience, or be current, i.e. the effect of interoceptive focusing caused by anxiety or depressive illness. In addition to these learned components, it is likely that there is also a constitutionally endowed level of interoceptive perceptual reactance which might cause some individuals to be predisposed to primary hypochondriasis.

The vagueness of the term makes estimation of the prevalence of hypochondriasis impossible. However cross-cultural studies suggest that depressive illness is present more commonly with hypochondriacal or somatic symptoms in non-European cultures (Kenyon, 1976). Iatrogenic factors are certainly involved but are notoriously difficult to clarify. Illness and abnormal illness behaviour in families produces hypochondriasis in individuals who identify the gains and model the behaviour. Generally, it is considered that hypochondriasis is more common in men, the young and the old, the lower socio-economic classes, and those close to disease, e.g. medical students (Kenyon, 1976).

Hypochondriasis presents clinically in many forms and Kenyon (1976) has provided a detailed review of common symptomatic areas such as pain, bodily appearance, smell, eye symptoms, sexual hypochondria, gastrointestinal, cardio-respiratory, ear, nose and throat symptoms. It is well known that there can be hypochondriacal elements in obsessional, phobic and anxiety states (see p. 215), and in hysteria (particularly in Briquet's syndrome). Hypochondriacal symptoms may reach delusional proportions in depressive and schizophrenic illnesses, and there may be a hypochondriacal component in acute (e.g. amphetamine psychosis) or chronic (e.g. arteriosclerotic dementia) organic psychotic syndromes.

The term hypochondriacal personality is often used pejoratively in medical practice to signify someone who irritates the doctor with his continuous over concern with physical and mental health. Often such patients are preoccupied with patent medicines, food fads, diets, keeping fit, bowel function, and trivial somatic phenomena, frequently make medical consultations about vague symptoms, and frustrate the doctor because they do not respond to any form of conventional treatment. Kenyon (1976) has suggested that a common trait of these personalities would be concern over avoiding disease, rather than a fear or conviction of having one. Premorbid personality characteristics of patients with hypochondriasis may include the classic Freudian triad of orderliness, obstinacy and parsimoniousness, may show mild hypochondriacal traits, or, as in the case of secondary hypochondriasis, there may be no clear premorbid type.

The prognosis, course and treatment of hypochondriacal illness clearly depends on its basis. Firstly, all efforts should be made to exclude the possibility of underlying organic pathology. Secondly, if the hypochondriasis is judged as secondary, the primary illness (e.g. depression) should be treated in the conventional manner. Often in affective disorders hypochondriacal symptoms fade as the primary illness remits. In cases of primary hypochondriasis, or where there is a markedly rigid personality, psychotherapeutic techniques have been disappointing, but some success has been reported with operant behavioural techniques (Bebbington, 1976). There is no identifiable natural history of hypochondriasis, and it is to be noted that in a follow-up of neurotic conditions hypochondriasis was least improved (Greer and Cawley, 1966).

It would appear then that hypochondriasis, like hysteria, is unlikely to disappear whilst ever an ill-defined group of patients present with multiple somatic symptomatology apparently unrelated to an underlying organic pathology. Avoidance of the term hypochondriasis, whether on academic grounds or just to evade being deprecatory, usually leads to equally unsatisfactory labels being taken up like Briquet's syndrome or personality disorder unspecified. The hypochondriac's propensity for production of unexplained and ill-defined symptoms is only matched by the psychiatrist's propensity for production of unexplained and ill-defined diagnostic labels.

Origins of the concept of psychopathic personality

The history of the concept and use of what is now allegedly recognized as psychopathic personality (see Chapter 16) is an intriguing history of confusion and inconsistency. Fundamentally it is the history of a concept; attached to the concept is a procession of causal theories each reflecting the fashionable outlook of their time. The concept is in essence a disorder, or group of disorders, which falls somewhere between normality and established recognizable madness, and at the same time is strongly associated with antisocial conduct (Walker and McCabe, 1973). Seen as a group of disorders it encompasses what we now recognize as personality disorder (and not a little neurosis) and so by examining the history of psychopathic personality in particular we are inevitably examining personality disorder in general.

The idea of a range or group of disorders falling between madness and sanity is probably much older than usually supposed, and Walker and McCabe (1973) and Craft (1966) have outlined its earliest history. In spite of these early ideas it is Pinel, in 1801, who is generally accredited with making the first major statement about a 'manie sans délire' (mania without confusion) which,

> may be either continued or intermittent. No sensible changes in the function of understanding, but perversions of the active faculties, marked by an abstract and sanguinary fury with a blind propensity to acts of violence.

Lewis (1974) points out that specific features of Pinel's condition were absence of any appreciable alterations in the intellectual functions—perception, judgement, imagination, memory—but pronounced disorder of the affective (i.e. emotional) functions. However, many of the cases described by Pinel would not now be recognized as psychopathic personality. Within a few years the American physician, Benjamin Rush (1812) emphasized the 'moral derangement' implicit in these cases and how the condition might be due to a congenital defect or disease, and therefore was worthy of medical treatment. Rush also appears to have been the first to give a description of those persons with sound reason and good intellect who from early days show irresponsibility or aggressiveness, without shame, being unaffected by the consequences or regard for others (Craft, 1966). This is a description much closer to modern views of psychopathic personality.

Initially in Britain the idea of insanity or disease without a defective understanding made little impact, but Prichard (1835) cast off an earlier scepticism, and made the first major statement regarding so-called 'moral insanity' in British psychiatry. Moral insanity was

> Madness, consisting in a morbid perversion of the natural feelings, affections, inclinations, temper, habits, moral dispositions, and natural impulses, without any remarkable (i.e. observable) disorder or defect of the interest of knowing and reasoning faculties, and particularly without any insane illusion or hallucinations.

Again Prichard's case descriptions barely accord with what a contemporary psychiatrist might call a psychopath, but more problematic was his use of the word moral. The mistaken idea grew that Prichard was describing a disorder which was necessarily characterized by sinful or antisocial conduct, whereas the term 'moral' may more probably have meant 'emotional' or 'psychological' (Walker and McCabe, 1973). Whatever its shortcomings and inconsistency, the concept of a disorder of madness not characterized by psychotic features, was a considerable step forward in extending medical responsibility and practice.

In the mid-nineteenth century two other influences made their contributions to the concept. First was the identification of life-long idiocy and mental deficiency, combined with moral insanity to emerge as the term: moral imbecility (see Chapter 6). Second was the very influential but vague concept of degeneracy and atavism developed by Morel and taken up by Maudsley and others. Under the wide umbrella of degeneracy were explained idiocy, epilepsy, insanity and criminality. Thus Maudsley (1874), who was in no doubt that 'there are some who are congenitally deprived of moral sense', wrote of their

> insane temperament which without being itself a disease may easily and abruptly break down into actual disease under a strain from without or within; moral feeling like any other feeling is a function of organisation; an absence of moral sense is an occasional result of descent from an insane family.

If, here, Maudsley utilized concepts of heredity and degeneracy to bridge the delicate gap between insane temperament and disease, he also appreciated criticisms of moral insanity as 'a form of mental alienation which has so much the look of vice or crime that many persons regard it as an unfounded medical invention' (Maudsley, 1874).

These confusions were typical in the latter half of the nineteenth century and it was not until 1891 that the German psychiatrist Koch attempted to clarify the area by introducing his concept of 'psychopathic inferiority'. Psychopathic inferiorities ('psychopathic' implying an underlying physical basis) included

> all mental irregularities whether congenital or acquired which influence a man in his personal life and cause him, even in the most favourable cases, to seem not fully in possession of normal mental capacity, though even in the bad cases the irregularities do not amount to mental disorder.

Koch included both deviations and eccentricities of behaviour, and symptomatic syndromes, which we would now call personality disorders and neuroses. German psychiatrists went on to describe elaborate lists of trait syndromes for recognition of those with psychopathic inferiority. The term 'inferiority' was abandoned and gradually the neutral and organically related term 'psychopath' collected the same approbrium and meaning of the older term 'moral insanity' (Lewis, 1974).

Lewis (1974) has shown how Kraepelin grappled with classification of psychopathic states in successive editions of his classic textbook, and how he finally admitted defeat. Schneider's (1950) contribution and its present influence has been described earlier (see p. 182). Most notable has been the failure of psychoanalytic theorists to provide any cogent and valuable contributions to the concept of psychopathic personality in particular whilst clearly making important contributions to personality and character disorders in general (Lewis, 1974).

It appears that recent English-speaking contributions to the concept are no more illuminating or clinically useful than those of their nineteenth century forebears. In 1939 Henderson described the predominantly inadequate, the predominantly aggressive, and the creative psychopath. In the creative group he instanced the unlikely bedfellows of Lawrence of Arabia and Joan of Arc, and not surprisingly this category has not been taken up by clinicians or theorists. The other two categories, however, have had some influence on modern practice (see for instance Walton's typology on p. 183) (Craft, 1966). Finally from the United States, an immensely impressive and richly detailed survey of psychopathy in all its forms, reminiscent of the early literary characterologists and the descriptions of Schneider, has been elaborated by Cleckley (1976). Here the use of the term psychopathic describes a specific personality syndrome and a trait cluster present in other personality disorders, whereas more generally in the United States the term sociopathic is applied to the common British view of psychopathic personality. It is notable that before the 1959 Mental Health Act and the official recognition of 'psychopathic disorder' in its more narrow sense, British psychiatrists, perhaps reflecting Cleckley's influence, often referred to all personality disorders as psychopaths.

The current status, academic background and forensic aspects of psychopathy are discussed in Chapter 16. We might therefore leave the final words of summary with Lewis (1974):

> The conclusion of the whole matter is somewhat gloomy. The diagnostic groupings of psychiatry seldom have sharp and definite limits. Some are worse than others in this respect. Worst of all is psychopathic personality, within its wavering confines. Its outline will not be firm until much more is known about its genetics, psychopathology and neuropathology.

Personality disorder: a final miscellany

Schizoid and paranoid personality

Kretschmer (1936) first clearly identified a characteristic premorbid personality in those patients with schizophrenia and coined the word schizoid. However, since his original description schizoid personalities have been described as including the pedant, the suspicious over-sensitive, the reckless and callous, the paranoid, the shy and delicate, the fanatic, the bigotedly pious and the eccentric! Not surprisingly, within this wide sweep Bleuler (1941) and others found that at least one-third of schizophrenic patients had 'schizoid' premorbid personalities. Today, at least in general psychiatry, schizoid personality is used in a much more restricted sense, and describes individuals with a marked degree of aloofness, shyness and reserve. Many schizoid personalities are socially phobic, and others show notable introspection or eccentricity of conduct. There is no strong evidence that these introverted individuals are particularly likely to develop a schizophrenic illness.

Paranoid personality is characterized by self reference, immense sensitivity to others, and an unreasonable degree of suspiciousness about their actions and motives. The key psychodynamic is the mechanism of projection. Some individuals react excessively to the average daily experiences of life with a sense of humiliation and subjection, and thus tend to blame others for their experiences. Others develop over valued ideas, *idée fixe*, or become exceedingly sensitive to their preserved rights, vulnerable to any violation of these, and develop great tenacity in defence of them. At one extreme such people may pursue endless and impoverishing law suits for the sake of some powerfully held principle. Many paranoid personalities do not come within the realm of psychiatric practice unless they are particularly handicapped by their attitudes. Occasionally, predisposed paranoid personalities under psychological stress or in the context of physical illness develop a 'paranoid reaction'. Here there is a florid and acute onset of paranoid symptoms including delusional ideas and even greater degrees of personal sensitivity. However, such patients do not usually go on to develop schizophrenic illness, are usually accessible to rational argument, and the psychogenic nature of the disorder is evidenced by its degree of modification by environmental factors. Usually the paranoid reaction fades to leave the paranoid personality intact, but in persistent cases with marked delusional ideas, phenothiazine medication can be of value. A useful account of the management of paranoid personalities has been given by Schapira (1973).

Personality disorder: a challenge for psychiatry

Personality disturbance involves some of an individual's most unique and intangible characteristics. For that reason, personality disorders produce some of the most interesting, and some of the most frustrating, work for the psychiatrist. The difficulty in generalizing from one patient to another makes clinical work difficult and hampers effective advances in research. The value of a categorical typology is limited and our knowledge is not increased by more and more use of the term personality disorder unspecified. It is probably significant that in spite of psychoanalytic typologies being developed (Kernberg, 1970), those who are perhaps closest to disturbed personality in their everyday work, the psychoanalyst and the forensic or prison psychiatrist, most recognize the part played by concomitant neurotic symptoms, and are least likely to describe specific personality types with any degree of confidence.

Treatment, if that is the right word or concept, of personality disorder is notoriously difficult. One of the reasons must be fixed ideas in doctors' minds about the inflexibility and ingrained nature of personality features, rather than regard for the potential of individual plasticity. Another must be the patient's passive adoption of a conventional sick role with its implicit loss of responsibility and accountability. A patient in a sick role expects something to be done to him to make him better, but the truth is that for personality disorder, little of meaning can be done *to* a patient which will make any difference. There is a fundamental dilemma here, because whilst in the passive sick role, the patient himself must be encouraged to develop personal accountability, to do things for himself, and so enter into an effective therapeutic contract based on shared responsibility.

Treatment has to attend to two related areas of personality activity: 'feeling' activities concerned with the intrapsychic world, and 'doing' activities concerned with the external world of action and purpose. Traditionally, the internal world of the individual has been approached by a psychotherapist within a classic psychoanalytic framework, but it is likely that the consistency of the framework is more important than which particular frame is used. As Sandler and his colleagues (1973) have written,

> therapeutic change . . . depends, to a large degree, on the provision of a structured and organised conceptual and affective framework within which the patient can effectively place himself and his subjective experience of himself and others.

Thus various psychoanalytic schools can each provide such a framework, as can pragmatic counselling techniques, and it is even arguable that non-medical belief systems, e.g. religion, politics or scientology, may provide an adequate basis for personality reorganization.

However, therapy aimed at altering intrapsychic structure and 'feelings' must spill over into 'doing' or external activity. Similarly, therapy designed to alter external behaviours and social functioning must alter or affect internal core constructs. If traditional psychotherapy concentrates on the feeling and behaviour therapy concentrates on the doing it is clear from any detailed analysis of these techniques that the overlap is very considerable (see Chapters 21 and 22). Personality disorders are often behaviourally handicapped or socially unskilled, or have concomitant neurotic symptoms, all of which are accessible to a functional analysis and subsequent behaviour therapy or social skills training (Liberman *et al.*, 1975). This is a fashionable area of therapeutic endeavour, but if combined with attention to the patient's internal constructs and dilemmas, it would seem to offer great potential (Argyle *et al.*, 1974; Falloon *et al.*, 1977).

Finally, as has become clear in this account, personality development based on a long-term complex interaction of nature and nurture, cannot be fundamentally changed by a short therapeutic contact, or by a prescription pad. Enabling a personality to change inevitably demands a consistent therapeutic approach, perhaps over several months or years, a preparedness on the part of both patient and physician to engage in a long-term high order re-learning process. Such long-term therapeutic programmes can have even more impact if they include within the model of consistency members of the patient's family, and more distantly, members of the wider multidisciplinary team.

Personality disorder, with or without neurosis, as a medical model of social deviance, presents psychiatry with one of its most complex and controversial challenges. This chapter has surveyed the immense richness of the field, indicated the complexity of the causal factors, and pointed to strengths and weakness of the clinical response. It is to be hoped that psychiatric contributions in the future remain both medically responsible and socially realistic.

References

Ackner, B. (1956). Emotions and the peripheral vasomotor system. A review of previous work. *J. Psychosom. Res.* **1**, 3–20.

Agras, W. S., Sylvester, D. and Oliveau, D. C. (1969). The epidemiology of common fears and phobias. *Comp. Psychiat.* **10**, 151–156.

Argyle, M., Trower, P. and Bryant, B. (1974). Explorations in the treatment of personality disorders and neuroses by social skills training. *Br. J. Med. Psychol.* **47**, 63–72.

Asher, R. (1951). Munchausen's Syndrome. *Lancet* **1**, 339–340.

Baruch, G. and Treacher, A. (1978). 'Psychiatry Observed'. Routledge and Kegan Paul, London.

Baum, M. (1970). Extinction and avoidance responding through response prevention (flooding). *Psychol. Bull.* **74**, 276–284.

Bebbington, P. E. (1976). Monosymptomatic hypochondriasis, abnormal illness behaviour and suicide. *Br. J. Psychiat.* **128**, 475–478.

Beech, H.R. (1974). 'Obsessional States'. Methuen, London.

Beech, H. R. (1978). Advances in the treatment of obsessional neurosis. *Br. J. Hosp. Med.* **19**, (1). 54–60.

Beech, H. R. and Perigault, J. (1974). Towards a theory of obsessional disorder. *In* 'Obsessional States' (Ed. H. R. Beech). Methuen, London.

Benaim, S., Horder, J. and Anderson, J. (1973). Hysterical epidemic in a classroom. *Psychol. Med.* **3**, 366–373.

Bianchi, G. N. (1973). Patterns of hypochondriasis: a principal components analysis. *Br. J. Psychiat.* **122**, 541–548.

Black, A. (1974). The natural history of obsessional neurosis. *In* 'Obsessional States' (Ed. H. R. Beech). Methuen, London.

Bleuler, M. (1941). 'Course of Illness, Personality and Family History in Schizophrenics'. Theime, Leipzig.

Bonn, J. A., Harrison, J., and Rees, W. L. (1971). Lactate infusion in the treatment of 'Free-Floating' Anxiety, p. 416. Abstracts of Papers presented to Fifth World Congress of Psychiatry. Prensa Medicana, Mexicana, Mexico City.

Bowlby, J. (1969). Psychopathology of anxiety; The role of affectional bonds. *In* 'Studies of Anxiety' (Ed. M. H. Lader). Royal Medico-Psychological Association, London.

Breuer, J. and Freud, S. (1893). 'Studies on Hysteria', standard edition. Hogarth, London, 1953.

Briquet, P. (1859). 'Traité clinique et thérapeutique de l'hystérie'. Paris.

Capstick, N. (1975). Clomipramine in the treatment of true obsessional states—a report on four patients. *Psychosomatics* **16**, (1), 21–25.

Carter, R. B. (1853). 'On the Pathology and Treatment of Hysteria'. John Churchill, London.

Cawley, R. (1974). Psychotherapy and obsessional disorders. *In* 'Obsessional States' (Ed. H. R. Beech). Methuen, London.

Chodoff, P. (1974). The diagnosis of hysteria: an overview. *Am. J. Psychiat.* **131**, 1073–1078.

Chodoff, P. and Lyons, H. (1958). Hysteria, the hysterical personality and hysterical conversion. *Am. J. Psychiat.* **114**, 734–740.

Clare, A. (1976). 'Psychiatry in Dissent: Controversial Issues in Thought and Practice'. Tavistock, London.

Cleckley, H. (1976). 'The Mask of Sanity: an Attempt to Clarify some Issues about the so-called Psychopathic Personality'. The C. V. Mosby Company, St Louis.

Cleghorn, R. A. (1969). Hysteria—multiple manifestations of somatic confusion. *Can. Psychiat. Ass. J.* **14**, 539–549.

Cloninger, C. R., Reich, T. and Guze, S. B. (1975). The multifactorial model of disease transmission: III. Family relationship between sociopathy and hysteria (Briquet's Syndrome). *Br. J. Psychiat.* **127**, 23–32.

Congdon, M. H., Hain, J. and Stevenson, I. (1961). A case of multiple personality illustrating the transition from role-playing. *J. Nerv. Ment. Dis.* **132**, 497–504.

Cooper, B. and Sylph, J. (1973). Life events and the onset of neurotic illness: an investigation in general practice. *Psychol. Med.* **3**, 421–435.

Corah, N. L., Anthony, E. J., Painter, P., Stern, J. A. and Thurston, D. (1965). Effects of perinatal anoxia after seven years. *Psychol. Monogr.* **79**, No. 3.

Corbett, J. A., Matthews, A. M., Connell, P. H. and Shapiro, D. A. (1969). Tics and Gilles de la Tourette's Syndrome: a follow up study and critical review. *Br. J. Psychiat.* **115**, 229–241.

Cox, A. (1976). The association between emotional disorders in childhood and neuroses in adult life. *In* 'Research in Neurosis' (Ed. H. M. van Praag). Bohn, Scheltema and Holkema, Utrecht.

Craft, M. (1966). 'Psychopathic Disorders'. Pergamon, Oxford.

Cramer, B., Gershberg, M. R. and Stern, M. (1971). Munchausen syndrome: its relationship to malingering, hysteria and the physician–patient relationship. *Arch. Gen. Psychiat.* **24**, 573–578.

Cutler, B. and Reed, J. (1975). Multiple personality: a single case study with a 15 year follow up. *Psychol. Med.* **5**, 18–26.

Drillien, C. M. (1969). School disposal and performance for children of different birth weight born 1953–60. *Archs Dis. Child.* **44**, 562–570.

Ellenberger, H. F. (1970). 'The Discovery of the Unconcious: the History and Evolution of Dynamic Psychiatry'. Allen Lane, London.

Enoch, M. D., Trethowan, W. H. and Barker, J. C. (1967). 'Some Uncommon Psychiatric Syndromes'. Wright, Bristol.

Eysenck, H. J. (1958). Hysterics and dysthymics as criterion groups in the study of introversion: extraversion: A reply. *J. Abnorm. Soc. Psychol.* **57**, 250.

Eysenck, H. J. (1969). Psychological aspects of anxiety. *In* 'Studies of Anxiety' (Ed. M.H. Lader). Royal Medico-Psychological Association, London.

Eysenck, H. J. (1976). The learning theory model of neurosis—a new approach. *Behav. Res. Ther.* **14**, 251–268.

Eysenck, H. J. (1977). 'You and Neurosis'. Fontana, London.

Falloon, I. R. H., Lindley, P., McDonald, R. and Marks, I. M. (1977). Social skills training of out patient groups: a controlled study of rehearsal and homework. *Br. J. Psychiat.* **(131)**, 599–605.

Fenichel, O. (1945). 'The Psychoanalytic Theory of Neurosis'. Routledge and Kegan Paul, London.

Fernando, S. J. M. (1976). Six cases of Gilles de la Tourette's Syndrome. *Br. J. Psychiat.* **128**, 436–441.

Foulds, G. A. (1965). 'Personality and Personal Illness'. Tavistock, London.

Foulds, G. A. (1976). 'The Hierarchical Nature of Personal Illness'. Academic Press, London and New York.

Fowlie, H. C. (1962). The physique of female psychiatric patients. *J. Ment. Sci.* **108**, 594–603.

Freud, S. (1894). 'On the Grounds for Detaching a Particular Syndrome from Neurasthenia Under the Description "Anxiety Neurosis"', Standard Edition, Vol. 3. Hogarth Press, London, 1962.

Freud, S. (1909). 'Notes upon a Case of Obsessional Neurosis', Standard Edition, Vol. 10. Hogarth, London, 1955.

Gillespie, R. D. (1928). Hypochondria: its definition, nosology and psychopathology. *Guy's Hospital Reports* **78**, 408–460.

Gittleson, N. L. (1966a). The effect of obsessions in depressive psychosis. *Br. J. Psychiat.* **112**, 253–259.

Gittleson, N. L. (1966b). The fate of obsessions in depressive psychosis. *Br. J. Psychiat.* **112**, 705–708.

Goktepe, E. O., Young, L. B. and Bridges, P. K. (1975). A further review of the results of stereotactic subcaudate tractotomy. *Br. J. Psyciat.* **126**, 270–280.

Goldstein, K. (1942). 'After Effects of Brain Injuries in War. Their Evaluation and Treatment'. Grune and Stratton, New York.

Goodwin, D. W., Guze, S. B. and Robins, E. (1969). Follow up studies in obsessional neurosis. *Arch. Gen. Psychiat.* **20**, 182–187.

Greer, S. (1969). The prognosis of anxiety states. *In* 'Studies of Anxiety' (Ed. M.H. Lader). Royal Medico-Psychological Association, London.

Greer, H. S. and Cawley, R. H. (1966). 'Some Observations on the Natural History of Neurotic Illness'. Archdall Medical Monograph No. 3. Australian Medical Publishing Co, Sydney.

Hagnell, O. (1970). Incidence and duration of episodes of mental illness in a total population. *In* 'Psychiatric Epidemiology' (Eds E. H. Hare and J. K. Wing). Oxford University Press, Oxford.

Hare, E.H. (1965). Triennial Statistical Report. Bethlem Royal and Maudsley Hospital, London.

Hare, E. H. and Shaw, G. K. (1965). 'Mental Health on a new Housing Estate'. Maudsley Monograph No. 12. Oxford University Press, Oxford.

Harper, M. and Roth, M. (1962). Temporal lobe epilepsy and the phobia-anxiety-depersonalisation syndrome. *Compr. Psychiat.* **3**, 129–151.

Harris, T. (1976). Social factors in neurosis, with special reference to depression. *In* 'Research in Neurosis' (Ed. H. M. van Praag). Bohn, Scheltema and Holkema, Utrecht.

Harvey-Smith, E. A. and Cooper, B. (1970). Patterns of neurotic illness in the community. *J. Roy. Coll. Gen. Pract.* **19**, 132–139.

Henderson, D. (1939). 'Psychopathic States'. W. W. Norton, New York.

Hill, D. and Watterson, D. (1942). Electroencephalographic studies of psychopathic personalities. *J. Neurol. Psychiat.* **5**, 47–52.

Hillbom, E. (1960) After effects of brain injuries. *Acta. Psychiat. Neurol. Scand.* **35**, Suppl. 142.

Huxley, A. (1952). 'The Devils of Loudun'. Chatto and Windus, London.

Ihda, S. (1965). Psychiatrische Zwillingsforschung in Japan. *Arch. Psychiat. Nervenk.* **207**, 209–220.

Ingham, J. and Robinson, J. O. (1964). Personality in the diagnosis of hysteria. *Br. J. Psychol.* **55**, 276–283.

Inouye, E. (1965). Similar and dissimilar manifestations of obsessive-compulsive neurosis in monozygotic twins. *Am. J. Psychiat.* **121**, 1171–1175.

Janet, P. (1925). 'Psychological Healing'. Trans. Eden and Cedar Paul. George Allen and Unwin, London.

Jaspers, K. (1923). 'General Psychopathology'. Trans. J. Hoenig and M.W. Hamilton, 1959. The University Press, Manchester.

Katschnig, H. and Shepherd, M. (1976). Neurosis: the epidemiological perspective. *In* 'Research in Neurosis' (Ed. H. M. van Praag). Bohn, Scheltema and Holkema, Utrecht.

Kedward, H. B. and Cooper, B. (1966). Neurotic disorders in urban practice: a 3 year follow up. *J. Roy. Coll. Gen. Pract.* **12**, 148–163.

Kendell, R. E. (1974). A new look at hysteria. *Medicine*, 1st Ser., No. 30, 1780–1783.

Kendell, R. E. (1976). 'The Role of Diagnosis in Psychiatry'. Blackwell, Oxford.

Kennedy, A. and Neville, J. (1957). Sudden loss of memory. *Br. Med. J.* **ii**, 428–432.

Kenyon, F. E. (1964). Hypochondriasis: a clinical study. *Br. J. Psychiat.* **110**, 478–488.

Kenyon, F. E. (1965). Hypochondriasis: a survey of some historical, clinical and social aspects. *Br. J. Med. Psychol.* **38**, 117–133.

Kenyon, F. E. (1976). Hypochondriacal States. *Br. J. Psychiat.* **129**, 1–14.

Kernberg, O. (1970). A psychoanalytic classification of character pathology. *J. Am. Psychoanal. Ass.* **18**, 800–822.

Kerr, T. A., Roth, M. and Schapira, K. (1974). Prediction of outcome in anxiety states and depressive illness. *Br. J. Psychiat.* **124**, 125–131.

Klein, D. F. (1964). Delineation of two drug responsive anxiety syndromes. *Psychopharmacologia* **5**, 397–408.

Kreitman, N. (1961). The reliability of psychiatric diagnosis. *J. Ment. Sci.* **107**, 876–886.

Kreitman, N., Collins, J., Nelson, B. and Troop, J. (1970). Neurosis and marital interaction. *Br. J. Psychiat.* **117**, 33–58.

Kreitman, N., Collins, J., Nelson, B. and Troop, J. (1971). Neurosis and marital interaction. *Br. J. Psychiat.* **119**, 223–252.

Kretschmer, E. (1936). 'Physique and Character', (2nd edn revised Miller). Routledge and Kegan Paul, London.

Kringlen, E. (1965). Obsessional neurosis—a long term follow up. *Br. J. Psychiat.* **112**, 709–722.

Kumar, R. (1976). Experimental neurosis in animals. *In* 'Research in Neurosis'. (Ed. H. M. van Praag). Bohn, Scheltema and Holkema, Utrecht.

Kumar, K. and Wilkinson, J. C. M. (1971). Thought-stopping: a useful treatment in phobias of 'internal stimuli'. *Br. J. Psychiat.* **119**, 305–307.

Lader, M. H. (1967). Palmar skin conductance measures in anxiety and phobic states. *J. Psychosom. Res.* **11**, 271–281.

Lader, M. H. (1974). 'The Psychophysiology of Mental Illness'. Routledge and Kegan Paul, London.

Lader, M. H. (1975a). Psychophysiology of clinical anxiety. *In* 'Contemporary Psychiatry' (Eds T. Silverstone and B. Barraclough). Royal College of Psychiatrists, London.

Lader, M. H. (1975b). Psychophysiological aspects of anxiety. *Medicine* 2nd Ser., No. 10, 429–432.

Lader, M. H. (1976). Physiological research in anxiety. *In* 'Research in Neurosis' (Ed. H. M. van Praag). Bohn, Scheltema and Holkema, Utrecht.

Lader, M. H. and Marks, I. M. (1971). 'Clinical Anxiety'. Heinemann, London.

Lader, M. H. and Sartorius, N. (1968). Anxiety in patients with hysterical conversion symptoms. *J. Neurol. Neurosurg. Psychiat.* **31**, 490–497.

Lader, M. H. and Wing, L. (1966). 'Physiological Measures, Sedative Drugs and Morbid Anxiety'. Oxford University Press, Oxford.

Lader, M. H., Gelder, M. G. and Marks, I. M. (1967). Palmar skin conductance measures as predictors of response to desensitisation. *J. Psychosom. Res.* **11**, 283–290.

Lancet (1977). Editorial: Briquet's Syndrome or hysteria? *Lancet* i,1138–1139.

Lazare, A. and Klerman, G. L. (1968). Hysteria and depression: the frequency and significance of hysterical personality features in hospitalised depressed women. *Am. J. Psychiat.* **124**, 48–56.

Lazare, A., Klerman, G. and Armor, D. (1966). Oral, obsessive and hysterical personality patterns. *Arch. Gen. Psychiat.* **14**, 624–630.

Leighton, A. H., Lambo, T. A., Hughes, C. C., Leighton, D. C., Murphy, J. M. and Macklin, D. B. (1963). 'Psychiatric Disorder among the Yoruba'. Cornell University Press, New York.

Leighton, D. C., Harding, J. S., Macklin, D. B., MacMillan, A. M. and Leighton, A. H. (1963). 'The Character of Danger: Psychiatric Symptoms in Selected Communities'. Basic Books, New York.

Lemert, E. (1967). 'Human Deviance, Social Problems and Social Control'. Prentice Hall, New Jersey.

Levy, R. and Meyer, V. (1971). Ritual prevention in obsessional patients. *Proc. Roy. Soc. Med.* **64**, 115–120.

Levy, R. and Mushin, J. (1973). Somatosensory evoked responses in patients with hysterical anaesthesia. *J. Psychosom. Res.* **17**, 81–84.

Lewis, A. (1936). Problems of obsessional illness. *Proc. Roy. Soc. Med.* **29**, 325–336.

Lewis, A. (1955). Health as a social concept. *Br. J. Sociol.* **4**, 109–124.

Lewis, A. (1967). Problems prescribed by the ambiguous word 'anxiety' as used in psychopathology. *Israel. Ann. Psychiat. Res. Discipl.* **5**, 105–107.

Lewis, A. (1974). Psychopathic personality: a most elusive category. *Psychol. Med.* **4**, 133–140.

Lewis, A. (1975). The survival of hysteria. *Psychol. Med.* **5**, 9–12.

Ley, P. (1972). The reliability of psychiatric diagnosis: some new thoughts. *Br. J. Psychiat.* **121**, 41–43.

Liberman, R. P., King, L. W., De Risi, W. J. and McCann, M. (1975). Personal effectiveness: guiding people to assert themselves and improve their social skills. Research Press, Champaign, Illinois.

Marks, I. M. (1969). 'Fears and Phobias'. Heinemann, London.

Marks, I. M. (1973). Research in neurosis: a selective review. 1. Causes and courses. *Psychol. Med.* **3**, 436–454.

Marks, I. M. (1974). Research in neurosis: a selective review. 2. Treatment. *Psychol. Med.* **4**, 89–109.

Marks, I. M. (1976). Neglected factors in neurosis. *In* 'Research in Neurosis' (Ed. H. M. van Praag). Bohn, Scheltema and Holkema, Utrecht.

Marks, I. M. and Gelder, M. G. (1966). Different ages of onset in varieties of phobia. *Am. J. Psychiat.* **123**, 218–221.

Marks, I. M., Crowe, M., Drewe, E., Young, J. and Dewhurst, W. G. (1969). Obsessive compulsive neurosis in identical twins. *Br. J. Psychiat.* **115**, 991–998.

Marks, I. M., Hodgson, R. and Rachman, S. (1975). Treatment of chronic obsessive compulsive neurosis by in vivo exposure. *Br. J. Psychiat.* **127**, 349–365.

Maudsley, H. (1874). 'Responsibility in Mental Disease'. King, London.

Mayer-Gross, W., Slater, E. and Roth, M. (1969). 'Clinical Psychiatry' (3rd edn). Balliere, Tindall and Cassell, London.

Meares, R. and Horvath, T. (1972). 'Acute' and 'chronic' hysteria. *Br. J. Psychiat.* **121**, 653–657.

Mechanic, D. (1962). The concept of illness behaviour. *J. Chron. Dis.* **15**, 189–194.

Melsopp, G. (1973). Adult psychiatric patients on whom information was recorded during childhood. *Br. J. Psychiat.* **123**, 617–646.

Merskey, H. (1978). Hysterical phenomena. *Br. J. Hosp. Med.* **19**, (4), 305–309.

Merskey, H. and Buhrich, N. A. (1975). Hysteria and organic brain disease. *Br. J. Med. Psychol.* **48**, 359–366.

Merskey, H. and Spear, F. G. (1967). 'Pain: Psychological and Psychiatric Aspects'. Balliere, London.

Miner, G. D. (1973). The evidence for genetic components in the neuroses. *Arch. Gen. Psychiat.* **29**, 111–118.

Mitchell-Heggs, N., Kelly, D. and Richardson, A. (1976). Stereotactic limbic leucotomy—a follow up at 16 months. *Br. J. Psychiat.* **128**, 226–240.

Moss, P. D. and McEvedy, C. P. (1966). An epidemic of overbreathing among schoolgirls. *Br. Med. J.* **ii**, 1295–1300.

Nelson, M. M. and Forfar, J. O. (1971). Associations between drugs administered during pregnancy and congenital abnormalities of the foetus. *Br. Med. J.* i, 523–527.

Noyes, A. P. and Kolb, L. C. (1958). 'Modern Clinical Psychiatry'. Saunders, London.

Orford, J. (1976). 'The Social Psychology of Mental Disorder'. Penguin, London.

Oswald, I. and Wolff, S. (1973). The biological roots of personality. *In* 'Companion to Psychiatric Studies' (Ed. A. Forrest) (1st edn). Churchill Livingstone, Edinburgh.

Ovenstone, I. M. K. (1973). The development of neurosis in the wives of neurotic men: Part II. Marital role functions and marital tension. *Br. J. Psychiat.* **122**, 711–717.

Parsons, T. (1951). 'The Social System'. Free Press, Chicago.

Pasamanick, B. and Knobloch, H. (1961). Epidemiologic studies on complications of pregnancy and the birth process. *In* 'Prevention of Mental Disorder in Children' (Ed. G. Caplan). Basic Books, New York.

Pearson, G. (1975). 'The Deviant Imagination: Psychiatry, Social Work and Social Change'. MacMillan, London.

Perley, M. J. and Guze, S. B. (1962). Hysteria: the stability and usefulness of clinical criteria. *New Engl. J. Med.* **266**, 429.

Petrie, A. (1967). 'Individuality in Pain and Suffering'. University of Chicago Press, Chicago.

Piaget, J. and Inhelder, B. (1970). 'The Psychology of the Child'. Routledge and Kegan Paul, London.

Pilowsky, I. (1967). Dimensions of hypochondriasis. *Br. J. Psychiat.* **113**, 89–93.

Pilowsky, I. (1969). Abnormal illness behaviour. *Br. J. Med. Psychol.* **42**, 347–351.

Pilowsky, I. (1970). Primary and secondary hypochondriasis. *Acta Psychiat. Scand.* **46**, 273–285.

Pilowsky, I. (1978). A general classification of abnormal illness behaviours. *Br. J. Med. Psychol.* **51**, 131–137.

Pinel, P. (1801). 'Traité Medico-philosophique sur l'alienation mentale, ou la manie'. Richard, Caille et Ravier, Paris.

Pollitt, J. (1957). Natural history of obsessional states. *Br. Med. J.* i, 194–198.

Presly, A. S. and Walton, H. J. (1973). Dimensions of abnormal personality. *Br. J. Psychiat.* **122**, 269–276.

Prichard, J. C. (1835). 'A Treatise on Insanity and other Disorders affecting the mind'. Sherwood, Gilbert and Piper, London.

Pritchard, M. and Graham, P. (1966). An investigation of a group of patients who have attended both the child and adult departments of the same psychiatric hospital. *Br. J. Psychiat.* **112**, 603–612.

Purtell, J. J., Robins, E. and Cohen, M. E. (1951). Observations on clinical aspects of hysteria: a quantitative study of 50 patients and 156 control subjects. *J. Am. Med. Ass.* **146**, 902–909.

Rachman, S. (1971). Obsessional ruminations. *Behav. Res. Ther.* **9**, 229–235.

Rachman, S., Hodgson, R. and Marks, I.M. (1971). Treatment of chronic obsessive compulsive neurosis. *Behav. Res. Ther.* **9**, 237–247.

Reed, J. L. (1975a). Hysteria. *In* 'Contemporary Psychiatry' (Eds T. Silverstone and B. Barraclough). Royal College of Psychiatrists, London.

Reed, J.L. (1975b). The diagnosis of 'hysteria'. *Psychol. Med.* **5**, 13–17.

Reed, J. L. (1977). Compensation neurosis and Munchausen syndrome. *Br. J. Hosp. Med.* **19**, (4), 314–321.

Robins, L. N. (1966). 'Deviant Children Grown Up'. Williams and Wilkins, Baltimore.

Rosen, I. (1957). The clinical significance of obsessions in schizophrenia. *J. Ment. Sci.* **103**, 773–786.

Rosenberg, C. M. (1968). Complications of obsessional neurosis. *Br. J. Psychiat.* **114**, 477–478.

Roth, M. (1959). The phobic-anxiety depersonalisation syndrome. *Proc. Roy. Soc. Med.* **52**, (8), 587–589.

Roth, M., Gurney, C., Garside, R. F. and Kerr, T. A. (1972). Studies in the classification of affective disorders. The relationship between anxiety states and depressive illness I. *Br. J. Psychiat.* **121**, 147–161.

Rüdin, E. (1953). Ein Beitrag zur Frage de Zwangskrankheit, insbesondre ihrer hereditaren Beziehungen. *Arch. Psychiat. Nervenk.* **191**, 14–54.

Rush, B. (1812). 'Medical Enquiries and Observations upon the Diseases of the Mind'. Philadelphia.

Rutter, M. (1972a). 'Maternal Deprivation Re-assessed'. Penguin, London.

Rutter, M. (1972b). Relationships between child and adult psychiatric disorders. *Acta. Psychiat. Scand.* **48**, 3–21.

Rutter, M., Birch, H. G., Thomas, A. and Chess, S. (1964). Temperamental characteristics in infancy and the later development of behavioural disorders. *Br. J. Psychiat.* **110**, 651–661.

Rycroft, C. (1972). 'A Critical Dictionary of Psychoanalysis'. Penguin, London.

Sainsbury, P. and Gibson, J. G. (1954). Symptoms of anxiety and tension and the accompanying physiological changes in the muscular system. *J. Neurol. Neurosurg. Psychiat.* **17**, 216–224.

Sandler, J., Dare, C. and Holder, A. (1973). 'The Patient and the Analyst: the Basis of the Psychoanalytic Process'. George Allen and Unwin, London.

Schachter, S. (1966). The interaction of cognitive and physiological determinants of emotional state. *In* 'Anxiety and Behavior' (Ed. C. D. Spielberger). Academic Press, New York and London.

Schaffer, H. R. (1971). 'The Growth of Sociability'. Penguin, London.

Schapira, K. (1973). The paranoid personality. *Practitioner* **210**, 38–43.

Scheff, T. (1968). Negotiating reality: notes on power in the assessment of responsibility. *Social Problems* **16**, 3–17.

Schepank, H. (1974). 'Erb—und Umweltfaktoren bei Neurosen'. Monographien aus dem Gesamtgebiete der Psychiatrie, Psychiatry Series, Band II. Springer-Verlag, Berlin.

Schneider, K. (1950). 'Psychopathic Personalities'. Translation of 9th edn by M. W. Hamilton, 1958. Cassell, London.

Schneider, K. (1959). 'Clinical Psychopathology'. Translation of 5th edn by M. W. Hamilton. Grune and Stratton, New York.

Schreiber, F. R. (1975). 'Sybil: the True Story of a Woman possessed by Sixteen Separate Personalities'. Penguin, London.

Shepherd, M. and Sartorius, N. (1974). Personality disorder and the International Classification of Diseases. *Psychol. Med.* **4**, 141–146.

Shepherd, M., Cooper, B., Brown, A. C. and Kalton, G. W. (1966). 'Psychiatric Illness in General Practice'. Oxford University Press, Oxford.

Shields, J. (1976). Genetic factors in neurosis. *In* 'Research in Neurosis'. (Ed. H. M. van Praag). Bohn, Scheltema and Holkema, Utrecht.

Sims, A. (1975). Factors predictive of outcome in neurosis. *Br. J. Psychiat.* **127**, 54–62.

Sirois, F. (1974). 'Epidemic Hysteria'. *Acta Psychiat. Scand.* Suppl. 252.

Slater, E. (1943). The neurotic constitution. *J. Neurol. Neurosurg. Psychiat.* **6**, 1.

Slater, E. (1961). 'Hysteria 311': 35th Maudsley Lecture. *J. Ment. Sci.* **107**, 359–381.

Slater, E. (1965). Diagnosis of 'Hysteria'. *Br. Med. J.* i, 1395–1399.

Slater, E. and Shields, J. (1969). Genetical studies of anxiety. *In* 'Studies of Anxiety' (Ed. M. H. Lader). Royal Medico-Psychological Association, London.

Slavney, P. R. and McHugh, P. (1974). The hysterical personality: a controlled study. *Arch. Gen. Psychiat.* **30**, 325–329.

Slavney, P. R. and McHugh, P. (1975). The hysterical personality: an attempt at validation with the M.M.P.I. *Arch. Gen. Psychiat.* **32**, 186–190.

Stefánsson, J. G., Messina, J. A. and Meyerowitz, S. (1976). Hysterical neurosis, conversion type: clinical and epidemiological considerations. *Acta. Psychiat. Scand.* **53**, 119–138.

Stern, R. S. (1970). Treatment of obsessional neurosis using thought stopping technique. *Br. J. Psychiat.* **117**, 441–442.

Stern, R. S. and Cobb, J. P. (1978). Phenomenology of obsessive-compulsive neurosis. *Br. J. Psychiat.* **132**, 233–239.

Sternberg, M. (1974). Physical treatments in obsessional disorders. *In* 'Obsessional States' (Ed. H. R. Beech). Methuen, London.

Sweet, R. D., Solomon, G. E., Wayne, H., Shapiro, E. and Shapiro, A. K. (1973). Neurological features of Gilles de la Tourette's Syndrome. *J. Neurol. Neurosurg. Psychiat.* **36**, 1–9.

Sykes, K. and Tredgold, R. F. (1964). Restricted orbital undercutting. A study of its effects on 350 patients over 10 years. *Br. J. Psychiat.* **110**, 609–640.

Szasz, T. S. (1961). The myth of mental illness. Secker and Warburg, London.

Tan, E., Marks, I. M. and Marset, P. (1971). Bimedial leucotomy in obsessive compulsive neurosis: a controlled enquiry. *Br. J. Psychiat.* **118**, 155–164.

Thomas, A., Birch, H. G., Chess, S., Hertig, M. E. and Korn, S. (1963) 'Behavioural Individuality in Early Childhood'. New York University Press, New York.

Thorley, A. P. (1974). A survey of the origins and derivation of the hysterical personality. Unpublished dissertation.

Tyrer, P., Candy, J. and Kelly, D. (1973). Phenelzine in phobic anxiety: a controlled trial. *Psychol. Med.* **3**, 120–124.

Veith, I. (1965). 'Hysteria: the History of a Disease'. University of Chicago Press, Chicago.

Walker, V. J. (1973). Explanation in obsessional neurosis. *Br. J. Psychiat.* **123**, 675–680.

Walker, N. and McCabe, S. (1973). 'Crime and Insanity in England', Vol. II: 'New Solutions and New Problems'. Edinburgh University Press, Edinburgh.

Walton, H. J., Foulds, G.A., Littmann, S. K. and Presly, A. S. (1970). Abnormal personality. *Br. J. Psychiat.* **116**, 497–510.

Walton, H. J. and Presly, A. S. (1973). Use of a category system in the diagnosis of abnormal personality. *Br. J. Psychiat.* **122**, 259–267.

Westphal, C. (1878). Zwangsvorstellungen. *Arch. Psychiat. Nervenk.* **8**, 734–750.

WHO (1971). 'Draft Glossary of Psychiatric Disorders'. World Health Organisation, Geneva.

WHO (1974). 'Glossary of Mental Disorders and Guide for their Classification'. For use with International Classification of Diseases, 8th revision. World Health Organisation, Geneva.

Wing, J. K. (1978). 'Reasoning about Madness'. Oxford University Press, Oxford.

Woerner, P. I. and Guze, S. B. (1968). A family and marital study of hysteria. *Br. J. Psychiat.* **114**, 161–168.

Woodruff, R. A., Clayton, P. J. and Guze, S. B. (1971). Hysteria: studies of diagnosis, outcome and prevalence. *J. Am. Med. Ass.* **215**, 425–428.

Wolpe, J. and Lazarus, A. A. (1966). 'Behavior Therapy Techniques'. Pergamon, New York.

Yamagami, T. (1971). The treatment of an obsession by thought stopping. *J. Behav. Ther. Exp. Psychiat.* **2**, 133–135.

8 Sexual disorders

Paul Bebbington

Sexual disorders comprise two disparate sets of conditions, the dysfunctions and the deviations. The same social climate which fostered an early, often forensic, interest in the study of the deviations inhibited the revelation and investigation of the dysfunctions. A fair amount was known about sexual deviation as much as eighty years ago (Krafft-Ebing, 1965; Schrenck-Nötzing, 1895; Moll, 1911) and we even have reports of treatment from that period which show success rates, and indeed techniques, comparable to those of today. The liberalization of values over the last twenty-five years has led to a lifting of the legal and cultural sanctions which define deviation and has induced people to question the ethic by which persons with a deviation so defined were persuaded towards treatment. As a result of relaxation of pressures from without and within, many more such people are happy (sometimes flamboyantly so) to live with their deviation.

Liberalization has at the same time opened the door to the frank and open discussion of the problems of dysfunction (Gagnon, 1975). Its proper study dates only from the pioneering work of Kinsey and his co-workers (1948, 1953) on the range of the human sexual response and from the therapeutic labours of Masters and Johnson (1970). It is very much an area of expansion and this appropriately reflects a demand. However, one should not thereby underestimate the importance that sexual deviations are likely to have for the clinical psychiatrist for the foreseeable future. There are still, after all, legal sanctions in the UK against homosexuality under certain circumstances.

The sexual dysfunctions

Sexual dysfunction may be defined as an absolute or relative deficit in sexual performance. It may be global or restricted to certain situations; the categories of primary and secondary dysfunction refer respectively to life-long conditions and to those which develop after a period of successful performance. Couched in these terms, the very large social element in the definition is apparent. The concept of proper sexual functioning must relate to our own expectations and those of our partner and these have become more stringent in response to and in line with recent social developments; this includes a contribution from the feminist movement. Treatments aimed at improving sexual function have become much more acceptable to the treating professions both in Europe and in the US. Increasing treatment expectations and prospects have interacted in producing a proliferation of new technologies.

The human sexual response

Any attempt at understanding dysfunction must emerge from our knowledge of the normal. Masters and Johnson (1966) have distinguished four phases of the physiological response cycle:
  (1) excitement
  (2) plateau
  (3) orgasm
  (4) resolution
This classification has been criticized (e.g. Kaplan, 1976) as it does not adequately emphasize the essentially *biphasic* nature of the response. Sharpe *et al.* (1976) stress that excitement and plateau both involve genital vasocongestion leading to erection in the male, to swelling and lubrication in the female. Both phases depend upon an intact parasympathetic system. The orgasm phase is mediated by the sympathetic branch of the autonomic nervous system. Masters and Johnson (1966) were well aware that, in the male, erection and orgasm could operate each without the necessary accompaniment of the other. Kaplan (1974a) feels that there has been an understatement of this biphasic character in the female response.

In the male, there are two orgasmic stages: emission involves the reflex clonic contraction of the internal male reproductive organs and ejaculation is produced by contraction of the perineal musculature. The female, lacking the Wolffian apparatus, does not experience the emission stage and her orgasm is anatomically and physiologically analogous to ejaculation.

Orgasm in both sexes probably involves analogous afferent and efferent limbs. The female orgasm, like the male, has a clitoral (penile) sensory component and a pelvic motor component. Unless a response solely to fantasy, the female orgasm probably always involves some kind of clitoral stimulation. The Freudian idea that the process of maturation in the female involved a transfer from clitoral to vaginal orgasm (i.e. from a clitoral to a vaginal afferent limb) is not supported by evidence: it carries an imputation of neuroticism which has proved to be scurrilous and the idea is roundly attacked by Kaplan (1974a).

Although these responses are autonomic, there is little doubt that they may be brought partially under voluntary control (Rosen, 1976).

Disorders of resolution after orgasm are rare, occur as acute medical emergencies (priapism) and have organic, vascular causes, often of serious import (for instance, leukaemia and sickle cell anaemia). Failure of resolution in the absence of orgasm is sometimes a female complaint and may lead to muscular tension and irritability for some time. This is, of course, primarily an orgasmic failure.

In addition to the process of actual physiological arousal, the pre-emptive phase of desire must also be considered. Little is known about the mediation of desire in either its psychological or physiological aspects. It seems likely that hypothalamic mechanisms are involved and the presence of testosterone appears a major determinant in both male and female.

The psychogenesis of disorders in the phases of desire, arousal and orgasm contains common elements: a detailed classification is required because the conditions very often occur independently and specific treatment strategies exist.

Classification

The classification adopted here (Table I) is based upon consideration of the stages of the sexual response and of recent discussion in the literature (Kaplan, 1974b; Sharpe *et al.*, 1976; Kaplan, 1976, 1977).

The Kinsey Reports (1948, 1953), notwithstanding the limitations of methodology, geography and time, provide some tentative norms. At the time of the first report, three-quarters of the American male population reached orgasm within two minutes of penetration. Erectile impotence increased in prevalance from 0·1% of men under 20 to 6·7% of 40-to 50-year-olds, rising to 75% of the over 70s. About 1·6% of Kinsey's total sample had lasting erectile impotence. Only 6 of his 4108 males had failure of ejaculation. Kinsey *et al.* (1953) recorded that 75% of women have achieved at least one orgasm by the end of the first year of marriage; this rose much more slowly thereafter to 90% by the fifteenth year.

Kaplan (1977) has recently turned her attention to the problem of the patient with desire phase disorders, and suggests this may often be the reason for failure of treatment. Indeed, she avers, hypoactive sexual desire may often be denied by the patient who may actually feel less impotent by admitting to arousal or orgasmic failure. This condition is also that most threatening to the partner.

Table I   *Classification of sexual dysfunction*

(A) *Desire phase*
  Hypoactive
  Hyperactive
  (Anaesthesias)

(B) *Physiological sexual response cycle*

	Male	Female
(i) Arousal phase	erectile dysfunction	vasocongestive dysfunction
(ii) Orgasmic phase	absence of ejaculation retarded ejaculation premature ejaculation	anorgasmia retarded orgasm premature orgasm

(C) *Vaginismus*

(D) *Diffuse sexual phobia*

(E) *Dyspareunia*

Low sex drive may or may not be associated with diminished function in the other phases. A primary disorder of this type is characteristically associated with low fantasy, low curiosity and rare or absent masturbation from an early age. The disorder may also be secondary and often dates in both sexes from a commitment to marriage or from childbirth. It may be situational rather than global: this is obviously not a problem where it is protective of a monogamous relationship but it is most certainly likely to become one when love and arousal are mutually exclusive. As men are responsible for most sexual initiations, low desire in a woman may never be revealed, particularly where there is no abnormality of excitement and orgasm.

Sharpe *et al.* (1976) point out that the term 'hypoactive sexual desire' can be used to cover cases where there is a consistent 'turnoff' after sexual activity has commenced—the act may proceed normally in physiological terms, but be perceived as mechanical. Something similar is involved in 'spectatoring', a term coined by Masters and Johnson (1970) to describe men so concerned with their sexual performance that they watched it as if from outside themselves and were dissociated from the emotional experience.

Hyperactive sexual desire is most liable to lead to personal difficulties by causing problems to society at large, as when the chosen outlet is socially unacceptable.

Sharpe *et al.* (1976) have included genital anaesthesias within the desire phase disorders. These are characterized by complaints of an inability to feel anything during sex—the man may say he cannot tell if and when he has ejaculated, the woman that she cannot feel the penis within her vagina. These appear to have more similarities to the hysterical anaesthesias than to sexual dysfunctions.

Dysfunction of arousal in the male is termed erectile dysfunction. It may be subdivided into primary and secondary, total or partial, global or situational, and such an exercise represents an important part of assessment. It signifies an impairment of the local mechanism of erection by dilatation of the penile blood vessels and blood trapping by the vascular valves, and therefore takes no account of less local physiological changes in the excitement phase. In the female we use the term vasocongestive dysfunction again to indicate the local emphasis. In this condition, the normal vaginal lubrication and colour changes of the labia and lower third of the vagina are absent or diminished. Once more the conditions can be divided into primary or secondary, total or partial, situational or global. A common example of situational dysfunction is the man who can erect, or the woman who can lubricate whilst masturbating, but not during coitus.

The symmetry of Table I for the orgasmic phase disorders is illusory: men present because their orgasmic response is too quick, women because it is too slow. Kaplan (1974a) has suggested that anorgasmia is one extreme of a normal distribution of responsivity, the other extreme being the ability to have orgasms in response to fantasy alone. Once more the primary and secondary, and generalized and situational dichotomies are very important. Retarded orgasm can be applied to cases where high states of arousal are accompanied by an unpleasant feeling of tension and require an inordinate time for orgasmic discharge.

Vaginismus is a prerogative of those who possess the Mullerian apparatus and as such has no analogue in the male. It is characterized by a conditioned spasm of the muscles surrounding the vaginal introitus and is independent of desire, excitement or orgasm. It is perfectly compatible with orgasm unaccompanied by penetration. Diffuse sexual phobia is another, but extremely rare, conditioned response which may be so generalized that the woman cannot bear to be touched, even by a child. Dyspareunia is genital pain during penetration and likewise is unrelated to the three phases of sexual response. It may occur in either sex and is very often the result of a physical illness or local inflammatory condition.

In this classification we have deliberately omitted three categories suggested by Sharpe *et al.* (1976), namely: (1) disturbance of sexual satisfaction; (2) distress concerning sexual functioning associated with false beliefs or lack of sexual knowledge; and (3) 'sociosexual distress'. Disturbances of sexual satisfaction cross all boundaries of dysfunction and are best looked upon as a necessary aspect for assessment for all sexual impairments. Where the second category co-exists with lowered sexual performance, it can be classified elsewhere, and where it does not it cannot really be held to be a disorder of sexual functioning. The third category includes sexual incompatibility between partners and the inability to form compatible affiliations or satisfying sexual relationships. It seems an unnecessary over-generalization to include cases where this does not absolutely relate to sexual functioning.

The importance of exercising such restrictions upon the domain of sexual disorders is that limitation to focal conditions comprehends dysfunctions with the common property of response to focal treatments. Moreover, there is evidence that their specific nature is not an imposed one: hence Munjack and Staples (1976) found that anorgasmic women attending a sex clinic could not be distinguished from normals on a battery of tests which included the MMPI, the EPI, and a symptom checklist, except in being more depressed. The primary and secondary groups were indistinguishable.

Aetiology

The distinction between orgasmic and psychological causes of sexual dysfunction is paramount for the sex therapist. The oft-quoted figure of 90% for the proportion of cases of psychogenic cause appears to date back to an unsubstantiated statement by Strauss (1950). As Levine (1976) sensibly points out, this figure will depend upon the population for which cases are drawn: organic causes are likely to preponderate, for instance, in a diabetic clinic. Sex therapy is obviously inappropriate for the organic causes listed in Table II: it may occasionally be used adjunctively in cases where the origin is a primary psychiatric disorder.

In many cases organic factors influence sexual functioning in a complex way, producing different patterns of disorder of desire, arousal and orgasm. Some organic causes specifically affect the arousal and orgasm phases, hence diabetes, an important contributor, may affect all phases by a temporary metabolic imbalance; through an autonomic neuropathy, it operates specifically on arousal and orgasm: this is usually a chronic complication, but may nevertheless be a presenting symptom. Many drugs affect the arousal and orgasm phases: adrenergic neurone blocking drugs like guanethidine produce a dissociated erectile dysfunction whilst ganglion blocking agents may lead only to failure of ejaculation. An

Table II *Organic and psychiatric causes of dysfunction*

	Chromosomal	Genetic	Congenital	Endocrine	Drugs	Drug Abuse
Desire phase	Klinefelter's Syndrome; Turner's Syndrome	Testicular feminization.		Acromegaly; Addison's Disease; primary and secondary hypogonadism; thyroid imbalance; diabetes.	Benperidol and neuroleptics; cyproterone; spironolactone; oestrogen; methadone; antabuse.	Opiates; alcohol; cocaine; amphetamines; barbiturates.
Arousal and orgasm	As above.	As above.	Local anatomical abnormalities.	As above plus diabetic autonomic neuropathy.	As above plus MAOIs; Tricyclic antidepressants; anticholinergic drugs; guanethidine; reserpine; methyldopa; ganglion blocking drugs.	As above.

(*continued*)

Table II *Organic and psychiatric causes of dysfunction (continued)*

	Surgery and radiotherapy	Trauma	Vascular	System failure	Neurological	Idiopathic	Pychiatric
Desire phase		Castration.		Cardiac; hepatic; renal; respiratory.	Epilepsy, particularly of temporal lobe.	Ageing.	Depression; agoraphobia; anxiety states; obsessional neurosis; hysterical personality; sexual deviations.
Arousal and orgasm	Perineal prostatectomy; aortofemoral by pass; sympathectomy; therapeutic irradiation of the pelvis.	Castration; cord fracture; pelvic fracture; penile trauma.	Disease of terminal aorta and iliac arteries.	As above.	Many including: B12 deficiency and multiple sclerosis.	Ageing.	As above.

extensive and detailed, albeit somewhat tentative list of organic causes and their particular supposed effects is given by Kaplan (1974a).

The psychological causes of sexual dysfunction have not been submitted to systematic study and are conjectural. Indirect and soft data arise from attempts at modification—the success of a technique suggests the analysis which led to its use is likely to be at least partially true, whilst failure may imply an inadequate formulation (Brady, 1976). In this way, the current powerful techniques enable us to make tentative aetiological suggestions.

The following schema owes much to Kaplan (1974a). The immediate causes of sexual dysfunction can be due to failure to engage in effective sexual behaviour, to anxiety or to perceptual or intellectual blocks. Ineffective sexual behaviour, that is, poor or insensitive technique, can arise from ignorance of what to do or of what one's partner likes or from actual avoidance of good sex for a variety of reasons. Sexual anxiety emerges essentially from fear of failure, whether due to inexperience, excessive demands or an excessive need to please the partner. This leads to a vicious circle of declining performance, but it should be emphasized that not all men respond to failure in this way. Perceptual and intellectual blocks against sexual functioning include the phenomenon of 'spectatoring' mentioned above.

These proximal causes of dysfunction in turn arise from distal elements. These may be characterized as due to trauma, difficulties with the current relationship or the result of early experience. Traumatic causes are often apparent in the history of those with dysfunction, ranging from rape to heavy sarcasm. The sexual and general aspects of any sexual relationship effect a powerful reciprocal influence, a situation in which causes become consequences and consequences causes—an appropriate allocation of significance is not always possible and there are both cases in which the sexual aspect can only be modified by change in the general interaction and those where the reverse pertains. It is of interest that McGovern *et al.* (1975) found that general problems with the relationship were more salient in cases of secondary as opposed to primary dysfunction.

The effect of early experiences can be convincing in individual cases of dysfunction. The obvious psychoanalytic interpretations rest upon the oedipus complex and preoedipal relations with the mother, offering an explanation in (infantile) sexual terms. It seems equally likely that nonsexual factors are important, that is, those factors which influence the development of trustful and committed relationships, for which an analogue may be perceived in the sexual difficulties of Harlow's isolated monkeys. Sex therapy does not illumine early learning, being directed essentially at the here and now, although Kaplan (1974a) uses the information arising from difficulties in therapy to explore early factors.

Assessment

Psychogenic causes are not admitted solely by exclusion of organic factors—the allocation of cause must be based on a total assessment of the patient's history (Levine, 1976). The nature and contingency of the impairment must be established: whether partial or total, constant or episodic, or restricted to certain circumstances. This information must be viewed in the context of the patient's total situation including any recent events of importance. Certain problems of dysfunction are highly suggestive of psychogenesis, for instance, the retained ability to obtain firm erections as in response to a full bladder on waking indicates intact vascular and neurological mechanisms. A detailed history of physical health and drug usage must be followed by a clinical examination. The full history leads the clinician to intelligent deployment of further investigation. The urine of every patient should be tested, although it is questionable whether a glucose tolerance test should always follow. Other endocrine investigations, karyotyping and vascular tests should be based on positive clinical findings. Autonomic neuropathy should not be blamed for diabetic impotence unless there are other signs of it. In the male adjuvant investigations are sometimes available, such as measurement of penile blood pressure (Gaskell, 1971) and strain gauge assessment of nocturnal erections (Karacan, 1970), and early results of psychometric discriminations have been published (Derogatis et al., 1976; Beutler et al., 1975). There remain, of course, cases in which organic and psychogenic factors are both major contributors.

If it becomes apparent that the dysfunction is caused by psychological factors, directive sex therapy may be advised. Usually this is aimed at people with a stable relationship although those without current partners can also be treated. Additional assessment is required of the following:

(1) The level of the subject's social skills
(2) The nature of the relationship. This must include patterns of behaviour and the 'covert contracts' which each partner makes, the private decisions about what each is prepared to give to the relationship and what each expects from it
(3) The causes of disagreement and its relationship to sexual activity
(4) The relationship of anxiety to sexual performance
(5) The extent of sexual knowledge of each partner
(6) The feelings and attitudes of each towards sexual activity
(7) Problems of technique: what is done, what each would like to do, and what each would like to have done

This information can be obtained in separate or joint interviews. Sex therapy, although in essence of pragmatic derivation, shares many aspects with behaviour therapy and likewise insists upon objectified measures of change. Obvious taboos normally preclude direct measures of change although these are available—vaginal photoplethysmography, for example. Obler (1973) argues for the use of direct measures casting the widest possible net, including psychophysiological criteria and the subjective accounts of both patient and partner. This does, of course, sometimes make for difficulties of interpretation where indices of change do not cohere. Assessment of treatment is probably less contaminated if structured instruments are used and these have been described, for instance by McGovern *et al.* (1975).

Treatment

Over the last twenty years, the directive approach to the therapy of psychogenic sexual dysfunction has become standard (Masters and Johnson, 1970; Kaplan, 1974a; Gillan and Gillan, 1976). Crowe's work (1973) suggests directive techniques are better for dealing with specific sexual difficulties. In the treatment of impotence and frigidity, the largest series is the uncontrolled one of Masters and Johnson (1970) of over 500 couples. They recommend that the couple is treated, rather than the individual, and two therapists are employed. The treatment is a complex package involving commitment to change, education and performance with feedback in a holiday atmosphere. Therapists act as referees and directors, mediators and educators.

The first part of treatment is an exploration of sexual attitudes which may need to be modified by education, interpretation and suggestion. This precedes sensate focus in which partners caress each other in the nude with a ban on intercourse. Then the partners go on to treatment of the specific dysfunction (see Table III). 'Graded stimulation' involves the gradual learning of a progression of sexual stimulation in a non-demanding and anxiety-free situation. Emphasis is placed upon the experience of sensation rather than a conscious progress towards orgasm. In the treatment of premature ejaculation the male withdraws as he feels

Table III   (*From Masters and Johnson, 1970*)

Problem	Specific treatment	Results
erectile impotence ⎱ anorgasmia ⎰	graded stimulation	1°–59%, 2°–74% 81%
premature ejaculation	squeeze technique	98%
vaginismus	graded dilators	100% for penetration 90% for orgasm
ejaculatory failure	superstimulation	82%

orgasm approaching and the female gives a firm squeeze to the glans penis which prevents the orgasm; intercourse is resumed and the time to orgasm is gradually built up. This is the so-called 'squeeze technique'. It is possible that biofeedback may add to the armamentarium against premature ejaculation. 'Superstimulation' in the treatment of ejaculatory failure requires the female partner firstly to masturbate the male to ejaculation, thus associating her with the event, and then proceeding to penetration at a point of near orgasm.

Since the work of Masters and Johnson (1970), there have been a number of developments. Hence both Lopiccolo and Lobitz (1972) and Annon (1975) describe the adjunctive use of masturbation in the treatment of dysfunction in slightly differing programmes. In most people the application of an 80 c.p.s. vibrator to the clitoris or to the underside of the penis at a point just proximal to the frenular attachment will produce arousal and orgasm. This is being investigated on an *ad hoc* basis in the treatment of dysfunction although the mechanisms of any improvement is likely to be complex, involving orgasmic facilitation, anxiety reduction and cognitive and attitudinal changes. 'Electricity has revolutionised housework; perhaps it will revolutionise sex' (Gillan and Gillan, 1976).

Low levels of sexual drive may be primary or secondary to disorders of arousal and orgasm. Certainly many clients with sexual problems have a poor fantasy life. Masters and Johnson (1970) describe 'stimulation therapy'—the use of pornography to increase drive and expand repertoire. Sexual Attitude Restructuring (SAR) is a similar programme, aimed mainly at sex professionals, in the National Sex Forum in California. For an hour the trainees watch eight to twelve films at a time cast onto the walls of a large room and displaying the whole range of sexually (relatively) normal activity.

Masters and Johnson (1970) describe the use of surrogates in the treatment of persons without a sexual partner and in some treatment centres these are used quite extensively. Surrogates work closely with sex therapists although there is debate over whether they should be vehicles of balm or of analysis. An interesting account of the difficulties and responsibilities of such work is given by Greene (1977). (One anticipates the early establishment of a professional body.)

Results of treatment

The magnum opus of Masters and Johnson (1970) was uncontrolled. Since that time there have been controlled studies which have established the efficacy of sex therapy and teased out the effective components (Obler, 1973; Kockott *et al.*, 1975; Wincze and Caird, 1976; Munjack *et al.*,

1976). There have also been strenuous attempts to resolve the confusion arising from the proliferation of strategies, heterogeneity of technique and an escalation of reports of varying calibre (Segraves, 1976; Munjack and Kanno, 1976, 1977).

Munjack and Kanno (1977) give a highly structured review of the prognosis of treatment in the female in which they attempt to quantify the weight which can be placed upon inferences from the literature. They put most faith in the opinion that behavioural approaches involving education, retraining and other strategies broadly based on learning principles have substantially improved prognosis and shortened therapy time. Some of their more modestly supported conclusions are listed in Table IV.

Table IV *Prognostic factors in female sexual inhibition (based on Munjack and Kanno, 1977)*

	Good prognosis	Bad prognosis	Not clearly indicative
Aetiology	Misinformation Acute situational stress		
Symptomatic factors	Mild symptoms Symptoms of short duration.	Extensive non-sexual psychopathology including anxiety phobias and obsessions.	
Marital	Good relationship	Hostility to spouse	Non-symptomatic spouse
Treatment factors		Hostility to therapist (!)	Treatment of individual *vs.* couple Presence of husband during treatment Dual-sex therapy team

Studies reporting pure systematic desensitization have very low or indeed non-existent success rates (Kockott *et al.*, 1975; Wincze and Caird, 1976) whilst broad-based programmes (Obler, 1973, Munjack *et al.*, 1976) report results as good as those of Masters and Johnson (1970). Segraves (1976) has concluded in his review of primary orgasmic dysfunction that systematic desensitization does not contribute to the efficacy of sex therapy and the essential component is likely to reside in a graded and a controlled progression towards anxiety free intercourse: 'homework'. The influence of the marital context upon treatment possibly underlies the finding of McGovern *et al.* (1975). These workers offered a flexible and time limited programme to women with primary and secondary anorgasmia. The primary group did very well; the sexual functioning of the secondary group did not improve in the time available for treatment although their overall marital relationship did. It would seem that the presence of the husband during treatment only aided those cases in which marital discord is an important factor in the dysfunction.

Sexual deviation

There is no succinct definition of sexual deviation as it is merely the list of sexual behaviours which are unacceptable to a given culture. Western attitudes have been particularly fluid in recent years. Moreover, acceptable sexual practices can contain elements which if extreme would be classed as deviant—mildly sadistic behaviour is not uncommon. A consensus would probably accede to the list in Table V, which covers both abnormalities of sexual orientation and disorders of gender role: however, the categories are not exhaustive and certainly not mutually exclusive. This becomes unimportant if the abnormalities of behaviour are precisely described under the separate headings of the eliciting circumstances of the response and the response itself. The response abnormality may follow inevitably from the controlling stimulus, as in homosexuality, or may be primary, as in exhibitionism.

The diagnosis of a sexual deviation should be based on an established anomaly of sexual fantasy or act. This issue has been somewhat confused by the central position of sexuality in analytical theory which leads to the labelling in sexual terms of behaviour not immediately sexual. To term someone a latent homosexual is to use the label in a radically different way.

Table V

(A) *Disorders of sexual orientation*
  (a) homosexuality (and lesbianism)
  (b) paedophilia
  (c) exhibitionism
  (d) voyeurism
  (e) sadomasochism
  (f) fetishism
  (g) symptomatic transvestism
  (h) others (frotteurism, bestiality, necrophilia)

(B) *Gender role abnormalities*
  (a) simple transvestism
  (b) transsexualism

Disorders of sexual orientation

Aetiology

Genetic factors are of no importance in the ontogenesis of deviation with the possible exception of male homosexuality. Kallman (1952) and Schlegel (1962) claim very high rates in MZ as opposed to DZ twins. Their data has been criticized (e.g. West, 1968) and current opinion favours a lesser genetic contribution (Heston and Shields, 1968).

Patients with Klinefelter's syndrome and temporal lobe epilepsy (TLE) of early onset (Kolarsky *et al.*, 1967) are somewhat more likely to be fetishists and transvestites, but such organic factors must have a tiny role in sexual deviation: virtually all homosexuals have normal sex chromation (Pare, 1956) and karyotypes (Pritchard, 1962). Patients with Turner's syndrome have normal gender role and sexual orientation. In cases of TLE, the deviation may be converted by temporal lobectomy. Physique in clinic homosexuals is slightly androgynous, but no more so than in a heterosexual clinic population (Coppen, 1959).

Acceptable assay techniques for testosterone have not clarified hormonal factors in homosexuality: Loraine *et al.* (1970), Kolodny *et al.* (1971) and Pillard *et al.* (1974) claimed lower levels than in normals; Barlow *et al.* (1974) and Dorner *et al.* (1975) have not confirmed these findings. Dorner *et al.* (1975) suggest that homosexuality may arise from lack of androgen only at a critical (perinatal) period and offer some indirect evidence.

Psychosocial explanations of sexual deviation are discussed in the two separate languages of psychoanalysis and of learning theory. Whatever the language, conjecture far outruns demonstration. Attempts at explanation may be an account of the circumstances precluding the approach to a sexual situation or they may describe the mechanism of association of stimulus and response.

Traumatic (sometimes single-trial) learning by association is suggested by many case histories and was first formalized by Binet (1888) and Schrenck-Nötzing (1895). Some behaviourists (e.g. Rachman, 1966) claim to have elicited mild sexual deviation in volunteers by classical conditioning. Others (Langevin and Martin, 1975) question this and in any case it is of doubtful relevance to the acquisition of clinical deviation. McGuire *et al.* (1965) extend the idea and suggest that the traumatic incident acts as a focus for future masturbation. This is difficult to prove: it is after all not surprising that sexual deviants masturbate to deviant fantasies.

Freud's (1909) postulate of infantile bisexuality requires an innate association which Rado (1940), for instance, has rejected. Rado (1940) prefers to leave the connection implicit.

Highly specific stimulus control occurs in some deviants, especially fetishists. This has been ascribed to a phylogenetic value of the fetish object (Krafft-Ebing, 1963; Marks, 1972; Epstein, 1975) or to a high degree of conditionability in fetishists akin to that of phobic subjects (Marks, 1969).

The issue is more complex because sexual activity can allay anxiety and this may be central to the deviation. This seems not uncommon in exhibitionism (Rooth, 1971) and cross-dressing can gradually cease to subserve a sexual gratification and become a non-sexual solace.

The psychoanalytic concept of bisexuality requires an explanation of deviation in terms of the obstruction of an innately available heterosexuality. The earlier literature on this issue has been admirably reviewed by Wiedeman (1962). Suggestions include mother fixation, whereby the subject (1) identifies with the mother, develops narcissistic self-love and proceeds narcissistically to love of a man like himself, or (2) remains faithful to the mother by abjuring heterosexuality. Other possibly pathogenic family circumstances comprise an absent mother, a cruel or feared father leading to oedipal renunciation of females, and an absent or weak father allowing inappropriate identification. Truly a wide net has been cast. It should be noted that behavioural explanations also require a codicil to account for the avoidance of and failure to develop freely available heterosexual outlets (McGuire et al., 1965).

Social learning theories (Bandura, 1969) sound very similar: it seems likely that the phenomenon of vicarious learning is largely applicable to the acquisition of appropriate approach behaviour. The quality of a model in terms of power, status, nurturance and similarity has an obvious bearing on the way in which a child acquires the sexual behaviour of its parents. Deviant sexual behaviour may arise from a deviant model or from an inappropriate one, e.g. from mother to son, when the father is absent or lacking in social power.

It can be seen from this résumé that the explanations of psychoanalysis and learning theory, albeit often mutually anathematous, are not necessarily mutually incompatible. Moreover, these ideas are open to scientific testing although there are difficulties of method to overcome. A number of studies have found a variety of abnormalities of parental relationships in homosexuality (Bieber et al., 1962; Bene, 1965; Robertson, 1972), lesbianism (Kenyon, 1968) and transvestism (Roth and Ball, 1964), although Siegelman's (1974) carefully conducted study suggests the reported abnormalities have more relationship to neuroticism than homosexuality. The issue remains sub judice.

Recently, Bell (1975) has argued forcibly that approaches which seek to explain homosexuality as the crystallized reflection of distant events and circumstances signally fail to recognize that the behaviours which constitute the homosexual identity are in dynamic equilibrium with the environment and this neglected interaction is likely to be of major importance in the maintenance of that identity.

Homosexuality

Homosexuality is the condition of being erotically attached towards members of the same sex. Kinsey (1948) in his study of 4108 adult American males showed that 4% were exclusively homosexual and over 37% had had adult sexual contact with another man leading to orgasm by age 45. Ten per cent of males were more or less exclusively homosexual for at least three consecutive years and 10% of married men admitted to concurrent homosexual experience. The incidence in European studies is lower, possibly because of differing methodology.

Psychopathology. Contrary to popular belief, effeminacy is not common among homosexuals. Freund *et al*. (1974b) showed only a slight tendency in homosexuals towards higher effeminacy compared with normals. Effeminacy may be related to the importance of self advertisement, or rarely to transvestite and transsexual feelings. Personality test studies reveal no consistent traits and are bedevilled by the bias caused by using patient populations. Siegelman (1972a) showed non-clinic homosexuals as well adjusted as normal controls on questionnaire measures.

Homosexual relationships tend to be impermanent and may be transient and promiscuous. The tendency to depression and suicide shown in a number of studies (e.g. Lambert, 1954) may be related to this impermanence of relationships. Certainly many present themselves for treatment of homosexuality at the time of waning attractiveness. Many express guilt about their deviance and exaggerate the animosity of others towards it. Recent liberalization of values parallels increased assertiveness amongst this minority. A major problem is to distinguish homosexual traits from the response of deviant minorities in general.

The commonest means of gratification are mutual masturbation, fellatio and anal intercourse. The idea of adherence to active and passive

Table VI *Kinsey ratings*

---

0 wholly heterosexual
1 predominantly heterosexual, only incidentally homosexual
2 predominantly heterosexual, more than incidentally homosexual
3 equally heterosexual and homosexual
4 predominantly homosexual, more than incidentally heterosexual
5 predominantly homosexual, only incidentally heterosexual
6 exclusively homosexual

---

roles is less than clear cut with individuals alternating or changing roles. Some do remain true to form.

Homosexuality and the law. The Sexual Offences Act (1967) was brought in following the Wolfenden Committee of 1958. Homosexual acts in private (i.e. two persons only present) between men over 21 are now legal. Acts between men over 21 with youths of 16–21 carry a penalty of up to five years imprisonment. Acts with boys under 16 carry penalties up to life imprisonment. Acts by youths aged 16–21 with anyone over 16 can incur up to two years imprisonment.

Lesbianism

This is homosexuality in the female (derived from Lesbos, the Greek island where Sappho, a homosexual poetess, lived). It is the only common sexual deviation of women—apart from sadomasochism, all other deviations are very rare indeed. Kinsey's (1953) study on 5940 American women revealed 15% had had homosexual contact with orgasm by age 45 and 4% were exclusively lesbian between 20 and 55. Cross-cultural studies reveal lesbianism to be much rarer in primitive communities than male homosexuality. Kenyon (1968) compared questionnaire answers from 125 members of a lesbian club with those of a normal control group. The club included an over-representation of the more exclusively homosexual. He found poor relationships with either parent much more common in the lesbians. There was a family history of homosexuality in a quarter and prudish family attitudes towards sex were the norm. Three times as many lesbians felt their parents would have preferred a boy and 20% thought they had been brought up like a boy. Early lesbian seduction did not appear to be important. Nearly twice as many lesbians had been frightened or disgusted by the sexual behaviour of a man. Many more lesbians rated themselves as poor performers in heterosexual situations. It seems as though heterophobia is important in homosexuality in women. However, about 60% of lesbians had had heterosexual intercourse, although only 10% with orgasm. More than half of the married lesbians were unhappily married. Compared with male homosexuals lesbians are less promiscuous and have longer relationships. Lesbian prostitution is almost unknown. The most common types of sexual gratification are mutual masturbation, orogenital contacts and genitogenital contact (tribadism). The use of prostheses is rare. Nineteen per cent of Kenyon's (1968) subjects had a psychiatric history compared with 6% of controls. This was usually of a depressive neurotic reaction. Depressive illness itself may release lesbian behaviour. However Siegelman (1972a) showed non clinic lesbians to be as well adjusted as normal controls.

Paedophilia

Paedophilia is the condition of being erotically attracted to pre-pubertal children. Paedophiliacs fall into three groups: heterosexual, homosexual and indiscriminate. The last group is rarer and tends to be more disturbed. Paedophilic acts rarely involve violence or coercion and usually take the form of immature sex play such as looking, showing, kissing and fondling. Coitus is uncommon. Other deviations which may have child objects include sadomasochism and exhibitionism. There are three age-groups of adult participants: the adolescent (who may be looked on as the upper end of a normal curve of immature sexual activity), the middle-aged and the elderly. The middle-aged group are mainly married, but with marital and social difficulties; the paedophilia may involve incest. The elderly paedophile is characterized by social isolation. Alcohol may be involved in releasing the behaviour in the latter two groups.

The adult partner is usually known to the child and in one study the child was an active participant in two-thirds of the cases (Gibbens and Prince, 1963). The age distribution of child partners is different for the two sexes. In boys, the distribution gradually phases into the curve for adult homosexual acts, but in girls it peaks at age seven to nine. As Mohr *et al.* (1964) point out, this age frequency distribution parallels that for early sexual exploration in female children given by Kinsey (1953) which reinforces the idea of child participation.

Management of the deviation includes proper and tactful handling of the turmoil aroused by a discovered paedophilic act and the protection of the child from that turmoil.

Voyeurism

Voyeurism is sexual gratification through looking and is characterized by a willingness to take risks in order to gratify. It is a solitary activity of adulthood and the voyeur never chooses people known to him. He may masturbate; he may be married and have normal heterosexual activity. About a third show other deviations and in an American study 10% were vagrants or vagrant alcoholics. The habitual voyeur virtually never proceeds to rape. The scanty literature on voyeurism has recently been reviewed by Smith (1976).

Sadomasochism

Sadism is sexual gratification involving fantasy or acts of cruelty and is named after the Marquis de Sade (1740–1814). Masochism is sexual gratification involving real or imaginary subjection to acts of cruelty or to the power of another. Krafft-Ebing coined the term after the Austrian novelist, Leopold von Sacher-Masoch (1836–1895). The two perversions may occur in the same individual but one usually predominates. Although initially he gave the phenomena equal standing, Freud later believed that masochism was primary and favoured the existence of the death instinct and would undergo reversal into sadism. Analysts regard sadism either as an infantile component instinct or possibly as a fusion of libidinal and aggressive instincts. In many case histories, a simpler explanation in terms of a traumatic association may be revealed.

Sadistic acts can be directed towards the self or towards others. Sadism may require a personal performance or merely watching others perform such acts. Some sadists inflict a general humiliation; others require a highly specific ritual. It sometimes demands the production of a specific stimulus such as bleeding. The condition is much commoner in men and may be directed towards females, males or animals. Krafft-Ebing emphasized that mild sadism is a normal variant and Kinsey (1953) records that about a quarter of male and female subjects are erotically aroused by biting. Sadistic acts may accompany or follow coitus or occasionally be used to induce ejaculation without coitus. The most extreme forms involve lust murder.

In some, sadism remains at the level of fantasy, and in others the act is symbolic as with a man who would defile a woman's hands with soot, or another who would cut a woman's fringe or clothes. Some of these symbolic acts may be committed in public with strangers and assume forensic importance.

Masochistic acts may also be a preamble or substitute for coitus and again can be vicarious or fantasied rather than direct and real. The acts tend to be generalized humiliations, but they may be highly specific and symbolic as with a patient of Krafft-Ebing who paid prostitutes to prepare him for shaving. Foot and shoe fetishism has obvious affinities with this type of symbolic masochism.

Fetishism

Normal men show preference for parts of the female form and for particular attire, but in them it is a focus of a general desire. Fetishism is a pathological variation in which the specific part or article becomes the sole or major object in itself. The term was coined by Binet and derives from feitico, the Portuguese for 'charm' or 'magic'.

Freud explained fetishism in terms of the mechanisms of condensation, splitting and symbolism: the fetish represents a female penis. Fenichel puts forward the idea of 'partial repression' to explain how the part becomes an acceptable representative of the whole. These theories have difficulty in explaining cases in which normal coitus alternates with fetishism.

Many histories of fetishists suggest the importance of an accidental association of sexual arousal and the fetish object. Fetishism may not exclude coitus and coitus may be possible even without the presence of the fetish; it may, however, be forced and accompanied by imagery of the fetish. Often the sexual end is attained by genital juxtaposition of the fetish, whether body part or object. It is probably best to regard fetishism as a graded phenomenon, through strong preference to necessity. Hand, and especially foot fetishisms are associated with masochism. Even bodily defects (lameness, amputation) may serve as fetish objects. (Rene Descartes had a squint fetish.) Occasionally the fetish may be an action, for instance, coughing or sneezing. Occasionally, there may be homosexual fetishism; fetishism in women is known, but very rare. Kinsey (1953) reports '2 or 3' cases amongst his 6000 women who were consistently aroused by objects.

Gender role abnormalities

The relationship between gender role and sexual orientation is complex and the interface of deviation of each occurs in the cross-dressing disorders. The usual classification follows Roth and Ball (1964):

(1) *Symptomatic transvestism*. This occurs either as a manifestation of homosexuality or as a form of fetishism in which the fetish objects are worn and cross-dressing leads to sexual arousal and orgasm. One sub-variety involves cross-dressing, bondage and partial self-asphyxiation (which occasionally misfires, becoming total).

(2) *Simple transvestism*. This is not uncommon—one estimate suggests there are 30,000 in the UK. It, like homosexuality, is a deviation with a sub-culture. Cross-dressing is associated with the relief of anxiety, not sexual gratification.

(3) *Transsexualism*. This is a deviation of gender role characterized by the strongly held conviction that, by a cruel stroke of fate, gender identity is misrepresented by anatomy. Transsexuals relentlessly pursue surgical and civil rectification. It is rare, occurring at an estimated rate of one per 34,000 males and one per 108,000 females in the UK (Hoenig and Kenna, 1974b).

Fetishistic transvestism is *per se* a sexual deviation, simple transvestism and transsexualism are abnormalities of gender role which may have homosexuality as a secondary sexual deviation. Nevertheless, as Bancroft

(1972) emphasizes, cross-dressing does form a continuum with some patients changing categories over the years: the sexual gratification afforded to the symptomatic transvestite may give way to an anxiety reducing function. Gradual acquisition of the transsexual role and status has been described also by Levine *et al.* (1975). The most consistent feature of early life is the relative or actual absence of the father. If present, he is usually devoid of social power compared with the mother (Lukianowicz, 1959). This would tie in with the modelling explanation. Fenichel's analytic explanation, that both transvestism and transsexualism represent a defence against castration fears by the creation of the 'phallic woman', falls down in those cases which actively seek castration.

Transvestism varies in severity, with increasingly prominent feminine traits, interests and hobbies. Cross-dressing may be surreptitious and continuous (e.g. wearing panties under normal male apparel) or sporadic and total. About 35% each of cases are homosexual and heterosexual. Others are autoerotic or asexual (Hirschfeld, 1930). Virtually all female transvestites are homosexual.

Transsexualism is a more profound disorder and the patients show a massive preoccupation with rectification of civil status and anatomy. To this end, they may use threats of suicide and actual self-mutilation (penectomy, castration). Despite above average ability, they obtain poor qualifications and show poor work records, mainly choosing feminine occupations. Quite a few marry, but the marriages tend to be unstable. They abhor homosexuality—they insist the men with whom they have sexual relations are normal heterosexuals (Freund *et al.*, 1974a).

Hoenig and Kenna (1974a) have reported on the sexual orientation of transsexual males and claim that nearly 10% were fetishistic, 40% homosexual and nearly 80% fetishistic transvestites before the full elaboration of their transsexualism. Only homosexuality persisted after the development of the syndrome. Nevertheless 15% remained in the most heterosexual category of Kinsey (see Table VI). Hoenig and Kenna (1974a) noted the low drive of transsexuals, correlating with a low incidence of masturbation.

Both transvestism and transsexualism are of early onset, with cross-dressing as early as perhaps five years old, often in the face of apparently strong adult sanctions. In childhood, transsexuals have no interest in gender-appropriate activity; not surprisingly they are maladjusted at school.

Surgery can give cosmetically acceptable results in males when combined with hormonal treatments. Results suggest that many, but not all, male transsexuals have improved post-operative adjustment (Money and Gaskin, 1970). Operation should not be offered unless the patient has lived successfully as a woman for at least two years.

Sexual deviance in the elderly

This occurs principally in the male. Some elderly deviants are merely young deviants grown old—the effect of ageing may be to reduce discretion or to allow covert behaviour to become overt. In others it may be a response to declining heterosexual potency which many of these men set particular store by. The common deviations are exhibitionism and paedophilia; violence is a rarity. There is often a loving emotional relationship which reflects social and emotional isolation. In one study of 15 geriatric sexual offenders, nine had some mild dementia.

Treatment of sexual deviation

This section will deal with treatments aimed at reorientation or suppression, although only a minority of sexual deviants seek this from the psychiatrist.

The results of such treatment are to be compared with the natural history of the disorders; for instance, Kinsey (1948) graded 81% of his male subjects in categories 1 and 2 at age 20. This rose to 93% by age 45. Pessimism regarding mutability of sexual deviation coincides with the classical period of analytical theory. Prior to this, for instance, Schrenck-Nötzing claimed a cure rate of 35% at follow-up in a mixed group of deviants treated by suggestion.

The results of dynamic psychotherapy are difficult to assess. Curran and Parr (1957) showed no change in treated homosexuals compared with untreated controls. However, they had a heavy loading of Kinsey rating 5 and 6. Mayerson and Lief (1965) reported a follow-up study on 19 homosexuals or bisexuals (five female) of average age 28 and claimed 47% had become exclusively heterosexual.

Bancroft (1974) has compared the results of 13 series treated by behavioural methods and two psychotherapeutic series offering adequate follow-up and shows that results are remarkably similar with about 40% of patients improved.

Therapeutic expertise in behavioural methods is rapidly advancing (see Table VII) and indeed has outrun controlled assessment.

Most sexual deviants have been treated by chemical and electrical aversion. The technique involves pairing deviant material (which may be photographic, verbal, imaginal or behavioural) with an aversive stimulus such as mild electric shock or apomorphine-induced nausea. If the patient can avoid the aversive stimulus, e.g. by turning off photographic material, the paradigm is of an avoidance response. Chemical and electrical methods are equally effective and the latter, being more convenient, are now favoured. There is good evidence that the technique does not operate by conditioning an aversion, since it in fact produces affective neutrality.

Table VII

Reduction of deviant sexuality
    (i) Aversion   Classical conditioning ⎫   Modalities: chemical
                       Paradigm   ⎬   electrical
                       Avoidance paradigm ⎭   covert
                                                    smell
                                                    shame

   (ii) Self-regulation

Increase in heterosexual behaviour
    (i) Aversion relief
   (ii) Operant shaping
  (iii) Desensitization
  (iv) Pairing (including fading and masturbatory conditioning)
   (v) Training deficient heterosexual skills

McConaghy and Barr (1973) report a study of electrical aversion in 46 subjects allocated to random groups treated by classical conditioning avoidance training or backwards conditioning (i.e. UCS precedes CS). Twenty sessions of treatment were given and the methods were equally effective. At one year follow-up about half the cases reported a reduction in homosexual feeling, half an increase in heterosexual feeling, a quarter increased frequency of heterosexual intercourse and a quarter ceased homosexual contacts.

The results of Feldman and MacCulloch (1971), using an avoidance paradigm of electrical aversion, are better. The technique also involved aversion relief as patients could switch to heterosexual slides and thus avoid the shock. There were 18–20 sessions of half an hour and 36 of 45 patients completed the treatment. Of these, 25 were significantly improved, most improvement occurring in those already having significant heterosexual interest.

Self-regulation is a technique involving the interruption of the response chain leading to deviant acts by switching to alternative thoughts of activities. A controlled study in exhibitionism suggests it was slightly less effective than electrical aversion (Rooth and Marks, 1974).

Pairing is a loose term covering techniques in which sexual arousal or orgasm is elicited either by masturbation or by deviant erotic stimuli (which may be fantasized or real) and paired with heterosexual stimuli. It has been effective at case-study level.

Desensitization would seem to be an obvious approach in those patients with high heterosexual anxiety, but has so far proved only moderately successful. The direct training of heterosexual skills would seem a hopeful area, but has been little reported.

The various sexual deviations respond differently to behavioural techniques. Bisexuals, fetishists and symptomatic transvestites do well; exhibitionists, homosexuals and simple transvestites do less well and transsexuals very badly. There are few reports on lesbians. The whole field is ably reviewed by Marks (1976).

The chemical suppression of sexual deviance may be acceptable in the more antisocial deviations. The drug of choice is cyproterone acetate which is an anti-androgen with none of the feminizing effects of stilboestrol. It reversibly reduces both desire and potency and has been used quite widely on the continent. It may not always be effective, particularly if deviation is associated with brain damage. The butyrophenone, benperidol has been shown to be more effective than placebo in the suppression of sexuality.

References

Annon, J. (1975). The behavioural treatment of sexual problems. Kapiolani Health Services, Honolulu.

Bancroft, J. H. J. (1970). Homosexuality in the male. *Br. J. Hosp. Med.* **5**, 168–181.

Bancroft, J. H. J. (1972). The relationship between gender identity and sexual behaviour: some clinical aspects. *In* 'Gender Differences: Their Ontogeny and Significance' (Ed. C. Ounsted and D. C. Taylor). Churchill-Livingstone, Edinburgh.

Bancroft, J. H. J. (1974). 'Deviant Sexual Behaviour: Modification and Assessment'. Clarendon Press, Oxford.

Bandura, A. (1969). 'Principles of Behaviour Modification'. Holt, Rinehart and Winston Inc., New York.

Barlow, B. H., Abel, G. G., Blanchard, E. B. and Mavissakalian, M. (1974). Plasma testosterone levels and male homosexuality: a failure to replicate. *Archs. Sex. Behav.* **3**, 571–575.

Bell, A. P. (1975). Research in homosexuality: back to the drawing board. *Archs. Sex. Behav.* **4**, 421–431.

Bene, E. (1965). On the genesis of male homosexuality: an attempt at clarifying the role of the parents. *Br. J. Psychiat.* **111**, 803–813.

Beutler, L. N., Karacan, I., Anch, A. M., Salis, R. J., Scott, F. B. and Williams, R. L. (1975). MMPI and MIT discriminations of biogenic and psychogenic impotence. *J. Consult. Clin. Psychol.* **43**, 899–903.

Bieber, I., Dain, H. J., Dince, P. R., Drellich, M. G., Grand, H. G., Gundlach, R. H., Kremer, M. W., Rifkin, A. H., Wilbur, C. B. and Bieber, T. B. (1962). 'Homosexuality: A Psychoanalytic Study'. Basic Books, New York.

Binet, A. (1888). 'Études de Psychologie Experimentale'. Paris.

Brady, J. P. (1976). Behaviour therapy and sex therapy. *Am. J. Psychiat.* **133**, 896–899.

Coppen, A. J. (1959). Body build of male homosexuals. *Br. Med. J.* **ii**, 1443–1445.

Crowe, M. J. (1973). Conjoint marital therapy: advice or interpretation. *J. Psychosom. Res.* **17**, 309–315.

Crowe, M. J. (1977). A comparison of directive and interpretative approaches in conjoint marital therapy. Paper read at Annual Conference of the British Psychological Society, Exeter.

Curran, D. and Parr, D. (1957). Homosexuality. An analysis of 100 male cases. *Br. Med. J.* **i**, 797–801.

Derogatis, L. R., Meyer, J. K. and Dupkin, C. N. (1976). Discrimination of organic versus psychogenic impotence with the DSFI. *J. Sex. Marital Ther.* **2**, 229–240.

Dorner, G., Rohde, W., Stahl, F., Krell, L. and Masius, W.G. (1975). A. Neuroendocrine predisposition for homosexuality in men. *Archs. Sex. Behav.* **4**, 1–8.

Epstein, A. W. (1975). The fetish object: phylogenetic considerations. *Archs. Sex. Behav.* **4**, 303–308.

Feldman, M. P. and MacCulloch, M. J. (1971). 'Homosexual Behaviour. Therapy and Assessment'. Pergamon, Oxford.

Fenichel, O. (1930). The psychology of transvestism. *Int. J. Psychoanal.* **II**, 211–227.

Freud, S. (1909). 'Five Lectures on Psychoanalysis', Standard Edition, Vol. II, pp. 3–56. Hogarth Press, London (1957).

Freund, K., Langevin, R., Zajac, Y., Steiner, B. and Zajac, A. (1974a). The transsexual syndrome in homosexual males. *J. Nerv. Ment. Dis.* **158**, 145–153.

Freund, K., Nagler, E., Langevin, R., Zajac, A. and Steiner, B. (1974b). Measuring female gender identity in homosexual males. *Archs. Sex. Behav.* **3**, 249–260.

Gagnon, J. H. (1975). Sex research and social change. *Archs. Sex. Behav.* **4**, 111–141.

Gaskell, P. (1971). The importance of penile blood pressure in cases of impotence. *Can. Med. Ass. J.* **105**, 1047–1051.

Gibbens, T. C. N. and Prince, J. (1963). 'Child Victims of Sex Offences'. I.S.T.D., London.

Gillan, P. and Gillan R. (1976). 'Sex Therapy Today'. Open Books, London.

Greene, S. (1977). Resisting the pressure to become a surrogate: A case study. *J. Sex Marital Ther.* **3**, 40–49.

Heston, L. L. and Shields, J. (1968). Homosexuality in twins. *Archs. Gen. Psychiat.* **18**, 149–160.

Hirschfeld, M. (1930). The homosexual as an intersex. *In* 'Homosexuality' (Eds C. Berg and A. M. Krich). Allen and Unwin, London (1958).

Hoenig, J. and Kenna, J. C. (1974a). The nosological position of transsexualism. *Archs. Sex. Behav.* **3**, 273–287.

Hoenig, J. and Kenna, J. C. (1974b). The prevalence of transsexualism in England and Wales. *Br. J. Psychiat.* **124**, 181–190.

Kallman, F. J. (1952). Comparative twin studies of the genetic aspects of male homosexuality. *J. Nerv. Ment. Dis.* **115**, 283–298.

Kaplan, H. S. (1974a). 'The New Sex Therapy'. Bruner/Mazel, New York.

Kaplan, H. S. (1974b). A new classification of the female sexual dysfunctions. *J. Sex. Marital Ther.* **1**, 124–138.

Kaplan, H. S. (1976). Editorial: towards a rational classification of the sexual dysfunctions. *J. Sex. Marital Ther.* **2**, 83–84.

Kaplan, H. S. (1977). Hypoactive sexual desire. *J. Sex. Marital Ther.* **3**, 3–9.

Karacan, I. (1970). Clinical value of nocturnal erection in the prognosis and diagnosis of impotence. *Med. Aspects Hum. Sex.* **4**, 27–34.

Kenyon, F. E. (1968). Studies in female homosexuality: IV Social and psychiatric aspects. V. Sexual development, attitudes and experience. *Br. J. Psychiat.* **114**, 1337–1350.

Kinsey, A. C., Pomeroy, W. B. and Martin, C. E. (1948). 'Sexual Behaviour in the Human Male'. Saunders, Philadelphia.

Kinsey, A. C. Pomeroy, W. B., Martin, C. E. and Gebhard, P. H. (1953). 'Sexual Behaviour in the Human Female'. Saunders, Philadelphia.

Kockott, G., Dittmar, F. and Nusselt, L. (1975). Systematic desensitisation of erectile impotence: a controlled study. *Archs. Sex. Behav.* **4**, 493–500.

Kolarsky, A., Freund, J., Machek, J. and Polak, O. (1967). Male sexual deviation. *Archs. Gen. Psychiat.* **17**, 735–743.

Kolodny, R. C., Masters, W. H., Hendry, J. and Toro, G. (1971). Plasma testosterone and semen analysis in male homosexuals. *New Eng. J. Med.* **285**, 1170–1174.

Krafft-Ebing, R. Von. (1965). 'Psychopathia sexualis; with special reference to the antipathic sexual instinct: a medicoforensic study'. Trans. F. S. Klaf. from 12th German edn. Stein and Day, New York.

Lambert, K. (1954). Homosexuals. *Med. Press.* **232**, 523–526.

Langevin, R. and Martin, M. (1975). Can erotic responses be classically conditioned? *Behav. Ther.* **6**, 350–355.

Levine, E. M., Shaiova, C. H. and Mihailovic, M. (1975). Male to female: The role transformation of transsexuals. *Archs. Sex. Behav.* **4**, 173–185.

Levine, S. B. (1976). Marital sexual dysfunction: erectile dysfunction. *Ann. Int. Med.* **85**, 342–350.

Lopiccolo, J. and Lobitz, W. C. (1972). The role of masturbation in the treatment of orgasmic dysfunction. *Archs. Sex. Behav.* **2**, 163–171.

Loraine, J. A., Ismail, A. A., Adamopaulos, D. A. and Dove, G. A. (1970). Endocrine functions in male and female homosexuals. *Br. Med. J.* **iv**, 406–409.

Marks, I. M. (1969). 'Fears and Phobias'. Heinemann Medical, London.

Marks, I. M. (1972). Phylogenesis and learning in the acquisition of fetishism. *Dan. Med. Bull.* **19**, 307–309.

Marks, I. M. (1976). Management of sexual disorders. *In* 'Handbook of Behaviour Modification' (Ed. H. Leitenberg). Prentice Hall, Englewood Cliffs, NJ.

Masters, W. H. and Johnson, V. E. (1966). 'Human Sexual Response'. Little, Brown, Boston.

Masters, W. H. and Johnson, V. E. (1970). 'Human Sexual Inadequacy'. Little, Brown, Boston.

Mayerson, P. and Lief, H. I. (1965). Psychotherapy of homosexuals. *In* 'Sexual Inversion' (Ed. J. Marmor). Basic Books, New York.

McConaghy, N. and Barr, R. F. (1973). Classical, avoidance and backward conditioning treatments of homosexuality. *Br. J. Psychiat.* **122**, 151–162.

McGovern, K. B., Stewart, R. C. and Lopiccolo, J. (1975). Secondary orgasmic dysfunction. I. Analysis and strategies for treatment. *Archs. Sex. Behav.* **4**, 265–275.

McGuire, R. J., Carlisle, J. M. and Young, B. G. (1965). Sexual deviations as conditioned behaviour: a hypothesis. *Behav. Res. Ther.* **2**, 185–190.

Moll, A. (1911). Die Behandlung sexueller Perversioner mit besonderer Beruchsichtigung der Assoziations Therapie. *Zeitschrift fur Psychotherapie* **3**, 1–29.

Mohr, J. W., Turner, R. E. and Jerry, M. B. (1964). 'Paedophilia and Exhibitionism'. Toronto University Press, Toronto.

Money, J. and Gaskin, R. J. (1970). Sex reassignment. *Int. J. Psychiat.* **9**, 249–269.

Munjack, D. and Kanno, P. (1976). An overview of outcome on frigidity: Treatment effects and effectiveness. *Comp. Psychiat.* **17**, 401–413.

Munjack, D. and Kanno, P. (1977). Prognosis in the treatment of female sexual inhibition. *Comp. Psychiat.* **18**, 481–488.

Munjack, D. J. and Staples, F. R. (1976). Psychological characteristics of women with sexual inhibition (frigidity) in sex clinics. *J. Nerv. Ment. Dis.* **163**, 117–123.

Munjack, D., Cristol, A., Goldstein, A., Phillips, D., Goldberg, A., Whipple, K., Staples, F. and Kanno, P. (1976). Behavioural treatment of orgasmic dysfunction: a controlled strudy. *Br. J. Psychiat.* **129**, 497–502.

Obler, M. (1973). Systematic desensitisation in sexual disorder. *J. Behav. Ther. Exp. Psychiat.* **4**, 93–101.

Pare, C. M. B. (1956). Homosexuality and chromosomal sex. *J. Psychosom. Res.* **1**, 247–251.

Parker, N. (1964). Homosexuality in twins: a report on three discordant pairs. *Br. J. Psychiat.* **110**, 489–495.

Pillard, R. C., Rose, R. M. and Sherwood, M. (1974). Plasma testosterone levels in homosexual men. *Archs. Sex. Behav.* **3**, 453–458.

Pritchard, M. (1962). Homosexuality and genetic sex. *J. Ment. Sci.* **108**, 616–623.

Rachman, S. (1966). Sexual fetishism: an experimental analogue. *Psychol. Rec.* **16**, 293–296.

Rado, S. (1940). A critical examination of the concept of bisexuality. *Psychosom. Med.* **2**, 459–467.

Robertson, G. (1972). Parent-child relationships and homosexuality. *Br. J. Psychiat.* **121**, 525–528.

Rooth, F. G. (1971). Indecent exposure and exhibitionism. *Br. J. Hosp. Med.* **5**, 521–533.

Rooth, F. G. and Marks, I. M. (1974). Persistent exhibitionism: short term responses to self regulation and relaxation treatment. *Archs. Sex. Behav.* **3**, 227–248.

Rosen, R. C. (1976). Biofeedback techniques in the treatment of sexual disorders. Paper read at International Congress of Sexology, Montreal.

Roth, M. and Ball, J. R. B. (1964). Psychiatric aspects of intersexuality. In 'Intersexuality in Vertebrates Including Man' (Eds C. N. Armstrong and A. J. Marshall). Academic Press, London and New York.

Schlegel, W. S. (1962). Die Konstitutionsbiologischen Grundlagen der Homosexuality. *Z. Menschl. Vererb. Konstitution-lehre.* **36**, 341–364.

Schrenck-Nötzing, A. Von. (1895). 'The Use of Hypnosis in Psychopathia Sexualis with Special Reference to Contrary Sexual Instinct'. Trans. C. G. Chaddock, 1956. Julian Press, New York.

Sharpe, L., Kuriansky, J. B. and O'Connor, J. F. (1976). A preliminary classification of human functional sexual disorders. *J. Sex. Marital Ther.* **2**, 106–114.

Siegelman, M. (1972a). Adjustment of male homosexuals and heterosexuals. *Archs. Sex. Behav.* **2**, 9–25.

Siegelman, M. (1972b). Adjustment of homosexual and heterosexual women. *Br. J. Psychiat.* **120**, 477–481.

Siegelman, M. (1974). Parental background of male homosexuals and heterosexuals. *Archs. Sex. Behav.* **3**, 3–18.

Smith, R. S. (1976). Voyeurism: a review of the literature. *Archs. Sex. Behav.* **5**, 585–608.

Strauss, E. B. (1950). Impotence from a psychiatric standpoint. *Br. Med. J.* **i**, 697–699.

West, D. J. (1968). 'Homosexuality' (2nd revised edn). Penguin Books, Harmondsworth.

Wiedeman, G. H. (1962). Survey of psychoanalytic literature on overt male homosexuality. *J. Am. Psychoanal. Ass.* **10**, 386–409.

Wincze, J. P. and Caird, W. K. (1976). The effects of systematic desensitisation and video desensitisation in the treatment of essential sexual dysfunction in women. *Behav. Ther.* **7**, 335–342.

9 Drug dependence

Anthony Thorley

Universally, in time and place, across cultures and throughout history man has taken substances which affect his mind and alter the quality of his consciousness. Acceptable drug taking and dependent behaviour are common features of stable society, but probably all societies have some degree of unacceptable drug taking. In the last hundred years this has been an increasing area of social concern. As medical opinion has been sought by the lawyer, politician and social planner, drug taking behaviour and its consequences have come into the province of medical and psychiatric illness. To what extent it is useful to continue to pursue an exclusively medical model of unacceptable drug taking is a moot question, and is as relevant here as it is to alcohol dependence.

The subject of drug dependence is not helped by the variety of substances which are misused, the variety of symptoms and behaviours which are produced and the variety of social and legal responses which ensue. If any order is possible through identifying and describing individual substance related dependence, it is thrown into confusion by the phenomena of multiple drug dependence. Here it becomes evident that it is not useful to separate drug dependence artificially from alcohol dependence, or to ignore related dependent behaviours such as over-eating and gambling. Consequently this chapter whilst pointing out the traditional distinctions in dependence disorders will attempt to draw attention to their commonalities.

Changing definitions and the concept of dependence

Changing definitions of drug dependence over the last thirty years reflect the concern of the politician, lawyer and doctor, changes in the pattern and types of drug taking, and developments in academic understanding. In 1950 the World Health Organization defined drug addiction as

> a state of periodic or chronic addiction detrimental to the individual and to society, produced by the repeated consumption of a drug (natural or synthetic). Characteristics include: (1) an overpowering desire or need (compulsion) to continue taking the drug and to obtain it by any means; (2) a tendency to increase the dose; (3) psychic (or psychological) and sometimes physical dependence on the effects of the drug; (4) a detrimental effect on the individual and on society.

Here the key word is addiction and the emphasis is on psychological dependence and individual and social damage. By 1957 the WHO reconsidered the definition and changed point (3) to 'generally a physical dependence'. In the United Kingdom the Brain Committee (Interdepartmental Committee, 1961) defined addiction very similarly laying stress on physical dependence, and then separately defined habituation as a less severe condition with 'some degree of psychological dependence' and 'detrimental effects, if any, primarily on the individual'. Thus amphetamine drugs were considered to be habituating and relatively harmless as compared with opiates. But as drug taking increased and multiple drug taking became more apparent, the distinction between habituation and addiction made less and less sense. In 1964 the WHO recommended that dependence was the preferred term and should be defined according to the drug used. In the current definitions addiction and habituation have disappeared but the mildly pejorative term 'drug abuse' has been introduced (WHO, 1969):

1. A drug is any substance that, when taken into the living organism, may modify one or more of its functions.
2. Drug abuse is persistent or sporadic excessive use of a drug inconsistent with, or unrelated to, acceptable medical practice.
3. Drug dependence is a state—psychic and sometimes also physical—resulting from the interaction between a living organism and a drug, characterised by behavioural and other responses that always include a compulsion to take the drug on a continuous or periodic basis in order to experience its psychic effects, and sometimes to avoid the discomfort of its absence. Tolerance may or may not be present. A person may be dependent on more than one drug.

What then is dependence, and if we are to insist that it is a fundamental concept drawing together heroin addiction, smoking and pathological gambling, can we identify its essential elements? In a seminal paper Russell (1976a) argues that it is not sufficient to remain fixated on the pharmacological aspects of drug taking. He believes that it is not frequent or continued use which denotes dependence, but rather the *difficulty in refraining* from further drug taking. He proposes a broad definition:

The notion of dependence on a drug, object, role, activity or any other stimulus-source requires the crucial feature of a negative affect experienced in its absence. The degree of dependence can be equated with the amount of this negative affect, which may range from mild discomfort to extreme distress, or it may be equated with the amount of difficulty or effort required to do without the drug, object etc.

This view of dependence brings it right into our everyday lives and so allows us to understand more easily the experience of those who are unacceptably dependent. Russell stresses that dependence is a normal part of human nature, for who has not felt a little sad (or experienced negative affect!) when denied their favourite beer or cigarettes, motor car, clothes, domestic pets, people, or activities like gardening or listening to music?

Dependence is most usefully seen as a continuum and not discontinuous from ordinary experience except in degree. It becomes arbitrary where degree of dependence becomes labelled as 'dependence disorder' or 'addiction'. Russell sees that pharmacological rewards are only one of a number of classes of reinforcer of dependent behaviour, and it is possible for strong psychological and social rewards to cause a higher degree of dependence than weak pharmacological ones.

Aetiology

The range of explanations and theories which account for syndromes of problem drug taking spans pharmacology to sociology, and it is increasingly clear that each drug dependence syndrome is the endpoint of a complex system of interrelated causal mechanisms. No single hypothesis can cover all the phenomena and there is a need to examine vertical explanations e.g. biochemical, psychological and social theories of opiate addiction, and integrate them with horizontal explanations, e.g. psychological theories of opiate, barbiturate, alcohol and multiple drug dependence (Fazey, 1976). Recent reviews of aetiology (Fazey, 1976; Bejerot, 1977; Plant, 1978) stress the breadth of factors involved and the lack of integration. In the sections that follow it is important to realize that whereas any single factor might account for drug dependence in the individual, it is more probable that the explanation lies with a group of factors working together.

Biological factors

1 *Pharmacological theories of tolerance and dependence*

It has long been recognized that the phenomenon of tolerance, i.e. a given and repeated dose of a drug having a decreasing effect, is a highly complex process and occurs at least at two levels: metabolic (e.g. liver enzyme induction destroying the drug) and cellular (reduction of cell sensitivity to the drug). The long acting barbiturates cause metabolic and cellular tolerance, whereas opiates only cause cellular tolerance. There is evidence that these cellular and metabolic changes can persist after complete withdrawal from some drugs in that tolerance is evident for weeks or months after abstinence.

Various general pharmacological theories of tolerance and dependence have been suggested but none satisfactorily explains the initiation of pharmacological dependence from a first dose. Opiates, for example, are known to affect the turnover of almost all CNS neurotransmitters and therefore Paton (1969) has suggested that there is a 'surfeit' effect of neurotransmitter in the terminal axon. Thus morphine reduces the effect of acetylcholine on isolated intestine, but morphine withdrawal causes a supramaximal release of acetylcholine, and hence the opiate abstinence symptoms of gut contractions. Collier (1969) has suggested that chronic opiate administration depresses neurotransmitter activity and induces a receptor 'supersensitivity'. Cessation of opiate leads to normal neurotransmitter release, but through the receptor supersensitivity, also to excessive stimulation and the appearance of withdrawal symptoms. Variations of these theories have been invoked by those wishing to describe the actions of opiates, opiate receptors and the endorphins (see below). Martin (1968) has proposed that there are at least two mechanistic channels of neuronal function, and that as one becomes blocked by a drug, another opens up and tolerance develops. On cessation of the drug, both routes are open and an excess of activity results. All of these hypothetical and generalized explanations may play a part and none has been convincingly demonstrated as a universal mechanism.

2   Animal studies

Evidence of drug dependence in animals presumes that cognitive and psychological functions are minimal and less important than some essential biological factor. Contrary to earlier impressions, it now appears that occasionally animals in the wild and in captivity can develop dependence to various plants and atypical foodstuffs (Leyhausen, 1973; Seevers, 1969). Laboratory studies with animals have shown that it is possible to establish drug dependence experimentally. Such studies, assuming that the animal dependence behaviour is validly applicable to man, theoretically allow new drugs to undergo preclinical assessment for 'abuse potential'. In spite of some animal/man inconsistencies, in general animal experiments must be accounted a particularly successful model (Kumar,

1974) and strongly suggest primary biological mechanisms of dependence.

3 Genetic and constitutional features

Biological evidence necessarily encourages the idea of genetic or constitutional predisposition to drug dependence whether based on pharmacological dysfunction, or more generally, on personality traits. Speculations that some opiate addicts may have a primary dysfunction of endorphin metabolism (Goldstein, 1978) are likely to increase in the future, but although there is considerable evidence of genetic factors affecting drug response and producing unwanted effects (Lader *et al.*, 1974), there is no specific evidence of a genetic component for drug dependence, as appears to have been established for alcohol dependence (see p. 331). Constitutional personality trait theories are never very satisfactory due to their over-simplistic application to human complexity, but Eysenck (1965) has argued that extroverted and introverted behaviour patterns may be due in large part to inherited characteristics of cerebral functioning. He predicts therefore that depressant drugs should enable introverts to become more extrovert (e.g. antidepressants for depression) and stimulant drugs should enable extroverts to become more introvert (e.g. stimulants for hyperactive children); but such a sweeping view would seem to be weakened by many pharmacological anomalies.

4 Physical illness and 'therapeutic addicts'

In the past pain and painful illnesses and iatrogenic factors have made a considerable contribution to the number of analgesic addicts. These so-called 'therapeutic addicts', mainly morphinists, once constituted a majority of British opiate addicts. Bejerot (1977) has described two types of therapeutic addict. (1) Addiction arising as a result of consciously accepted risk during medical treatment. This type mainly applies to the use of analgesics in terminal illness, and some doctors in fact tend to deny appropriate doses of opiates even when the element of dependence has been shown to be minimal and the effects most beneficial (Twycross, 1975). (2) Addiction inadvertently caused by medical treatment. Although iatrogenic opiate addiction is much less likely today, certain illnesses still create at risk populations, e.g. haemophilia, where home therapy provides patients with injection equipment and powerful opiate analgesics for painful bleeds. However, it is far more significant that in the last ten years thousands of people have inadvertently become dependent on hypnotics and tranquillizers owing to less than cautious psychotropic drug prescribing.

Psychological factors

1   Psychological theories

Psychological theory has been used to illuminate drug taking and dependence at several levels. Wikler (1971, 1973) stresses the role of reinforcement. *Primary direct reinforcement* is pharmacological and refers to the direct pleasure, thrill, reduction in anxiety or pain, caused by the drug. Drug taking is likely to be repeated for this direct reward: psychological dependence. *Primary indirect reinforcement*, mainly refers to the removal by the drug of uncomfortable withdrawal symptoms or their anticipation: physical dependence. *Secondary reinforcement* relies on classical conditioning linking external stimuli (objects, places, people, etc.) or internal stimuli (body changes after one drug dose) with the pharmacological effects of the drug when addicted. Wikler (1973) believes secondary reinforcement helps to explain how in abstinent, non tolerant ex-addicts one drug dose in a drug taking environment so commonly initiates a relapse into drug taking and dependence. *Social reinforcement*, e.g. personal acceptance and encouragement of a drug taking subgroup, may be in important factor in the initiation of drug taking (Wikler, 1973). Solomon and Marshall (1973) have argued in a comprehensive psychological theory of drug taking that acquisition is facilitated by social reinforcement contingent upon drug taking, as well as by primary pharmacological reinforcement. These authors point out the need to explain how, despite initial unpleasant and aversive effects, drug taking is continued, and suggest that the unpleasant effects (e.g. pain from needle, nausea) serve as discriminate stimuli for the occurrence of positive social reinforcement (e.g. approval from drug taking girlfriend) or other components of direct primary reinforcement (e.g. analgesia, relaxation). It is well known that addicts gain some relief by pricking themselves with needles, injecting saline, or 'flushing' venous blood in and out of the syringe.

At a more cognitive level, Orford (1976) has proposed that drug taking and dependence are essentially problems in decision making, and that the drug taker sets up values and probabilities against various outcomes of continuing or ceasing drug use. Thus treatment, which is concerned with changing attitudes and effecting decisions, must consider the whole range of contingencies and should admit the positive as well as the negative value of continuing drug use. Oppenheim (1976) has interpreted drug taking in terms of cognitive dissonance theory, and notes the way some individuals reduce intolerable cognitive dissonance by shifting from interdependence on people to dependence on drugs.

2 Psychoanalysis and personality characteristics

There has been a long search for specific personality disturbances associated with drug dependence. Psychoanalytic theory considers drug takers as fixated at or regressed to an oral level of psychosexual development. However, as Einstein (1977) has noted, oral personality does not necessarily impute drug taking as there are known to be various alternatives for such personalities: eating, love making, talking, playing the clarinet, etc! More valuable perhaps are the kinds of observations and insights developed by Bowlby (1977) into normal dependence and separation phenomena. Long-term abstinence phenomena and bereavement reactions have much in common.

The wide variety of types of drug taker seems to deny the discovery of a specific 'addictive personality'. Mott (1972) found that opiate addicts are more likely than norms to be above average intelligence and to have high neuroticism scores, but they fail to satisfy Eysenck's criteria of a psychopath, namely high neuroticism and extraversion scores. More recently in a population of British in-patient addicts, Gossop (1976) has shown that such patients are likely to show higher than normal hostility and intropunitiveness. To what extent it is fair to generalize from these in-patient populations to all drug takers remains a moot question.

3 Psychiatric illness

There is little doubt that mood altering drugs are taken to modify the unpleasant sensations of depression and anxiety, and that this causes some people to develop dependence. Some of these mood changes are a normal part of adolescent development, and this may partly explain why young people are associated with drug taking. The relationship between frank psychiatric illness and drug taking is more complex. As a diagnosis present in glossaries and classifications of mental disorders drug dependence constitutes psychiatric illness in itself, but even when substance-specific this is little more than empty labelling rather than explanatory diagnosis. It is evident, however, that hospitalized drug addicts (overlapping as they do with the delinquent population) are often psychiatrically disturbed, with anxiety and depressive symptoms to the fore, or are considered to have unspecified abnormal personalities (James, 1971). Although a common personality dysfunction appears elusive there remains a strong clinical impression that hospitalized drug takers are particularly handicapped in the social skills necessary to initiate and maintain close and meaningful interpersonal relations, and that the self gratification from drugs becomes a surrogate relationship in its own right. In a 12-year follow-up study of hospitalized patients (Sims, 1975) has shown that pre-existing neurotic illnesses predispose the development of alcohol or drug dependence. Findings from studies of British drug takers who are free agents in society vary widely, but it appears that a majority do not have any obvious psychiatric morbidity (Stevenson and Carney, 1971; Plant, 1975). Finally, it must be noted that some drugs, e.g. amphetamines and hallucinogens, may in themselves generate varying degrees of psychiatric disturbance.

Demographic and socio-environmental factors

1 Age and sex

It is a general finding that males outnumber females in populations of drug takers. Stimson's representative sample of 128 British heroin addicts found a sex ratio, males to females of 4:1 (Stimson, 1973). Plant's non-representative sample of 200 regular drug takers identified by personal contact methods in a small British town had a ratio of 3:1 (Plant, 1975). There is no adequate single explanation of this marked sex difference.

Although drug taking occurs at all ages, Hindmarch (1972) has drawn attention to the fact that those who are commonly involved in identity crises, adolescents and the middle-aged, are particularly associated with drug dependence. Blumberg (1977) has provided a detailed review of drug taking in young people.

2 Ethnicity and social class

Patterns of drug taking in the United States vary widely between ethnic groups but there is a strong association between opiate use and urban minority groups (e.g. blacks and Puertoricans) living in areas character-ized by poverty, poor housing, crime and delinquency (Chein et al., 1964). In contrast, in the United Kingdom, minority groups are not especially associated with drug taking. It is a general observation that cannabis smoking amongst black West Indians is not uncommon, whereas opiate dependence is rare. Before the increase in opiate dependence in the 1960s the majority of white British opiate addicts were middle-aged and middle class (Spear, 1969). Socio-economic analysis of recent British drug takers is difficult because of age and unemployment, but the evidence suggests that addicts are drawn from every kind of class background.

3 Family background and social deprivation

There is considerable evidence that a high proportion of institutionalized British drug takers come from homes where there has been parental disturbance and family disruption, although it is to be noted that this is commonly associated with other psychiatric populations. Stimson (1973) found 47% of his sample of heroin addicts had been separated from both parents for at least a year before the age of 16. There is an association between high levels of drug involvement and parental alcoholism (Plant, 1978). However the broad range of social deprivation described by Chein *et al.* (1964) in the United States does not appear to apply to drug takers in the United Kingdom.

4 Delinquency and criminality

Delinquency and drug taking are very closely associated and Cockett (1971) has pointed out that young delinquent drug takers have much in common with non-drug-taking delinquents, particularly in institutional settings. d'Orban (1973) considers that delinquency and drug taking are parallel phenomena, not causally related, but often an expression of similar underlying personality traits leading to deviance.

Although there is general agreement that there is some association between opiate drug taking and criminality, the nature, extent and significance of the association remains controversial. Drug related offences can clearly be within the Drugs Acts, e.g. possession, or without, e.g. theft of goods to sell in order to buy illicit drugs. Mott (1975) has reviewed the criminal histories of male opiate addicts in the United Kingdom and finds that pre-drug-taking conviction rates are somewhat higher than the general population. Criminal histories after identification as opiate addicts showed a decrease in the number of convictions for theft and other non-drug offences, and an increase in the number of offences under the Drugs Act. However, for men, pre-drug-taking conviction rates did not strongly predict levels of conviction rates during drug taking. In 1969 Stimson and Ogborne (1970) reported that 79% of their sample of heroin addicts had a previous conviction, 34% reported an offence outside the Drug Acts and 80% reported some undetected criminal activity in the three months preceding the interview. When subsequent annual conviction rates were analysed for this sample between 1969 and 1976 it was found that conviction rates of abstinent ex-addicts average one-third those of addicts who continue to use drugs, suggesting that abstinence and criminality are strongly related (Stimson *et al.*, 1978).

5 Access and availability

Access and availability of drugs are major factors in the production of problem drug takers, as is clearly evidenced by changing patterns of drug dependence in the United Kingdom in the last forty years. It also appears that unlike a disease like schizophrenia, there is no biologically based natural prevalence of any specific drug dependence found in all societies. Broadly speaking, as more and more drugs are available, more and more people become involved. Thus in Hong Kong, where heroin is relatively cheap and plentiful, the prevalence of opiate addiction in the adult male population is 8–10% (Singer, 1975), some thousand times greater than the estimated prevalence in the United Kingdom.

At a more specific level, occupations and professions like nursing, medicine, dentistry and pharmacy, with special access to addictive drugs, run high risks of drug dependence (Plant, 1978). The particular risks run by doctors have been described by Murray (1974a).

Initial access and further availability is often facilitated by a subgroup which condones drug taking and even makes it prestigious. Peer pressures are a very important influence, and young people, particularly with problems of social affiliation, are likely to identify with such a subgroup, and become persuaded that drug taking is a safe and valued type of behaviour (Plant and Reeves, 1974).

6   Sociological theories

Sociological theory and insights have much to offer in understanding drug dependence, but only two broadly based theories deserve our attention in a brief review. An influential theory has been that of Merton (1957) who has refined Durkheim's concept of anomie to account for deviant forms of behaviour including drug taking. It is proposed that if people in society fail to achieve their ambitions and objectives by legitimate means, e.g. conventional employment, they may resort to illegal or deviant methods instead. Drug taking becomes a retreat from social processes, and groups with poor educational and employment prospects opt out and establish a subgroup culture of their own. Merton has argued that this opting out tends to happen when society fails to meet the requirements of all those within it.

More recently, the process of deviancy amplification has been invoked as applying to drug taking (Young, 1971). Thus a small group become identified in society as drug takers. This identification of deviancy, it is postulated, is an essential process by which society clarifies and refines its own normalcy. Society views the deviant group as an example or cause of its own inherent and universal difficulties, i.e. drug takers are experimenters, radicals, hedonists, work shy, morally inferior, and insists on social controls to deal with this emerging problem. Controls and restraints lead to increased public awareness of the deviance, and a recruitment of deviants. This increase in the number of drug takers leads to increased social control and so on in a circular process of deviancy amplification. It is perhaps debatable that control measures inevitably create drug takers, but there appears little doubt that calls from the media for 'something to be done' and the hysteria of the press contributed to the size of the drug epidemic in the late 1960s (Cohen, 1972).

The control of drugs: a brief legislative history

To understand the relevance of current drug legislation it is necessary to briefly survey its historical development in the last one hundred and fifty years. A general social history of drug use has been provided by Inglis (1975) and more detailed accounts of opiate legislation in the USA (Musto, 1973) and the UK (Judson, 1974; Teff, 1975; Lydiate, 1977) are recommended.

Although at one stage Britain had a thriving homegrown opium industry (Berridge, 1977), drugs did not become a significant international issue until the despicable affair of British Indian opium pressured on to an unwilling Imperial China, resulted in the Opium Wars of the 1840s. If for the sake of tax savings to pay for its Indian colony, Britain part-addicted China over a hundred years ago, it is a massive irony that current taxes have to now be used by the authorities to keep 'Chinese' heroin out of the United Kingdom!

Eventually the health risk and social disturbance associated with opiates became a matter of international concern, and with the United States in the forefront, restrictions were called for in the traffic of narcotics. In 1909 the USA banned the import of opium for smoking and in 1911 the international Hague Convention called for measures of opiate control which were adopted by many countries. The USA passed the Harrison Narcotics Bill in 1914 which tightened the medical prescription of narcotic drugs, until in a one-sentence amendment of the Act in 1924, heroin prescription was totally prohibited (Musto, 1973). The influential Harrison Act, and its related 'criminal' approach to opiate possession and addiction, was not replaced until 1970 when, in a series of new acts of drug control, heroin along with LSD became theoretically prescribable in approved clinical research programmes. Practically, in terms of any movement towards a heroin maintenance programme, the psychological and political prohibition remains intact (Judson, 1974).

As a signatory of the Hague Convention the United Kingdom introduced the Dangerous Drugs Act in 1920 and established the Home Office as responsible for the control of opiates and cocaine. However, as further legislation was required, a drift towards the problematic Harrison Act kind of legislation was avoided by the medically dominated Rolleston

Committee Report in 1926. This Report established the principle whereby physicians could use their discretion to prescribe opiates on an indefinite basis to addicts who were 'capable of leading a fairly normal life so long as they take a certain quantity, usually small, of their drug of addiction' (Judson, 1974). This important principle underpins the subsequent British approach to maintenance opiate prescription for the stable addict.

Soon after 1934, newly suspected or confirmed cases of addiction were listed in an index at the Home Office. In 1936, there were 616 known addicts, of which the majority were morphinists and 146 were doctors! By 1953, with the law substantially the same, drug smuggling was insignificant and the number of known addicts, mainly therapeutic, had dropped to 290. Very gradually in the late 1950s the number of non-therapeutic addicts grew until by 1961 the total had risen to 470. However this growth in opiate dependence was not an isolated phenomenon for in the same period there was a massive increase in legal amphetamine and barbiturate prescribing.

The precise reasons for the British epidemic of drug taking in the 1960s remain obscure (Spear, 1969) but the irresponsibility or misplaced charity of a handful of generous general practitioners exercising Rolleston-derived prescribing rights ensured cheap and legal supplies of opiates and amphetamines for hundreds of new addicts. The second Inter-departmental Brain Committee (1965) recommended tighter control of prescribing and a compulsory Home Office notification procedure for addicts. In 1968 the right of prescribing heroin and cocaine to addicts was restricted to only those doctors granted a Home Office licence. In spring of the same year drug dependence clinics were set up to provide a facility for legal maintenance prescribing and appropriate treatment for drug takers. A series of drug acts reflecting a hasty response to an epidemic situation culminated in the comprehensive Misuse of Drugs Act 1971 (Lydiate, 1977).

The Act gives powers to the Home Secretary to introduce legal procedures to investigate and control irresponsible prescribing and also to place new drugs of misuse into a controlled category. Most significantly it places drugs into three classes with regard to severity of penalty for production, supplying, possession etc.

Class A: Heroin, cocaine, morphine, methadone, LSD, mescalin, opium, psilocybin, cannabinol and all derivatives of these.
Class B: Amphetamines (various kinds), codeine, dihydrocodeine, cannabis.
Class C: Amphetamines (various kinds), methaqualone (mandrax).

The 1973 Notification and Supply to Addicts regulation of the Act lists fourteen opiate drugs and cocaine, and states that any person addicted or suspected of addiction (in terms of the Act addiction means 'as a result of repeated administration [the individual] becomes so dependent upon the drug that he has an overpowering desire for the administration to be continued') has to be notified by all practitioners to the Home Office Drugs Branch. There is evidence that there is failure amongst practitioners to satisfy this statutory requirement (Ghodse, 1977). At present (1978) only doctors issued with a Home Office Licence may prescribe heroin and/or cocaine to an addict. In practice the vast majority of licensed doctors are psychiatrists working in drug dependence clinics.

In 1977 the Advisory Council on the Misuse of Drugs recommended that along with other services in general medicine and psychiatry, drug dependence clinics, hitherto rather associated with opiate addicts, attempt to be more therapeutically active with the growing problem of non-opiate dependent multiple drug takers.

The opiates

Opium has been extracted from varieties of wild and cultivated poppy for thousands of years. However, morphine, a constituent of opium was not isolated until 1804, and morphinism did not become a significant problem until the invention of the hypodermic needle in 1853. Diacetylmorphine, or heroin, was synthesized at St Mary's Hospital, London, in 1874 and introduced clinically as treatment for morphine addiction in 1898. Today, legal heroin production is confined to a handful of countries, and most heroin contributing to the international drug problem is illegally produced and comes from the 'Golden Triangle' area of the far east, or from regions in and around Turkey (Newsday Staff, 1974). Elaborate smuggling arrangements guarantee supplies of illegal heroin to most of Western Europe and North America and international attempts to curtail this traffic have largely been ineffective. Opiates in the United Kingdom come from three sources: (1) legal prescriptions; (2) the proceeds of burgled chemists and pharmacies; (3) smuggled oriental heroin, often containing diluents and adulterants and therefore of varying opiate content.

Most countries are not able to report reliably the prevalence of opiate addiction (Moser, 1974) but many European countries estimate numbers in the tens of thousands, and the number in the USA is estimated in excess of 100,000. Bewley (1968) estimated the United Kingdom prevalence to be 4–8 per 100,000, and the Home Office records for the 1970s have never reported a total number of addicts in excess of 3000. At the end of 1976 the official number was 1881 (Home Office, 1977) but due to addicts not being detected by the notification system the actual number who are physically dependent may be closer to 5000 (Blumberg, 1977; Teff, 1975). For the last few years the number of notified addicts has remained stable and there has been a significant reduction in the number of newly notified addicts under 18 (Home Office, 1977).

What kind of people are British opiate addicts?

Several studies have found that the standard caricature of the addict as a lying, long haired, ill-kempt, social drop-out covered in abcesses and needle marks, may be true for a minority, but is essentially a gross and misleading exaggeration. Stimson (1973) found that his representative sample of British heroin addicts divided broadly into four types. 'Stables' (33%) were employed, tended to avoid other addicts, had few social and medical complications and were low in criminal activity. 'Junkies' (17%) by contrast, were unemployed and supported themselves by drug related criminal activity, were highly involved in the drug sub-culture and had high rates of medical morbidity. 'Loners' (29%) had low involvement in the drug sub-culture, unstable living arrangements and low rates of criminal activity. 'Two-worlders' (21%), like 'Junkies', had a high rate of criminal activity and drug culture involvement, but like 'Stables' they were also employed and had few medical complications of addiction.

Is there a natural history of opiate dependence?

For some years there have been attempts to chart a natural history of opiate addiction, as if it were a biologically based disease process, so that as time went by there would be predictable amounts of morbidity, mortality and abstinence. Longitudinal studies have established that each year 2–3% of a sample will die of drug related causes, and that after one year's follow-up 10% will be abstinent, after five years 25% and after ten years 40% will be drug free (Vaillant, 1973; Thorley, 1978). Stimson and his colleagues have carried out a seven-year follow-up of 128 British heroin addicts with a 97% contact rate and found that 36% are no longer taking opiates (Stimson et al., 1978). Winick (1962) has suggested that as addicts reach their mid-thirties they will tend to naturally 'mature out' of their addiction and broadly speaking it appears as if the majority of an eventually abstinent group become abstinent in the first five years, and that subsequent abstinence comes in a steady trickle and may reflect a hard core maturing out (Thorley, 1978).

However, there are doubts to be cast on an inexorable biologically based natural history process as some intermittent opiate drug takers (chippers) never develop physical dependence (J.C. Blackwell, 1975, personal communication) and special circumstances like leaving a stressful war zone and returning home apparently caused 95% of Vietnam soldier addicts to become abstinent and only a minority to continue intermittent use (Robins *et al.*, 1974). Similarly, although it has been commonly reported that abstinent opiate addicts transfer their dependence to alcohol or other drugs, this kind of transfer was found only rarely in a seven-year follow-up of British addicts (Stimson *et al.*, 1978). These variations from predicted findings and the influence of circumstantial changes make it important to develop career studies which study the processes of social interaction as well as the biological processes which shape addict lives (Thorley, 1978).

Opiates and endorphins

Important developments have taken place in the neurochemistry of opiate substances leading to renewed speculation about the nature of opiate dependence. The long suspected opiate receptors were discovered in the brain in the early 1970s and found to be particularly distributed in the limbic system, suggesting a connection between opiates and the emotional content of pain (Snyder, 1977). In 1975 a team in Aberdeen identified the first endogenous opiate neurotransmitters, methionine enkephalin and leucine enkephalin (Hughes, 1976). Soon afterwards a more complex series of opiate related pituitary peptide hormones were identified of which the most common is β-endorphin, but at present the relationship between these pituitary hormones and the enkephalins is not known.

The function of enkephalin neurotransmitters is speculated as mediating the integration of sensory information associated with pain and emotional behaviour. It is suggested that enkephalin neurones release enkephalins and so reduce the production or release of conventional neurotransmitters, e.g. acetylcholine from the presynaptic neurone. Thus exogenous opiates, e.g. morphine, suppress the release of conventional neurotransmitters and slow down neuronal activity, and to maintain normal function there is a compensatory hypertrophy of enzymic systems producing neurotransmitters, and thus increased amounts of exogenous opiates are required to inhibit neuronal function (tolerance). Cessation or abrupt reduction of opiates causes a sudden release of conventional neurotransmitter on to a supersensitive post-synaptic receptor and a massive rise in neuronal activity translated into withdrawal phenomena. Clarification of these processes constitutes a major world wide research endeavour (Snyder, 1977).

The effects of opiates and the withdrawal syndrome

The addict may take his opiate by mouth (dropping), smoke it in a cigarette, inhale the fumes of burning heroin (chasing the dragon), inject it (fix), intramuscularly or subcutaneously (skin pop) or intravenously (mainline). The effects of this powerful and mythical group of drugs are in fact very variable and the curious are recommended to explore the many personal accounts by writers and artists. However, amongst the first sensations experienced after intravenous heroin injection is a 'rush', 'thrill', 'kick' or 'flash', characterized by a tingling sensation, a metal-like taste in the back of the throat, and a pervasive sense of warmth and intense pleasure. This experience of the 'buzz' is often compared to a rather superior sexual orgasm and not surprisingly it is greatly sought after by addicts. However, many addicts initially experience dysphoria and unpleasant nausea, and it may well be that much of the euphoria is learnt. There is some release of histamine causing itching, reddening of the eyes and hypotension. Within a few hours the CNS depressant effects begin to show. Although there is meiosis, visual acuity is reduced and there is mental clouding and often mild sleepiness. Often there is an intense feeling of detached relaxation and euphoria; appetite and sexual desire are reduced and there is little interest in social contact. Interference with gut motility makes constipation a very common side-effect.

It is unlikely that anyone has ever become addicted immediately after a first injection, but psychological dependence can develop rapidly as dysphoric sensations are overcome, and physical dependence can develop within a few weeks of high dose regular injecting. It is not uncommon, however, to come across addicts who have taken six months between their first injection and physical dependence. In this period tolerance increases rapidly and eventually a point is reached where the initial injection thrill and subsequent euphoria almost totally disappear. Now the drug is taken only to 'straighten out', to remain normal in affect, and to avoid withdrawal symptoms. Almost all chronic opiate addicts are trapped in this paradoxical and experiential limbo of energetically chasing the 'buzz' with higher and higher doses only to find the pleasure receding further and further away.

Sensitivity over the elusive euphoria means that addicts will describe fine distinctions between 'chinese' and the NHS heroin, morphine, pethidine and methadone. Although these distinctions are not usually recognized in textbooks, they are not to be disregarded (like distinctions between wines, teas and beers). In the United Kingdom dipipanone (Diconal) appears to be a highly regarded opiate drug.

The withdrawal syndrome is a compounding of psychological and physical manifestations in which many of the former anticipate the latter.

Thus anxiety in all its forms may merely be evidence of presumed future withdrawal rather than actual withdrawal. There is considerable evidence that every addict involved in the drug subculture has learned exactly what the withdrawal will bring as florid accounts of 'cold turkey' withdrawal experiences are widely circulated. Judson (1974) has described an experiment of Connell's in which hospitalized opiate addicts were gradually withdrawn over 28 days randomly allocated to one of two oral methadone dilution schedules. In one schedule methadone ceased on day 10 and in the other on day 21, and for both subsequent doses were of placebo which looked and tasted the same. Addicts and staff were blind to the allocation and staff observed withdrawal symptoms throughout the 28 days. There was no distinction between the groups and withdrawal symptoms for both were associated with the nearness of the twenty-eighth day, suggesting that psychological rather than physiological mechanisms were paramount in this hospital situation. Other experiments have produced withdrawal symptoms in hypnotized ex-addicts (Ludwig and Lyle, 1964).

In spite of these psychological observations there is a copious literature on the traditional withdrawal symptoms. Within 8 to 10 hours of the last dose the addict may develop rhinorrhoea, lacrimation, yawning, perspiration as well as craving. He may sleep but wakes unrefreshed and miserable, feeling restless and irritable. As time goes by he may become chilly and develop 'goose flesh', and develop nausea, anorexia, vomiting, diarrhoea, cramps and muscle pains. Central nervous system rebound excitability is shown by mydriasis, tachycardia, hypertension, flushing and involuntary movements. There may be a leucocytosis and fluid loss may lead to electrolyte imbalance, and very rarely cardiovascular collapse. However, in the absence of profound organic disease it is extremely rare for withdrawal to significantly endanger life. After 72 hours the symptoms recede in intensity and the severity of the entire syndrome is probably related to the degree of physical dependence (Hofmann, 1975). Gross disturbance has disappeared after 14 days although conditioned psychological and cognitive elements of addiction may persist for some time. It is now apparent that as well as tolerance, certain mild physiological changes including hypertension, hyperthermia and tachycardia may be evident for several months, the so-called 'protracted abstinence' (Martin *et al.*, 1969).

Morbidity and mortality

There is no convincing evidence that opiates in themselves cause any primary pathological or structural abnormality, and almost the whole of the morbidity associated with opiates is due to other drugs, adulterants and infections arising from contaminated injection equipment, or related to the social and physical deterioration secondary, in some individuals, to the addiction.

The morbidity associated with opiates is very wide and recent reviews have been made by Richter (1975) and Ghodse (1978). Although opiates are not directly hepatotoxic, many addicts have abnormal liver function tests, often associated with serum hepatitis and dirty injection technique. There is some evidence that between 1969 and 1977 British addicts have improved their aseptic technique (Stimson, 1978). Septic complications are found in up to 40% of some samples and other chronic complications include endocarditis, nephrotic syndrome, tuberculosis, transverse myelitis, finger gangrene and muscle fibrosis and contractures associated with chronic intramuscular injection trauma.

Mortality rates in opiate addicts are high and almost fifteen times that of non drug taking populations. Estimates from the USA and the UK range between 16 and 30 per 1000 per year (Ghodse, 1978; Hofmann, 1975). The excessive mortality is most commonly drug related, and death is usually due to respiratory failure due to multiple drug overdose. Suicide rates are certainly in excess of normal but are very difficult to reliably establish. Some deaths appear to occur within minutes of injection and an immunological hypersensitivity reaction to an adulterant has been postulated (Ghodse, 1978).

Treatment

The treatment of opiate drug taking falls into three areas. Firstly, there is the assessment and management of ongoing opiate requirements and related withdrawal phenomena. Secondly, there is the management of drug related medical morbidity which is more appropriate to medical textbooks and will not be pursued here. Thirdly, there is long-term management and rehabilitation.

To do his individuality justice and to escape caricature the new or suspected addict must be fully assessed, broadly under the headings described in the aetiology section of this chapter. In the UK this is usually best done at a drug dependence clinic, where a detailed clinical history and examination can be supplemented by evidence from out-patient urine tests. Assessment of degree of dependence and the decision to give an opiate maintenance prescription is better made by admitting the patient for 72 hours so that his drug requirements can be monitored. As withdrawal symptoms arise they can be ameliorated with small doses of oral methadone until a 24-hour drug requirement is established. This daily dose should be sufficient to prevent physical withdrawal and enable stable functioning. Profound psychological dependence is not best responded to with opiate maintenance as other drugs, e.g. benzodiazepines, if essential, can be used to allay anxiety for limited periods. Fundamentally, both assessment and treatment should see drug prescription requirements as very secondary to an opportunity to work on the personal and social problems which emerge from the history. This longer-term clinical work should be seen in a perspective of months rather than weeks, and should be aimed at minimizing the negative aspects of the sick role and encouraging personal responsibility. Thus out-patient and community-based counselling and skilled social work is probably more value than long-term in-patient treatment.

The acute management of opiate withdrawal symptoms, often much feared by drug takers, can take the form of oral methadone titration as a preliminary to a short-term daily reduction programme, either in hospital or as an out-patient depending on the severity and circumstances. Cover by tranquillizers may be required. Multiple drug withdrawal symptoms, especially when barbiturates are involved, may require acute medical in-patient treatment. There is increasing evidence that acupuncture techniques moderate the severity of withdrawal symptoms (Bourne, 1977).

The long-term treatment of the opiate addict is more controversial. In the USA, prison sentences, parole and enforced abstinence have been supplemented in the last ten years by oral methadone maintenance programmes. These programmes, which have had some success in reducing participants' criminality, have been controversial (Peck and Beckett, 1976; Gossop, 1978) and opiate prescription restrictions have led others to examine alternative approaches, e.g. allegedly safer artificial opiates, opiate antagonists (e.g. apomorphine), biofeedback techniques, meditation and acupuncture (Bourne, 1977).

Opiate maintenance in the UK has been based on drug dependency clinics since 1968 and its advantages and disadvantages have been reviewed by Edwards and Busch (1978). Every clinic has its stable addicts who lead conventional and productive lives, but it is the chaotic 'junkie' type addict who commands the attention of medical and psychiatric services. Most British clinics provide injectables and oral doses, heroin and methadone, often in combination, and broadly speaking the clinical atmosphere encourages the patient to gradually reduce his dose. The precise nature of the non-prescribing treatment of British clinics has never been assessed and no study since 1968 has shown that the 'British System' is clearly effective, and one seven-year follow-up shows abstinence and death rates very similar to USA studies (Thorley, 1978). Mitcheson and Hartnoll (1977, personal communication) have evaluated the advantages of prescribing oral methadone against injected heroin, and whilst oral methadone is more effective than heroin in reducing doses for a majority, a significant minority will increase their criminality to illegally service an injection habit. Rathod (1977) has shown how many addicts, particularly those less severely dependent, can benefit from a non-prescribing clinic which offers counselling and medical facilities.

Therapeutic communities and 'concept house' treatment and rehabilitation programmes such as Synanon, Phoenix House and Daytop Village in the USA and Phoenix House and Alpha House in the UK, have received wide publicity. Their effectiveness is difficult to evaluate, but a follow-up study of a British therapeutic community has established that this treatment method is effective for a significant minority of addicts (Ogborne and Melotte, 1977).

In summary, there are a wide variety and type of addict, and effective treatment may require a combination of medical, psychiatric, social and legal services. Each individual will need a specific response and perhaps a long-term perspective. Short-term prison or hospital based enforced abstinence almost always leads to relapse whereas long-term out-patient treatment allowing the growth of personal responsibility and choice seems to be more associated with eventual abstinence (Stimson, 1978).

Barbiturates and other hypnotic and sedative drugs

Barbiturates first came into use in 1903 and cases of dependence were reported in Germany as early as 1912. As treatment for insomnia, depression and anxiety, barbiturates rapidly became one of the most prescribed and abused drugs in medicine, but it was not until 1950 that Isbell and his colleagues established that physical dependence to barbiturates could be experimentally produced. Today, barbiturates probably cause more serious drug dependence than any other group of drugs.

In 1966 Bewley estimated that there were 100,000 persons in the UK dependent on barbiturates and a further 500,000 who were regular drug takers but probably not dependent. Surveys in general practice established that 4% of patients were receiving prescribed barbiturates and 58% had been taking them for over a year (Adams et al., 1966). A majority of these practice patients were female and over 40 and this group constitutes the majority of barbiturate addicts. A second group, more clearly identifiable as addicts, but numerically much smaller, are young multiple drug users. Here, men outnumber women, some may inject barbiturates or use opiates, and their broad characteristics are closer to the opiate addict population. In Britain the problem of unnecessary barbiturate prescribing has been tackled by a campaign to encourage practitioners to introduce voluntary controls and to transfer dependent patients on to safer hypnotic drugs (Connell, 1976; d'Orban, 1976; Wells, 1976). However, before this campaign there was evidence that between 1968 and 1973 the ratio of prescribed barbiturates to benzodiazapines had declined from 9·7:1 to 1·5:1 (Howie, 1975). This reassuring change in the prescribing pattern and a reduction in the 'middle-aged housewife addict' has unfortunately been matched by an increasing problem of barbiturate abuse by young multiple drug takers. Some of the supplies for this non-medical use come from burgled pharmacies but a significant proportion still comes from general practitioners (d'Orban, 1976).

The most commonly abused barbiturates are the short acting types like pentobarbitone (Nembutal), secobarbitone (Seconal) and amylobarbitone (Amytal) and a mixture of the last two (Tuinal). However other non-barbiturates may also lead to dependence disorders and should be prescribed with great caution, e.g. chloralhydrate, glutethimide (Doriden), methaqualone (a controlled drug in Mandrax), meprobromate (Equanil), chlormethiazole (Heminevrin) and benzodiazepines (e.g. Valium and Mogadon). Daily dose levels at which some of these drugs are considered to produce physical dependence are shown in Table I.

Table I *Minimal doses of hypnotic and sedative drugs required for establishment of physical dependence*

Drug	Minimal dose (mg/day)
Pentobarbitone (Nembutal)	400
Secobarbitone (Seconal)	400
Glutethimide (Doriden)	2500
Chlordiazepoxide (Librium)	300
Diazepam (Valium)	100
Chloremethiazole (Heminevrin)	5000

The effects of barbiturates are very little distinguishable from other CNS depressants. A state of intoxication is produced which in early cases may produce such minor impairment of functioning that it goes virtually undetected. Higher doses may lead to increasing ataxia, stupor and eventual unconsciousness. During sleep moderate doses reduce dreaming, suppress REM as judged by rapid eye movements, and reduce the vividness of dreams (Oswald, 1970). Barbiturate addicts may develop physical dependence and tolerance equivalent to a daily dose of 2000–2500 mg (10–12 capsules of Tuinal) but as there is little tolerance developed to the respiratory depressant effects, the chronic user is always at risk for a fatal overdose. Some individuals appear to develop a paradoxical reaction of excitation and activity which may be associated with violence, but whether this is a rare but direct effect of the drug or an interaction of the drug in predisposed personalities is not known (Hofmann, 1975).

Isbell *et al.* (1950) established that abrupt cessation led to withdrawal symptoms very similar to those of alcohol dependence: initial tremulousness and agitation followed by *grand mal* convulsions, perceptual disturbances and a psychotic delirium. Convulsions and delirium are much more common than in alcohol withdrawal and may occur in up to three-quarters of cases. It is worth noting that after withdrawal, short acting barbiturates convulsions occur within two or three days whereas after long acting barbiturates they may not appear for ten days. In the first few weeks following cessation of barbiturates there is an increase in levels of anxiety and insomnia, and during sleep, REM and dreaming are more prominent (Oswald, 1970).

The morbidity and mortality of barbiturate and related drug dependence are very considerable. Acute or chronic intoxication leads to defective judgement and there is a risk of traffic accidents and other kinds of physical trauma. Individuals who inject barbiturates run a risk of direct chemical injury to tissue as well as the complications due to infection, e.g. thrombophlebitis, ulcers, lymphoedema, abscesses, muscle ischaemia and gangrene due to intra-arterial injection. Barbiturates are especially associated with severe and fatal overdoses. In a survey in London, Ghodse (1976) found that barbiturates were used in 54% of overdoses taken by drug dependent individuals compared with 9% of overdoses taken by non drug dependent individuals. Moreover, 52% of the drug dependent patients had been taking barbiturates during the past 12 months.

Treatment of the overdosed barbiturate addict is a matter for acute medical care and a general physician. Treatment of barbiturate withdrawal requires in-patient care and close supervision. In order to control the withdrawal symptoms, a short acting barbiturate, e.g. pentobarbitone, should be given four to six hourly. Then after stabilization a very gradual reduction can be initiated with 10% of the total barbiturate dose being removed each day to minimize the likelihood of convulsions. Some physicians also provide cover with an anticonvulsant such as Phenytoin, and withdrawal may take up to three weeks. Treatment of the underlying basis of the dependence is along the lines described in the section on opiates.

Amphetamines and stimulant drugs

Amphetamines originated in the early part of the century and were introduced into clinical practice in 1935. During the 1940s and 1950s amphetamines were widely prescribed for depression, fatigue and obesity and many susceptible individuals were observed to develop handicapping psychological dependence.

In the 1960s various studies established the prevalence of amphetamine prescribing and misuse. Kiloh and Brandon (1962) in a survey of general practices in Newcastle upon Tyne found 1% of the population to be receiving amphetamines and 20% of these were psychologically dependent. The majority of amphetamine misusers were women over 30 initially prescribed amphetamines for depression and obesity. By the end of the 1960s it became apparent that amphetamines were increasingly being misused by young multiple drug takers and that this constituted a second area of problematic amphetamine dependence. Hawks *et al.* (1969) surveyed 74 regular injectors of methylamphetamine, and found that they were predominantly British, under 25, and had a history of parental separation, or family disturbance. A considerable proportion had criminal histories, and 30% were regularly using non-amphetamine drugs.

The epidemic of amphetamine injecting was curtailed in 1968, six months after drug dependency clinics opened, when the manufacturers by arrangements with the DHSS and the BMA withdrew methylamphetamine from retail chemists. Injection practice diminished rapidly, and soon afterwards, following a successful experiment in which practitioners in Ipswich agreed to refrain from prescribing, the BMA adopted as official policy a similar voluntary ban. There are few defensible indications for prescribing amphetamines and today most countries make some attempt to control legal prescribing. However, for the determined addict these restrictions matter little as amphetamines are easily made in illegal 'back kitchen' factories. Although the amphetamine dependent 'housewife addict' has virtually disappeared, great care must be taken when prescribing other non amphetamine stimulants like methylphenidate (Ritalin) and various slimming drugs.

Many amphetamine addicts (speed freaks) commence with oral use and primary effects quickly produce psychological dependence in susceptible individuals. Progression to regular continuous use orally or intravenously may be rapid, and as there is no substantial physical dependence, there may be drug free periods of days or weeks. Injecting continuously on a 'run' may go on for 10–12 days before the individual collapses with fatigue. Barbiturates are often used at this time to sleep and upon waking the user is hungry, lethargic and often profoundly depressed. Some authorities have argued that these symptoms are not simply to be regarded as physiological compensations after a protracted period of wakeful activity and starvation, but are in fact evidence of a withdrawal syndrome, implying physical dependence (Hofmann, 1975).

The effects of amphetamines are related to dose and to individual tolerance. Essentially, hunger and fatigue are reduced, the individual becomes more talkative with heightened awareness, greater energy and an increased capacity for concentration. The picture of restless activity is not unlike a mild hypomanic illness. As the effects increase, the pupils are dilated, there is a tachycardia and hyper-reflexia. Finally, there may be fine tremor, slurred speech and accompanying ataxia, nausea and headache. Moderate amphetamine use does not result in the headache or hangover. Intravenous injection produces a 'rush' or 'flash' and for some addicts an intense sensation of pleasure. It is not surprising that methylamphetamine has always been a popular adjuvant for those who inject opiates.

Connell (1958) drew attention to the amphetamine psychosis, and showed that whilst it is not absolutely dose frequency related, and may rarely be precipitated by low 'therapeutic' doses, it is relatively common in chronic high dose users. Paranoid symptoms and ideations are not uncommon in regular amphetamine drug takers, but occasionally the paranoid symptoms take on a frank delusional quality. Visual, tactile and auditory hallucinations, ideas of reference, and persecutory delusions can occur in a setting of clear consciousness, so that the syndrome is indistinguishable from acute or chronic schizophrenia of a paranoid type. The potential role of amphetamines in such psychosis can be investigated with urinalysis. Usually the psychosis fades over five to seven days as the amphetamines are excreted, but rarely, individuals fail to recover completely and may manifest psychotic disturbance for months after cessation of the drug. It is not known whether this extended psychotic illness is directly due to the drug or represents the appearance of a schizophrenic illness in predisposed individuals. It is usual to treat persistent symptoms with phenothiazines.

Amphetamines in high doses have been reported as producing toxic symptoms which may threaten life, and cerebro-vascular accidents (occlusion or haemorrhage) leading to sub-acute onset of focal neurological deficits, or coma (Yatsu et al., 1975).

Cocaine

Cocaine ('snow' or 'coke') has figured prominently in the folklore of drug taking from the late nineteenth century onwards, and will always be considered an aristocrat amongst stimulant drugs. Its association with Sigmund Freud and his fictional contemporary, Sherlock Holmes, bear witness to the vicarious in middle class life at the turn of the century. For centuries indigenous groups in South America have chewed the leaves of the coca shrub so as to benefit from its stimulant effects. In 1858 cocaine was isolated from coca extracts and its local anaesthetic properties were first described in 1862 (Hofmann, 1975). Although clearly not a narcotic, cocaine has always been closely associated with opiate drug taking and consequently both in the USA and UK it has been legislated for alongside heroin.

In the drug epidemic of the 1960s cocaine was widely used as an intravenous adjuvant to heroin. Since 1968 cocaine has been in the same legal category as heroin, and clinical prescribing as a stimulant is extremely rare. Most supplies are illegal and imported from South America. The powder is sniffed or 'snorted' using a small spoon, or tube into the nostril, and absorption is direct through the nasal mucosae. The psychic effects and general characteristics are similar to amphetamines but are said to have a less sharp and more subtle quality. As cocaine is inactivated fairly rapidly a new dose is needed within 20–30 minutes, and sprees of cocaine snorting are unlikely to last for more than a few hours. Another restricting aspect, certainly in the UK, is its relative rarity and extreme expense, but there is some evidence of a current vogue with middle class occasional users on both sides of the Atlantic (Gay, 1975).

Cocaine can cause a paranoid psychosis like amphetamines, but tactile hallucinations tend to be more prominent. Chronic 'snorting' can lead to ulceration of the nasal mucosae. Essentially the cocaine taker is exposed to the same range of acute and toxic effects as already described for the amphetamine user.

Hallucinogenic drugs

The use of hallucinatory plants stretches back into antiquity and classic accounts of mushroom cults have been provided by Wasson (Ebin, 1961). More recently western experimenters have described their experiences with mescalin (Ebin, 1961) derived from the peyote cactus *Lophophora williamsii*. Mescalin was synthesized in 1918, and in 1938 lysergic acid diethylamide (LSD) was discovered in Switzerland by Hofmann whilst engaged on a study of ergot derivatives (Cohen, 1964).

In spite of the variety of hallucinogenic substances now known, including psilocybin, dimethyl tryptamine, DOM (2,5–dimethoxy–4–methyl amphetamine), and mescalin, only one, LSD, is produced in quantities which make it a significant drug of misuse. During the late 1950s and 1960s LSD was legally prescribed for the investigation and treatment of psychotic illnesses, but startling or unequivocal benefits were not evident, and since 1968 this substance has virtually ceased to be prescribed in the UK. The illicit use of LSD on a massive scale began in the USA around 1965 and is associated historically, but not necessarily causally, with the advocacy of Dr Timothy Leary. A world wide epidemic of LSD use soon followed, and fears of its effects for society partly explain why it is a Class A drug in the 1971 Misuse of Drugs Act. The prevalence of hallucinogen use in the UK is impossible to measure, but relates directly to price and availability of the drug. It is unlikely that drug control measures will ever be successful in removing hallucinogen use in the UK as several species of commonly growing fungi are hallucinogenic and LSD can be synthesized by amateur chemists at home.

Hallucinogenic drugs taken orally cause perceptual changes which are noticeable within 40 minutes. Physiological effects peak at three and disappear by six hours. Commonly these include mild hypertension, tachycardia, mydriasis, cutaneous flushing, increased salivation and lacrimation, hyper-reflexia and occasionally a mild ataxia. The psychological changes, usually categorized as a good or bad 'trip', last eight to 12 hours. Clinical and phenomenological accounts cannot do justice to the complex and rich experience which can ensue, and poetry and metaphor are necessarily invoked (Ebin, 1961). Visual, spacial and colour, sound and touch sensations and perceptions are all effected, often heightened, and experiences associated with one sensory modality may be translated to another: synaesthesia. Thus colours may be smelled and sounds may be seen. The perceptual disturbances may be described as pseudo-hallucinations, illusions and visions since the LSD taker usually retains insight that his experience is drug induced. Occasionally time is distorted, a few seconds seem like a life-time, and experiences bordering on the mystical are commonly reported. Whilst this journey into 'inner space' is superficially attractive, the perceptual distortions and experience can become delusional so that the drug taker may believe that he can fly or walk on water, only to find traumatically that he cannot. Less predictably there may be marked emotional changes ranging from a giggling ecstatic euphoria to a terrifying sense of despair, anxiety or doom (Cohen, 1964). Effects gradually fade away over 24 hours, but a heightened perception may remain for some days.

There is no evidence of physical dependence on LSD and psychological dependence may not be a valid concept for enthusiastic but very infrequent users. Few drug takers take LSD on a daily basis. If they do, tolerance develops after five days but will disappear after a few days of abstinence.

It is very difficult to assess the adverse reactions, morbidity and mortality due to LSD as many individuals take other drugs. There are no deaths reported as being directly due to the drug, but accidental death or suicide whilst affected by its perceptual effects is not uncommon. Bad trips are associated with naïve use, predisposing personality disturbance or unresolved difficulties, excessive LSD doses and additional amphetamines

(Hofmann, 1975). The most common features of a bad trip are acute anxiety and loss of control of psychological function, and a consequent terror of imminent insanity.

Occasionally LSD does seem to be associated with prolonged psychotic reactions which may last from one week to several years. Schizophreniform reactions are the most common and usually self limiting. When not, treatment is along conventional lines. Flash back experiences are to be distinguished from prolonged psychotic phenomena. Here non-psychotic, and more rarely, psychotic components of the LSD experience recur spontaneously as long as a year after the last dose. The flash back may be triggered by stress, fatigue or the use of other drugs such as barbiturates, and occur more commonly in those who have had prolonged heavy LSD use. Visual images predominate and the precise aetiology of these episodes remains unknown.

Several authorities have described a 'psychedelic syndrome' of long-term changes in patterns of thought and behaviour following repeated LSD trips (Blacker *et al.*, 1968), but it is very difficult to clarify these phenomena in such a way that the drug is unequivocally implicated. In high doses LSD has been shown to cause *in vitro* chromosomal damage, and stillbirths and malformations in animal studies, but there is little evidence that these effects occur in human LSD drug takers (Hofmann, 1975).

Cannabis

The hemp plant (*Cannabis sativa*) grows freely in the temperate and tropical zones of the world. In the East the leaves and flowers have been used for medicinal purposes for centuries. In the West the stalk fibres have been twisted into rope and cord and the seeds have been fed to poultry and caged birds! Over the last twenty-five years, as cannabis has become widely used as a drug in the West, a vast literature has developed, principally because of the division between those who hold it to be a dangerous drug and those who believe that for the vast majority of users it is harmless. At a pragmatic level cannabis related morbidity cannot be held to greatly occupy the time of the average psychiatrist.

The concern about cannabis and observations of its growth of use in the West has led to many studies being carried out into the prevalence of cannabis use in society and more specifically in allegedly at risk sub-groups. Prevalence studies in the UK have not been entirely satisfactory and rates vary between 2 and 40%, with about 10% of young people emerging as having tried cannabis at some time (Kosviner, 1976). Studies on UK students reveal that between 10 and 40% have ever used cannabis and that 20 to 25% are using once a week or more. Characteristics of those who have 'ever used' show that they are more hedonistic, non-conformist, non-religious, politically left wing, neurotic and frustrated than those who have 'never used' (Kosviner, 1976). Clearly absolute prevalences remain elusive.

The essential effective chemicals are extracted from the cannabis plant in two forms. Marijuana is the vegetable substance from dried flowering tops, leaves and stems. It is known as Ganja in India, Kif in North Africa, Bhang in the Middle East and Dagga in South Africa. Hashish, the other form, is cannabis resin, an extract of resinous secretions (especially from the male and female flowers) boiled in solvents, and usually sold in the form of cubes or pellets. There are at least twenty cannabinoid substances in the extract, but only two exert hallucinogenic and sedative action. Tetrahydrocannibol (THC) the main active substance was isolated in 1964, and it is estimated that hashish has a THC content of 5 to 12% and potent marijuana a content of 4 to 8%. Varieties of the plant in different parts of the world and varying qualities and concentrations of cannabis extracted are of great significance to regular users.

Cannabis is smoked, mixed usually with tobacco in a cigarette or 'joint', or in a pipe as in the Middle East. In India, food or drinks containing cannabis are taken. The effects are noticeable within minutes (smoking), or within an hour (ingestion), and will last for about six hours. Cannabis does not appear to cause physical dependence, but some degree of psychological dependence can occur in susceptible individuals. Tolerance to the drug is not very apparent in infrequent low dose use, but is clearly present in high dose users (Graham, 1977). The drug causes tachycardia, increased peripheral blood flow and conjunctival injection, and these effects are broadly dose related. Psychological effects vary widely, but inhalation of a marihuana cigarette is followed within minutes in most people by feelings of well being, relaxation and tranquillity. However, those who are noticeably apprehensive, angry or depressed may become more so. External circumstances and ambience play an important part and naïve smokers have probably to learn the best experiences from a drug taking peer group (Becker, 1953). Cannabis tends, like alcohol, to be a social drug. Perceptual disturbances of time, sight and sound occur but as with hallucinogens these are not commonly psychotic. Occasionally disturbances of cognitive and psychomotor function occur. A broad range of experiences and phenomena from a group of British cannabis enthusiasts has been presented and analysed by Berke (1976).

The morbidity surrounding cannabis use has been the subject of many recent reviews (Graham, 1976, 1977; Petersen, 1976; Ghodse, 1978). In the psychiatric area there seems little doubt that cannabis can produce an acute psychotic syndrome as this has been demonstrated in experimental subjects (Isbell et al., 1967). Psychotic episodes tend to clear up spontaneously and rarely last more than 48 hours. The relationship between cannabis and chronic psychotic illness has been more controversial although Edwards (1974, 1976) believes that a causal connection remains extremely dubious. As with more potent hallucinogens, e.g. LSD, cannabis produces, although rarely, transient flash back experiences after cessation of the drug.

Reports from the East have suggested a cannabis induced 'amotivational syndrome', characterized by loss of ambition, slothfulness and apathy. However, there is no firm evidence of this syndrome in the West; it has not been satisfactorily produced under experimental conditions and further research is required (Ghodse, 1978; Graham, 1977). Similarly, early reports of cannabis induced brain damage characterized by enlarged cerebral ventricles have not been confirmed in more recent studies (Ghodse, 1978).

Edwards (1974) and Graham (1977) have discussed cannabis and the alleged escalation to more serious drug use and in particular opiates. There can be no reasonable doubt that most cannabis users in most parts of the world will not progress to opiates, but an uncertain proportion will have a minor experience of some other illicit drug, e.g. amphetamines or LSD. Equally, there can also be no doubt that a great majority of young opiate addicts will have had prior experience of cannabis, but the two drugs are sufficiently different in their actions to give little support to the idea that the use of one produces a compulsion to use the other (Graham, 1977).

All this evidence and much else besides has been used in a long-term debate as to whether the legal restrictions on the use of cannabis should be relaxed. The universal presence of cannabis in Western societies is evidence of a failure to control supply. At present possession and personal use of small amounts of cannabis is permitted in several states of the USA and to date there does not appear to have been a significant increase in cannabis consumption (Graham, 1977). Thus, although there may be deep reservations about legalization of cannabis, as well as enthusiastic and informed advocacy, it seems likely, at least in a historical perspective, that very gradually legal relaxation will take place.

Solvent sniffing

Over the past few years there have been reports from both sides of the Atlantic of solvent and glue sniffing, their psychological effects and related damage. The range of products employed is extensive and includes petrol, cleaning solvents, various aerosols, paint and lacquer cleaners as well as the more common household glues and modelling cements (Hofmann, 1975). Toluene and acetone are two commonly used organic base substances found in such products and they both have a generalized CNS depressant effect.

Much concern arises because sniffers are often young children, and in the UK, to buy or possess such domestic products, is not in any way illegal. Some sniffers remain isolated, sometimes undetected by their own families, but occasionally localized epidemics of sniffing break out in peer groups. There is some evidence that sniffers come from disturbed and deprived backgrounds (Watson, 1977).

In general the solvent fumes are inhaled from a milk bottle, paper or plastic bag. Initial effects are euphoria, and if inhalation continues, stupor and loss of consciousness. Perceptual disturbances can occur, but they may be confined to predisposed individuals. Physical dependence is rare but psychological dependence occurs quite commonly, and compulsive repeated sniffing has been reported. Tolerance occurs gradually, but data concerning cross tolerance to different solvents is not available.

The toxic effects of many of these substances is profound, and include hepato-renal damage, cerebral damage, polyneuropathy and aplastic anaemia. Fatalities due to cardiac arrhythmias have been reported. Legal restriction of access to these substances appears unlikely and the major response to this problem must lie in preventive and educational measures.

Non-opiate analgesic abuse

Non-opiate analgesics are the most widely consumed medicines in our society, and in 1970 9% of UK adults took them weekly and almost 3% took them daily (Murray, 1974b). Drugs of the aspirin, phenacetin and paracetamol type have unfounded pharmacological and medical actions attributed to them by the general public under the influence of dubious advertising, and are commonly taken not only for pain relief, but for insomnia, anxiety, and mental disorders. Some individuals indubitably develop psychological dependence on these drugs and authors have drawn attention to an analgesic abuse syndrome.

Commonly, this syndrome is characterized not only by the drug dependence but also by the associated analgesic induced morbidity. Most significant is analgesic nephropathy apparently caused by phenacetin in combination with aspirin, phenazone or caffeine. World wide prevalence of analgesic nephropathy correlates well with national per capita consumption of phenacetin, but aspirin and other salycilate drugs also have a direct nephrotoxic action. Murray has adopted as a criterion of abuse analgesic consumption of at least one gram daily for three years, and has drawn attention to the high incidence of analgesic nephropathy in the west of Scotland (Murray, 1973, 1974b). Heavy analgesic use is also associated with peptic ulceration, various anaemias, and neurological manifestations.

Characteristics of those with analgesic dependence show many shared features with other forms of drug dependence. Patients are secretive about their drug taking, and in one study one-third totally denied analgesic use and up to one-third continued their drug taking with knowledge of the consequences and against medical advice (Murray, 1973). Murrary (1973) has shown that patients with analgesic nephropathy are more likely to occasionally abuse other drugs or alcohol, have psychiatric histories, and to come from disturbed family backgrounds with associated psychiatric morbidity. Complementary studies of psychiatric hospital populations have shown that women with chronic neurosis, reactive depression and personality disturbance are particularly prone to analgesic abuse (Murray, 1974b).

Multiple drug dependence

All of the preceding sections have dealt with single substance dependence so as to mask the reality and significance of multiple drug dependence. It is very common for those who are physically dependent on one drug to be concurrently psychologically dependent on others. Similarly it is common to be psychologically dependent on a variety of drugs including alcohol but not physically dependent on any single drug. The range of substances taken relates more to availability and drug fashions than to any logic dictated by the pharmacological effect of the drugs.

In 1970 Mitcheson and his colleagues showed that in a sample of UK heroin addicts, 95% had used barbiturates, 99% had used intravenous methylamphetamines or oral amphetamine-barbiturate mixtures, 77% had used cocaine, 74% had used hallucinogens and all had smoked cannabis. Similarly an analysis of drug taking in methylamphetamine addicts showed that 24% had a history of heavy drinking and 56% were currently using cannabis, 50% were using heroin, 28% sedatives and tranquillizers and 21% were using hallucinogens (Hawks *et al.*, 1969).

In the last ten years patterns of drug use have changed but multiple drug dependence has remained the predominant form. There is an impression that in the United Kingdom, as illicit opiate supplies have become prohibitively expensive, potential opiate addicts have turned to multiple drug taking without necessarily developing physical dependence. Thus a 'drug addict' in the late 1970s may be taking tranquillizers, barbiturates, cannabis and excessively drinking alcohol. At present very little is known about the new multiple drug taker in the UK as he is more likely to be seen as an overdose in a casualty department rather than a patient in a drug dependence clinic. Ghodse (1976) analysed drug problems dealt with by 62 casualty departments in London in the month of October, 1975. The vast majority of the cases were of self poisoning, three-quarters were under 40, and more than a quarter were considered to be drug dependent. In cases of self poisoning 45% had used more than one drug. Although this study only reflects drug dependent individuals attending casualty departments in one city, it does suggest a large number of multiple drug takers in London virtually unknown to the medical authorities.

The expansion of multiple drug use has several implications. Firstly, it makes it difficult to explain drug taking as wholly in accordance with the pharmacological action of drugs. Secondly, it requires that we carefully monitor and take into account drug availability and changing fashions in drug taking. Finally it reminds us that treatment or prevention directed at specific drugs or limited groups may be of little consequence, and challenges the clinician to reconsider the complexities of an underlying and more generalized dependence concept.

Nicotine dependence and tobacco smoking

Russell has stated that 'cigarette smoking is probably the most addictive and dependence producing form of object specific gratification known to man' and argues that tobacco smoking is a form of drug dependence different but no less significant than that of other addictive drugs (Russell, 1976b). The medical hazards and increased mortality associated with tobacco consumption are widely acknowledged and accounts are available in standard medical texts, thus in this brief section only aspects of tobacco dependence and their implications will be discussed.

Russell (1971) has surveyed the 'natural history' of cigarette smoking and shown that 70% of those who have more than one cigarette in their teens are likely to be smoking in middle age. The causes of cigarette smoking, the process of initiation and maintenance are all complex and multifactorial but Russell argues that insufficient attention has been paid in the past to the major pharmacological feature of tobacco dependence: nicotine.

Nicotine is rapidly absorbed through skin, buccal and nasal mucosae as well as lung alveoli, and inhaled cigarette smoke nicotine takes only 7·5 seconds to reach the brain. It is an immensely toxic drug and two or three drops placed on the tongue would speedily kill an adult, as would the nicotine content of a cigar (about 60 mg) if injected intravenously.

Ingested nicotine is rapidly converted in the liver to inert cotinine which explains why tobacco chewers do not swallow tobacco, and why there are rarely fatalities when children and animals eat cigarettes.

Nicotine has many complex actions but principally affects the brain, the cardiovascular system and the adrenals. Its major effect is to raise the level of cerebral arousal, and to prime the cardiovascular system for activity. These stimulatory effects may well be rewarding to the smoker especially in situations of boredom. Nicotine also directly stimulates the production of adrenalin which may be beneficial in situations of stress. Paradoxically, nicotine also relaxes skeletal muscle and increases the rate of habituation to unimportant stimuli, features which smokers may perceive and value as relaxing. This combination of increased arousal with relaxation makes nicotine from tobacco a particularly valued drug (Russell, 1976b).

Dependence on smoking is usually regarded as psychological, but Russell (1976b) has argued that in heavy smokers there is also a physical dependence on nicotine. Firstly, it is clear that tolerance occurs, initial smoking experience gives rise to palpitations, dizziness, sweating, nausea or vomiting and it is some time before the smoking pattern allows a high nicotine intake. Secondly, there is a clearly identifiable tobacco withdrawal syndrome. Apart from intense craving, depression, tension, restlessness and difficulty in concentration, there are more specific physical effects of brachycardia, hypotension, constipation and sleep disturbance with EEG changes.

Historical evidence shows that in the past societies and individuals have been able to easily switch from pipe smoking to snuff or tobacco smoking, but at present there is great difficulty for individuals to change from cigarette smoking to other forms. Russell (1976b) suggests this is because air cured tobacco as used in cigars and pipe tobacco produces an alkaline smoke and nicotine which is easily absorbed from the buccal mucosa and therefore makes deep inhalation unnecessary. Consequently, there is a slow steady increase to relatively low blood nicotine levels. In contrast flue cured tobacco as used in cigarettes produces an acid smoke with poor buccal mucosa absorption and so encourages the smoker to inhale to absorb nicotine through the alveoli. Each inhalation, seven to ten for an average cigarette, produces a potent bolus of highly concentrated nicotine in the bloodstream. The brain equilibrates with these high concentration boli and smokers titrate their nicotine levels by adjusting their depth and rates. Russell (1976b) considers that these intermittent nicotine boli are powerful units of reinforcement in their own right, and together with physical dependence in heavy smokers, and more general social and psychological aspects of dependence, explain why cigarette smoking is so particularly addictive and so difficult to give up.

Attempts to reduce the health risk associated with cigarette smoking and tobacco consumption have been made in two main areas. Anti-smoking clinics have concentrated on the individual smokers and have not been very successful. Thirty to 40% of patients stop smoking at the end of various forms of clinic treatment, but at follow-up the success rate dwindles to 12 to 28%. In spite of various optimistic claims the most successful treatments have progressed little further than exercises of self-discipline, enthusiastic support from a doctor or peer non-smoking group, and attempts to transfer elements of the smoking dependence behaviour to more acceptable dependence activities, e.g. spending the money saved not smoking on a regular buy of records or hire purchase committment (Raw, 1976; Russell, 1977). Anti-smoking propaganda and judicious fiscal control has been taken very seriously by statutory authorities in recent years and there has been a significant reduction in annual tobacco consumption. Consumers are now encouraged to move from more dangerous high tar to low tar brands, but as Russell (1976c) has pointed out whilst ever dependence producing nicotine levels correlate highly ($+0.93$) with tar levels, such changes are very difficult. Ideally what is required is a low tar (to minimize health risk) medium nicotine (to satisfy dependence needs) cigarette and it is likely that attempts will be made to develop such a cigarette in the future.

Dependent over-eating

The relationship between over-eating and obesity is highly complicated (Burland et al., 1974; Silverstone, 1975; Bruch, 1973) and only the basic elements of eating dependence will be considered here. Thus although the majority of individuals who suffer from dependent over-eating may be obese, the converse that a majority of obese people have an eating dependence is not true.

Assessing the dependent elements in over-eating and obesity necessitates a detailed history of eating habits, variations, and external circumstances. The relationship of eating to subjective hunger and satiety is particularly important. Episodes of over-eating may be obviously pathological as in the bulimia of anorexia nervosa (see Chapter 5) but they are more likely to be related to more general emotional states or specific external cues. Thus whilst it is clear that the excessive eater does not necessarily have social or unconscious forces which drive him to persistent eating, many obese people do eat to reduce unpleasant feelings of boredom, anxiety or altered mood states. Removal of the unpleasant experience or emotion becomes a powerful reinforcement for further eating, and people learn to take solace in food whenever they become anxious or upset. Further internal cues such as physciological effects of ingested calories have been found to be less important than external factors such as palatability, social and cognitive cues, in contributing to a psychological model of dependent over-eating (Wooley and Wooley, 1975).

The role of the practitioner in helping an obese patient lose weight is often to manipulate the various factors evident from the assessment. Basic weight loss can be initiated and successful in a variety of ways which depend essentially on calorie controlled diets, and perhaps the support from a weight reduction peer group. However, for the more severely dependent over-eater, attention must be given first to the underlying affective state and level of emotional functioning, and then to the cognitive elements and most significant external cues. In theory, the strength of the dependence can be reduced by avoiding the most salient cues, e.g. stopping purchase of problematic foods, or where this is impossible, by cue exposure, e.g. practice in resisting favourite foods, so as to reduce cue saliency. The role of anorectic drugs has been discussed by Silverstone (1975).

Pathological gambling

Risk taking is an essential human trait closely bound up with personal survival. One of its particular elaborations, gambling, is a universal activity present in all societies. Excessive gambling, gambling dependence, or more medically, pathological gambling is a generic term for gambling behaviour which leads to personal and social problems. The impact of gambling in all its forms, its moral status, its aetiology and economic and social consequences have been reviewed in detail by Cornish (1978). Newman (1972) has indicated that sociological contributions to an understanding of gambling have been concerned with the causes and functions of gambling within the social structure, and the factors which impel individuals and sub-cultural groups to indulge in gambling activities. Newman's study of gambling behaviour in 500 people in London's East End led him to conclude that only a small and insignificant minority can be regarded as pathological gamblers, and that normal gambling plays a part in holding together the structure of society. This view is far from those who regard gambling with a degree of moral condemnation (Moody, 1974). Moran (1975) has developed an influential view of pathological gambling, but the most thoughtful and eloquent account of the phenomenology and experience of gambling, informed by psychodynamic and cross-cultural insights, has been provided by Halliday and Fuller (1974).

Moran (1975) has described a syndrome of pathological gambling characterized by any of the following:

(1) Concern on the part of the gambler and/or the family about the amount of gambling which is considered to be excessive.

(2) The presence of an overpowering urge to gamble so that the individual may be intermittently or continuously preoccupied with thoughts of gambling; this is usually associated with a feeling of tension which is found to be relieved only by further gambling.

(3) The subjective experience of an inability to control the amount once gambling has started, in spite of the realization that damage is resulting from this.

(4) Disturbances of economic, social and/or psychological functioning of the gambler and/or the family as a result of persistent gambling.

Moran (1975) has further suggested the following varieties of the syndrome.

Symptomatic gambling is seen as secondary to a primary mental disorder, usually a depressive illness. Gambling is resorted to in an attempt to obtain relief from anxiety and depression.

Psychopathic gambling is part of a generalized disturbance of behaviour which may include criminality unrelated to gambling, sexual disorders, poor work record and personal relationships.

Neurotic gambling is a response to some stressful situation or emotional problem. Often it is used instrumentally to hurt a spouse or parent, but when the interpersonal difficulty is resolved, the gambling stops.

Impulsive gambling is characterized by loss of control so that gambling continues until circumstances prevent it or money runs out. The similarities with a traditional concept of alcohol dependence are unavoidable.

Sub-cultural gambling arises out of the person's social and cultural background which is one of excessive gambling with little abstention.

The limitations to this categorical approach are similar to Jellinek's traditional varieties of alcoholism (see Chapter 10). Rarely do patients or clients fit into any one category and the temporal variations within any category, i.e. the variety of gambling career, make the value of such a categorical approach somewhat dubious.

It becomes essential in the treatment of any individual with pathological gambling to take a careful history and assessment, eliciting factors derived from an aetiology of pathological gambling. Factors which are important include the psychology of probability and risk taking, operant learning and in particular intermittent reinforcement, psychodynamic and personality characteristics, associated psychiatric illnesses and other dependence disorders, and social and economic aspects relating to access and control of gambling, e.g. betting shops (Halliday and Fuller, 1974; Moran, 1975; Cornish, 1978).

It has fallen to the doctor and psychiatrist to treat pathological gambling and it has apparently necessitated considering this form of social deviance within a disease model. There are grave disadvantages in this approach, partly because it implies reductionist thinking which militates against the necessary contributions of the lawyer, social scientist and even the psychologist. In practice, as with other dependence disorders, only a multidisciplinary approach can lead to a fuller understanding of the problem and the most relevant and effective responses.

Response to the pathological or problem gambler and his family lies in several areas. First one should establish a relationship and carry out a full assessment. It is useful to involve the gambler's spouse or family as early as possible. Secondly, counselling should be provided along with advice and information about how to deal with practical aspects of money management and debt. Thirdly, any underlying psychiatric illness should be given appropriate treatment. There may be need for a forensic psychiatric response, or separate support and counsel for the family. More significant emotional problems of the gambler can be approached with further counselling or psychotherapy. Finally a full psychological analysis of various aspects of the gambling behaviour may lead to a programme of behavioural treatment. Long-term support is often essential and a minority of pathological gamblers affiliate with the Gamblers Anonymous organization. Although this teaches that pathological gambling is a disease and encourages abstinence, it is an important self-help and social support system which has been a means to order and self-respect for many individuals.

References

Adams, B. G., Horder, E. J., Horder, J. P., Modell, M., Steen, C. A. and Wigg, J. W. (1966). Patients receiving barbiturates in an urban general practice. *J. Coll. Gen. Pract.* **12**, 24–31.

Advisory Council on the Misuse of Drugs (1977). First Interim Report of Treatment and Rehabilitation Working Group. September, 1977. DHSS, London.

Becker, H. S. (1953). Becoming a marijuana user. *Am. J. Sociol.* **59**, 235–242.

Bejerot, N. (1977). The nature of addiction. *In* 'Drug Dependence: Current Problems and Issues' (Ed. M. M. Glatt). MTP, London.

Berridge, V. (1977). Our own opium: cultivation of the opium poppy in Britain, 1740–1823. *Br. J. Addict.* **72**, 90–94.

Bewley, T. H. (1966). Recent changes in the pattern of drug abuse in the United Kingdom. *Bull. Narcotics* **18**, (4), 1–13.

Bewley, T. H. (1968). Recent changes in the incidence of all types of drug dependence in Great Britain. *Proc. Roy. Soc. Med.* **62**, 175–177.

Blacker, K. H., Jones, R. T., Stone, G. C. and Pfefferbaum (1968). Chronic users of L.S.D.: The 'acid heads'. *Am. J. Psychiat.* **125**, 341–348.

Blumberg, H. H. (1977). Drug taking among children and adolescents. *In* 'Recent Developments in Child Psychiatry' (Eds M. Rutter and L. Hersov), Blackwell, Oxford.

Bourne, P. G. (1977). New and innovative techniques in the treatment of drug abuse. *In* 'Drug Dependence: Current Problems and Issues' (Ed. M. M. Glatt). MTP, London.

Bowlby, J. (1977). The making and breaking of affectional bonds: I Aetiology and psychopathology in the light of attachment theory. *Br. J. Psychiat.* **130**, 201–210.

Burland, W. L., Samuel, P. D. and Yudkin, J. (Eds.) (1974). 'Obesity Symposium'. Churchill-Livingstone, Edinburgh.

Bruch, H. (1973). 'Eating Disorders: Obesity, Anorexia Nervosa, and the Person Within'. Basic Books, New York.

Chein, I., Gerard, D. I., Lee, R. S. and Rosenfeld, E. (1964). 'The Road to H'. Basic Books, New York.

Cockett, R. (1971). 'Drug Abuse and Personality in Young Offenders'. Butterworths, London.

Cohen, S. (1964). 'Drugs of Hallucination'. Secker and Warburg, London.

Cohen, S. (1972). 'Folk Devils and Moral Panics'. McGibbon and Kee, London.

Collier, H. O. J. (1969). Humoral transmitters, supersensitivity, receptors and dependence. *In* 'Scientific Basis of Drug Dependence' (Ed. H. Steinberg). Churchill, London.

Connell, P. H. (1958). 'Amphetamine Psychosis', Maudsley Monograph No. 5. Oxford University Press, Oxford.

Connell, P. H. (1976). What is barbiturate dependence and who is at risk? *J. Med. Ethics* **2**, 58–62,

Cornish, D. B. (1978). Gambling: a review of the literature and its implications for policy and research. Home Office Research Study No. 42. HMSO, London.

Ebin, D. (Ed.) (1961). 'The Drug Experience: First person accounts of addicts, scientists, and others'. Grove Press, New York.

Edwards, G. (1974). Cannabis and the criteria for legislation of a currently prohibited recreational drugs: ground work for a debate. *Acta. Psych. Scand.*, Suppl. 251.

Edwards, G. (1976). Cannabis and the psychiatric position. *In* 'Cannabis and Health' (Ed. J. D. P. Graham). Academic Press, London and New York.

Edwards, G. and Busch, C. (Eds.) (1978) 'The British Drug Problem and the Responses: 1966–1977. (in press).

Einstein, S. (1977). Alcohol and drug misuse treatment: problems and issues. *In* 'Drug Dependence: Current Problems and Issues' (Ed. M. M. Glatt). MTP, London.

Eysenck, H. J. (1965). 'Smoking, Health and Personality'. Wiedenfeld and Nicholson, London.

Fazey, C. (1976). 'The Aetiology of Non-medical Drug Use'. UNESCO, New York.

Gay, G. R. (1975). Cocaine in perspective. *In* 'Medical Aspects of Drug Abuse' (Ed. R. W. Richter). Harper and Row, New York.

Ghodse, A. H. (1976). Drug problems dealt with by 62 London casualty departments. *Br. J. Prev. Soc. Med.* **30**, 251–256.

Ghodse, A. H. (1977). Casualty departments and the monitoring of drug dependence. *Br. Med. J.* **i**, 1381–1382.

Ghodse, A. H. (1978). Morbidity and mortality. *In* 'The British Drug Problem and the Responses: 1966–1977' (Eds G. Edwards and C. Busch) (in press).

Goldstein, A. (1978). Are some heroin addicts self treating a metabolic disease? *World Medicine* February 22, 33–34.

Gossop, M. (1976). Drug dependence and self esteem. *Int. J. Addict.* **11**, (5), 741–753.

Gossop, M. (1978). A review of the evidence for methadone maintenance as a treatment for narcotic addiction. *Lancet* **i**, 812–815.

Graham, J. D. P. (Ed.) (1976) 'Cannabis and Health'. Academic Press, London and New York.

Graham, J. D. P. (1977). 'Cannabis Now'. HM and M. Publishers, London.

Halliday, J. and Fuller, P. (1974). 'The Psychology of Gambling'. Allen Lane, London.

Hawks, D., Mitcheson, M., Ogborne, A. and Edwards, G. (1969). Abuse of methylamphetamine. *Br. Med. J.* **ii**, 715–721.

Hindmarch, I. (1972). Drugs and their abuse: age groups particularly at risk. *Br. J. Addict.* **67**, 209–214.

Hofmann, F. G. (1975). 'A Handbook on Drug and Alcohol Abuse: The Biomedical Aspects'. Oxford University Press, Oxford.

Home Office (1977). 1976 Statistics of the Misuse of Drugs in the United Kingdom. Home Office News Release, London.

Howie, J. G. (1975). Psychotropic drugs in general practice. *Br. Med. J.* **ii**, 177–179.

Hughes, J. (1976). Enkephalin and Drug Dependence. *Br. J. Addict.* **71**, 199–209.

Interdepartmental Committee on Drug Addiction (1961) (The Brain Committee) HMSO, London.

Interdepartmental Committee on Drug Addiction (1965) (The Brain Committee's second Report) HMSO, London.

Inglis, B. (1975). 'The Forbidden Game: A Social History of Drugs'. Hodder and Stoughton, London.

Isbell, H., Altschul, S., Kornetsky, C. H. Eisenman, A. J., Flanary, H. G. and Fraser, H. F. (1950). Chronic barbiturate intoxication. *Archs Neurol Psychiat.* **64**, i. 416–418.

Isbell, H., Gorodetsky, G. W., Jasinski, D., Claussen, U., Spulack. F. and Korte, F. (1967). Effects of delta-9-transtetrahydrocannibinol in man. *Psychopharmacologia* **ii**, 184–188.

James, I. P. (1971) The changing pattern of narcotic addiction in Britain. *Int. J. Addict.* **6**, 119–134.

Judson, H. F. (1974). 'Heroin Addiction in Britain'. Harcourt Brace Jovanovich, New York.

Kiloh, L. G. and Brandon, S. (1962). Habituation and addiction to amphetamines. *Br. Med. J.* **ii**, 40–43.

Kosviner, A. (1976). Social science and cannabis use. *In* 'Cannabis and Health' (Ed. J. D. P. Graham). Academic Press, London and New York.

Kumar, R. (1974). Animal models for evaluating psychotropic drugs. *Psychol. Med.* **4**, 353–359.

Lader, M., Kendell, R. and Kasriel, J. (1974). The genetic contribution to unwanted drug effects. *Clin. Pharmacol. Ther.* **16**, 343–347.

Leyhausen, P. (1973). Addictive behaviour in free ranging animals. *In* 'Psychic Dependence: Definition, Assessment in Animals and Man, Theoretical and Clinical Implications' (Eds L. Goldberg and F. Hoffmeister). Springer-Verlag, New York.

Ludwig, A. M. and Lyle, W. H. (1964). The experimental production of narcotic drug effects and withdrawal symptoms through hypnosis. *Int. J. Clin. Exp. Hypnosis* **12**, i, 1–17.

Lydiate, P. W. H. (1977). 'The Law Relating to the Misuse of Drugs'. Butterworths, London.

Martin, W. R. (1968). A homeostatic and redundancy theory of tolerance to and dependence on narcotic analgesics. *Res. Publ. Ass. Res. Ment. Dis.* **46**, 206–223.

Martin, W. R. and Jasinski, D. R. (1969). Physiological parameters of morphine dependence in man—tolerance, early abstinence, protracted abstinence. *J. Psychiat. Res.* **7**, 9–12.

Merton, B. K. (1957). 'Social Theory and Social Structure'. Collier-MacMillan, Toronto.

Misuse of Drugs Act (1973). Notification of and Supply to Addicts Regulations Statutory Instruments. Dangerous Drugs No. 799. HMSO, London.

Moody, G. E. (1974). 'Social Control of Gambling: an independent view of gambling in Britain now'. The Churches Council on Gambling, London.

Moran, E. (1975). Pathological gambling. *In* 'Contemporary Psychiatry' (Eds T. Silverstone and B. Barraclough). Royal College of Psychiatrists, London.

Moser, J. (1974). 'Problems and Programmes related to Alcohol and Drug Dependence in 33 Countries'. WHO, Geneva.

Mott, J. (1972). The psychological basis of drug dependence: The intellectual and personality characteristics of opiate users. *Br. J. Addict.* **67**, 89–99.

Mott, J. (1975). The criminal histories of male non-medical opiate users in the United Kingdom. *Bull. Narcotics* **27**, (4), 41–48.

Murray, R. M. (1973). The origins of analgesic nephropathy. *Br. J. Psychiat.* **123**, 99–106.

Murray, R. M. (1974a). Psychiatric illness in doctors. *Lancet* i, 1211–1213.

Murray, R. M. (1974b). Analgesic abuse. *Br. J. Hosp. Med.* **2**, (5), 772–780.

Musto, D. F. (1973). 'The American Disease: Origins of Narcotics Control'. Yale University Press, New Haven.

Newman, O. (1972). 'Gambling: Hazard and Reward'. Athlone Press, London.

Newsday Staff (1974). 'The Heroin Trail'. Souvenir Press, London.

Ogborne, A. C. and Melotte, C. (1977). An Evaluation of a therapeutic community for former drug users. *Br. J. Addict.* **72**, 75–82.

d'Orban, P. T. (1973). Female narcotic addicts: a follow up study of criminal and addiction careers. *Br. Med. J.* **iv**, 345–347.

d'Orban, P. T. (1976). Barbiturate abuse. *J. Med. Ethics* **2**, 63–67.

Oppenheim, A. N. (1976). Towards a social psychology of dependence. *In* 'Drugs and Drug Dependence' (Eds G. Edwards, M. A. H. Russell, D. Hawks and M. MacCafferty). Saxon House/Lexington Books, London.

Orford, J. (1976). Aspects of the relationship between alcohol and drug abuse. *In* 'Drugs and Drug Dependence' (Eds G. Edwards, M. A. H. Russell, D. Hawks and M. MacCafferty). Saxon House/Lexington Books, London.

Oswald, I. (1970). Dependence upon hypnotic and sedative drugs. *Br. J. Hosp. Med.* August, 168–172.

Paton, W. D. M. (1969). A pharmacological approach to drug dependence and drug tolerance. *In* 'Scientific Basis of Drug Dependence' (Ed. H. Steinberg). Churchill, London.

Petersen, R. C. (1976). Marijuana and Health. Sixth Annual Report to the U.S. Congress from the Secretary of Health, Education and Welfare. National Institute of Drug Abuse, Rockville.

Plant, M. A. (1975). 'Drugtakers in an English Town'. Tavistock Publications, London.

Plant, M. A. (1978). What aetiologies? *In* 'The British Drug Problem and the Responses 1966–1977' (Eds G. Edwards and C. Busch) (in press).

Plant, M. A. and Reeves, C. E. (1974). The group dynamics of becoming a drug taker. *Interpersonal Development* **4**, 99–106.

Peck, D. G. and Beckett, W. (1976). Methadone maintenance: a review and critique. *Br. J. Addict.* **71**, 369–376.

Rathod, N. H. (1977). Follow up study of injectors in a provicial town. *Drug and Alcohol Dependence* **2**, 1–21.

Raw, M. (1976). Persuading people to stop smoking. *Behav. Res. Ther.* **14**, 97–101.

Richter, R. W. (Ed.) (1975) 'Medical Aspects of Drug Abuse'. Harper and Row, New York.

Robins, L. N., Davis, D. H. and Goodwin, D. W. (1974). Drug use by U. S. Army enlisted men in Vietnam: a follow-up on their return home. *Am. J. Epidemiol.* **99**, 4, 235–249.

Russell, M. A. H. (1971). Cigarette smoking: natural history of a dependence disorder. *Br. J. Med. Psychol.* **44**, 1–16.

Russell, M. A. H. (1976a). What is dependence? *In* 'Drugs and Drug Dependence' (Eds G., Edwards, M. A. H. Russell, D. Hawks and M. MacCafferty). Saxon House/Lexington Books, London.

Russell, M. A. H. (1976b). Tobacco smoking and nicotine dependence. *In* 'Research Advances in Alcohol and Drug Dependence' (Ed. Gibbins *et al.*), vol. 3. John Wiley, New York.

Russell, M. A. H. (1976c). Low-tar medium-nicotine cigarettes: a new approach to safer smoking. *Br. Med. J.* **i**, 1430–1433.

Russell, M. A. H. (1977). Stopping patients smoking. *General Practitioner* April 15, 16.

Seevers, M. (1969). Drugs, monkeys and man. *Michigan Q. Rev.* **1**, 3–7.

Silverstone, T. (1975). Anorectic drugs. *In* 'Obesity: Pathogenesis and Management' (Ed. T. Silverstone). MTP, London.

Sims, A. (1975). Dependence on alcohol and drugs following treatment for neurosis. *Br. J. Addict* **70**, 33–40.

Singer, K. (1975). 'The Prognosis of Narcotic Addiction'. Butterworths, London.

Snyder, S. H. (1977). Opiate receptors and internal opiates. *Scientific American* March, 44–56.

Solomon, E. and Marshall, W. L. (1973). A comprehensive model for the acquisition, maintenance and treatment of drug taking behaviour. *Br. J. Addict.* **63**, 215–220.

Spear, H. B. (1969). The growth of heroin addiction in the United Kingdom. *Br. J. Addict.* **64**, 245–255.

Stevenson, R. D. and Carney, A. (1971). Social and psychological background of drug addicts interviewed in Dublin. *J. Irish Med. Ass.* **64**, 372–375.

Stimson, G. V. (1973). 'Heroin and Behaviour: diversity among addicts attending London clinics'. Irish University Press, Shannon.

Stimson, G. V. and Ogborne, A. C. (1970). Survey of addicts prescribed heroin at London clinics. *Lancet* **i**, 1163–1166.

Stimson, G. V., Oppenheimer, E. and Thorley, A. (1978). Seven year followed up of heroin addicts: drug use and outcome. *Br. Med. J.* **i**, 1190–1192.

Teff, H. (1975). 'Drugs, Society and the Law'. Saxon House/Lexington Books, London.

Thorley, A. (1978). Longitudinal studies of drug dependence. *In* 'The British Drug Problem and the Responses: 1966–1977' (Eds G. Edwards and C. Busch) (in press).

Twycross, R. G. (1975). The use of narcotic analgesics in terminal illness. *J. Med. Ethics* **1**, 10–17.

Vaillant, G. (1973). A 20 year follow-up of New York narcotic addicts. *Arch. Gen. Psychiat* **29**, 237–241.

Watson, J. M. (1977). Glue-sniffing in profile. *Practitioner* **218**, 255–259.

Wells, F. (1976). The moral choice in prescribing barbiturates. *J. Med. Ethics* **2**, 68–70.

WHO (1950). Report of Expert Committee on Addiction-producing Drugs. WHO Technical Report Series **21**, 6.

WHO (1957). Report of Expert Committee on Addiction-producing Drugs. WHO Technical Report Series **116**.

WHO (1964). Report of Expert Committee on Addiction-producing Drugs. WHO Technical Report Series **273**, 13.

WHO (1969). Report of Expert Committee on Addiction-producing Drugs. WHO Technical Report Series **407**, 11.

Wikler, A. (1971). Present status of the concept of drug dependence. *Psychol. Med.* **1**, 377–380.

Wikler, A. (1973). Sources of reinforcement for drug using behaviour-a theoretical formulation. *In* 'Pharmacology and the Future of Man'. Proceedings of 5th International Congress of Pharmacology, San Francisco 1972, **1**, 18–30. Karger, Basel.

Winick, C. (1962). Maturing out of narcotic addiction. *Bull. Narcotics* **14**, 1–7.

Wooley, O. W. and Wooley, S. C. (1975). The experimental psychology of obesity. *In* 'Obesity: Its Pathogenesis and Management' (Ed. T. Silverstone,). MTP, London.

Yatsu, F. M., Wesson, D. R. and Smith, D. E. (1975). Amphetamine abuse. *In* 'Medical Aspects of Drug Abuse' (Ed. R. W. Richter). Harper and Row, New York.

Young, J. (1971). 'The Drugtakers: The Social Meaning of Drug Use'. McGibbon and Kee, London.

10 Alcoholism

Robin Murray

Alcohol as a drug

Ethyl alcohol (C_2H_5OH) is produced by the action of yeast fungi in fermenting sugars, a process which continues until the sugar supply is exhausted or the alcohol level reaches about 14% by volume at which concentration the yeast can no longer survive. Thereafter, more potent beverages can be produced by distilling off and isolating the volatile alcohol from the other fluids. The alcohol content of beer varies between 3 and 6%, that of table wines between 8 and 14%, and most distilled spirits (whisky, rum, brandy) contain 37 to 40% alcohol.

Alcohol is absorbed relatively slowly from the stomach, but rapidly from the small intestine. Food, particularly milk, delays absorption mainly by slowing stomach emptying. Ninety-five per cent or more of ingested alcohol is broken down by oxidation in the presence of the enzyme alcohol dehydrogenase. The acetaldehyde formed is then further oxidized to acetate and eventually carbon dioxide and water (Wallgren and Barry, 1970). Although only 2–5% of alcohol is excreted unchanged via the kidneys and lungs, the quantity of alcohol in expired air correlates well with concentrations in the tissues providing the basis for the breathalyser test. Metabolism can increase when large amounts of alcohol are ingested, and heavy drinkers usually oxidize alcohol more rapidly than light drinkers (Badawy, 1978).

The effect of alcohol on the functioning of the nervous system is, of course, the primary reason for its widespread consumption. Contrary to the layman's view, alcohol is a central nervous depressant. The apparent stimulation arises from the activity of parts of the brain freed from restraint as a result of depression of inhibitory control systems. At a blood level of about 50 mg% most people feel carefree and released from many of their ordinary anxieties. Emotional lability and clumsiness follow from a level of 100 mg%, and at a concentration of 300 mg% nine out of ten individuals are obviously intoxicated. Confusion, progressive stupor and anaesthesia ensue, and the fatal level lies between 500 and 800 mg%.

Fine tests of discrimination, memory, and arithmetic ability all show that impairment begins with the commencement of drinking. Memory for words, fluency in their use and the quality of word association become impaired, communication becomes more disorganized and the conventional rules of speech etiquette are likely to be flouted (Smith *et al.*, 1975). Interestingly, information learned while intoxicated is often recalled better during a similar state, a phenomenon known as state dependent learning (Weingarter *et al.*, 1976). Many people under the influence of alcohol falsely believe that their performance is normal or even improved. Alcohol, therefore, tends to increase risk taking. Bus drivers given several drinks are more likely to try and drive their buses through spaces that are too small (Cohen *et al.*, 1958).

The pharmacological effect of alcohol on mood is difficult to disentangle from the effect of both the circumstances in which the alcohol is taken, and the effect which the drinker expects it to have. Nevertheless, when experimental subjects are given alcohol the observed alterations in mood largely confirm every day experience with contentment, cheerfulness and euphoria being prominent. Alcohol is widely thought to be an aphrodisiac, but while a few drinks can help to overcome shyness, lack of confidence and feelings of guilt, large doses spoil the capacity to perform. The disinhibiting effects of alcohol may also release suppressed feelings of aggression and hostility, and numerous studies have associated intoxication with impulsive violence (Tinkleberg, 1972).

Alcoholism

Over the last century there has been a change in society's attitude towards the abuse of alcohol, from regarding it as a vice or a sign of moral degeneracy to considering it a disease (Paredes, 1976; Tarter and Schneider, 1976). On the whole the change has benefited the excessive drinker who is usually more appropriately dealt with by doctors than prison officers. This 'disease model' of alcoholism has enabled wives to see their drinking husbands as ill rather than merely bad, and it has also been a useful concept in educating the public to the dangers of alcohol abuse.

But is alcoholism a true disease? Undoubtedly, chronic alcohol abuse can cause physical damage, but it is illogical to call it a disease for this reason alone; on this basis promiscuity and bad driving would also qualify! Furthermore, Robinson (1972) has pointed out that labelling alcoholics as diseased can have unfortunate consequences; it may make doctors associate the condition with physical disorder and cause them to miss early cases, and it supplies the alcoholic with a 'sick role' which he may consider absolves him from responsibility for his drinking.

The evidence necessary to determine whether alcoholism is a disease is not yet available and the answer will in any case depend on the definition of alcoholism employed (Edwards, 1970). Although the word alcoholism is in common use almost everyone is puzzled as to its exact meaning. As Keller (1962) states, 'The definition of alcoholism (and alcoholics) has long been marked by uncertainty, conflict and ambiguity'. The most widely accepted current definition is that of the World Health Organization (1952) which described alcoholics as

> those excessive drinkers whose dependence upon alcohol has attained such a degree that it shows a noticeable mental disturbance or an interference with their bodily and mental health, their interpersonal relations and their smooth social functioning; or those who show the prodromal signs of such developments.

Implicit in this definition are the concepts of (i) dependence on alcohol, (ii) damaging drinking, and (iii) excessive drinking (Davies, 1976). These usually, but not invariably, occur together. All those individuals who are dependent on alcohol may without difficulty be regarded as alcoholic. However, definitions such as this which take not only physical and mental, but also social damage as diagnostic criteria are somewhat unsatisfactory (Seeley, 1959). What is regarded as abnormal drinking varies between cultures, and consequently what is socially damaging and therefore indicative of alcoholism in one country may be tolerated in another. A variety of attempts have been made to clarify the relationship between excessive drinking and damaging drinking. de Lindt and Schmidt (1971) found that the typical daily consumption of patients admitted to alcoholic units were in excess of 15 centilitres of absolute alcohol (the equivalent of 8 pints of beer or 15 single whiskies). However, individuals who drink considerably less may still incur consequent problems.

Jellinek's (1960) solution to such problems of classification was to describe various types of alcoholism. In Jellinek's scheme the following types are most common: *Alpha* (symptomatic) alcoholism, drinking as an attempt to relieve psychological and physical pain; in *Beta* alcoholism physical complications result from a combination of cultural drinking patterns and poor nutrition; *Gamma* (Anglo-Saxon) alcoholism consists of craving for alcohol, loss of control of drinking and withdrawal symptoms; *Delta* (continental) alcoholism is characterized by inability to abstain and causes comparatively little social disruption. Bout drinking is known as dipsomania or *Epsilon* alcoholism. These were formerly regarded as distinct entities, but there is now evidence that an individual drinker may present with different types at different times, and that cases do not inevitably progress from prodromal signs to full blown cases in the classical pattern. Jellinek's classification is, therefore, falling into disuse.

Nevertheless, there remains a need for an operational definition of alcoholism. In an effort to standardize diagnostic habits the American National Council on Alcoholism (1972) set out a series of criteria upon which the diagnosis can be made. The presence of some, e.g. evidence of physiological dependence, make the diagnosis obligatory, while others by themselves, e.g. suicidal gestures while drinking, are merely suggestive.

Dependence on alcohol

Another way of classifying heavy drinkers is to ascertain whether or not they are dependent on alcohol. The 'alcohol dependence syndrome' has been clearly described by Edwards and Gross (1976). They consider the main features:

(1) Narrowing of the drinking repertoire. The ordinary drinker drinks because of a variety of internal and external cues, and consequently his consumption varies from day to day. The dependent drinker drinks to relieve or avoid withdrawal and can often describe within fairly narrow limits his daily routine of drinking. The more dependent he is, the more stereotyped his schedule becomes.

(2) Salience of drinking over other activities. Drinking increasingly takes priority over other activities, and unpleasant consequences fail to deter further consumption. In the same way that a dependent monkey will work hard for its alcohol (Meisch *et al.*, 1975), the dependent human will beg, borrow or steal for a drink.

(3) Alcohol is a drug to which the central nervous system develops tolerance (Kalant *et al.*, 1971) possibly through some changes at the synaptic junction. Tolerance is shown by the dependent person being able to sustain an alcohol intake which would incapacitate the average man. The fact that an individual can still conduct his business on such an intake is not proof of some special strength or immunity, but rather an indicator of the seriousness of his dependence.

(4) Repeated withdrawal symptoms. Experiments on animals and men have amply confirmed the reality of the withdrawal syndrome (Hershon, 1973). This was first delineated by Isbell *et al.* (1955) who gave 10 ex-morphine addicts 250–400 ml of alcohol daily for up to 87 days. Abrupt

cessation led to lethargy, tremor, vomiting and intense fear with poor sleep punctuated by terrifying nightmares and both visual and auditory hallucinations; two subjects had fits and two became confused and disorientated. Only a few hours of abstinence (8–12 hours usually) are necessary for the development of withdrawal symptoms. Thus, common morning symptoms are sweating, tremor, gagging, retching and vomiting, agitation, anxiety, and 'the shakes'.

(5) Relief of withdrawal symptoms by further drinking. The patient recognizes his withdrawal symptoms as such. It is not only the severe morning symptoms which have to be 'cured', but if he is severely dependent he will react to mild warning symptoms throughout the day; he may also wake during the night for the drink which will abort incipient withdrawal.

(6) Subjective awareness of a compulsion to drink. The dependent drinker reports a subjective experience of impaired control over his drinking; he can no longer be sure of drinking in the way he wishes to drink or of stopping once he has started.

(7) Reinstatement after abstinence. The alcohol dependent person may find initial abstinence surprisingly easy to maintain. However, if he experimentally drinks again he is likely to relapse to his previous degree of dependence. The severely dependent person is likely to relapse explosively while the mildly dependent individual may take weeks or months before he again experiences withdrawal symptoms.

Alcohol related disabilities

Thus, there exists in society people who have incurred such damage from drinking that they are termed alcoholics, and many of these suffer from a clearly definable alcohol dependence syndrome. Such individuals usually have a variety of alcohol related disabilities, but these disabilities are by no means confined to alcoholics or alcohol dependent individuals. To disregard this fact is to ignore a great mass of people with difficulties resulting from the excessive use of alcohol. Alcohol related disabilities can be conveniently discussed under the headings of social, psychological and physical disabilities. They may occur singly, but the more serious a drinking problem then the more likely they are to co-exist and interact.

Social disabilities

The notion of social disability implies either (a) failure of an individual to perform in a role expected of him, e.g. as husband or father, or to adequately meet expected obligations, e.g. to go to work, or (b) transgressing social rules, e.g. crime or sexual deviation. Social disabilities may precede psychological and physical disabilities by several years. However, it must be stressed that the judgements as to what constitutes social disability are arbitrary. Society is the rule maker and referee.

Family problems: Marital problems are all too frequently a consequence of heavy drinking (Orford, 1977). A wife may complain that her husband tends to be stupidly embarrassing at parties; she is fed-up with his boastfulness, silly stories, pseudo-sexuality, and repeated sulks. The impact of this chronic wear and tear may cause emotional withdrawal or marital breakdown. One survey of AA members (Edwards *et al.*, 1967) revealed that 35% of men and 28% of women believed that drinking had broken up their marriage. In another study 52 out of 100 battered wives reported that their partners indulged in frequent heavy drinking. There is also evidence that parental alcoholism can be a powerful damaging influence on the personalities of children (Orford, 1977).

Employment problems: Alcoholics lose at least two and a half times as many days off work as their more sober workmates (reviewed by Murray), 1975). In the study of Alcoholics Anonymous to which reference has already been made (Edwards *et al.*, 1967) 63% of men had at some time been sacked because of their drinking. Edwards and his colleagues also interviewed 300 men who sought help at offices of the National Council on Alcoholism. All but 2% had lost time from work, 45% were either unemployed or off sick, and 12% had been sacked at least five times.

Accidents: Wechsler *et al.* (1969) found a positive breathalyser reading in 15·5% of patients admitted to an emergency hospital because of accidents at work, while Kirkpatrick and Taubenhaus (1967) detected blood levels greater than 50 mg% in one-third of home accident patients. Moser (1974) reported that 'excessive alcohol intake is stated to be the cause of a varying percentage of traffic accidents, estimated at least 30% in France and 3–10% in several other countries'. In the United Kingdom in 1974 one in three drivers killed in road accidents had blood alcohol levels above the statutory limit of 80 mg%: the proportion reached 71% on Saturday nights (Royal College of Psychiatrists, 1979).

Crime: In many countries being drunk and disorderly constitutes an offence. Relatively few such offenders are casual roisterers. The majority have had previous arrests for drunkenness, and in one study (Gath *et al.*, 1968) 50% were considered chemically dependent on alcohol. The bulk of other alcohol-related crime consists of petty offences committed by relatively unstable, unskilled and socially handicapped individuals. Gibbens and Silberman (1970) interviewed 400 representative London prisoners and classified 40% as excessive drinkers. Edwards *et al.* (1971) found that amongst prisoners serving sentences of three months or less, 43% recognized that they had a drinking problem, and 56% believed that they were drunk at the time of the offence. Recidivists are especially likely to be heavy drinkers as are those who turn to crime in their thirties or later. Drinking may allow the acting out of previously controlled fantasies, e.g. the 'respectable' citizen arrested for soliciting in a public toilet. In England and Wales approximately 20% of sexual offenders and up to 42% of murder offenders have been drinking before their offence (Zacune and Hensman, 1971).

Vagrancy: The destitute man on 'Skid Row' is not necessarily an alcoholic; he may be an eccentric, a schizophrenic, or someone with multiple social handicaps. However, a considerable proportion of homeless men are alcohol dependent, and the sight of a couple of ragged men sharing a bottle on a park bench is a familiar one in many large cities, e.g. the Bowery in New York (Myerson and Mayer, 1966; Moser, 1974).

Psychological disabilities

Dysphoria: Heavy drinking itself can produce a very depressing effect on mood, and the drinker may become prey to all sorts of doubts, miseries, suspicions and gloom. All this is likely to be exacerbated by his failing health and the accumulation of social problems, and may be wrongly diagnosed as primary depression or anxiety.

Personality deterioration: It can be difficult to distinguish personality features consequent on excessive drinking from those which were previously present. However, Kammier *et al.* (1973) compared profiles on the MMPI (p. 94) of alcoholics entering treatment with their previous scores at college. The early scores were not deviant; the later ones indicated excessive dependency. As the severity and chronicity of a drinking problem advance, a person's personality may apparently coarsen and he may be labelled as suffering from psychopathy.

Sexual problems: Failure of sexual interest or functioning may result from chronic heavy alcohol use. Sometimes the heavy drinker will act out otherwise controlled or subconscious sexual problems and, for instance, find himself involved in homosexual behaviour. A substantial minority of those with morbid jealousy are heavy drinkers (Shepherd, 1961). In some cases the development can be understood as being due to a combination of the patient's decreasing sexual competence and his spouse's revulsion at his drunken invitations to intercourse.

Delirium tremens describes the toxic confusional state which may complicate withdrawal from alcohol. Typically it begins at night, lasts for 48–96 hours and is accompanied by intense fear and restlessness. Other features include illusions, vivid visual hallucinations and delusions.

Tremor and ataxia are marked and autonomic disturbances include tachycardia, increase in blood pressure and fever (Gross, 1973, 1975). There was formerly a considerable mortality rate, but tranquillizers, correction of electrolyte disturbances (particularly hypoglycaemia and hypomagnesaemia), and treatment of intercurrent infection have greatly reduced this.

Alcoholic hallucinosis: Rarely hallucinations occur in the context of clear consciousness. They can occur at times of both relative increase and decrease in alcohol intake and may be distinct from delirium tremens. Voices are frequently offensive, accusing the sufferer of sexual perversions and the patient may become secondarily paranoid (see Cutting, 1978). Although the condition usually improves after cessation of drinking, a minority prove to be schizophrenic.

Amnesias: Most alcoholics experience 'black-outs'. These usually occur at times of severe intoxication and reflect the acquisition of tolerance to high blood alcohol levels. They range from fragmentary memory lapses to total amnesias for many hours (Goodwin *et al.*, 1969). They are not diagnostic of alcoholism since 15–20% of men who drink have experienced short-term amnesia.

Intellectual impairment: A proportion of alcoholics develop detectable 'intellectual impairment' even though at first glance they appear normal. A degree of recovery takes place after alcohol withdrawal, but psychomotor speed, problem solving ability and long-term memory may be permanently impaired (Ron, 1977).

Suicide: Approximately 6 to 10% of hospitalized alcoholics commit suicide. Kessel and Grossman (1961) found the suicide rate of ex-Maudsley inpatients to be 75 times that expected. Kessel (1965) found that 39% of men and 8% of women who attempted suicide in Edinburgh were alcoholics. Alcohol may also be taken as false courage before an attempt and in one Glasgow study (Patel *et al.*, 1972) heavy drinking preceded taking an overdose in 70% of men and 40% of women. Adverse life events such as loss of job or family are especially likely to precipitate self-poisoning.

Physical disabilities

Alcohol may adversely affect physical health directly, through secondary nutritional deficiencies or through a general lowering of resistance to infection. As might be expected mortality studies have consistently revealed elevated death rates in samples of alcoholics and other heavy drinkers, usually at least twice as high (Bruun *et al.*, 1975). These individuals die particularly from accidents, suicide, cirrhosis, lung cancer and heart disease (Chafetz *et al.*, 1974; Nicholls *et al.*, 1974).

Liver damage can be expected to ensue if ingestion of sufficiently large quantities of alcohol is maintained for sufficiently long. Nutritional deficiencies greatly enhance the deleterious effects of alcohol, but their absence does not prevent liver damage which is generally related to 'life-time' intake (Lelbach, 1974; Chafetz *et al.*, 1974). The earliest pathological change is fatty infiltration. Liver function tests, e.g. SGOT and SGPT, are often abnormal after an acute drinking bout, but soon revert to normal. If alcohol consumption continues hepatitis may supervene, and after some years cirrhosis which occurs in about 10% of alcoholics. The incidence of cirrhosis is increasing in most countries, and it is now the third commonest cause of death in New York males between the ages of 25 and 64 years (Schmidt, 1977). A small minority of patients develop oesophageal varices, hepatoma, or Zieve's Syndrome of transient hyperlipidaemia, jaundice, and haemolytic anaemia.

Other gastro-intestinal disorders: Non-specific gastritis is a common consequence of excessive drinking, and pancreatitis may also ensue (Cogbill and Song, 1970) although more commonly in the USA than Britain. Up to 20% of alcoholics give a history of peptic ulcer; half of these have had gastric surgery which may exacerbate dependence. Upper alimentary bleeding may result from gastritis, peptic ulcer, or varices, and bleeding may be exacerbated by the failure of the liver to produce vitamin K.

Anaemia may result from nutritional folate deficiency, failure of absorption of vitamin B_{12}, or from iron deficiency consequent upon gastro-intestinal dysfunction with poor absorption or blood loss. Excessive alcohol may itself cause thrombocytopenia and macrocytosis and their otherwise unexplained occurrence may be a useful pointer towards alcohol abuse (Wu *et al.*, 1974).

Cancer: Heavy drinkers are especially liable to cancers of the lung and upper digestive and respiratory tracts, but although hepatoma is associated with cirrhosis it has rarely been reported as a significant cause of mortality. Since heavy drinkers tend to be heavy smokers it is highly probable that the excess mortality from lung cancer is due to smoking. In the case of carcinoma of the larynx and oesophagus it seems that alcohol consumption and cigarette smoking each have an independent effect, but are synergistic when combined (Kissin and Kaley, 1974).

Heart disease: Drinkers do not have more coronary artery disease than abstainers and there have even been some suggestions that alcohol may have a protective effect. Alcohol abuse has, however, been conclusively linked to cardiomyopathy (Sanders, 1970). 'Beer drinkers' heart' although rare may cause severe cardiac failure; this usually improves with bed rest, routine medical treatment and absolute abstinence from alcohol.

Infection: Tuberculosis and pneumonia may result from a combination of poor nutrition, lowered resistance and poor hygiene.

Foetal Alcohol Syndrome: In 1972 Ulleland reported the occurrence of low birth weight and retarded development in some children of alcohol dependent mothers. This report was followed by that of Jones *et al*. (1976) describing 16 children of alcohol dependent women with similar patterns of retarded growth and development, and craniofacial, limb and cardiovascular defects. This constellation of anomalies was termed the Foetal Alcohol Syndrome. It is likely that such infants lie at the severe end of a spectrum of children disadvantaged by their mother's abuse of alcohol.

Drug-alcohol interactions: As befits a powerful pharmacological agent alcohol may interact with other drugs. It potentiates the effects of other CNS depressants such as barbiturates and benzodiazepines thus making coma from a combined overdosage deeper and more dangerous. Since alcohol competes for the liver enzymes which break down some anticoagulants, an acute drinking bout may precipitate bleeding in an individual on warfarin. Paradoxically as prolonged heavy drinking leads to induction of these same enzymes it may greatly increase drug breakdown, e.g. phenytoin breakdown may be doubled thus threatening control of epilepsy (Chakraborty, 1978).

Neurological disorders

Acute intoxication with disturbance of gait, balance and speech may progress to coma. Intravenous fructose can enhance the metabolism of alcohol and consequently in comatose patients with a possible complicating head injury fructose may help to reveal underlying pathology by shortening the period of intoxication.

The Wernicke-Korsakoff Syndrome: The term Wernicke's Encephalopathy refers to a condition characterized by acute onset of nystagmus, ocular palsies and ataxia, and usually accompanied by polyneuropathy. Ninety per cent show mental changes which generally take the form of global confusion, dullness and apathy, but may sometimes be more like delirium tremens. Pathological changes include damage to the thalamus, hypothalamus and mammillary bodies. This acute condition is frequently followed by Korsakoff's Psychosis which consists of (a) inability to form new memories and a retrograde amnesia extending back for days or years, (b) mild impairment of conceptual and perceptual functions, and (c) apathy. Patients may be disorientated and confabulate. Wernicke's Encephalopathy and Korsakoff's Psychosis are simply successive states in one disease process (Victor *et al.*, 1971). The underlying cause is thiamine depletion and this can be confirmed by finding a marked reduction of blood transketolase. It is usually associated with alcoholism, but may occasionally follow hyperemesis gravidarum or other conditions of mal-nutrition and prolonged vomiting. Untreated most patients with Wer-nicke's Encephalopathy die, but with large doses of thiamine ocular palsies generally recover within a week or so, although nystagmus and ataxia diminish more slowly. In the acute state the administration of glucose or a high carbohydrate diet may precipitate rapid deterioration by exhausting thiamine stores. If thiamine is given before the development of confusion and apathy it may prevent Korsakoff's Syndrome, but once that has developed recovery is incomplete in 80%.

Peripheral neuropathy develops to a greater or lesser degree in some 10% of chronic alcoholics. It can cause impotence, and in severe cases is very painful ('burning feet').

Epilepsy: At least 10% of alcoholics have had convulsions. These may occur in acute intoxication, withdrawal ('rum fits'), hypoglycaemia or in association with cerebral damage.

Conditions of unknown pathogenesis which occasionally occur in alcoholics include *Marchiafava-Bignami disease* (primary degeneration of the corpus callosum), *central pontine myelinolysis* and *cerebellar degeneration*. Retrobulbar neuritis and optic atrophy may follow methanol poisoning. These rare disorders are discussed by Pearce (1977).

Epidemiology

The frequency of excessive drinking may be estimated indirectly by means of indices having some indirect relationship to its occurrence, or more directly by field surveys.

Indirect indices

Mortality from cirrhosis of the liver: Although not all cirrhosis is due to heavy drinking the two are closely related, and Jellinek (1960) devised a formula for deriving the prevalence of alcoholism from the mortality rate for cirrhosis. Using this formulae France heads the international league with the United States in the middle category while England and Wales have a relatively low mortality rate from cirrhosis. Deaths from cirrhosis are rising steadily in most countries (Schmidt, 1977).

Per capita consumption of alcohol: A close relationship obtains between national *per capita* alcohol consumption and liver cirrhosis mortality, and thus between *per capita* consumption and alcoholism prevalence (Popham, 1970; de Lindt and Schmidt, 1971). The latter authors have further demonstrated for a variety of populations that the distribution of drinkers by consumption closely approximates to a smooth skewed normal curve known as the 'logarithmic normal curve'. If *per capita* consumption in any country increases, then the percentage of very heavy drinkers increases at least proportionately. This finding has considerable public health importance particularly since Chafetz *et al.* (1974) reported alcohol consumption to be rising in 16 out of the 17 countries for which data was available. In the United Kingdom the *per capita* alcohol consumption rose by 87% between 1950 and 1976.

In countries such as France, Italy and Portugal where alcohol is inexpensive and readily available both *per capita* alcohol consumption and cirrhosis mortality rates are high (de Lindt and Schmidt, 1971). Conversely, deaths from cirrhosis fell in the USA during prohibition, and in France during the extreme shortages of alcohol which occurred during both World Wars (Bruun *et al.*, 1975).

Hospital admissions for alcoholism: Although these are partly determined by the numbers of beds available and by admission policies, they can provide useful indices. In Scotland hospital admissions for alcoholism are seven times as high for males and five times as high for females as in England and Wales; this is a clear reflection of Scotland's greater problem (*British Medical Journal*, 1973; Sclare, 1975). Nevertheless, admissions to NHS psychiatric hospitals have increased in England and Wales 25-fold over the past 20 years, and the annual cost is reckoned to be over £4,000,000.

Drunkenness convictions: After falling for much of the earlier part of this century convictions in England and Wales have been rising, especially amongst juveniles, since the post-war period. The annual figure for drunkenness arrests rose from 47,717 in 1950 to 103,203 in 1974.

Drunken driving convictions: Like drunkenness convictions these are greatly influenced by legal changes, e.g. convictions in England and Wales doubled in 1968 following the introduction of a breath test for alcohol. But, while the total number of drivers involved in all accidents rose at an annual rate of 2·3% between 1968 and 1973, the proportion of those accidents in which a positive breath test was found rose by 27%.

Field surveys

Identifying problem drinkers by field surveys has largely been confined to North America and Western Europe. Two methods have been used:
1 *Case reporting surveys.* In this method one or more medical or social agencies are used to spot alcoholics. The most ambitious of those carried

out by general practitioners is that of Wilkins (1974) who surveyed a Manchester general practice (p. 336).

2 *Normal population surveys.* Well known 'house to house' surveys have been carried out in Iowa and Manhattan. American resources have been combined into a national ongoing project which is examining the whole range of drinking practices and attitudes (Cahalan and Room, 1974). Results so far have indicated increasing numbers of women both drinking and drinking abnormally.

Edwards *et al.* (1973) used both the agency method and house to house interviewing to survey a South London borough, and concluded that less than one-quarter of 'needful cases' were known to any agency. Although only 14% of men owned themselves to be heavy drinkers, 25% had suffered some social or economic disruption through drinking.

In spite of the wide national variations in the prevalence of problem drinking and alcoholism (Moser, 1974), certain broad trends emerge. Heavy drinking tends to be a male pursuit while abstinence is more common in women (10% of English women are abstainers rising to over 30% in the USA, and 70% in Japan) and in Church attenders. Although the mean age of hospitalized alcoholics is in the mid-forties, population surveys have found that the highest rates of alcohol-related problems are amongst men under 25 years old; older age groups have a diminishing proportion of heavy drinkers.

In the USA, heavy drinking is less common in the South and in rural areas (Chafetz *et al.*, 1971). In Britain the upper social classes have a pattern of frequent light drinking while the lower social classes show more heavy drinking at the weekend, and the middle classes have the lowest prevalence of alcoholism. Clinical studies invariably report a high proportion of the divorced and separated; this may be consequent rather than causal to alcoholism.

Aetiology

Genetic theories. The prevalence of alcoholism amongst the parents and siblings of alcoholics is about two and a half times that of the general population, and the morbidity risk of alcoholism for an individual with one alcoholic parent is approximately 25% (reviewed by Shields, 1977). This may be partly due to imitation rather than inheritance, and suggestions that dependence on alcohol is associated with colour blindness (an X-linked trait) have not been substantiated (Edwards, 1970). The conclusion to an elaborate study of 902 male twin pairs by Partanen *et al.* (1966) was that heredity influences the use of alcohol, but not its social consequences. Kaij (1960) found 71% of monozygotic twins to be concordant for drinking habits compared with 32% of dizygotic twins. Five pairs of monozygotic twins reared apart have also been reported and in four of these drinking habits were similar (Shields, 1977).

The most impressive evidence in favour of a genetic component has come from Goodwin and his colleagues (1973) who found that sons of Danish alcoholics who were adopted in early life were four times more likely to become alcoholic than adoptees without alcoholic biological parents. A further study comparing adopted sons of alcoholics with brothers raised by the alcoholic parent revealed rates of alcoholism of 25% and 17% respectively (Goodwin et al., 1974). The more severe the father's alcoholism the more likely was the son to become alcoholic. The authors conclude that 'environmental factors contributed little, if anything, to the development of alcoholism in sons of severe alcoholics in this sample'.

The balance of evidence is that genetic factors do make a contribution to alcohol dependence, but not such an overwhelming one as Goodwin's study suggests. Such a contribution could be through some pharmacogenetic means, and studies of alcohol elimination in twins have shown it to be partly under genetic control. An alternative mechanism would be a general predisposition to psychiatric disorder. Winokur et al. (1971) found that 35% of the male relatives of alcoholics they studied were also alcoholics; amongst female relations only 9% were alcoholic, but depression was very common. These authors consider that alcoholism, sociopathy and early onset unipolar depression constitute 'depressive spectrum disorder', and that this is most frequently expressed in males as alcoholism and in women as depression.

Biochemical theories. Some alcoholics relate such difficulties with alcohol from their earliest drinking experiences that it is tempting to postulate that they have a chemical predisposition to dependence. However, metabolic differences so far demonstrated between alcoholics and non-alcoholics are mainly the consequence rather than the cause of the dependence (Dietrich, 1976). The existence of an atypically active form of the enzyme alcohol dehydrogenase has aroused much interest. Only a small percentage of Europeans have this enzyme, but it is found in 85% of the Japanese population. Ewing et al. (1974) have shown that Oriental people are most likely to develop facial flushing when given alcohol and suggested that this is due to their developing higher acetaldehyde levels than Europeans. This could result from their having the more active alcohol dehydrogenase; as a consequence drinking might be less attractive to Asian people.

Until recently biochemical research was hampered by the lack of a suitable model of alcohol dependence (Mello, 1976). Most animals dislike the taste of alcohol, but rhesus monkeys can be induced to inject sufficient alcohol into themselves to produce sustained intoxication and a subsequent physical withdrawal syndrome. Littleton (1975, 1977) gave alcohol to mice by inhalation for 10 days and discovered that cessation produced a withdrawal syndrome lasting about 10 hours. It was easier to induce the dependence in mice if (a) they had a form of metabolism which predisposed to the accumulation of aldehydes in the brain, (b) if monoamine turnover was high during the alcohol administration, and (c) the mice were subjected to concurrent environmental stress. Those animals with more severely damaged livers had more severe withdrawal symptoms.

Littleton (1979) postulates that the acute effects of alcohol are caused by a biophysical effect on neuronal cell membranes, and the tolerance and dependence result from an adaptive change in the lipid or protein composition of the synaptic membrane with secondary alterations in monoamine receptor sensitivity.

Personality. The personality traits which have been suggested as underlying alcoholism range through oral fixation, latent homosexuality, immaturity to self-destruction. There is no evidence to support the existence of a universal unique alcoholic personality although pathological drinking can be one expression of long-standing personality disturbance (Kessel and Walton, 1969).

McCord and McCord (1960) examined social work records of over 200 boys who attended the Cambridge-Somerville Youth Study in the 1930s. The 29 who became alcoholic in later life were more likely to have shown unrestrained aggression, hyperactivity and denial of fears and feelings of inferiority. Their fathers were frequently deviant, and the McCords suggested that the absence of a suitable adult male on which to model their behaviour led these boys to adopt a façade of intense masculinity of which heavy drinking was a part.

Robins (1966) compared adults who had, as children, attended a child psychiatric clinic with control subjects. The clinic attenders were much more prone to develop alcoholism in later life, and anti-social traits in childhood such as theft or running away were more predictive of later alcoholism than neurotic traits.

Men with younger onset of alcohol misuse show greater antisocial behaviour (Foulds and Hassall, 1969). Evidence has also been advanced that there are personality differences according to the type of drinking pattern. Walton (1968) claims that typical loss of control alcoholics tend to be more aggressive, and more fearful of not being able to control aggressive tendencies and more easily depressed over losses and disappointments than typical 'inability to abstain' alcoholics.

Other psychiatric disorders. Excessive drinking may be symptomatic of other psychiatric disorders. Agoraphobics, social phobics and other neurotics may use alcohol as a tranquillizer, and occasionally alcohol abuse may herald dementia or schizophrenia. It is said that mania may be accompanied by increased consumption of alcohol while depressed patients may drink to allay their misery.

Psychological theories consider alcoholism as a form of learned behaviour, and the development of abnormal drinking as being influenced by three different types of learning (Orford, 1977).

(1) Imitation learning (modelling) determines the tendency for an individual's attitude to drink and drinking habits to be in line with those of his parents and immediate peer group.

(2) Operant learning. Alcohol produces pleasant states of feeling and relieves anxiety and guilt; thus each time a subject drinks he reinforces his drinking.

(3) Classical conditioning. The repeated association of the taste and smell of alcoholic beverages and sights and sounds of drinking occasions with pleasant alcohol-induced feelings can lead to these associated factors becoming pleasurable for their own sake.

Cultural factors. Wherever rates of alcoholism have been analysed by ethnic groups the rates for those of Irish origin have been found to be high and the rates for Jews to be low (Bales, 1959). The high Irish rates have been attributed to the ambivalence shown to alcohol in Irish culture—heavy drinking is condemned as immoral by one major section of society and lauded as intensely masculine by the remainder. In contrast Jews are introduced early to alcohol, taught to drink in moderation, but subject to a strict taboo against drunkenness. Thus, Jewish society avoids establishing attitudes—common elsewhere—equating the ability to drink heavily with the achievement of manhood.

Occupational factors. Certain occupations have more than their fair share of alcoholics. At risk are those concerned in the manufacture, distribution and sale of alcohol, company directors and commercial travellers, seamen and those in the armed forces, plus journalists, entertainers and doctors (Murray, 1975, 1976). Three factors appear to be particularly important.

(1) Ready availability of cheap or free alcohol.

(2) Mobility and consequent estrangement from the stabilizing influences of home life.

(3) Absence of supervision at work.

A multifactorial model. Since the aetiology of alcoholism is likely to be multifactorial, the various theories reviewed above are not all necessarily incompatible. Indeed Plaut (1967) has put forward a model which incorporates elements of several hypotheses. An individual who (i) responds to alcohol, perhaps in a physiologically determined way, by experiencing relief and relaxation, and who (ii) has difficulty in overcoming depression, frustration and anxiety, and who (iii) is a member of a culture that induces guilt and confusion about drinking behaviour, is more likely to develop problem drinking than most people.

Detection of problem drinkers

A number of attempts have been made to apply mass screening techniques to the identification of individuals with alcohol related disabilities (see Murray, 1977). These have mainly involved the use of questionnaires, but the only one with any promise has been the Michegan Alcoholism Screening Test (MAST). This 25-item questionnaire has been shown to separate out alcoholics from both normal individuals and other psychiatric patients with only minimal misclassification (Selzer, 1971; Moore, 1972). Since a proportion of hospitalized alcoholics have evidence of hypomagnesaemia, hyperlipidaemia, or hyperuricaemia and others are deficient in folic acid or vitamin B_{12}, some investigators have used a battery of laboratory tests in an effort to find characteristic patterns of abnormalities; as yet such efforts have not been rewarded.

Transaminase elevation is common in the alcoholic who requires hospitalization, but is much less frequent in the less seriously ill. However, Rosalki and Rau (1972) have drawn attention to the frequency of raised levels of serum gamma glutamyl transpeptidase (GGTP) amongst problem drinkers. Another simple investigation which may be of value as a routine screening test is macrocytosis without anaemia (Wu *et al.*, 1974; Unger and Johnson, 1974). Surprisingly, high blood alcohol levels have been little used as a screening test outside the legal sphere.

In the absence of a simple diagnostic test a high index of suspicion particularly towards 'high risk groups' remains the most valuable tool. These groups include:

General hospital patients especially with disorders associated with heavy drinking (p. 326). Nolan (1965) judged alcoholism to be a significant factor in 13·8% of admissions to a New Haven hospital, while Green (1965) found that 19% of men and 4% of women in the medical wards of an Australian hospital were alcoholics. Moser (1974) reported that up to 45% of men in some French general wards were alcoholic.

Psychiatric patients particularly men presenting relatively late with seeming psychopathic personality, depression and attempted suicide.

Patients attending Emergency Services since heavy drinkers are prone to accidents at home, at work, and on the roads.

Patients attending general practitioners: The family doctor is uniquely placed to detect problem drinkers, but singlehanded practitioners and those with small patients lists report much higher rates than those whose practices encourage anonymity. The most thorough investigation has been that of Wilkins (1974) who first identified individuals in his practice whom he considered 'at risk' by virtue of having some factor associated with alcohol dependence, e.g. working as a publican or late onset epilepsy. He then interviewed all those with at least one 'at risk' factor, and from a practice of some 12,000 patients found some 250 abnormal drinkers of whom he rated 155 as problem drinkers or alcohol addicts.

'High risk' occupational groups: Workers in those occupations associated with heavy drinking deserve special attention. In the United States programmes to combat alcoholism have been developed in many industries. Such programmes are based on the twin beliefs that the problem drinker will be detected earlier and that fear of losing his job will motivate him towards recovery (Murray, 1975). Emphasis has been placed on teaching supervisors useful signs of alcoholism, e.g. absenteeism especially on Mondays and on treating all alcoholic employees alike in a non-vindictive manner. Results from some programmes have been very encouraging.

Criminals, particularly drunkenness offenders, short-term prisoners and recidivists.

Vagrants and those in hostels for the destitute.

Treatment

To understand an individual's drinking problem it is necessary to ascertain: (a) whether he is alcohol-dependent or not, and how severe any dependence is; (b) what kinds and degrees of alcohol-related disabilities he suffers from; (c) what important personal or environmental factors underlie, exacerbate or ameliorate the dependence or disabilities. One's initial contact with a patient should be devoted to the dual task of eliciting this information and establishing a therapeutic relationship. It is often valuable to reconstruct with the patient a 'typical drinking day' starting with how he feels when he wakes up, and working through where he drinks, what he drinks and how much he drinks in the course of 24 hours. It is useless to become involved in an argument with the patient over whether he is an alcoholic or not, particularly since Cartwright *et al.* (1975) found that only a minority of those attending an alcoholism outpatient clinic were prepared to call themselves 'alcoholics'. Neither does it help to deliver lectures on the evils of drinking. The alcoholic lives with the pain of self-loathing and humiliation, of loss of family and friends, and of knowing he is gradually destroying his body and soul. He knows only too well that his formerly pleasurable drinking has become a nightmare of retching, shakes and lost memories.

Psychotherapy

Although the results of investigations into the effects of psychotherapy are either equivocal or contradictory (Baekeland *et al.*, 1975), most studies agree that it is essential to give the alcoholic the opportunity to develop a trusting relationship with a therapist. A long-term supportive relationship can be invaluable in dealing with the recurrent life problems which tend to afflict alcoholics. Group therapy is widely employed, although the evidence of its effectiveness is inconclusive (Baekeland *et al.*, 1975). At its best group therapy can permit the alcoholic to see himself more honestly, to analyse his relationships with others, and to feel an integral part of a social group. Because of the effects of alcoholism on the patient's spouse and vice versa, there is a growing trend to involve spouses and other members of the immediate family in therapy (Steinglass *et al.*, 1971). Rae (1972) reported that an alcoholic's prognosis is to some extent related to the degree of psychopathy his spouse exhibits.

Drug treatment

Mild or moderate withdrawal symptoms can be dealt with on an in- or out-patient basis using drugs which show cross-tolerance with alcohol, e.g. diazepam or chlormethiazole; these can usually be tailed off over 5–7 days. A useful regime is chlormethiazole 6 g daily for 2 days, 4 g daily for a further 2 days, and 2 g daily for a final 2 days. Although the majority of alcoholics are not vitamin depleted, oral or intramuscular vitamins are often given. Delirium tremens is best treated in hospital or in a detoxification unit.

Hypnotics, tranquillizers and antidepressants should be prescribed only when specifically indicated and then with caution because of the dangers of dependence.

Drugs such as disulfiram (Antabuse) and citrated calcium carbimide (Abstem) react with alcohol to cause very unpleasant acetaldehyde intoxication and histamine release. A daily maintenance dose means that an alcoholic with an overwhelming urge for alcohol must wait until the Antabuse or Abstem is eliminated from the body before he can drink safely; thus, it provides a 'chemical fence' around the alcoholic for at least 24 hours. Disulfiram implantation has recently been employed, but it is uncertain whether the blood levels achieved are sufficiently high to act as a pharmacological deterrent or whether the effects are mainly psychological (Malcolm *et al.*, 1974).

Treatment facilities. Specialized in-patient units generally admit patients for periods of 4 to 12 weeks and provide a non-authoritarian milieu incorporating group therapy with occupational therapy and education about alcoholism. These function most effectively as part of an integrated system of community facilities. The essence of such a system is that it should be able to respond rapidly to individual need with appropriate action. This may involve brief hospitalization for detoxification, attendance at a day hospital or a place in a half-way house (Cartwright *et al.*, 1975). In the latter the alcoholic may have the opportunity to continue group therapy and take a breather while he job hunts; the hostel also provides the lonely alcoholic with built-in acquaintances with whom he can relate. Voluntary organizations often play a vital role in providing a variety of community facilities.

Alcoholics Anonymous. This self-help organization provides its members with a social structure to fill the gap previously occupied by drinking, and gives their lives purpose through aiding others to achieve abstinence. Alanon, the organization for wives and husbands of alcoholics, can give important support to families. For those who can accept its 'Twelve Steps to Sobriety' AA is invaluable, but unfortunately not all alcoholics welcome its spiritual ethic and others, particularly younger and skid-row alcoholics, tend to be less easily integrated into its fellowship. As a consequence of its anonymous nature there have been relatively few controlled studies of AA (Leach, 1973). Thus, its considerable reputation for effectiveness is largely based on its own claims (Bebbington, 1976).

Outcome of treatment

Unfortunately little is known of what happens to untreated alcoholics. In one of the few such studies Lemere (1953) concluded that 50% would either drink themselves to death or only stop drinking during a terminal illness, 29% would continue to have a problem, while 11% would abstain successfully and 10% would regain at least partial control over their drinking.

Davies *et al.* (1956) followed up 50 alcoholics for two years after in-patient treatment: 36% were either totally or largely abstinent, a further

42% had maintained their social efficacy in spite of drinking while 22% had deteriorated. Subsequent studies have reported abstinence rates ranging from 5 to 50% and largely reflecting their selection criteria. To avoid such bias Edwards and Guthrie (1967) allocated 40 patients at random to either 8–9 weeks in-patient treatment or intensive out-patient care. No difference in outcome was found after one year follow-up.

Recently Costello (1975) analysed the combined results of some 58 studies involving more than 11,000 patients. One year following treatment 1% had died, 53% had a continuing drinking problem, 25% had no current drinking problem and 21% had been lost to follow-up. In a personal series followed-up for eight years he found that 27% had died, 37% had a continuing problem, 37% had been lost. Costello concluded that the treatment programmes with the best results were those in which (a) patients were carefully selected; (b) intense active therapy was employed; (c) there was effective follow-up; the use of Antabuse, behaviour therapy and social workers all appeared beneficial, but the length of in-patient care was not crucial. Armor *et al.* (1976) have also reported a multicentre study. Fewer than 25% of the patients had abstained for the six months before the 18 month follow-up. The more therapy patients had, the better they appeared to do, and regular AA attendance also increased the likelihood of abstinence. On the other hand, Orford and Edwards (1977) compared the progress of 50 patients who received a comprehensive programme of psychiatric and social therapy with 50 patients (randomly selected) who were given only an initial session of counselling. One year later there was no evidence that the patients offered the comprehensive care had fared much better. These authors conclude that 'alcoholism treatment should in general be less interventionist than has been the fashion'.

In general, the outcome of alcoholism depends not so much on the treatment given as on personal and environmental factors affecting individual patients (McCance and McCance, 1969). Well motivated patients with a stable background and supportive family have the best prognosis while younger patients and those with major personality disorders do worst. Condition at six months is a fairly reliable guide to drinking behaviour at a later date.

Experimental treatment programmes

If alcoholism is seen as an irreversible disease then the idea of a patient returning to controlled drinking becomes a practical impossibility and total abstinence the goal of all therapy. This is, of course, the view of Alcoholics Anonymous and until recently was the basis of all treatment

offered to alcoholics. The first serious challenge to this 'abstinence concept' came in 1962 when Davies reported that seven out of 93 alcoholic
patients returned to social drinking after a short period of abstinence in
hospital. Since then many other investigations have confirmed that between 5 and 15% of alcohol addicts are subsequently able to control their
drinking. Since the majority of these studies had goals of abstinence
the authors cannot be accused of confirming their own prejudice.
Epidemiological studies have uncovered a similar tendency for men to
move in and out of an addictive drinking pattern (Bailey and Stewart,
1967; Edwards *et al.*, 1973).

Pattison (1968, 1976) has pointed out that it is simplistic to take abstinence as the sole criterion of successful treatment since some abstinent
alcoholics can be more disturbed than others who are drinking. Alcoholics who take one drink do not inevitably trigger off physiological craving
and addictive drinking, and telling patients that they are only one drink
away from becoming a drunk may constitute a self-fulfilling prophecy; an
alcoholic imbued with this philosophy who takes one drink may proceed
to binge drinking because he believes that will inevitably occur. Furthermore, demanding total abstinence from patients may deter some from
seeking help.

Consequently, experiments have been undertaken to try and teach
alcoholics to drink in a controlled fashion. Sobell and Sobell (1973) using a
simulated bar-room, found that they could modify drinking habits by
giving painful stimuli when the alcoholic drank too much or too fast, or
took excessively large gulps of his drink. One year follow-up demonstrated that a group of patients treated by these behavioural means did as
well as a control group treated on the 'abstinence model'.

It would be a foolhardy psychiatrist who would recommend to all his
alcoholic patients that they attempt to return to social drinking, and
unfortunately it is at present impossible to tell which patients are most
likely to be able to control their drinking. Nevertheless, the possibility of
teaching controlled drinking can no longer be dismissed. It may be that in
the future different types of alcoholics will be offered different treatment
programmes with goals varying from total abstinence to social drinking.

Special problems

'The skid-row alcoholic'

A well recognized stereotype has emerged from the extensive literature
on 'the skid-row alcoholic'. He is middle-aged, maritally unattached and

lives in hostels, shelters or 'rough' in the decaying areas of large cities, and has had frequent arrests mainly for drunkenness (Myerson and Mayer, 1966). He is poorly educated, relatively unskilled, often an immigrant to the city and may be using its anonymity as a hiding place. Such individuals have a distinct medical as well as social profile with a high prevalence of physical disorder especially malnutrition, fatty liver, peptic ulceration and bleeding, and tuberculosis (Ashley *et al.*, 1976).

Although this group accounts for less than 5% of alcoholics, it provides the greatest therapeutic challenge (Blumberg *et al.*, 1971). Since amongst this group abstinence is rare without the achievement of some social stability, therapy aimed exclusively at alcoholism does not fulfil the rehabilitation needs of this population. They may be reached best by very committed workers and by the provision of 'shop-front' centres, day shelters and unpretentious night hostels. In Eastern Europe and in North America detoxification units have also been developed as an alternative to going in and out of jail for drunkenness offences (Siegel, 1973). These may either be hospital based or community based with only minimal medical involvement; the rationale for the latter is that the major need is rarely for intensive medical care and more frequently for rehabilitation and social support. The case for the cost-effectiveness of either type of unit remains to be made convincingly. In Toronto a major system of such units has had little effect in the overall problem; only 10% of those admitted to the units were referred for psychiatric treatment, and of those referred the percentage who improved was relatively small (Smart, 1976).

The female alcoholic

With a few exceptions (e.g. Sclare, 1970; Greenblatt and Schukitt, 1976) the problems of the female alcoholic have been neglected. Until recently, and in many cultures even now, moderate drinking by women has been considered 'un-ladylike' and alcoholism as totally reprehensible. Consequently female alcoholics try hard to conceal their drinking—50% drink alone—and their dependence can be very difficult to detect.

The 'typical' female alcoholic begins drinking excessively in her early thirties, increases her consumption as her children grow away from her and comes to treatment in her mid-forties. Women alcoholics give a family history of alcoholism more frequently than their male counterparts, and are said to show greater personality disintegration; depression and attempted suicide are common.

Alcoholism in women often follows a 'telescoped' course with more rapid deterioration. Alcoholic wives get less support from their spouses than do alcoholic husbands, and a proportion end up homeless with multiple convictions for drunkenness and prostitution.

Prevention

Prevalence studies suggest that there are at least 300,000 alcoholics in England and Wales. Admissions to hospital for alcoholism are now running at about 13,500 per year, and even including the contribution to treatment of out-patient clinics, general practitioners, social workers and Alcoholics Anonymous, it is obvious that the treatment system reaches only a small proportion of alcoholics. Since the cost, to say nothing of cost-effectiveness, of offering help to all those in need would be prohibitive, attention has recently turned to the possibility of prevention.

Since there is a direct relationship between national *per capita* alcohol consumption and alcoholism prevalence (p. 329), preventive strategy has focused on means of influencing *per capita* consumption; these means include Pricing Policy and Licensing Laws. A mass of evidence from many countries suggests that there is an inverse correlation between the 'real' price of drink (as a percentage of average disposable income) and national *per capita* consumption of alcohol. When the 'real' price of drink goes up, consumption falls; when the 'real' price goes down, consumption rises (Bruun *et al.*, 1975). There is also evidence that the more available alcohol is, the more consumption rises. For instance, in 1969 the Finnish Government abruptly relaxed their previously restrictive licensing laws. The number of licensed outlets for alcohol increased from 1600 in 1968 to over 21,000 in 1970, and as a result the *per capita* alcohol consumption rose by 50% over these two years.

Since pricing and licensing are subject to government policy, the Royal College of Psychiatrists (1979) has suggested that they should be manipulated to ensure that the national *per capita* alcohol consumption and therefore alcoholism prevalence should not rise and if possible decline. In addition, the College requested a greatly increased government commitment to public education to the dangers of alcohol abuse.

References

Armor, D. J., Polich, J. M. and Stambul, H. B. (1976). 'Alcoholism and Treatment. National Institute of Alcohol Abuse and Alcoholism'. The Rand Corporation, Santa Monica, California.
Ashley, M. J., Olin, J. S., Harding Le Riche, W., Kornaczewski, A., Schmidt, W. and Rankin, J. G. (1976). Skid row alcoholism: a distinct sociomedical entity. *Arch. Int. Med.* **136**, 272–278.

Badawy, A. A. (1978). The metabolism of alcohol. *Clin. Endocrin. Metab.* **7**, 247–272.

Baekeland, F., Lundwall, L., and Kissin, B. (1975). Methods for the treatment of chronic alcoholism. *In* 'Research Advances in Alcohol and Drug Problems' (Ed. R. J. Gibbins *et al.*), Vol. 2. Wiley, London.

Bailey, M. B. and Steward, J. (1967). Normal drinking by persons reporting previous problem drinking. *Q. J. Stud. Alcohol* **28**, 305–319.

Bales, R. F. (1959). Cultural differences in rates of alcoholism. *In* 'Drinking and Intoxication' (Ed. R. G. McCarthy). Free Press, New York.

Bebbington, P. E. (1976). The efficacy of alcoholics anonymous: the elusiveness of hard data. *Br. J. Psychiat.* **128**, 572–580.

Blumberg, L. V., Shirley, T. W., Jnr. and Moor, J. D., Jnr. (1971). The skid row man and the skid row status community. *Br. J. Stud. Alc.* **32**, 909–941.

British Medical Journal (1973). Editorial on Scotland's drink problem. **4**, 64.

Brunn, K., Edwards, G., Lumio, M., Makela, K. *et al.* (1976). 'Alcohol Control Policies in Public Health Perspective'. The Finnish Foundation for Alcohol Studies, Vol. 25. Helsinki.

Cahalan, D. and Room, R. (1974). 'Problem Drinking Among American Men'. Rutgers Centre of Alcohol Studies, New Brunswick.

Cartwright, A. K. J., Shaw, S. J. and Spratley, T. A. (1975). Designing a Comprehensive Community Response to Problems of Alcohol Abuse. Report to the Department of Health and Social Security, London.

Chafetz, M. E. *et al.* (1971). First Special Report to the US Congress on Alcohol and Health, National Institute of Alcohol Abuse and Alcoholism, Washington.

Chafetz, M. E. *et al.* (1974). Second Special Report to the US Congress on Alcohol and Health, National Institute on Alcohol Abuse and Alcoholism, Washington.

Chakraborty, J. (1978). Alcohol and its interactions with other drugs. *Clin. Endocrin. Metab.* **7**, 273–296.

Cogbill, C. L. and Song, K. I. (1970). Acute pancreatitis. *Arch. Surg.* **100**, 673–676.

Cohen, J., Dearnaley, E. J. and Hansel, L. E. M. (1958). The risk taken in driving under the influence of alcohol. *Br. Med. J.* **1**, 1438–1442.

Costello, R. (1975). Alcoholism treatment and evaluation, I and II. *Int. J. Addict.* **10**, 251–275, 857–867.

Cutting, J. (1978). A reappraisal of alcoholic hallucinosis. *Psychol. Med.* **8** (in press).

Davies, D. L. (1962). Normal drinking in recovered alcoholics. *Q. Jl. Stud. Alc.* **23**, 94–104.

Davies, D. L. (1976). Definitional issues. *In* 'Alcoholism, Interdisciplinary Approaches to an Enduring Problem' (Eds R. E. Tarfur and A. A. Sugerman). Addison-Wesley, Reading, Massachusetts.

Davies, D. L., Shepherd M. and Myers, E. (1956). The two year prognosis of 50 alcohol addicts after treatment in hospital. *Q. Jl. Stud. Alc.* **17**, 485–502.

de Lindt, J. and Schmidt W. (1971). Consumption averages and alcoholism prevalence. *Br. J. Addict.* **66**, 97–107.

Dietrich. R. A. (1976). Biochemical aspects of alcoholism. *Psychoneuroendocrinology* **1**, 325–346.

Edwards, G. (1970). The status of alcoholism as a disease. *In* 'Modern Trends in Drug Dependence and Alcoholism' (Ed. R. V. Phillipson). Butterworths, London.

Edwards, G. and Gross, M. M. (1976). Alcohol dependence: provisional description of a clinical syndrome. *Br. Med. J.* **1**, 1058–1061.

Edwards, G. and Guthrie, S. (1967). A controlled trial of inpatient and outpatient treatment of alcohol dependency. *Lancet* **i**, 555–559.

Edwards, G., Hensman, C., Hawker, A. and Williamson, V. (1967). Alcoholics Anonymous: the anatomy of a self-help group. *Soc. Psychiat.* **1**, 195–204.

Edwards, G., Hensman, C. and Peto, J. (1971). Drinking problems among prisoners. *Psychol. Med.* **1**, 388–399.

Edwards, G., Hawker, A., Hensman, C., Peto, J. and Williamson, V. (1973). Alcoholics known or unknown to Agencies. *Br. J. Psychiat* **123**, 169–184.

Ewing, J. A., Rouse, B. A. and Pellizzari, E. D. (1974). Alcohol sensitivity and ethnic background. *Am. J. Psychiat.* **131**, 206–210.

Foulds, G. A. and Hassel, C. (1969). The significance of age of onset of excessive drinking in male alcoholics. *Br. J. Psychiat.* **115**, 1027–1032.

Gath, D., Hensman, C., Hawker, A., Kelly, M. and Edwards, G. (1968). The drunk in court. *Br. Med. J.* **4**, 808–811.

Gibbens, T. C. N. and Silberman, M. (1970). Alcoholism among prisoners. *Psychol. Med.* **1**, 73–78.

Goodwin, D. W., Crane, J. B. and Guze, S. B. (1969). Alcoholic 'blackouts'. A review and clinical study of 100 alcoholics. *Am. J. Psychiat.* **126**, 191–198.

Goodwin, D. W., Schulsinger, F., Hermansen, L., Guze, S. B. and Winokur, G. (1973). Alcoholic problems in adoptees raised apart from alcoholic biological parents. *Arch. Gen. Psychiat.* **28**, 238–243.

Goodwin, D. W., Schulsinger, F., Moller, N., Hermansen, L., Winokur, G. and Guze, S. B. (1974). Drinking problems in adopted and non-adopted sons of alcoholics. *Arch. Gen. Psychiat.* **31**, 164–169.

Green, J. R. (1965). The incidence of alcoholism in patients admitted to medical wards. *Med. J. Aust.* **1**, 465–466.

Greenblatt, M. and Schuckit, M. A. (1976). 'Alcoholism Problems in Women and Children'. Grune and Stratton, New York.

Gross, M. M. (1973 and 1975). 'Alcohol Intoxication and Withdrawal: Experimental Studies', Vols I and II. Plenum Press, New York.

Hershon, H. (1973). Alcohol withdrawal symptoms. *Br. J. Addict.* **68**, 295–302.

Isbell, H., Fraser, H., Wikler, A., Belleville, R. and Eisenman, A. (1955). An experimental study of the etiology of 'rum fits' and 'delirium tremens'. *Q. Jl. Stud. Alc.* **16**, 1–33.

Jellinek, E. M. (1960). 'The Disease Concept of Alcoholism'. Hillhouse Press, New Jersey.

Jones, K. J., Smith, D. W. and Ulleland, C. N. (1976). Fetal alcohol syndrome—clinical delineation. *Ann. N. Y. Acad. Sci.* **273**, 130–137.

Kaij, L. (1960). 'Alcoholism in Twins'. Alonquist and Wiksell, Stockholm.

Kalant, H., Le Blanc, A. E. and Gibbens, R. J. (1971). *In* 'Biological Basis of Alcoholism' (Eds Y. Israel and J. Mardones). Wiley, New York.

Kammier, M. L., Hoffman, H. and Loper, R. G. (1973). Personality characteristics of alcoholics as college freshmen and at the time of treatment. *Q. Jl. Stud. Alc.* **34**, 390–399.

Keller, M. (1962). The definition of alcoholism and its prevalence. *In* 'Society, Culture and Drinking Patterns' (Eds D. J. Pittman and C. R. Snyder). Wiley, New York.

Kessel, W. I. N. (1965). Self poisoning. *Br. Med. J.* **2**, 1265–1270.

Kessel, W. I. N. and Granville-Grossman, G. (1961). Suicide in alcoholics. *Br. Med. J.* **2**, 773–774.

Kessel, N. and Walton, H. (1969). 'Alcoholism'. Penguin Books, London.

Kilpatrick, J. R. and Tanbenhaus, L. J. (1967). Blood alcohol levels of home accident patients. *Q. Jl. Stud. Alc.* **28**, 734–737.

Kissin, B. and Kaley, M. M. (1974). Alcoholism and cancer. *In* 'The Biology of Alcoholism' (Eds B. Kissin and H. Begleiter) Vol. 3. Plenum Press, New York.

Leach, B. (1973). Alcoholics anonymous. *In* 'Alcoholism: Progress in Research and Treatment' (Eds P. Bourne and R. Fox). Academic Press, New York and London.

Lelbach, W. K. (1974). Organic pathology related to volume and pattern of alcohol use. *In* 'Research Advances in Alcohol and Drug Problems', (Eds R. J. Gibbens *et al.*), Vol. 1. Wiley, New York.

Lemere, F. (1953). What happens to alcoholics. *Am. J. Psychiat.* **109**, 674–676.

Littleton, J. M. (1975). The experimental approach to alcoholism. *Br. J. Addict.* **70**, 99–102.

Littleton, J. M. (1977). The biological basis of alcoholism. *In* 'Alcoholism, New Knowledge and New Responses' (Eds G. Edwards and M. Grant). Croom Helm, London.

McCance, C. and McCance, P. F. (1969). Alcoholism in north-east Scotland; its treatment and outcome. *Br. J. Psychiat.* **115**, 189–198.

McCord, W. and McCord, J. (1960). 'The Origins of Alcoholism'. Tavistock, London.

Malcolm, M. J., Madden, J. S. and Williams, A. E. (1974). Disulfiram implantation critically evaluated. *Br. J. Psychiat.* **125**, 485–489.

Mello N. K. (1976). Animal models for the study of alcohol addiction. *Psychoneuroendocrinology* **1**, 347–357.

Meisch, R. A., Henningfield, J. E. and Thompson, T. (1975). *In* 'Alcohol Intoxication and Withdrawal' (Ed. M. M. Gross). Plenum Press, New York.

Moore, R. A. (1972). The diagnosis of alcoholism in a psychiatric hospital. *Am. J. Psychiat.* **128**, 1565–1569.

Moser. J. (1974). 'Problems and Programmes Related to Alcohol and Drug Dependence in 33 Countries'. World Health Organization, Geneva.

Murray, R. M. (1975). Alcoholism and employment. *J. Alcoholism* **10**, 23–26.

Murray, R. M. (1976). The characteristics and prognosis of alcoholic doctors. *Br. Med. J.* **2**, 1537–1539.

Murray, R. M. (1977). Screening and early detection instruments for alcoholism. *In* 'Alcohol Related Disabilities'. World Health Organization, Geneva.

Myerson, D. J. and Mayer, J. (1966). Origins, treatment and destiny of skid-row alcoholic men. *New Eng. J. Med.* **275**, 419–425.

National Council on Alcoholism (1972). Criteria for the diagnosis of alcoholism. *Am. J. Psychiat.* **129**, 127–131.

Nicholls, P., Edwards, G. and Kyle, E. (1974). Alcoholics admitted to four hospitals in England, II general and cause—specific mortality. *Q. Jl. Stud. Alc.* **35**, 841–855.

Nolan, J. P. (1965). Alcohol as a factor in the illness of university service patients. *Am. J. Med. Sci.* **249**, 135–139.

Orford, J. (1977). Impact of alcoholism on family and home, and Alcoholism; what psychology offers. *In* 'Alcoholism; New Knowledge and New Responses' (Eds G. Edwards and M. Grant). Croom Helm, London.

Orford, J. and Edwards, G. (1977). 'Alcoholism'. Oxford University Press, Oxford.

Paredes, A. (1976). The history of the concept of alcoholism. *In* 'Alcoholism:

Interdisciplinary Approaches to an Enduring Problem' (Eds R. E. Tarter and A. A. Sugerman). Addison-Wesley, Reading, Massachusetts.

Partanen, J., Bruun, K. and Markkanen, T. (1966). 'Inheritance of Drinking Behaviour'. Finnish Foundation for Alcohol Studies, Helsinki.

Patel, A. R., Roy, M. and Wilson, G. M. (1972). Self poisoning and alcohol. *Lancet* ii, 1099–1102.

Pattison, E. M. (1968). A critique of abstinence criteria in the treatment of alcoholism. *Int. J. Soc. Psychiat.* 14, 268–276.

Pattison, E. M. (1976). Nonabstinent drinking goals in the treatment of alcoholism. *Arch. Gen. Psychiat.* 33, 923–931.

Pearce, J. M. S. (1977). Neurological aspects of alcoholism. *Br. J. Hosp. Med.* 18, 132–142.

Plaut, T. F. (1967). 'Alcohol Problems: A Report to the Nation'. Oxford University Press, New York.

Popham, R. E. (1970). Indirect methods of alcoholism prevalence estimation. *In* 'Alcohol and Alcoholism' (Ed. R. E. Popham). Toronto University Press, Toronto.

Rae, J. B. (1972). The influence of wives on the treatment outcome of alcoholics. *Br. J. Psychiat.* 120, 601–613.

Robins, L. N. (1966). 'Deviant Children Grown Up'. Williams and Wilkins, Baltimore.

Robinson, D. (1972). The alcohologists' addiction. *Q. Jl. Alc.* 33, 1028–1042.

Ron, M. A. (1977). Brain damage in chronic alcoholism: a neuropathological, neuroradiological and psychological review. *Psychol. Med.* 7, 103–112.

Rosalki, S. B. and Rau (1972). Serum glutamyl transpeptidase activity in alcoholism. *Clin. Chim. Acta.* 39, 41–44.

Royal College of Psychiatrists (1978). Report of the Special Committee on Alcohol and Alcoholism.

Saunders, M. G. (1970). Alcoholic cardiomyopathy: a critical review. *Q. Jl. Stud. Alc.* , 324–368.

Schmidt, W. (1977). Cirrhosis and alcohol consumption. *In* 'Alcoholism: New Knowledge and New Responses' (Eds G. Edwards and M. Grant). Croom Helm, London.

Sclare, A. B. (1970). The female alcoholic. *Br. J. Addict.* 65, 99–107.

Sclare, A. B. (1975). Drinking habits in Scotland. *Int. J. Offend. Ther. Comp. Criminol.* 18, 241–249.

Seeley, J. R. (1959). The WHO definition of alcoholism. *Q. Jl. Stud. Alc.* 20, 352–356.

Selzer, M. L. (1971). The Michegan alcoholism screening test. *Am. J. Psychiat.* 127, 1653–1658.

Shepherd, M. (1961). Morbid jealousy: some clinical and social aspects of a psychiatric symptom. *J. Ment. Sci.* 107, 687–400.

Shields, J. (1977). Genetics and alcoholism. *In* 'Alcoholism; New Knowledge and New Responses' (Eds G. Edwards and M. Grant). Croom Helm, London.

Smart, R. (1976). The Ontario Detoxification System. Paper read at the 3rd International Conference on Alcohol and Drug Dependence, Liverpool.

Smith, R. C., Parker, E. S. and Noble, E. P. (1975). Alcohol's effect on some formal aspects of verbal social communication. *Arch. Gen. Psychiat.* 32, 1294–1402.

Sobell, M. B. and Sobell, L. C. (1973). Alcoholics treated by individual behaviour therapy—one year treatment outcome. *Behav. Res. Ther.* 11, 599–618.

Steinglass, P., Weiner, S. and Mendelson, J. H. (1971). Interactional issues as determinants of alcoholism. *Am. J. Psychiat.* **128**, 275–280.
Tarter, R. E. and Schneider, D. U. (1976). Models and theories of alcoholism. *In* 'Alcoholism: Interdisciplinary Approaches to an Enduring Problem' (Eds R. E. Tarter and A. A. Sugerman). Addison-Wesley, Reading, Massachusetts.
Tinckleberg, J. R. (1972). Alcohol and violence. *In* 'Alcoholism: Progress in Research and Treatment' (Eds R. Fox and P. Bourne). Academic Press, New York and London.
Unger, K. W., and Johnson, D., Jnr. (1974). Red cell mean corpuscular volume: a potential indicator of alcohol usage in a working population. *Am. J. Med. Sci.* **267**, 281–289.
Victor, M., Adams, R. D. and Collins, G. M. (1971). 'The Wernicke-Korsakoff Syndrome'. Blackwell, Oxford.
Wallgren, H. and Barry, H. (1970). 'Actions of Alcohol', Vols I, II and III. Elsevier, New York.
Walton, H. J. (1968). Personality as a determinant of the form of alcoholism. *Br. J. Psychiat.* **114**, 761–766.
Weingarter, H., Adefris, W., Eich, J. E. and Murphy, D. L. (1976). Encoding—imagery specificity in alcohol state-dependent learning. *J. Exp. Psychol.* **2**, 83–87.
Weschler, H., Kasey, E. H., Thurn, D. and Demone, H. W. (1969). Alcohol level and home accidents. *Pub. Hlth* Rep. (Washington) **84**, 1043–1050.
Wilkins, R. W. (1974). 'The Hidden Alcoholic in General Practice'. Elek Science, London.
Winokur, G., Rimmer, J. and Reich, T. (1971). Is there more than one type of alcoholism? *Br. J. Psychiat.* **118**, 525–532.
World Health Organization (1952). Expert Committee on Mental Health, Alcoholism Subcommittee, Second Report. Technical Report Series No. 48, Geneva.
Wu, A., Chanarin I. and Levi, A. J. (1974). Macrocytosis of chronic alcoholism. *Lancet* **i**, 829–830.
Zacune, J. and Hensman, C. (1971). 'Drugs, Alcohol and Tobacco in Britain'. Heinemann, London.

11 Schizophrenia

Robin Murray

The concept of schizophrenia

The development of the concept

Haslam offered one of the first clear pictures of a schizophrenic psychosis in 1809, but gave the disorder no name, and many psychiatrists of the time continued to believe in a single psychosis 'the Einheitpsychose' which could manifest itself in various forms (see Scharfetter, 1975). Then, in 1851 the French psychiatrist Falret delineated *'folie circulaire'* or manic depressive psychosis, and shortly thereafter his compatriot Morel applied the term *'démence précoce'* to a deteriorating psychosis in a patient whose withdrawal, bizarre mannerisms and personal neglect had begun in adolescence. Kahlbaum subsequently employed the term hebephrenia for a similar picture, and in 1874 published a monograph on catatonia which he described as a cyclical condition characterized by stereotyped movement, mannerisms, and occasional outbursts of intense excitement, automatic obedience, negativism and stupor. Kahlbaum considered hebephrenia and catatonia quite distinct from one another and also from paranoia, a term which he reserved for those with primary systematized delusions (see Altschule, 1975).

In 1898 Emil Kraepelin brought hebephrenia, catatonia and paranoia together into the single entity of dementia praecox, and to these he later added a fourth type dementia simplex. Regardless of the type Kraepelin considered the following symptoms characteristic of dementia praecox: hallucinations, a decrease in attention towards the outside world, lack of curiosity, disorder of thought, lack of insight and judgement, delusions, emotional blunting, negativism and stereotypies. Kraepelin believed that the four conditions were similar not only in their symptomatology, but also in their usual onset in early adult life, and in their frequent progression to a 'demented' end stage. He did, however, recognize that the breakdown was not an intellectual one, that it did not necessarily occur in adolescence, and that the prognosis was not invariably poor.

The Swiss psychiatrist Eugene Bleuler (1911) did not consider dementia praecox as a disease *per se*, but spoke instead of 'the schizophrenias', a term he used since 'the disconnection or splitting of the psychic functions is an outstanding feature of the whole group'. Bleuler attempted to separate primary symptoms caused directly by a supposed aetiological agent, from secondary symptoms which he considered merely a reaction to the primary changes. The primary symptoms which he believed were characteristic and present during all stages of schizophrenia, are often called the four As—altered associations, altered affectivity, ambivalence and autism. Even when secondary symptoms such as delusions and hallucinations predominated Bleuler regarded them as non-specific since they could occur in non-schizophrenic disorders. Bleuler is generally regarded as having widened the concept of dementia praecox, but his intention was the opposite. His primary symptoms were an attempt to strengthen the unity which Kraepelin had created, but unfortunately these symptoms were themselves so difficult to define that they allowed clinicians a great deal of diagnostic latitude. As the World Health Organization (1973) commented 'diversity re-entered through the door which should have shut it out'.

Schneider's criteria

Since the foundations of the concept of schizophrenia were laid by Kraepelin and Bleuler much detailed knowledge has been added, but no external validating factors have been discovered to guide clinicians in refining the diagnosis. The problem as Kendell (1972) puts it is that

> the only defining characteristic available to us is the syndrome itself. In our present state of knowledge, our criteria for a diagnosis can only be the typical clinical features of schizophenia.

The most influential attempt at a phenomenological definition has been that of Kurt Schneider (1959) who described a number of symptoms which he regarded as being of *first rank* importance in differentiating schizophrenia from other conditions. Schneider made no theoretical claims for his first rank symptoms, but empirically considered that whenever any were found in the absence of organic disease or drug intoxication one could make a diagnosis of schizophrenia. First rank symptoms are: having audible thoughts *'echo de la pensée'*; hearing voices talking to each other or commenting on oneself; somatic passivity feelings; thought insertion, withdrawal or communication to others; delusional perception; feelings of external control over one's emotions, drives and volition—'made' feelings, drives and acts.

Schneider's criteria have been criticized as being both too narrow and insufficiently specific. Mellor (1970) for instance, studied chronic patients in an English hospital who had been originally diagnosed as schizophrenic, and found that only 79% were known to have ever had any first rank symptoms. In the much wider International Pilot Study on Schizophrenia (IPSS) 1202 patients were studied in nine different countries; only 58% of acute patients with a hospital diagnosis of schizophrenia had one or more first rank symptoms (World Health Organization, 1973). Unfortunately, first rank symptoms do also occasionally occur in non-schizophrenic states; they were present in 7·5% of non-schizophrenic patients in the IPSS. This had led to suggestions that the use of first rank symptoms may cause diagnostic error, but as Wing and Nixon (1975) point out 'the term pathogenic if interpreted to mean 100% accuracy, cannot at the present time be used of any symptom known to medicine'.

A further technique used in the IPSS was to identify a group of patients who were diagnosed as schizophrenic not only by local psychiatrists, but also by the Catego Computer programme based on the Present State Examination (Chapter 4), and also by cluster analysis. The frequency of different symptoms in these 306 patients is shown in Table I.

Table I *Frequency of symptoms in 306 concordant schizophrenics in the International Pilot Study on Schizophrenia*

	%
Lack of insight	97
Auditory hallucinations	74
Ideas of reference	70
Suspiciousness	66
Flatness of affect	66
Delusional mood	64
Delusions of persecution	64
Thought alienation	52
Thoughts spoken aloud	50

Nuclear and peripheral schizophrenia

A great deal of controversy has focused on whether patients with both schizophrenic and affective symptoms should be considered within the limits of schizophrenia. Kasanin coined the term 'schizoaffective-psychosis' for such cases while Langfeldt distinguished between process schizophrenia (roughly equivalent to Kraepelin's dementia praecox) and 'schizophreniform illness' with precipitating factors, a strong affective component, often disturbance of consciousness and on the whole a good prognosis. Numerous other terms have been used, but the status of such individuals remains a persistent enigma. Because of the frequency of affective disorder in their families and their remitting course Winokur regards these patients as having a variant of affective disorder. Leonard believes that they constitute a distinct third group of 'cycloid psychoses' while others consider them on a transitional spectrum between schizophrenia and affective disorders (see Procci, 1976).

Similar difficulties have been encountered with those patients on the borderland between schizophrenia and neurosis and personality disorder. In many cases of simple schizophrenia the diagnosis is based not so much on positive symptoms as on a gradual deterioration in personality with increasing emotional bluntness; occasional brief psychotic episodes help to confirm the diagnosis. A similar course may characterize what Hoch and Polatin (1949) called 'pseudoneurotic schizophrenia' because of a predominance of anxiety, hypochondriasis and anancastic mechanisms. A 'borderline syndrome' has also been proposed by Grinker and his colleagues (1968) to describe young patients without delusions who have repeated histrionic episodes and who show 'an ego alien quality to any transient psychotic-like behaviour'. Neither pseudoneurotic schizophrenia nor the borderline syndrome have been accepted outside the USA, but the genetic studies of Rosenthal and Kety (p. 361) have suggested that borderline schizophrenia may be a real entity.

Criticism of the concept

The term schizophrenia has numerous critics including Thomas Szasz and R. D. Laing, both of whom regard schizophrenia as a medical fiction invented for the needs of society, relatives and psychiatrists rather than patients. Their arguments are essentially political and have been admirably dissected by Clare (1976). More serious criticism has come from sociologists like Scheff (1963) who drew attention to the negative aspects of receiving a diagnosis of schizophrenia, and considered that many of the symptoms were a consequence of being labelled as mad. Certainly once an individual is diagnosed as schizophrenic his relations with family, employers and doctors can be considerably altered, and the adverse effects of long-term hospitalization are well established (Wing and Brown, 1970). It is easy to conceive how a societal reaction might pressurize an individual into deviancy but as Wing (1974) states 'it is difficult to imagine how a similar reaction would force him to adopt the central schizophrenic syndrome since this would need special coaching from an expert'.

Psychologists have also made serious assaults on the concept of schizophrenia. Rosenhan and his colleagues (1973) managed to get themselves admitted to 12 American mental hospitals merely by declaring that they heard voices saying 'empty', 'hollow' and 'thud'. Despite ceasing to simulate any psychiatric abnormality once admitted to hospital they were diagnosed as schizophrenic. This study is often quoted as establishing the arbitrariness of the label schizophrenia, but others more realistically (e.g. Spitzer, 1976) regard it as a vivid and useful polemic against the practice of bad psychiatry. Some psychiatrists react to criticism by totally denying its validity, and by reasserting the medical disease model of schizophrenia. But this is less than satisfactory since the issue of whether schizophrenic symptoms are qualitatively different from normal human behaviour has not been resolved. Indeed, the supposed discontinuity of schizophrenic phenomena from normal function has been increasingly challenged. The Eysencks (p. 94) have proposed a dimensional hypothesis for psychosis, as has Claridge (1972) who regards the schizophrenic predisposition as a continuously variable personality dimension.

Current position

There remains widespread confusion regarding the meaning, boundaries and even value of the term schizophrenia (Shepherd, 1976; Pope and Lipinski, 1978). Some authorities define schizophrenia on the basis of symptomatology and some by characteristic course, while some consider it merely a syndrome and others regard it as a disease process not necessarily revealed in overt behaviour. The origin of the confusion is that we have failed to discover the aetiology of the conditions referred to under the term schizophrenia, and it is likely that our confusion will continue until we have a better understanding of the pathogenesis of schizophrenia.

Currently the most widely employed system of psychiatric classification is the International Classification of Diseases. Unfortunately, this classification leaves unresolved a number of problems including the fact that the major categories are neither mutually exclusive nor jointly exhaustive. As a consequence there has been a proliferation of operational definitions of schizophrenia including the computerized systems of Wing and of Spitzer which are described in Chapter 4. Brockington *et al.* (1978) who recently compared ten different operational definitions of schizophrenia, found wide variations in their reliability, concordance and predictive powers. Wherever a wide concept of schizophrenia has been applied one can separate off atypical types that differ essentially from nuclear schizophrenia. But attempts at subdividing nuclear schizophrenia have not been successful. Even the differences between the classical groups of hebephrenic, catatonic, paranoid and simple schizophrenia appear to be of a pathoplastic nature determined by age of onset and by cultural and environmental factors (Carpenter *et al.*, 1976).

The author's view is that the current classification of the functional psychoses is extremely unsatisfactory, but there is no viable alternative to the use of the term schizophrenia. In the absence of evidence to the contrary schizophrenia is best considered as a syndrome which may cover several different conditions. A relatively restrictive concept should be applied conservatively both in the interests of diagnostic homogeneity and because of the adverse consequences of labelling doubtful cases as schizophrenic. Schneider's first rank symptoms are the most useful criteria for achieving this although they are by no means infallible and do not appear to carry implications for the prognosis (Brockington *et al.*, 1978; Pope and Lipinski, 1978).

Differential diagnosis

The definition and elucidation of many of the clinical phenomena of schizophrenia have been described in Chapter 2, and the various criteria for making the diagnosis have just been outlined. But, given the rudimentary state of current psychiatric knowledge the diagnosis often cannot be made simply on positive findings of schizophrenia, but must include an absence of features more characteristic of other syndromes. The conditions to be considered in the differential diagnosis include the following:

Drug-induced psychosis. Drugs such as amphetamine, LSD, cocaine and cannabis may produce a psychosis mimicking schizophrenia (Davison, 1976). Of these amphetamine psychosis may be the most difficult to distinguish since the symptoms can be identical with those of paranoid schizophrenia (Connell, 1958). While LSD and the other hallucinogens tend to cause visual rather than auditory hallucinations, cannabis is said by some to produce the 'amotivational syndrome'. Debate continues over whether individuals who develop drug psychoses are constitutionally predisposed, and there is some evidence that patients who develop apparently genuine schizophrenia following drug abuse break down at an earlier age than those who have not taken drugs (Breakey *et al.*, 1974). Alcoholic hallucinosis may also be mistaken for schizophrenia and once again there is dispute over whether this arises in those who have a genetic predisposition to schizophrenia (Cutting, 1978).

Organic conditions. Distinction can usually be made from psychosis associated with gross cerebral pathology, infection or metabolic disorder because of the presence of clouding of consciousness, physical signs or laboratory abnormalities in such conditions (Lishman, 1978), but any newly presenting schizophrenic should receive a careful workup including skull X-ray and EEG and where relevant EMI scan. In a small proportion temporal lobe epilepsy or other organic pathology will be found (Flor-Henry, 1976). Most puerperal psychoses are not schizophrenic, but a minority are, or later clearly become so.

Paranoid states. The exact classification of the paranoid states has been a matter of controversy for years (Forrest, 1975) and some authorities regard the differences between paranoid personality, paranoia and paranoid schizophrenia as merely a matter of degree. Individuals with *paranoid personality* are generally rigid and inflexible, suspicious and morbidly sensitive. They may be of rather dominant nature and their friendships of short duration. The so-called overvalued idea or *idée fixe* may be prominent. *Paranoia* is a relatively rare condition (Winokur, 1977), characterized by an intricate, complex and logically elaborated delusional system without hallucinations. The delusions are systematized, firmly knit and more or less isolated so that the rest of the personality remains relatively intact. Paranoia is rare before 30 years of age and appears especially common in migrants. Many paranoiacs are single, and few people bother with them provided they are not dangerous to themselves or others. But occasionally a paranoiac may consider that he has unique abilities and may seek political expression of his views.

In erotomania, also known as de Clerambault's Syndrome (Enoch *et al.*, 1967), a patient, usually female, presents ideas that she is loved by another person who does not make a direct avowal, but indicates his love in many indirect ways. The individual cast in the role of lover is often a person of some status who is pestered by the patient with letters or visits. In some cases symptoms persist for many years without disintegration of the personality, but in others deterioration typical of nuclear schizophrenia occurs.

Morbid jealousy is characterized by delusions of marital infidelity and a search for evidence of adultery. Spouses may be followed or their underwear repeatedly examined for seminal stains. Improbable accusations may be succeeded by violence and occasional homicide of the wife or her supposed lover. Morbid jealousy is a symptom which may occur in paranoid states, schizophrenia, alcoholism or depressive psychosis (Shepherd, 1961).

In *folie à deux* a delusion is transmitted from one person to another so that the second comes to share the psychopathology of the first. Usually the two persons are living together, perhaps as husband and wife, or mother and daughter. The person to whom the delusions are transmitted is often passive and dependent, and usually recovers within a few months if the two are separated. *Folie à deux* and the other eponymous conditions have been well reviewed by Enoch *et al.* (1967).

Other psychiatric conditions. The boundaries between schizophrenia and affective disorder are vague. One should be particularly aware of the intensification of affect which may be an early symptom of schizophrenia, and of the occasional occurrence of first rank symptoms and of over-inclusive thinking in manics. Even when the greatest care is taken patients diagnosed on their initial hospitalization as schizophrenic will sometimes need to be re-classified as having affective disorder and vice versa (Sheldrick *et al.*, 1977).

It may at times be difficult to differentiate between schizoid personality and schizophrenia, and obsessional neurosis may also be wrongly diagnosed as schizophrenia. A careful history should demonstrate that even the most persistent or bizarre obsessional thought does not have the quality of absolute certainty of a delusion.

Cultural differences. Migrants are particularly likely to be diagnosed as schizophrenic. Part of this may be a consequence of psychiatrists considering unfamiliar beliefs (e.g. believing in spells or evil spirits) as delusions. Similar considerations apply to sub-cultural groups in Western society such as spiritualists.

Many features of adolescent crises—exultation, preoccupation with abstract ideas, unpredictability, introspection, extreme shyness—can occur in schizophrenia. The diagnostic problem can be compounded if the young person belongs to a youth counterculture with whose norms the psychiatrist is unfamiliar. Because of the serious implications of a diagnosis of schizophrenia and the spontaneous improvement of adolescent turbulence, one should be very cautious before diagnosing any doubtful adolescent as schizophrenic.

Epidemiology

Cross cultural differences

Although early anthropological studies failed to report schizophrenia among primitive peoples, many subsequent investigators have acknowledged its occurrence. Murphy (1978), for instance, has reported that typical schizophrenia occurs among primitive Eskimos in a frequency comparable to that in developed countries. However, Fuller-Torrey (1973) claims that most of the anthropological studies have been carried out among peoples with significant contact with Western technology, and Cooper and Sartorius (1977) report that schizophrenia in less developed countries tends to have a more acute onset, but more benign prognosis. Thus while there is general agreement that schizophrenia is a universal phenomena there remains some doubt as to whether its frequency and characteristics are the same in more primitive peoples.

Most developed countries report life-time expectancies of about 1% with a slightly higher risk among men than women. But within countries there may be sub-cultural groups with a different expectation. Two early surveys appeared to differ markedly in their results. Eaton and Weil (1955) studied the Hutterites, a North American anabaptist sect who lived in a close-knit farming community and whose every-day life was simple, austere and pious. They found a rather low prevalence of schizophrenia, but a second study (Murphy, 1968) failed to confirm this. Böök (1953) carried out a very careful survey in Northern Sweden where the climate was severe and the population lived very isolated lives. He found the expectation of schizophrenia at 2·85% to be three times as high as in other Scandinavian studies. Böök's explanation was in terms of genetics and selective migration; he believed a schizoid personality was an advantage for survival in such an area.

Murphy (1968) has reviewed the statistics of people receiving psychiatric treatment. There appears to be significantly higher expectations of schizophrenia among four peoples—the Tamils of southern India and Ceylon, the people of north-west Croatia, Roman Catholics in Canada, and the Southern Irish. The reasons for these high risk groups remain uncertain. One explanation often given for the high rate in Southern Ireland concerns the long continued emigration from this area; perhaps mentally healthy people tended to emigrate leaving behind a high proportion of schizophrenia-prone people. On the other hand, several studies have suggested that those who migrate are more susceptible to schizophrenia. Ødegaard (1932) found that schizophrenia occurred more commonly among Norwegians who emigrated to America than among those who remained behind. Mezey (1960) also found a higher rate among those who left Hungary during the 1956 uprising, especially those who did not give political reasons for leaving.

International variations in diagnosis

In 1961 Kramer drew attention to the fact that the first admission rate for schizophrenia was considerably higher in the United States than in England and Wales, while the reverse was true for affective disorder. The suspicion that these differences were not due to genuine variation in the incidence of the condition, but rather to different diagnostic practices prompted the establishment of the US–UK Diagnostic Project. Samples of newly admitted patients in New York and London were interviewed by researchers using the Present State Examination (p. 89). The results were clear-cut. Hospital psychiatrists in New York did, as expected, diagnose schizophrenia more frequently and affective disorder less frequently than their counterparts in London. However, the project psychiatrists employing the standardized interviews diagnosed the disorders in much the same proportions in each city. These researchers (Cooper et al., 1972) concluded that the New York concept of schizophrenia embraced almost all of what British psychiatrists would call mania plus a good proportion of what they would call depressive illness and neurosis. The transatlantic differences appear to arise from the fact that the British concept of schizophrenia is firmly rooted in the teaching of Kraepelin and Schneider while in the United States the more analytically oriented views of Bleuler prevailed. The latter was partly due to the influence of Adolf Meyer who regarded schizophrenia as a collection of habit patterns often developed in response to chronic environmental stress, and also due to Sullivan who emphasized the importance of disturbed interpersonal relationships.

A wider study of international variations in diagnostic practice was carried out under the auspices of the World Health Organization (1973).This International Pilot Study on Schizophrenia involved 1202 patients examined using the Present State Examination in nine different countries. The three European (Czechoslovakia, Denmark and Britain) and four developing countries (Columbia, India, Nigeria and Taiwan) had similar criteria for diagnosing schizophrenia, but once again the prevailing concept was broader in the United States, and also in Russia where categories such as sluggish and periodic schizophrenia were employed.

Social and economic differences

One of the most consistent findings of psychiatric epidemiology has been the detection of a disproportionate number of schizophrenics in certain districts of large cities. In the original study Faris and Dunham (1939) found higher admission rates for schizophrenia in the central areas of lowest socio-economic status in Chicago than in the higher status suburbs. This pattern has been confirmed in other large cities in the United States and Europe, but does not appear to hold for smaller towns and those where the poorer areas are not characterized by social isolation.

Two main explanations have been proposed for these findings. The first 'the social causation hypothesis' assumes that a poor social environment either causes schizophrenia or favours its onset in the predisposed by exposing them to social isolation, economic deprivation, poor health care and education. The second 'the drift hypothesis' claims that low occupational status and poor environment are a consequence of psychopathology and that schizophrenics and pre-schizophrenics are downwardly mobile either because of their social and occupational incompetence, or because they actively seek out anonymity and isolation in the decaying areas of large cities. Goldberg and Morrison (1963) provided support for the drift hypothesis by finding that hospitalized schizophrenics were in lower status occupations than their fathers. Hare (1967) and almost all of his British colleagues have concluded that the bulk of evidence favours the drift hypothesis, but a few Americans such as Kohn (1976) are not yet convinced.

Genetics

The evidence for a genetic predisposition to schizophrenia is well reviewed by Gottesman and Shields, 1976, and comes from three main sources listed below.

Studies of relatives

The life-time expectancy for schizophrenia in the general population is of the order of 0·3 to 2·8%, but much higher figures have been found in relatives of schizophrenic patients (Zerbin-Rudin, 1972). Children, both of whose parents have had schizophrenia, have at least a 25% chance of developing the condition, but where only one parent was affected the average risk is 12%. Siblings of a person with schizophrenia show an expected risk of between 8 and 14%, while the risk for parents is 5 to 10%, and that for second degree relatives varies around 2·5%. Thus, as the degree of relatedness weakens, so the risk diminishes until it approximates to that of the general population.

Studies of twins

The increased frequency of schizophrenia in the families of patients is compatible with either genetic or environmental transmission of the disorder. The significance of twin studies lies in the fact that monozygotic (MZ) twins have exactly the same heredity while dizygotic (DZ) twins share only half their genes. If, therefore, pairs of MZ twins share the same psychopathology more often than DZ twins, this can be taken as evidence of a genetic contribution to the disorder. Early twin studies appeared to amply confirm the genetic hypothesis, since MZ twins were much more often concordant (i.e. both twins schizophrenic) than DZ pairs. Rosenthal (1962) criticized these studies on the grounds that the samples were biased in various ways, and the diagnosis of probands and co-twins could have been biased by knowledge of zygosity. He concluded that the concordance rates for MZ twins—86% in one study—were misleadingly high. Subsequent studies based on population registers or consecutive hospital admissions have tended to diminish concordance rates; the rates for MZ twins have ranged from 35% in Tienari's study to 58% in Gottesman and Shields', and for DZ twins from the 9% reported by Pollin to the 26% found by Fischer (quoted from Gottesman and Shields, 1972).

There have been criticisms of twin strategy. Jackson (1960) claimed that MZ twins may be at special risk for schizophrenia on account of problems such as confusion of identity and weak ego formation. Parents and other close relatives do apparently confuse identical twins with each other, but if this is of causal significance in schizophrenia, MZ twins should show higher rates of illness than the general population and they do not (Allen and Pollin, 1970). It has also been suggested that MZ twins might be more likely to be exposed to the same predisposing environmental factors than DZ twins. The strongest evidence against such an explanation is derived from studies of twins reared apart. Gottesman and Shields (1972) collected from the literature 17 such pairs of whom 11 were concordant for schizophrenia, a remarkably high figure.

Studies of adoptees

Since an individual receives his genetic environment from one family, but his life experiences as a member of another, adoptive studies have been extensively used to disentangle genetic and environmental effects. Heston and Denney (1968) followed up 47 adopted away offspring of chronically hospitalized schizophrenic mothers and a well matched control group of 50 adoptees born to mothers without psychiatric disorder; all the children had been separated from their mothers by the age of two weeks. The findings were striking! The offspring of the schizophrenic mothers were significantly more disordered on each of six indices: a mental health rating scale, the number of schizophrenics (five in the experimental group, none in the controls), the numbers of mental defectives, sociopaths and neurotics, and the number who had spent two years in jail.

The past decade has seen the publication of a series of papers from a large Danish-American study of adoptees and their relatives. Rosenthal and his colleagues (1971) searched the psychiatric register for the names of all 5500 children put up for non-familial adoption in the Greater Copenhagen area between 1923 and 1947. These investigators then studied the frequency of schizophrenia among the offspring of parents who were known to have been psychotic, and among a carefully matched control group of adoptees whose biological parents were free of known psychiatric illness. Diagnoses were made in a 'blind' fashion from case abstracts prepared by workers unaware of the purpose or design of this study. Subjects could be rated as having acute or chronic schizophrenia, borderline state, or personality disorder, and all these diagnoses were included under the rubric 'schizophrenia spectrum disorder'. Of the index cases 31·6% received the latter label compared with 17·8% of control adoptees. Three of the index offspring were definitely schizophrenic whereas not one of the 67 controls was so diagnosed. Thus, Rosenthal's studies strongly support the view that genetic factors are of considerable importance in the transmission of schizophrenia.

As part of the same fruitful collaboration Kety and his colleagues (1975) 'blindly' rated extensive psychiatric assessments of the biological and adoptive relatives of 33 schizophrenic adoptees. There was a 'statistically significant concentration of definite schizophrenics in the biological relatives of adopted index cases but not in the adoptive relatives'; 21% of the biological relatives fell into the schizophrenia spectrum compared to 5% of the adoptive relatives. Among the relatives of a control group of healthy adoptees the figures were 11% and 8% respectively.

Genetic models

All experts are agreed that what is inherited is not a certainty of developing schizophrenia but a vulnerability to the condition. For most if not all cases genetic factors are insufficient to cause frank schizophrenia; environmental factors are also necessary. But now that the existence of a genetic contribution has been established it becomes important to provide a theory for its mode of transmission. Genetic models can be divided into three broad categories; monogenic, genetic heterogeneity, and polygenic. Monogenic theories involve a dominant gene. Heston (1970) suggests that such a gene expresses itself either as classical schizophrenia or if the full disorder does not appear as schizoid personality. Pollin (1972) tested this theory by studying 15 MZ twin pairs who were discordant for schizophrenia; the non-schizophrenic co-twins were not particularly characterized by schizoid features.

Theories of genetic heterogeneity propose that schizophrenia can be divided into different conditions each with a different heredity. The most fully developed theory of this kind is probably that of Mitsuda (1967), but a genetic distinction between typical and atypical schizophrenia is also proposed by many others. The third genetic model suggests that inheritance is by polygenic means. It has been proposed (e.g. Gottesman and Shields, 1972) since no single gene hypothesis whether dominant, recessive or intermediate can account for the observed data without the supplementary hypothesis of a reduced manifestation rate. However, this third model has been no more successful than the previous two in achieving universal acceptance.

Biochemical approaches

The notion that schizophrenia might have a biochemical basis has attracted a great deal of attention, but as yet no biochemical abnormalities have been consistently and exclusively associated with schizophrenia. The serum of schizophrenics has been claimed to cause rats to behave strangely, to induce irregularities in spiders' web spinning and to drive normal volunteers mad. There have also been reports of a 'psychotogenic' globulin (tarexin), circulating anti-brain antibodies, an altered lipoprotein (the S-globulin), and an allergy to dietary glutens. These findings have generally been based on methodologically unsound observations and remain unconfirmed. As Rodnight (1971) states, 'Biochemists in this field tend to divide their time between disproving the research of their less vigorous colleagues and adding to an increasingly long catalogue of essentially negative results'.

Three factors persuade biochemists to continue their efforts. These are (a) the evidence that liability to schizophrenia is partly inherited and the implication that what is transmitted may be a biochemical predisposition; (b) the existence of drugs which can produce psychotic states bearing some resemblance to schizophrenia; (c) the knowledge that some drugs can ameliorate schizophrenia, and attendant curiosity as to their mode and site of action.

The dopamine hypothesis

This is partly based on the evidence that amphetamine abuse can produce a syndrome consisting primarily of ideas of reference, delusions of persecution and auditory and visual hallucinations (Connell, 1958). Amphetamine psychosis is most frequently observed in addicts who have consumed enormous quantities of the drug over prolonged periods, and usually resolves within a few days of ceasing the abuse. But when large oral doses are given to subjects without evidence of schizoid traits, psychosis invariably results within one to five days (Griffiths *et al.*, 1972); indeed, intravenous amphetamine can produce the psychosis within a matter of hours. Small 'therapeutic' doses of amphetamine rapidly and reproducibly exacerbate schizophrenic symptoms (Janowsky *et al.*, 1973) and schizophrenic patients are reportedly unable to differentiate an amphetamine psychosis from their usual symptoms.

Amphetamines enhance the effects of noradrenaline and dopamine through directly releasing them into the synaptic cleft and by preventing their inactivation through re-uptake into the nerve terminal that released them. The actions of amphetamine in eliciting psychosis appear to involve an increase in synaptic dopamine rather than noradrenaline.

The second strand of the dopamine hypothesis rests on the well known tendency of the antipsychotic drugs to cause Parkinsonism. With the discovery that dopamine was deficient in the caudate nucleus in Parkinson's disease, it appeared likely that the Parkinsonian effects of the antipsychotics were due to their producing a functional dopamine deficiency. Carlsson and Lindquist (1963) then suggested that the antipsychotic effects were also due to the drugs blockading dopamine receptors on the post synaptic membrane. This is now accepted. With a few exceptions the antipsychotic potency of the various neuroleptics correlates closely with their tendency to produce extrapyramidal effects, and with their ability to inhibit dopamine-sensitive adenylate cyclase (see Crow *et al.*, 1976).

If blocking dopamine receptors relieves schizophrenic symptoms, and amphetamines which flood the receptors with dopamine can cause psychosis, then could overactivity of central dopaminergic neurones underlie the symptomatology of schizophrenia (Snyder *et al.*, 1974)? Until recently there was no evidence for any increased brain synthesis or release of dopamine in schizophrenia, but now Bird *et al.* (1977) claim to

have found increased dopamine in limbic areas of the brains of schizophrenics at post mortem. This could be a consequence of medication
rather than schizophrenia, and there are other defects in the dopamine hypothesis (Crow *et al.*, 1976), but it is an area of great potential
advance.

The transmethylation hypothesis

This proposes that some schizophrenic symptoms may be caused by the
abnormal accumulation of a methylated biogenic amine. This hypothesis,
originally suggested twenty-five years ago, gained impetus from the
demonstration by Pollin *et al.* (1961) that when chronic schizophrenic
patients are given a monoamine oxidase inhibitor plus a methyl group
donor such as methionine, some will develop an acute psychosis.

In the search for methylated compounds which might mediate this
clinical deterioration, attention was focused throughout the 1960s on 3,
4-Dimethoxyphenylethylamine (Freidhoff and van Winkle, 1962). However, this substance is not hallucinogenic in man and initial suggestions
that it appeared selectively in the urine of schizophrenics have not been
substantiated. Indeed, the 'pink spot' seen in chromatographic studies
reportedly representing dimethoxyphenylethylamine was found to be
produced by phenothiazine metabolites and tea drinking.

More recently methylated indoleamines have re-emerged as possible
hallucinogenic products of transmethylation. The most intriguing of
these is dimethyltryptamine (DMT), which was first isolated from the
snuff used by Haitian natives to produce mystical states. When injected
into human volunteers DMT does induce a short lasting psychosis in
which some of the symptoms of schizophrenia can be discerned.
Dimethyltryptamine is the first human hallucinogen for which there is a
known biosynthetic mechanism. Several groups of workers have
examined the blood of mentally ill subjects for DMT, but the results have
been contradictory. Murray *et al.* (1979) found DMT in the urine of both
patients and normal subjects, but the level of excretion was much higher
for psychotic patients than normals and neurotics. Whether increased
DMT excretion is a cause or consequence of psychosis remains uncertain.

Other hypotheses

In 1972 Murphy and Wyatt reported finding reduced levels of monoamine oxidase (MAO) in the platelets of schizophrenics. This reduction

was also observed in the identical twins of schizophrenics whether or not they had the illness, indicating that it might be a genetic marker for the disorder. Subsequent studies have not been conclusive, with low platelet MAO being found more often in chronic than in acute schizophrenia. But it has also been reported in non-schizophrenic conditions suggesting that it may be a factor predisposing to psychiatric illness in general (Murphy and Buchsbaum, 1978).

Creatine Phosphokinase (CPK) is elevated in plasma in association with various tissue injuries and also, unaccountably, in acute psychotic states, especially schizophrenia (Meltzer, 1976). Chronic schizophrenic patients and non-psychotic psychiatric patients do not manifest these abnormalities. As the source of the CPK is skeletal muscle it is unlikely that the abnormalities are of aetiological significance.

Neurological abnormality

One of the dogmas of schizophrenia is embodied in its description as a functional psychosis. It has been assumed that schizophrenia has no demonstrable neuropathology, an assertion that Bliss (1976) has questioned in view of reports scattered throughout the literature of dilated ventricles in some schizophrenics, particularly the more refractory cases. The most recent demonstration of this was by Johnstone and her colleagues (1976) who using computerized axial tomography (EMI scan) found that a minority of institutionalized schizophrenics showed evidence of increased ventricular size in association with impaired cognitive functioning. This could have been a consequence of the long-term phenothiazines or ECT to which many of these patients had been subjected.

Davison and Bagley (1969) have exhaustively reviewed the literature on the occurrence of psychosis in individuals with neurological disorders. They conclude that 'in many organic CNS disorders the association of "schizophrenia" exceeds chance expectation. Lesions in the temporal lobe and diencephalon are particularly significant in the genesis of these psychoses'. Schizophrenia may follow brain injury, and may be mimicked by brain tumours and encephalitis, but particular attention has been directed towards temporal lobe epilepsy. The incidence of schizophrenia in temporal lobe epilepsy is only about 2%, but among epileptics with psychosis 70 to 85% have a temporal lobe focus (Flor-Henry, 1976). In 1963 Slater and his colleagues published a very detailed account of 69 patients with both temporal lobe epilepsy and schizophrenia and demonstrated that the two were causally related.

Flor-Henry has gone on to suggest that in temporal lobe epilepsy schizophrenic psychosis is significantly associated with dominant lobe lesions, while affective psychosis tends to be related to epilepsy of the non-dominant hemisphere. When schizophrenics are asked to cross-match two stimuli flashed simultaneously to the two hemispheres, they show a significant deficit in matching letters presented to the left hemisphere. Gur (1977) compared 200 schizophrenics to 200 normal controls on measures of laterality that included handedness, footedness and eye dominance. Schizophrenics showed more left handedness, appearing to corroborate previous findings that schizophrenia may be related to left hemisphere dysfunction.

Recently a great deal of interest has centred on the demonstration by Holzman and his colleagues (1976) that schizophrenics show an abnormally jagged eye tracking pattern both when ill and when in remission. This trait also appears more frequently in the families of schizophrenics. These findings have been successfully replicated, but there is controversy over whether the eye tracking abnormality is indicative of an underlying neurophysiological abnormality or of an attentional deficit.

The influence of family life

Since 1948 when Fromm-Reichman coined the term 'schizophrenogenic mother', many investigations have examined the question of whether the mothers of schizophrenics are abnormal or peculiar people. There appears to be a general consensus (Hirsch and Leff, 1975) that the mothers are more concerned, more protective and possibly more intrusive than control mothers. These attitudes are present both before and after the child has developed schizophrenia, but they may have developed as a response to an already abnormal child. Alanen (1968) has produced results supporting the concept of the 'schizophrenogenic mother'. He found that compared with the mothers of neurotics and normals the mothers of schizophrenics were less able to understand their children's needs or feelings, and were both overprotective and hostile to them. This is one of the few scientific studies to have come to such a conclusion, and other well conducted enquiries (see Hirsch and Leff, 1975) have suggested that the characterization of the mothers of schizophrenics as exhibiting a combination of overprotection and hostile rejection cannot be sustained.

In studies of parents, mothers have borne the brunt of the investigation and also regrettably the blame. Much less interest has been shown in fathers and this has been reflected in a dearth of experimental work. In one typically poorly controlled study Lidz *et al*. (1957) described five different types of personality in attempting to characterize the fathers of only 14 schizophrenics. Lidz and his colleagues have also advocated the idea of atypical dominance patterns between the parents of schizophrenics. Two interesting concepts utilized in this approach are those of marital 'skew' and 'schism'. In marital 'skew' one parent is inadequate in his role, e.g. passive, withdrawn or weak, and the other excessively dominant, e.g. demanding, possessive and overwhelming. 'Schism' refers to a relationship in which there is an emotional divorce between the parents, but they remain together despite disharmony because one depends on the other. Lidz (1968) claims that such distorted relationships 'create a strange family milieu filled with inconsistencies, contradictory meanings and a denial of what should be obvious', and consequently contribute to the genesis of schizophrenia.

Lidz and his co-workers never tested their theories experimentally but others have done so, with the overwhelming conclusion that the dominance patterns shown by the parents of schizophrenics do not differ from those of normal families. There has, however, been a consistent finding that the parents of schizophrenics show more marital disharmony than normals as indicated by open or tacit conflict and expressed hostility; this is particularly so for chronic schizophrenics and those with a poor premorbid personality (Waring and Ricks, 1965).

Another group of workers headed by Bateson concentrated on the parent–child relationship, and in particular on the concept of the 'double-bind' (Bateson *et al.*, 1956). They hypothesized that the pathogenic parent habitually presents a paradoxical communication containing contradictory messages to the child. In this a superficial injunction suggests one response and a deeper message the opposite. The theory was that a child repeatedly exposed to this impossible situation would respond either by withdrawing from the interaction (perhaps into a fantasy world) or by himself behaving in an ambiguous and irrational fashion. The 'double-bind hypothesis' has had a considerable impact upon both mental health professionals and interested laymen, but since it has not been experimentally tested there is no conclusive evidence that double-bind interactions are, indeed, particularly common in the families of schizophrenics.

The work which comes closest to supporting a theory of disordered communication in the families of schizophrenics is that carried out by Singer and Wynne (1966) at the National Institute of Mental Health. These authors studied family interaction patterns using taped interviews and a battery of psychological tests in a series of controlled experiments. When these were analysed by an independent observer, there was a clear-cut difference in the number of deviant responses between the parents of schizophrenics and those of normal children with practically no overlap between them. The patients' parents showed amorphous and fragmented styles of thought, inability to focus attention selectively and difficulties in showing feelings. Singer and Wynne's studies were sufficiently impressive to stimulate Hirsch and Leff (1975) to attempt to replicate their work under even more rigorously controlled conditions. This British work offered no support for Singer and Wynne's hypothesis possibly because the British group was studying nuclear schizophrenics, and Singer and Wynne more borderline schizophrenics.

Some analysts hold that the contemporary family is a pathogenic institution which scapegoats children and drives them mad. Indeed, Laing and Esterson (1964) do not view the individual schizophrenic as the unit of illness but rather the family or even society at large. Laing suggests not only that the source of the schizophrenic's difficulties is the family, but also embraces the sociological model in which schizophrenia is seen as a label pinned on certain people as a result of a social process. A third and more messianic thread through his later work is that in which the schizophrenic process is valued as a therapeutic experience through which the patient should be guided. The work of Laing and his colleagues has achieved considerable acclaim among both lay and professional workers, but few of their theories have stood the light of critical examination (Clare, 1976).

Problems concerning family studies

Even where abnormalities have been shown in the families of schizophrenics it cannot be assumed that these are necessarily causative to schizophrenia. As early as 1934 Kasanin reported an excess of birth injuries, malnutrition, physical illness and poor development among schizophrenics and concluded that such anomalies caused overprotectiveness in their mothers. More recent evidence has come from follow-up studies of Child Guidance Clinic referrals in which children who subsequently became schizophrenic were compared with matched controls who did not. In O'Neal and Robins' (1958) study the pre-schizophrenic group had more severe infections, disfigurements, and locomotor problems, as well as more eating disorders, sleep problems, tics and antisocial behaviour; not surprisingly 38% of the pre-schizophrenics against 2% of the controls were overdependent on their mother.

Another question which family theorists have to answer relates to the 'selection' of one child to develop psychopathology; if a family is schizophrenogenic then why does only one of several children become psychotic. In a study of twins discordant for schizophrenia Mosher and his colleagues suggested that as a result of an initial constitutional difference such as low birth weight, the pre-schizophrenic twin may attract an excess of attention from the more pathogenic parent. An alternative view was proposed by Hoover and Franz (1972) who examined the siblings of 30 schizophrenics and found that 59% were without significant psychopathology; they suggested that the healthier sibs were less entangled in the family, and had used outside relationships and activities as a source of growing strength and ease in human contact.

Further problems for family theories of schizophrenia come from the mounting evidence that being raised by a schizophrenic parent does not induce schizophrenia. The Danish-American cross-fostering study of Wender *et al.* (1974) included an examination of the effect on children with normal biological parents of being raised by parents one of whom had received a diagnosis in the schizophrenia spectrum. When followed-up these children showed no more psychopathology than children with psychiatrically well biological parents and normal adopting parents. This study does not rule out the possibility of an additive effect of rearing by a schizophrenic parent on a child with a genetic predisposition. Higgins (1976) has examined this possibility by studying two groups of offspring born to schizophrenic mothers, one group mother-reared and the other reared apart. Intensive investigation of these two groups found that the coaction of a genetic predisposition plus rearing by a schizophrenic parent was not greater than the effects of genetic predisposition alone.

Current stress and family life

The role of early experience in the aetiology of schizophrenia remains difficult to evaluate, but there is less doubt about the part played by current stress in precipitating schizophrenic illness. Brown and Birley (1968) studied consecutively admitted acute onset schizophrenics, and in a systematized fashion charted the occurrence of life events for the preceding three months. They found that the schizophrenic patients experienced a significantly higher frequency of such events during the three-week period prior to the onset of their symptoms than did a matched group of non-schizophrenic controls. This was true even of independent events which could not have been caused by the patient becoming ill. Brown *et al.* (1972) suggest that most life events serve to trigger the florid onset and re-appearance of symptoms 'in those who are predisposed and are experiencing tense and difficult situations'.

Psychological theories

Thought disorder

Those interested in psychology have published a number of interesting theories regarding the genesis of schizophrenic thought disorder (see Payne, 1973). Goldstein, for instance, considered that in schizophrenia the ability to form normal abstract concepts is lost and instead concrete ones are formed. Certainly much of the schizophrenics's thinking is in very literal terms as can be demonstrated by asking him to interpret a well known proverb. Another line of investigation stems from Bleuler's description of loosening of associations as underlying schizophrenic thought disorder. Cameron's explanation of this was that schizophrenics had difficulty in maintaining the boundaries of concepts so that each concept spreads into other concepts and each thus becomes over-inclusive.

Payne and Friedlander (1962) adopted over-inclusion as the basic disorder of schizophrenic thought, and put together a battery of three tests of over-inclusiveness. The first, the Payne object classification test, involved classifying a number of small objects of different shapes, materials, thickness and colours. Payne found that acute schizophrenics tended to classify the objects in unusual and idiosyncratic ways. The other two tests in the battery are the Goldstein-Scheerer Object Sorting Test designed to measure concreteness and the Benjamin Proverbs Test. Payne (1973) has found that chronic schizophrenics are less likely than acute to have over-inclusive thinking, and believes consequently that patients who show over-inclusive thinking when they are admitted to hospital have a better prognosis than those who do not.

Personal construct theory

A different approach to the problem of schizophrenic thought disorder has been that made by Bannister (1962) in terms of Kelly's personal construct theory. Construct theory asserts that on the basis of his personal experience an individual develops his own repertoire of constructs and of relationships between such constructs; by means of these he is able to comprehend his environment and interrelate with it in a meaningful and consistent fashion. Thus, if an individual's construct of honest–dishonest is interlinked with other constructs such as punctual–unpunctual or trustworthy–untrustworthy then he may assume that an acquaintance he knows to be honest will also be punctual and trustworthy.

In 1966 Bannister and Fransella published a test in which the subject had to rate eight photographs of unknown people on a variety of constructs such as how kind, selfish or honest they seemed. In a series of experiments these workers then found that schizophrenics differed from normal people in that they had low correlations between the different constructs (low 'intensity') as well as low 'consistency' if the test were repeated. Bannister theorizes that as a result of being repeatedly invalidated in their attempts to develop a meaningful personal construct system schizophrenics may end up with a very loose construct system. If true this theory would provide a mechanism whereby abnormal family interaction such as 'double-bind' communication might by weakening a child's construct system eventually lead to thought disorder. This is an attractive theory, but as yet, scores on the Bannister-Fransella test have not been highly correlated with other measures of schizophrenic thought disorder.

Attention and perception

Freedman (1974) has reviewed the perceptual abnormalities which many schizophrenics experience. In some cases perceptions may become more direct, vivid and alert while in others sensory awareness becomes muted and the world may appear flat, artificial or unreal; once familiar objects may seem different and people may shrink, grow or become distorted in a terrifying manner. McGhie and Chapman's patients (1961) described many subjective experiences of being bombarded by stimuli, and these authors quote a patient as saying 'the sounds are coming through to me but I feel my mind cannot cope with everything. It is difficult to concentrate on any one sound. It's like trying to do two or three different things at one time'. McGhie and Chapman interpreted these findings in the light of Broadbent's 'filter' theory of input limitation which suggests that schizophrenics or at least certain subgroups of schizophrenics may have a deficit in the filter mechanism which limits sensory input to a level which the brain can deal with.

Many studies have attempted to link schizophrenic pathology with a hypothesized attention deficit by means of dichotic listening and signal detection tasks (see Hemsley, 1975). While firm conclusions have yet to be drawn it appears that filtering is less efficient in acute schizophrenics, but chronic patients do have the capacity to ignore or attenuate some types of sensory ones and concentrate on others. Attentional data does also appear to give support to those who would separate the paranoid group from other forms of schizophrenia. Paranoid patients demonstrate a highly selective type of attention that enables them to screen out extraneous stimulation more efficiently than normal subjects. Indeed it seems as if the filter mechanism of the paranoid patient is set to selectively screen out events which might interfere with the rationale of his delusional system.

Arousal

Several groups have suggested that a disorder of the arousal mechanism might be a feature of schizophrenia. As is usual in schizophrenia research findings are confusing, but the bulk of both the autonomic and elec-trophysiological evidence suggests that in the situations which most closely approximate a true 'resting' state schizophrenic patients are on the average more aroused than normal subjects; this appears to be particularly true for chronic and non-paranoid patients. However, it may be that arousal is not a unitary entity since measures of 'cortical arousal' do not appear to be linearly related to measures of autonomic arousal. Claridge (1972), who has summarized much of the literature on arousal, suggests that there are at least two arousal systems, and that those predisposed to schizophrenia show an abnormality in the way their attention and arousal covary.

High risk studies

It is not possible to conclude from studies of already manifest schizophrenics whether any positive findings reflect a cause or result of the illness. Consequently, interest has turned to the study of individuals at high risk of the condition such as the children of schizophrenics. The best known of these 'high risk' studies is that of Mednick and Schulsinger (1968) in Denmark. These authors chose 200 pre-adolescent and teenage offspring of schizophrenic mothers and matched them with 100 low risk children; the average age of both groups was 15 years and they were followed up for six years. By that time 20 of the high risk children had had a psychiatric breakdown; this 'sick' group were distinguished particularly by a history of birth and pregnancy complications, and on the original testing had shown more deviant autonomic responsivity. A second study by Mednick et al. (1973) found lowered birth weights in high risk children.

However, these findings have not been consistently replicated, a common problem in this field of study. Garmezy and Streitman (1974) point out that the characteristics claimed as occurring more frequently in high risk children include not only pregnancy complications and psychophysiological abnormalities, but also deficits in attention, poor motor coordination, soft neurological signs, and disturbance of interpersonal relationships. One report of considerable interest (Rieder *et al.*, 1975) has indicated an increase of foetal and neonatal deaths among the offspring of schizophrenics including some with neurological abnormalities. Reider and his colleagues consider three possible explanations for these findings—genetic influence, adverse uterine environment or medication toxicity. By contrast, Hanson *et al.* (1976) studied a series of children of schizophrenics from birth to age seven, and found them remarkably normal on a host of pregnancy and delivery variables, neurological examinations and psychological tests; but 17% showed enduring patterns of maladjustment and were more often described as emotionally flat, withdrawn, distractible, passive, irritable and negativistic.

A major problem with high risk studies is that only a minority of schizophrenics have parents with schizophrenia, i.e. the majority of schizophrenics to be would not qualify as 'high risk'.

One very strange epidemiological finding has been that schizophrenic patients are born significantly more often in winter and spring than the general population. Although the excess is only some 8% more than expected it has been confirmed in Scandinavia and Britain (Hare, 1975) and also in the USA (Torrey *et al.*, 1977). Genetic, nutritional, viral and other environmental explanations have been put forward but none are convincing (Torrey *et al.*, 1977).

Management

Admission to hospital

Most young adults presenting schizophrenic symptoms for the first time should initially be admitted to a psychiatric unit. The aims are five-fold. Firstly, given the serious personal implications of receiving a diagnosis of schizophrenia, it is vital to exclude conditions which may be mistaken for it. Secondly, a thorough investigation of the patient's psychological, social and physical status must be undertaken to elucidate possible aetiological or exacerbating factors. Thirdly, only after a comprehensive assessment of a patient's assets and liabilities can an individually tailored treatment programme be instigated. Fourthly, although the dangers of institutional dependence are now well known, overtly disturbed patients need an environment which will not penalize them for a period of abnormal behaviour. Lastly, perhaps because of the absorbing nature of their internal experiences or because of feelings of paranoia, many patients are unwilling to undergo treatment unless supervision and reassurance on a scale only possible in hospital are available.

There are two essential principles of treatment. Antipsychotic drugs should be used to induce an initial remission, and in some cases to maintain that remission over prolonged periods. In addition, a variety of social measures should be used to provide a social and work environment to suit the patient's particular needs. The fact that the two principles are complementary has at times been obscured by debate over whether drug or social treatment has contributed more to the decline in the number of chronically hospitalized schizophrenics since the early 1950s. The protagonists of extreme positions ignore the evidence that the antipsychotic drugs not only lessen florid symptoms, but also produce change in the ward atmosphere, and that a therapeutic milieu may not only improve a patient's will to recover, but also increase his compliance in medicine taking.

Antipsychotic drugs

Electroconvulsive therapy is only very occasionally indicated in catatonia (Chapter 20) while insulin coma and leucotomy have no place in the current somatic management of schizophrenia which instead relies on the antipsychotic drugs. These have now been studied in literally hundreds of double blind trials, the vast majority of which indicate that the neuroleptics are superior to placebo in the treatment of both acute and chronic schizophrenia (Davis, 1976). When the phenothiazines were introduced to psychiatry they were initially considered as major tranquillizers rather than specifically antipsychotic agents. The latter property was attributed to them in the 1960s for two reasons. Firstly, a number of studies revealed that phenothiazines were significantly superior to phenobarbitone in the treatment of schizophrenia, and that although some phenothiazines had sedative properties, these effects did not appear to be central to their benefit. Secondly, a very influential study by Goldberg et al. (1965) demonstrated the effectiveness of phenothiazines against what were considered particularly 'fundamental' symptoms such as slowed speech and movement, hebephrenic symptoms, lack of self care and indifference to the environment. In retrospect there can be little doubt that the neuroleptics are antipsychotic rather than mere tranquillizers, but there must remain some scepticism about whether they have a specific anti-schizophrenic action.

There are three major types of phenothiazines: (a) aliphatics such as chlorpromazine; (b) piperidines such as thioridazine and (c) piperazines such as trifluperazine and fluphenazine. Several other classes of anti-psychotics have also been developed including the thioxanthine derivatives (e.g. thiothixene) which are close structural analogues of the phenothiazines, and the butyrophenones such as haloperidol. None of these drugs has been shown to be more effective than chlorpromazine and consequently many psychiatrists prefer to commence treatment with chlorpromazine. It is usually necessary to reach at least 500 mg of chlorpromazine daily to achieve adequate effect, and occasionally the dose may be up to 800 or 1000 mg for a short time. In a very excited patient 100 mg intramuscularly two or three times per day may be necessary. The majority of patients begin to respond within two to three weeks and most of the therapeutic gain occurs within the first six weeks of treatment. The magnitude of improvement which the antipsychotics produce is considerable. In one large NIMH study about two-thirds of the patients improved significantly on phenothiazines, only 10% failed to be helped to some degree and none worsened; in contrast only one-quarter of the placebo group showed significant improvement.

Thioridazine, trifluoperazine, fluphenazine and haloperidol although differing in dosage and side-effects are approximately equal to chlorpromazine in therapeutic effect. There has been a great deal of investigation into whether specific subgroups of patients would respond to particular drugs, but in spite of some interesting leads the notion that different 'antipsychotic' drugs affect target symptoms selectively has failed to find experimental support (Hollister, 1974). It is, however, useful when a patient develops side-effects or fails to respond to one drug to change to another.

Maintenance treatment

During the resolving phase of schizophrenia it is usually possible to reduce the dose of medication to between one-half and two-thirds of that necessary during the acute phase. But once patients have recovered from their psychotic episode should they remain on neuroleptic medication? There have already been 24 controlled studies comparing the relapse rate of patients on placebo and on maintenance therapy, and in each one many more patients relapsed on placebo than on drugs. For example, Hogarty et al. (1974) followed-up 374 schizophrenics discharged from three American State hospitals; at the end of two years 84% of placebo-treated patients had relapsed compared with 48% of the drug maintenance group.

Whether all schizophrenics should receive maintenance therapy is more controversial. Leff and Wing (1971) suggested that patients with very poor prognostic signs relapse despite receiving drugs while those with very good prognostic signs do not relapse even without drugs. Goldberg and his colleagues (1977) agreed that the poor prognosis group benefits little from long-term medication but produced evidence that the good prognosis group profits most from maintenance therapy. In practice, since the greatest risk appears to be in the year following discharge the majority of schizophrenics should receive medication over this period. Then, they should be re-assessed and a trial of decreased dosage or cessation of drugs should be considered.

A major problem in maintenance therapy is ensuring that patients take their medication. Renton et al. (1963) reported that 46% of schizophrenic out-patients failed to take their tablets as prescribed and Hare and Wilcox (1967) found that one-fifth of psychiatric in-patients did not take the medication given by the nursing staff. Van Putten and his colleagues (1976) compared drug compliers with habitual defaulters and found that when the former decompensated they tended to develop dysphoric symptoms while the latter were more likely to develop ego syntonic grandiose psychoses which they preferred to relative drug-induced normality. It is possible to check whether patients are taking some, at least, of their drugs by measuring their plasma prolactin, but a simpler method of ensuring compliance is to use long-acting injectable preparations.

Three depot neuroleptics are now in common use—fluphenazine enanthate and decanoate, and flupenthixol decanoate. The fluphenazines are roughly equipotent, but the decanoate causes fewer extrapyramidal side-effects (Groves and Mandel, 1976), while flupenthixol is said to have some antidepressant as well as antipsychotic actions. In a double-blind trial of fluphenazine decanoate, Hirsch and Leff (1975) found that 66% of patients on placebo relapsed within nine months compared with only 8% of those on active drugs. The active injections significantly aided family relationships and decreased delusions and socially embarrassing behaviour. Because of their administrative convenience some psychiatrists routinely prescribe depot rather than oral preparations even for in-patients and drug compliers. Such a practice ignores the evidence that toxicity is higher with depot preparations (Rifkin et al., 1977; Falloon et al., 1978).

Unfortunately a minority of schizophrenics fail to respond significantly to all standard neuroleptic drugs, and as yet there appears no proven way of predicting response. It may be that some of those who fail to respond do not absorb sufficient of the drugs, or metabolize them in a different manner. Some workers have suggested that extremely high doses of phenothiazines might produce a remission in some previously resistant patients. This does not seem to be the case for most drug resistant patients, but a few young acute schizophrenics may derive some benefit (Davis, 1976). A number of other antipsychotic drugs are available in some countries, and should be considered in otherwise resistant patients. Pimozide is widely used in Britain (Falloon *et al.*, 1978) and sulpiride in France, while loxapine and the depot preparation fluspirilene are still being evaluated. A recent alternative, that of very high doses of pro-pranolol, has been used with success by Yorkston *et al.* (1977), but their findings await confirmation.

Side-effects

The most obvious of the side-effects of the neuroleptics are extrapyrami-dal symptoms; they are commonest with haloperidol and fluphenazine and least common with thioridazine. Van Praag and Korf (1976) have shown that patients with low CSF pre-therapeutic homovanillic acid (HVA) response to probenecid are especially liable to Parkinsonian side-effects. Dystonic spasms usually affect the muscles of the neck, face, and tongue and include torticolis, oculogyric crises, and rarely opisthotonus. They tend to occur within a few days of treatment and are most frequent with piperazine drugs. Akathisia is sometimes known as the 'restless legs syndrome'; in it the patient has a great urge to move about and considerable difficulty in sitting still.

Parkinsonian symptoms, dystonia and akathisia can all usually be relieved by antiparkinsonian agents orally or occasionally in an emergency intramuscularly, but there is controversy over whether one should routinely administer these agents to all patients on neuroleptics. Certainly, the side-effects of neuroleptics may be very distressing, and physical immobility and mask-like faces may be misdiagnosed as worsen-ing of the psychosis. On the other hand, there is no clear evidence that antiparkinsonian drugs are prophylactic, and they may themselves cause side-effects. Furthermore, not all patients develop side-effects on the neuroleptics and there have been suggestions that the antiparkinsonian drugs may lessen the blood levels and effectiveness of the neuroleptics.

The most troublesome side-effect of prolonged high dosage neurolep-tic medication is tardive dyskinesia which is characterized by slow rhythmical movements in the region of the mouth—grimacing, smacking of the lips, side to side movements of the chin, and protrusion of the tongue. The frequency of this condition in the chronic wards of mental hospitals has been overlooked for many years (Crane, 1973). Unfortu-nately, stopping the medication does not necessarily lead to the dis-appearance of the dyskinesia and may sometimes make it worse (Kobayashi, 1977).

When chlorpromazine was first introduced cholestatic jaundice used to occur in about one in every 100 patients, but for some reason the incidence has now dropped to about one case per 1000 patients treated. On the other hand, weight gain is very common and may be gross and disturbing to patients. Breast engorgement is also frequent but less than 5% of women complain of overt lactation. The dosage should be carefully monitored and the possibility of having 'drug holidays'—missing the drug one day a week—should be considered.

Social treatment

The idea that schizophrenics could benefit from social therapy achieved prominence through the development of the concept of the therapeutic community in the post war years. Now 'milieu therapy' is often prescribed for all in-patient schizophrenics on the supposition that such an environment will exert a therapeutic effect on all who are exposed to it. To this end schizophrenics are often expected to participate in a programme which includes varying degrees and combinations of occupational therapy, group activity, recreational therapy, group psychotherapy, therapeutic community, resocialization, vocational rehabilitation and industrial therapy. The case for indiscriminate milieu therapy rests more on general humanitarian grounds than on demonstrated therapeutic effect. Its proponents take its effectiveness for granted but with a few prominent exceptions controlled outcome studies are lacking (Van Putten and May, 1976).

Handicaps

Wing, Brown and their colleagues at the Institute of Psychiatry have adopted a much more scientifically rigorous approach to social treatment. They have emphasized that before the treatment plan for any individual schizophrenic is instigated it is essential to make a careful assessment of the assets and liabilities both of the patient and of significant others in his life; only then can one develop an informed definition of treatment goals and the appropriate therapeutic means to achieve them. In this context it is useful to review the three forms of handicap to which Wing and Brown (1970) consider schizophrenics are particularly liable. First there is premorbid handicap due to factors which precede the illness *per se*, such as poverty, lack of education, and of working skills; all of these may impede resettlement into the community.

Next there is primary handicap which arises as a direct consequence of the illness and takes the form of either negative or positive symptoms. Negative symptoms are characterized by decrease of function and include slowness, social withdrawal, flatness of affect, poverty of speech, lack of initiative, underactivity and poor motivation. These negative symptoms become particularly evident in an under-stimulating environment such as the chronic wards of a large mental hospital. In a carefully controlled evaluation Wing and Brown (1970) studied the progress of long-stay schizophrenics in three hospitals which differed in the amount of environmental stimulation they offered, the length of time patients were restricted on the ward, and the time which patients spent doing nothing. The hospital with the most barren under-stimulating wards contained patients who were the most withdrawn, most silent and most affectively blunted. There was a high correlation between low social stimulation and the severity of negative symptoms.

Positive symptoms are the florid symptoms of schizophrenia such as delusions and hallucinations which are often seen in an acute illness or with an exacerbation in chronic patients. Too vigorous an attempt at rehabilitation can be a source of excessive stimulation and lead to the re-emergence of dormant delusions and hallucinations. In one study this occurred among a group of chronic patients put directly into an industrial rehabilitation unit, but not among a similar group who had first experienced a period of graded preparation (Wing *et al.*, 1964). Such relapse can be prevented by beginning with work periods on the ward and then graduating the patient to a hospital occupational training unit before going on to outside work in sheltered employment or an industrial therapy unit. Another kind of over-stimulation may result from over-enthusiastic milieu therapy. Van Putten and May (1976) believe that lively, intense group meetings, searches for hidden meanings and role diffusion may constitute a toxic environment for schizophrenics with deficits in perception, attention and information processing. For schizophrenics living outside hospital not only the family milieu but also the occurrence of independent life events provide a potential source of excessive stimulation leading to the re-emergence of positive symptoms. Thus, the primary handicaps of schizophrenia can be seen as an extraordinary vulnerability, like walking a tight-rope with the dangers of an under-stimulating environment leading to negative symptoms on one side and the dangers of over-stimulation leading to florid symptoms on the other.

Secondary handicaps occur as a result of being ill, but are not a direct product of the illness itself. Institutionalization, for example, is a major handicap to rehabilitating schizophrenics. It was in 1959 that Barton first drew attention to a syndrome characterized by apathy, loss of interest and initiative, submissiveness, lack of individuality, and deterioration of personal habits, among the inmates of institutions like mental hospitals and prisons. Even before the introduction of phenothiazines and Parkinsonian side-effects, chronic mental hospital patients and particularly schizophrenics were noted for their cowed and passive stance, their shuffling gait, and their resigned acceptance that things will go on as they are—unchanging, inevitably and indefinitely. Barton (1976) identified this syndrome as stemming from the attitudes and social structure of the institutional setting: asocialization, loss of responsibility and basic rights, sedation and authoritarian staff attitudes.

In Wing and Brown's (1970) comparative study of three hospitals, the strongest determinant of the patient's attitude to discharge was how long he or she had been in hospital; the longer a patient had been in hospital the less likely that he would want to leave. The vulnerability of the schizophrenic to institutionalization is often reinforced by the attitudes of hospital staff who restrict patients' liberty and take over large areas of their decision making. In wards where patients had the fewest personal possessions and nurses were most pessimistic about the hope for social recovery, Wing and Brown found that the wish to remain in hospital was most prevalent. Improvement in patients' clinical and social responses were most highly correlated with increase in work activity and decrease in unoccupied time.

Rehabilitation

For the effective rehabilitation of schizophrenics a wide range of facilities within and without hospital are necessary. These should include occupational therapy units of graded complexity, a day hospital, an industrial therapy unit, sheltered workshops, good links with sympathetic employers and with government re-training units, hostels, boarding houses, group houses and flats. An effective registration and follow-up system is also essential to ensure that patients do not drop out of the system. As yet few places have a full range of facilities or staff and voluntary agencies often play a vital role in filling the deficiencies.

Rehabilitation should proceed on two fronts, the first social and domestic and the second employment; the two do not necessarily go together and so are best dealt with separately. Thus, a severely handicapped patient may be started on a ward where simple occupational tasks are brought in for a few hours each day. Then, he may go to a supervised work unit where a simple repetitive task is carried out for increasingly long periods. Thereafter, he may progress through a series of steps involving increasing responsibility, simulated industrial experience inside the hospital, a sheltered workshop outside and eventually return to normal employment. Conversely some patients may progress through open wards to an on-site patient managed hostel, then a supervised group home outside the hospital, but still have to attend the hospital rehabilitation unit.

Brown and his colleagues (1972) have demonstrated that schizophrenics are highly responsive to the quality of the emotional relationship between them and the relative with whom they live. These workers found that they could predict relapse by using an index of the emotions shown by the relative which expressed the amount of critical comment, hostility and emotional over-involvement of that relative; during the nine months after discharge from hospital 58% of patients from houses with high 'expressed emotion' relapsed as against only 16% from low 'expressed emotion' homes. Vaughn and Leff (1976) have almost exactly replicated these results, and demonstrated that patients from homes with high 'expressed emotion' do better if they have little face-to-face contact with their relatives. These authors suggest that patients in high expressed emotion homes constitute a 'high risk' group, especially if male and unmarried, and consider that a major effort should be made to ensure that such patients continue to receive medication and see as little of their relatives as possible.

Consequences of out-patient management

Inherent in the idea of the out-patient management of schizophrenics is the notion that schizophrenics can lead a more productive and contented life in the community than in the chronic wards of a mental hospital. This notion of community care has been behind the drive both in Europe and America to reduce the size of mental hospitals and discharge many patients. This approach has many advantages. Families are less disrupted when a spouse, parent or child is only away for brief periods, and when care is given locally the family can continue to function as a unit despite one member being hospitalized. Successful community care demands extensive community facilities and unfortunately the development of these facilities has only rarely kept pace with the decrease in size of the mental hospitals.

Relatively little is known of the overall quality of life of discharged schizophrenics. Indeed Hirsch (1976) states that social and community psychiatry have become

> euphemisms for the undesirable process by which a group of persons are converted from their former status as chronic institutionalised patients to a new equally undesirable status as lonely, single persons, homeless or

inadequately housed often residing in flop homes, prisons or the park bench with a high prevalence of unemployment and self neglect.

Thus, modern treatment makes it possible for large numbers of schizophrenics to be managed in the community at relatively low cost, but this may mean depriving them of many of the facilities that a good psychiatric hospital provides. Brown *et al.* (1966) found that chronic unemployed schizophrenics living outside the hospital spent about 30% of their time doing nothing—i.e. approximately the same as one would observe in the back wards of a bad mental hospital.

Another consequence of community care is the effect which caring for a schizophrenic may have on the health and way of life of family members. Brown *et al.* (1966) found that the relatives of 29% of first admitted and 60% of previously admitted patients who were not in hospital five years later had one or more problems which the relatives attributed to the patients. The investigators considered that far from exaggerating their problems the relatives in fact underestimated their hardships.

Combined drug and social therapy

Hogarty *et al.* (1974) have studied the relationship between drug and social treatment in the after-care of 374 patients discharged from hospital. In addition to confirming the well-known benefits of maintenance drug treatment they demonstrated that social therapy had little effect on the overall relapse rate. But a combination of intensive social casework and vocational rehabilitation counselling improved adjustment and interpersonal relationships in relatively asymptomatic patients, while in patients with severe symptomatology this variant of social therapy actually hastened relapse. These authors hypothesized that in severe patients with an inability to manage a complex cognitive field a treatment that encourages the patient to expand his horizons may actually induce a state with which he cannot cope. Hogarty and his colleagues recommended that such treatment should be deferred until the patient is essentially asymptomatic.

There is some evidence that phenothiazines can provide some protection against such over-stimulation. Leff *et al.* (1973) looked at the proportion of patients experiencing life events in the five weeks preceding relapse on either placebo or phenothiazine. There had been no increase over the expected number of life events among patients who relapsed on placebo, but among those who relapsed on active medication 89% had undergone a significant preceding life event. This result strongly supports the theory that phenothiazines raise the threshold of vulnerability to ordinary experiences so that a patient on medication requires a particu-larly stressful experience before he will relapse while a schizophrenic not on medication can relapse without the additional stimulus of a significant life event. Neuroleptics also appear to decrease vulnerability to the over-arousing effects of living at home with hostile emotionally over-involved relatives (Vaughn and Leff, 1976).

Psychological treatment

There is little evidence that classical psychoanalysis is of any value in schizophrenia, but a long-term supportive relationship is of help both to patients and their relatives. In such a relationship the therapist may see himself as an 'ambassador of reality', giving understanding and advice and helping the patient to learn new techniques of adaption. Surpris-ingly little is known of which approaches are most helpful to the schizo-phrenic. For instance, it is uncertain whether it is better to encourage a patient on recovery from an acute psychotic episode to integrate this period into his general life experience, or to deny and gloss over the psychotic episode.

In recent years behaviour therapy has also been used, particularly in the treatment of chronic schizophrenia. In the behavioural paradigm mental hospitals are seen as places which condition long-term patients to be compliant, passive and socially incompetent. This model considers that patients are rewarded for causing no trouble while staff are rewarded by their compliant patients having few emotional outbursts, and enabling staff to easily complete their routine duties. Institutionalism is thus seen as being produced by the contingencies of reinforcement that impinge on both patients and staff in large mental hospitals.

One response to the self-defeating results of the above process has been the token economy. Instead of receiving food, bed, privileges and small luxuries like cigarettes free of charge patients must work to earn tokens which can be exchanged for these things. The idea is to make patients' actions have clear-cut consequences. Presenting a shaved face in the morning, helping to clean the ward, wearing a tie, etc., mean that the patient earns cigarettes, TV or a more comfortable bed. Ayllon and Azrin (1968) have described their pioneering efforts with this system, while others (reviewed by Liberman, 1976) have documented how token economies can increase work activity and self-care, and improve dis-charge rates. But there remains doubt over whether behaviour therapy can improve primary rather than secondary handicaps in schizophrenia, and how far its effects generalize outside the treatment ward.

Outcome

In 1932 Meyer-Gross reported a 16-year follow-up in which about 35% of hospitalized schizophrenics made social recoveries. A study by Harris of patients admitted to the Maudsley Hospital between 1945 and 1950 revealed that 45% had socially recovered after five years and another 21% had left hospital although they remained quite socially incompetent. By 1966 Brown *et al.* were able to report that after five years 56% of initially hospitalized schizophrenics made a social recovery, 35% were socially damaged but in the community, and only 11% were still chronically hospitalized.

Manfred Bleuler (1974) who has followed up a cohort of 208 patients over a 22-year period has made the important observation that on average schizophrenics show little further deterioration after five years, but rather tend to improve. He claims that schizophrenia cannot be considered a progressive disease since 20 years after the event the proportion of recovered patients remains the same as five years after the onset. At five years about one-quarter of the schizophrenics who were alive were in hospital; thereafter although individual patients were admitted or discharged the percentage in hospital remained roughly similar. Bleuler concludes that over this century schizophrenia has become milder and a course of acute episodes followed by improvement has become more frequent.

Prognostic indicators

There have been many studies of the factors which influence outcome in schizophrenia. There is unanimity that the outlook is bad if the illness leads to hospitalization before age 15 years. This may be because earlier breakdown is indicative of more severe illness, or because the younger patient has not had sufficient time to build up social and occupational skills and supports to aid his rehabilitation. Other ominous features include a history of schizophrenia in a first degree relative, low social class, and an IQ below 90 (*British Medical Journal*, 1977). Women have a slightly better prognosis than men, and marriage appears to have a protective role against future relapse (Vaughn and Leff, 1976).

There is a high correlation between poor premorbid personality and bad outcome, and also, as Offord and Gross (1969) suggest, with scholastic and other difficulties in childhood. A history of good adjustment in social, sexual and occupational functioning indicates a more favourable prognosis, as do catatonic features, and a family history of affective disorder (Wittenborn *et al.*, 1977). Thought disorder, delusions and hallucinations are not of prognostic importance and neither apparently are Schneider's first rank symptoms (Hawk *et al.*, 1975; Brockington *et al.*, 1978). The latter authors did, however, confirm the value of Langfeldt's criteria for poor prognosis schizophrenia. The more acute the onset of the psychosis and the more obvious the precipitants the greater the chances of recovery, while not surprisingly chronicity tends to predict chronicity. Lack of insight, emotional withdrawal and blunting of affect are bad signs.

References

Alanen, Y. O. (1968). From the mothers of schizophrenic patients to interactional family dynamics. *In* 'The Transmission of Schizophrenia' (Eds D. Rosenthal and S. Kety). Pergamon Press, Oxford.

Allen, M. G. and Pollin, W. (1970). Schizophrenia in twins and the diffuse ego boundary hypothesis. *Am. J. Psychiat.* **127**, 437–442.

Altschule, M. D. (1975). Evolution of the concept of schizophrenia. *In* 'The Biology of the Schizophrenic Process' (Eds S. Wolf and B. B. Berle). Plenum Press, New York and London.

Ayllon, T. and Azrin, N. H. (1968). 'The Token Economy'. Appleton-Century-Crofts, New York.

Bateson, G., Jackson, D. D., Haley J. and Weakland, J. H. (1956). Toward a theory of schizophrenia. *Behav. Sci.* **1**, 251–264.

Bannister, D. (1962). The nature and measurement of schizophrenic thought disorder. *J. Ment. Sci.* **108**, 825–842.

Bannister, D. and Fransella, F. (1966). A grid test of schizophrenic thought disorder. *Br. J. Soc. Clin. Psychol.* **5**, 95–102.

Barton, R. (1976). 'Institutional Neurosis'. Wright, Bristol.

Bird, E. D., Spokes, E. G., Barnes, J., Mackay, A. V. P., Iversen, L. and Shepherd, M. (1977). Increased dopamine and reduced glutamic acid decarboxylase and choline acetyl transferase activity in schizophrenia. *Lancet* **2**, 1157–1158.

Bleuler, E. (1911). 'Dementia Praecox or the Group of Schizophrenias'. Trans. J. Zinkin, 1950. International Universities Press, New York.

Bleuler, M. (1974). The long-term course of the schizophrenic psychoses. *Psychol. Med.* **4**, 244–254.

Bliss, E. L. (1975). Neural substrates. *In* 'The Biology of the Schizophrenic Process' (Eds S. Wolf and B. B. Berle). Plenum Press, New York and London.

Böök, J. A. (1953). A genetic and neuropsychiatric investigation of a north-Swedish population. *Acta. Genet. Stat. Med.* **4**, 1–15.

Breakey, W. R., Goodell, H., Lorenz, P. C. and McHugh, P. (1974). Hallucinogenic drugs as precipitants of schizophrenia. *Psychol. Med.* **4**, 255–261.

British Medical Journal (Editorial) (1977). First attacks of schizophrenia, i, 733–734.

Brockington, I. F., Kendell, R. E. and Leff, J. P. (1978). Definitions of schizophrenia: concordance and prediction of outcome. *Psychol. Med.* **8**, 387–398.

Brown, G. W. and Birley, J. L. T. (1968). Crises and life changes and the onset of schizophrenia. *J. Hlth Soc. Behav.* **9**, 203–214.

Brown, G. W., Bone, M., Dalinson, B. M. and Wing, J. K. (1966). 'Schizophrenia and Social Care'. Maudsley Monograph No. 17. Oxford University Press, Oxford.

Brown, G. W., Birley, J. L. T. and Wing, J. K. (1972). Influence of family life on the source of schizophrenic disorders: a replication. Br. J. Psychiat. 121, 241–258.

Carlsson, A. and Lindquist, M. (1963). Effect of chlorpromazine or haloperidol on formation of 3 methoxytryptamine and normetanephrine in mouse brain. Acta. Pharmacol. 20, 140–144.

Carpenter, W. T., Bartko, J. J., Langsner, C. and Strauss, J. (1976). Another view of schizophrenic subtypes. Arch. Gen. Psychiat. 33, 508–516.

Clare, A. W. (1976). 'Psychiatry in Dissent'. Controversial Issues in Thought and Practice'. Tavistock, London.

Claridge, G. (1972). The schizophrenics as nervous types. Br. J. Psychiat. 121, 1–17.

Cohen, S., Nichols, A. Wyatt, R. J. and Pollin, W. (1974). The administration of methionine to chronic schizophrenic patients: a review of ten studies. Biol. Psychiat. 8, 209–225.

Cooper, J. E. and Sartorius, N. (1977). Cultural and temporal variations in schizophrenia. Br. J. Psychiat. 130, 50–57.

Cooper, J. E., Kendell, R. E., Gurland, B. J., Sharpe, L., Copeland, J. R. M. and Simon, R. (1972). 'Psychiatric Diagnosis in New York and London'. Maudsley Monograph No. 20. Oxford University Press, Oxford.

Connell, P. H. (1958). 'Amphetamine Psychosis'. Maudsley Monograph. Oxford University Press, Oxford.

Cutting, J. (1978). A reappraisal of alcoholic psychoses. Psychol. Med. 8, 285–296.

Crane, G. E. (1973). Persistent dyskinesia. Br. J. Psychiat. 122, 395.

Crow, T. J., Deakin, J. F. W., Johnstone, E. C. and Longden, A. (1976). Dopamine and schizophrenia. Lancet i, 563–566.

Davis, J. M. (1976). Recent developments in the drug treatments of schizophrenia. Am. J. Psychiat. 133, 208–214.

Davison, K. (1976). Drug-induced psychoses and their relationship to schizophrenia. In 'Schizophrenia Today' (Eds D. Kemali, G. Bartholini and D. Richter). Pergamon Press, Oxford.

Davison, K. and Bagley, C. R. (1969). Schizophrenia-like psychoses associated with organic disorder of the central nervous system. In 'Current Problems in Neuropsychiatry' (Ed. R. Herrington). Headley Brothers, Ashford, Kent.

Eaton, J. W. and Weil, R. J. (1955). 'Culture and Mental Disorders'. The Free Press, Glencoe, Illinois.

Enoch, M. D., Trethowan, W. H. and Barker, J. C. (1967). 'Some Uncommon Psychiatric Syndromes'. Wright, Bristol.

Falloon, I., Watt, D. C. and Shepherd, M. (1978). A comparative controlled trial of pimozide and flupenazine decanoate in schizophrenia. Psychol. Med. 8, 59–70.

Faris, R. E. L. and Dunham, H. W. (1939). 'Mental Disorders in Urban Areas. An Ecological Study of Schizophrenia and Other Psychoses'. University of Chicago Press, Chicago.

Flor-Henry, P. (1976). Epilepsy and psychopathology. In 'Recent Advances in Clinical Psychiatry' (Ed. K. Granville-Grossman), Vol. 2. Churchill Livingstone, Edinburgh.

Forrest, A. (1975). Paranoid states and paranoid psychosis. In 'New Perspectives in Schizophrenia' (Eds A. Forrest and J. Affleck). Churchill Livingstone, Edinburgh.

Freedman, B. J. (1974). The subjective experience of perceptual and cognitive disturbances in schizophrenia. *Arch. Gen. Psychiat.* **30**, 333–340.

Friedhoff, A. J. and Van Winkle, E. (1962). Isolation and characterisation of a compound from the urine of schizophrenics. *Nature* **194**, 897–898.

Fuller-Torrey, E. (1973). Is schizophrenia universal? An open question. *Schizophrenia Bull.* **7**, 53–58.

Garmezy, N. and Streitman, S. (1974). Children at risk: the search for the antecedents of schizophrenia. *Schizophrenia Bull.* **8**, 13–90; **9**, 55–125.

Goldberg, E. M. and Morrison, S. L. (1963). Schizophrenia and social class. *Br. J. Psychiat.* **109**, 785.

Goldberg, S. C., Klerman, G. L. and Cole, J. O. (1965). Changes in schizophrenic psychopathology and ward behaviour as a function of phenothiazine treatment. *Br. J. Psychiat.* **116**, 107–117.

Goldberg, S. C., Schooler, N. R., Hogarty, H. E. and Roper, M. (1977). Prediction of relapse in schizophrenia outpatients treated by drug and sociotherapy. *Arch. Gen. Psychiat.* **34**, 171–184.

Gottesman, I. I. and Shields, J. (1972). 'Schizophrenia and Genetics: A Twin Study Vantage Point'. Academic Press, New York and London.

Gottesman, I. I. and Shields, J. (1976). Critical review of recent adoption, twin and family studies. *Schizophrenia Bull.* **2**, 360–400.

Griffiths, J. D., Cavanagh, J., Held, J. and Oates, J. A. (1972). Dextroamphetamine: evaluation of psychomimetic properties in man. *Arch. Gen. Psychiat.* **26**, 97–100.

Grinker, R., Werble, B. and Drye, R. (1968). 'The Borderline Syndrome'. Basic Books, New York.

Groves, J. E. and Mandel, M. (1975). The long acting phenothiazines. *Arch. Gen. Psychiat.* **32**, 893–900.

Gur, R. E. (1977). Motoric laterality imbalance in schizophrenia. *Arch. Gen. Psychiat.* **34**, 33–37.

Hanson, D. R., Gottesman, I. and Heston, L. L. (1976). Some possible childhood indicators of adult schizophrenia inferred from children of schizophrenics. *Br. J. Psychiat.* **129**, 142–154.

Hare, E. H. (1967). The epidemiology of schizophrenia. *In* 'Developments in Schizophrenia' (Eds A. Coppen and A. Walk). Headley Brothers, Ashford, Kent.

Hare, E. H. (1975). Season of birth in schizophrenia and neurosis. *Am. J. Psychiat.* **132**, 1168–1171.

Hare, E. H. and Wilcox, D. R. C. (1967). Do psychiatric inpatients take their pills? *Br. J. Psychiat.* **113**, 1435–1439.

Hawk, A. B., Carpenter, W. T. and Strauss, J. S. (1975). Diagnostic criteria and five year outcome in schizophrenia. *Arch. Gen. Psychiat.* **32**, 343–347.

Hemsley, D. R. (1975). A two-stage model of attention in schizophrenia research. *Br. J. Soc. Clin. Psychol.* **14**, 81–89.

Heston, L. L. (1970). The genetics of schizophrenic and schizoid disease. *Science* **167**. 249–256.

Heston, L. L. and Denney, D. (1968). Interactions between early life experience and biological factors in schizophrenics. *In* 'The Transmission of Schizophrenia' (Eds D. Rosenthal and S. Kety). Pergamon Press, Oxford.

Higgins, J. (1976). Effects of child rearing by schizophrenic mothers: a follow-up. *J. Psychiat. Res.* **13**, 1–9.

Hirsch, S. R. (1976). Interacting social and biological factors determining prognosis in the rehabilitation and management of persons with schizophrenia. *In* Annual Review of the Schizophrenic Syndrome 1974–5' (Ed. R. Cancro). Brunner/Mazel, New York.

Hirsch, S. R., and Leff, J. P. (1975). 'Abnormalities in the Parents of Schizophrenics'. Maudsley Monograph No. 22. Oxford University Press, Oxford.

Hirsch, S. R., Gaind, R. Rohde, P. D. *et al.* (1973). Outpatient maintenance of chronic schizophrenic patients with long acting fluphenazine. *Br. Med. J.* **1**, 633–637.

Hoch, P. H. and Polatin, P. (1949). Pseudoneurotic forms of schizophrenia. *Psychiat. Q. 23*, 248.

Hogarty, G. E., Goldberg, S. C., Schoolar, N. R. and Ulrich, R. F. (1974). Drugs and sociotherapy in the aftercare of schizophrenic patients. *Arch. Gen. Psychiat.* **31**, 603–608.

Hollister, L. E. (1974). Clinical differences among phenothiazines in schizophrenics. *In* 'Phenothiazines and Structurally Related Drugs' (Ed. Forest). Raven Press, New York.

Holzman, P. S., Levy, D. and Proctor, L. R. (1976). Smooth pursuit eye movements, attention, and schizophrenia. *Arch. Gen. Psychiat.* **33**, 1415–1420.

Hoover, C. F. and Franz, J. D. (1972). Siblings in the families of schizophrenics. *Arch. Gen. Psychiat.* **26**, 334–342.

Jackson, D. D. (1960). 'The Aetiology of Schizophrenia'. Basic Books, New York.

Janowsky, D. S., el-Yousef, M. K. and Davis, J. M. (1973). Provocation of schizophrenic symptoms by intravenous administration of methylphenidate. *Arch. Gen. Psychiat.* **28**, 185–191.

Johnstone, E. C., Crow, T. J., Frith, C. D., Husband, J. and Kreel, L. (1976). Cerebral ventricular size and cognitive impairment in chronic schizophrenia. *Lancet* **ii**, 924–926.

Kendell, R. E. (1972). Schizophrenia: the remedy for diagnostic confusion. *Br. J. Hosp. Med.* **8**, 383–390.

Kety, S. S., Rosenthal, D. and Wender P. H. (1973). Mental illness in the biological and adoptive families of adopted individuals who have become schizophrenic. *Proc. Am. Psychopathol. Ass.* **63**, 147–165.

Kobayashi, R. M. (1977). Drug therapy of tardive dyskinesia. *New Eng. J. Med.* **296**, 257–260.

Kohn, M. L. (1976). The interaction of social class and other factors in the etiology of schizophrenia. *Am. J. Psychiat.* **133**, 177–180.

Laing, R. D. and Esterson, A. (1964). 'Sanity, Madness and the Family'. Tavistock, London.

Leff, J. P. and Wing, J. K. (1971). Trial of maintenance therapy in schizophrenics. *Br. Med. J.* **3**, 599–604.

Leff, J. P., Hirsch, S. R., Rohde, P., Gaind, R. and Stevens, B. C. (1973). Life events and maintenance therapy in schizophrenic relapse. *Br. J. Psychiat.* **123**, 659–660.

Liberman, R. P. (1976). Behaviour therapy for schizophrenia. *In* 'Treatment of Schizophrenia: Progress and Prospects' (Eds L. J. West and D. E. Flinn). Grune and Stratton, New York.

Lidz, T. (1968). The family, language and transmission of schizophrenia. *In* 'The Transmission of Schizophrenia' (Eds D. Rosenthal and S. Kety). Pergamon Press, Oxford.

Lidz, T., Cornelison, A. R., Fleck, S. and Terry, D. (1957). The intrafamilial environment of the schizophrenic patient I. *Psychiatry* **20**, 329–342.

Lishman, A. (1978). 'Organic Psychiatry'. Blackwell, Oxford.

McGhie, A. and Chapman, J. (1961). Disorders of attention and perception in early schizophrenia. *Br. J. Med. Psychol.* **34**, 103–116.

Mednick, S. A. and Schulsinger, F. (1968). Some premorbid characteristics related to breakdown in children with schizophrenic mothers. *J. Psychiat. Res.* **6**, 267–291 (Suppl. 1).

Mednick, S. A. Miora, E., Schulsinger, F. *et al.* (1963). Erratum and further analysis: perinatal conditions and infant development in children with schizophrenic parents. *Social Biology* **20**, 111–112.

Mellor, C. S. (1970). First rank symptoms of schizophrenia. *Br. J. Psychiat.* **117**, 15.

Meltzer, H. Y. (1976). Serum creatine phosphokinase in schizophrenia. *Am. J. Psychiat.* **133**, 192–196.

Mezey, A. G. (1960). Psychiatric aspects of human migrations. *Int. J. Soc. Psychiat.* **5**, 245–260.

Mitsuda, H. (1967). 'Clinical Genetics in Psychiatry'. Igaku-Shoin, Tokyo.

Murphy, D. L. and Wyatt, R. J. (1972). Reduced MAO activity in blood platelets from schizophrenic patients. *Nature* **238**, 225–226.

Murphy, H. B. M. (1968). Cultural factors in the genesis of schizophrenia. *In* 'The Transmission of Schizophrenia' (Eds D. Rosenthal and S. Kety). Pergamon, Oxford.

Murphy, J. (1978). Recognition of psychosis in non-western societies. *In* 'Current Issues in Psychiatric Diagnosis'. Raven Press, New York.

Murray, R. M., Don, M. C. H., Smith, A. L., Birley, J. L. Y. and Rodnight, R. (1979). A possible association between raised urinary DMT and certain psychotic symptoms. *Arch. Gen. Psychiat.* (in press).

Odegaard, O. (1932). Emigration and insanity. *Acta. Psychiat.*, Suppl. 4.

Offord, D. R. and Gross, L. A. (1969). Behavioural antecedents of adult schizophrenia. *Arch. Gen. Psychiat.* **21**, 267–283.

O'Neal, P. and Robins, L. N. (1958). Childhood patterns predictive of adult schizophrenia. *Am. J. Psychiat.* **115**, 385–391.

Payne, R. W. (1973). Cognitive abnormalities. *In* 'Handbook of Abnormal Psychology' (Ed. H. J. Eysenck) (2nd edn). Pitman Medical, London.

Payne, R. W. and Friedlander, D. (1962). A short battery of simple tests for measuring over inclusive thinking. *J. Ment. Sci.* **108**, 362–367.

Pollin, W, (1972). The pathogenesis of schizophrenia. *Arch. Gen. Psychiat.* **27**, 29–37.

Pollin, W., Cardon, P. and Kety, S. (1961). Effects of amino acid feedings in schizophrenic patients treated with iproniazide. *Science* **133**, 104–105.

Procci, W. R. (1976). Schizo-affective psychosis: fact or fiction. *Arch. Gen. Psychiat.* **33**, 1167–1178.

Rieder, R., Rosenthal, D., Wender, P. and Blumental, H. (1975). The offspring of schizophrenics: fetal and neonatal deaths. *Arch. Gen. Psychiat.* **32**, 200–211.

Renton, C. A., Affleck, J. W., Carstairs, G. M. and Forrest, A. D. (1963). A follow-up of schizophrenic patients in Edinburgh. *Acta Psychiat. Scand.* **39**, 548–600.

Rifkin, A., Quitkin, F., Rabiner, C. and Klein, D. F. (1977). Fluphenazine decanoate, fluphenazine hydrochloride and placebo in remitted schizophrenics. *Arch. Gen. Psychiat.* **34**, 43–47.

Rodnight, R. (1971). Biochemical research in psychiatry (Editorial). *Psychol. Med.* **1**, 353–355.

Rosenhan, D. (1973). On being sane in insane places. *Science* **179**, 250–258.

Rosenthal, D. (1962). Problems of sampling and diagnosis in the major twin studies of schizophrenia. *J. Psychiat. Res.* **1**, 116–134.

Rosenthal, D., Wender, P., Kety, S., Welner, J. and Schulsinger, F. (1971). The adopted-away offspring of schizophrenics. *Am. J. Psychiat.* **128**, 307–311.

Scharfetter, C. (1975). The historical development of the concept of schizophrenia. *In* 'Studies of Schizophrenia' (Ed. M. H. Lader). Headley Brothers, Ashford, Kent.

Schneider, K. (1959). 'Clinical Psychopathology'. Trans. M. W. Hamilton. Grune and Stratton, New York.

Scheff, T. F. (1963). The role of the mentally ill and the dynamics of mental disorder: a research framework. *Sociometry* **26**, 436–453.

Sheldrick, C., Jablensky, A., Sartorius N. and Shepherd M. (1977). Schizophrenia succeeded by affective illness. *Psychol. Med.* **7**, 619–624.

Shepherd, M. (1961). Morbid jealousy. *J. Ment. Sci.* **107**.

Shepherd, M. (1976). Definition, classification and nomenclature: a clinical overview. *In* 'Schizophrenia Today' (Eds D. Kemali, G. Bartholini and D. Richter). Pergamon Press, Oxford.

Singer, M. T. and Wynne, L. C. (1966). Communication styles in parents of normals, neurotics and schizophrenics. *Psychiat. Res. Rep.* **20**, 25–38.

Snyder, S. H., Bannerjee, S. P., Yamamura, H. I. and Greenberg, D. (1974). Drugs, neurotransmitters and schizophrenia. *Science* **184**, 1234–1253.

Spitzer, R. L. (1976). More on pseudoscience in science and the case for psychiatric diagnosis. *Arch. Gen. Psychiat.* **33**, 458–470.

Torrey, E. F., Torrey, B. B. and Peterson, M. R., (1977). Seasonality of schizophrenic births in the United States. *Arch. Gen. Psychiat.* **34**, 1065–1070.

Van Putten, T. V. and May, P. R. A. (1976). Milieu therapy of the schizophrenias. *In* 'Treatment of Schizophrenia: Progress and Prospects' (Eds L. J. West and D. E. Flinn). Grune and Stratton, New York.

Van Putten, T. V., Crumpton, E. and Yale, C. (1976). Drug refusal in schizophrenia and the wish to be crazy. *Arch. Gen. Psychiat.* **33**, 1443–1447.

Van Praag, H. M. and Korf, J. (1976). Importance of dopamine metabolism for clinical effects and side effects of neuroleptics. *Am. J. Psychiat.* **133**, 1171–1177.

Vaughn, C. and Leff, J. P. (1976). The influence of family and social factors on the course of psychiatric illness. *Br. J. Psychiat.* **129**, 125–137.

Waring, M. and Ricks, D. (1965). Family patterns of children who become adult schizophrenics. *J. Nerv. Ment. Dis.* **140**, 351–364.

Wender, P. H., Rosenthal, D., Kety, S. S., Schulsinger, F. and Welner, J. (1974). Crossfostering: a research strategy for clarifying the role of genetic and experiential factors in the aetiology of schizophrenia. *Am. J. Psychiat.* **30**, 121–128.

Wing, J. K. (1973). Unpublished, quoted by Clare, 1976.

Wing, J. K. and Brown, G. W. (1970). 'Institutionalism and Schizophrenia'. Cambridge University Press, Cambridge.

Wing, J. K. and Nixon, J. (1975). Discriminating symptoms in schizophrenia. *Arch. Gen. Psychiat.* **32**, 853–859.

Wing, J. K., Bennett, D. H. and Denham, J. (1964). The Industrial Rehabilitation of Long-Stay Schizophrenic Patients. Medical Research Council Memo No. 42. London, HMSO.

Winokur, G. (1977). Delusional disorder (paranoia) *Compr. Psychiat.* **18**, 511–521.

Wittenborn, R., McDonald, D. C. and Maurer, H. S. (1977). Persisting symptoms in schizophrenia predicted by background factors. *Arch. Gen. Psychiat.* **34**, 1057–1061.

World Health Organization (1973). 'The International Pilot Study of Schizophrenia', Vol. 1. Geneva.

12 Affective disorder

Sadrudin Bhanji

Introduction

The affective disorders are characterized by inappropriate depression or elation. Abnormalities in perception and cognition may also occur, but arise out of the mood disturbance. In most cases the aetiology is unknown, but some affective disorders appear to bear a close relationship to external or internal stress. However, even when this is clearly so, the mechanisms whereby symptoms arise are largely unknown.

Epidemiology

There are a number of pitfalls in the epidemiological study of the affective disorders, not least of which is the fact that the term depression may describe an appropriate mood state, a symptom, or an illness. There are thus two necessary steps in defining depressive illness. Firstly, a distinction must be made between normal and morbid depression: secondly, depression as a symptom must be distinguished from depression as an illness. The latter step, and the subsequent one of subdividing the depressive illnesses are discussed in the section on classification.

There is little agreement over the relationship between normal and morbid depressions. Some regard these as distinct states, others as merging imperceptibly with each other. Thus many psychiatrists regard depression as pathological if its cause appears insufficient and its duration and severity exceed that normally expected in a given population. By contrast, others (e.g. Zung, 1973) define abnormal depression on the basis of physiological, psychomotor and attitudinal changes in addition to the mood disturbance.

Unfortunately, even where depression refers to an illness, selection criteria vary from study to study. Some authors have included all depressives, others have selected only those with manic depressive disease or have subdivided their sample according to their preferred classification. International comparisons of incidence and prevalence are particularly difficult to interpret as diagnostic criteria may differ considerably. For some time it was believed that first admission rates for manic depressive psychosis were lower in the United States than in England and Wales. However, Cooper et al. (1972) demonstrated that such differences were apparent rather than real and derived largely from the broad American concept of schizophrenia, which included patients who in England and Wales would be classified as suffering from depressive illness, neurosis, personality disorder, or mania. Further problems arise as not all depressed subjects are willing or able to draw attention to themselves. Hence incidence and prevalence estimates depend upon whether the sample studied is drawn from hospitals, out-patient clinics, general practice, or selected populations (e.g. the relatives of affected probands, or populations chosen according to geographical distribution, sex, age, religion, social class, or nativity). Brown et al. (1975) conducted a community survey in a London borough and found that a significant proportion of depressed working class women had not sought professional help. Such cases would clearly not be detected in studies carried out on patients. The position as regards mania is more satisfactory in that the term has a more circumscribed usage, and cases are more likely to attract notice. However, chronic forms of hypomania may be misclassified as personality disorders, and acute episodes as schizophrenic psychoses.

Perris (1976) has discussed a number of epidemiological studies in terms of the results obtained using different selection criteria and populations. Thus one day point prevalence estimates ranged from 0·2 to 10·4/1000 for psychotic depressives and from 1·4 to 26·5/1000 for neurotic depressives. Life-time expectancy rates obtained from population studies showed less variation (9·0 to 18·0/1000 for males; 22·4 to 28·0/1000 for females). Using first admission rates much lower figures were obtained, but a prospective population survey of all types of depression revealed expectancy rates of 85·0/1000 and 177·0/1000 for males and females respectively (Essen-Moller and Haguell, 1961).

A more succinct view is that of Lehmann (1971) who has estimated the prevalence of depressive illness in Western society as between 3 and 4% of the general population. Of these one in five seek treatment (though not always from a psychiatrist), one in 50 enter hospital, and one in 200 commit suicide. The majority will experience further attacks of depression, and approximately a quarter will suffer from mania. This last figure, however, may be an overestimate. A study of over 200 psychotic depressives followed up for up to 20 years showed that less than 5% became manic (Winokur and Morrison, 1973).

Psychotic depression is generally regarded as being more common beyond middle-age, but it is possible that much adolescent and childhood depression goes unrecognized. Spicer *et al.* (1973) have compared the age incidence curves for psychotic depression, mania and neurotic depression. For male psychotic depressives the peak first admission rate was around 60 years, for females between 50 and 70 years. First admission rates for mania showed a steady increase with age. Neurotic depression reached its peak in males between 25 and 40 years, and in females at around 25 years. In Europe and North America the incidence of depression in females is twice that in males. This may not apply on the Indian subcontinent, where male depressives predominate (Rao, 1970), nor amongst lower economic groups in Western society (Schwab *et al.*, 1967a). The long-held belief that depression is less common amongst American negroes than whites was not supported by Tonks *et al.* (1970). However, Hemsi (1967) found the incidence of affective disorder amongst West Indian immigrants in two London boroughs was three times that of the native population. More recently Leff *et al.* (1976) have found a six-fold increase in the incidence of mania amongst West Indian as opposed to native-born inhabitants of one of these boroughs.

The relationship between social class and affective illness has yet to be established. Hare *et al.* (1972) found the parental social class distribution among manic depressives to be no different from that among the general population. Nystrom and Lindegard (1975) found no differences in social conditions and income between 37 depressives and 370 healthy controls. However, as the subjects of this prospective study were drawn from a population of male car-owners their socio-economic distribution may have been unrepresentative of the general population. An interesting finding, which just failed to reach statistical significance, was an excess of depressives amongst those who had previously received financial support from social welfare agencies. Others have found that depression is commoner in the upper socio-economic groups. Bagley (1973) has suggested that this may be due to a tendency, amongst American psychiatrists in particular, to empathize more readily with members of the upper and middle classes. Other possibilities, he suggests, are that particular personalities predispose not only to a rise up the social scale, but also to depression, or that the stresses of achieving, or coping with, upper class life are responsible. A study of women in a London suburb, however, suggests that those from the working classes are more likely to develop a depressive illness (Brown *et al.*, 1975).

The possibility that cultural background may influence the incidence of affective illness derives some support from studies of the American Hutterites and a northern Swedish population (Odegaard, 1961). The former lived in small cohesive groups in which outward display of aggression was proscribed and guilt accepted rather than displaced on to others. In contrast, the Swedish population lived in conditions of low population density and poor communication. The ratio of schizophrenic to manic depressive illness amongst the Hutterites was 0·23, whilst among the north Swedish population it was 46·0. Further evidence suggesting that depressive illness is less likely to occur under conditions where aggression may be freely expressed is provided by a study of psychiatric morbidity during the disturbances in Northern Ireland (Lyons, 1971).

There is some evidence that the incidence of depressive illness is higher during the spring and autumn than at other times of the year.

Symptomatology

In the absence of any generally accepted aetiological theory the affective disorders can be diagnosed only on the basis of symptomatology. Most psychiatrists recognize three major syndromes—psychotic depression, neurotic depression and mania. Unfortunately there is little consistency in the way these terms have been applied. Thus, psychotic depression has been regarded as (a) inappropriate depression of mood occurring concurrently with certain physiological symptoms, (b) primary depression occurring in the presence of impaired reality testing, (c) primary depression accompanied by delusions or hallucinations, and (d) depression when it occurs as a symptom of any psychotic illness. Some psychiatrists do not employ the terms psychotic or neurotic, but instead describe the illness as respectively endogenous or reactive. However, psychotic depression may follow external stress, and, depending on the definition employed, an apparently endogenous mood disturbance need not necessarily be psychotic. On balance the adjectives psychotic and neurotic are to be preferred as at least they do not imply an aetiology that is by no means proven. The term mania is used in a more uniform fashion. The major disagreement amongst clinicians concerns the value of classifying manic states according to severity, and the criteria employed for so doing. In particular there is no generally accepted dividing line between hypomania and mania.

Psychotic depression

Otherwise termed as endogenous or manic depressive depression, this condition typically commences in middle age in persons of adequate premorbid personality and often with a family history of depressive illness. The term endogenous implies the absence of any external pre- cipitant, but some psychiatrists assert that with careful searching one can always ascribe the illness to real or symbolic trauma (Lewis, 1934).

The major symptom, though not necessarily the presenting complaint, is of a persistent sad despairing mood qualitatively different from normal unhappiness. This feeling is usually regarded as most marked on waking. However, Stallone *et al.* (1973) observed 10 patients for over 60 days and reported that they exhibited such a diurnal variation in mood less than 50% of the time. Others have stated that the diurnal mood swing disappears when the illness is at its height (van Praag *et al.*, 1965).

Agitation or retardation may be present; the latter may occasionally progress into stupor. Auditory and visual hallucinations are not uncom- mon and are usually depressive in content. Ideas of inadequacy, unworthiness, guilt and persecution are frequently elicited and may assume a delusional nature. Where hypochondriacal beliefs are promin- ent, the depressed affect may be less in evidence (Kreitman *et al.*, 1965). Obsessional ideas, when they occur, are usually aggressive in content (Kendell and Discipio, 1970). Cognitive functioning may be impaired— depressive pseudo-dementia (Madden *et al.*, 1952)—as may psychomotor speed. The current consensus is that these changes reflect lack of motiva- tion, confidence, concentration and interest rather than psychological deficits specific to depression (Miller, 1975). Lloyd and Lishman (1975) have demonstrated that depressed patients recall unpleasant experiences more readily than pleasant.

Vegetative disturbances are the rule, anorexia, weight loss, loss of libido, and amenorrhoea frequently occur. Insomnia is common and classically affects the last third of the night.

The above symptomatology is often modified by the patient's sex, personality, social class, nationality and age. Palpitations, nausea and crying spells are more common in female patients, whereas males are more likely to show increased alcohol consumption and loss of libido (Cassidy *et al.*, 1957). Patients with premorbid hysterical personalities exhibit more hypochondriacal and hysterical conversion symptoms, appear less depressed, and feel less hopeless and unworthy. They are also less retarded, and display fewer paranoid and obsessional symptoms (Lazare and Klerman, 1968). Gittleson (1966) found that obsessional neurotics who develop depression do so at a younger age and have a greater incidence of obsessional symptoms, nihilism and depersonalization during the illness. His finding, however, that the risk of suicide is diminished in such patients was not confirmed by a more recent study (Videbech, 1975) in which anancastic endogenous depressives were compared with non-anancastic cases. The former tended to be more anxious, agitated and depersonalized, and more likely to exhibit a diurnal mood swing, early morning waking and a seasonal variation in their symptoms. Non-anancastic depressives were found to be more retarded, deluded and hallucinated, and more likely to have experienced episodes of mania.

Schwab et al. (1967b) discerned three class-related syndromes amongst American depressives. In the upper classes loss of interest in social life was the major symptom. The middle classes exhibited more loneliness and guilt, and cried more. Finally, lower class depressives were likely to present with feelings of powerlessness and hopelessness. However, these findings were obtained from only 29 patients, over half of whom came from the middle classes.

Cross-national comparisons of depressive symptomatology have yielded contradictory findings, as regards, for example, the notion that guilt feelings are rarely encountered amongst Asian depressives (Teja et al., 1971). Hashmi (1970) has suggested that male immigrants from patriarchal societies, such as Pakistan, tend to complain of a fear of loss of potency when depressed. By contrast, West Indian men, who hold physical fitness in high regard, complain of loss of strength and inability to work. Tonks et al. (1970) compared primary depression as seen in American negroes with that of whites. When the two groups were matched for social class and for severity of illness the only significant difference was that the whites felt more helpless.

For many years there existed the belief that depressive illnesses arising for the first time in later life took on a distinctive character. Classical involutional melancholia arises in patients of obsessional over-anxious nature in the absence of any emotional precipitant. The symptomatology is dominated by marked agitation and florid delusions. The latter tend to consist of grandiose convictions of guilt and hypochondriacal notions of a bizarre nihilistic nature (Cotard's syndrome). Most authors (e.g. Stenstedt, 1959; Kendell, 1976) now believe that involutional melancholia consists of a heterogeneous mixture of psychotic and neurotic depression occurring in later life.

It has been estimated that approximately a quarter of depressives experience a major degree of social and personal disruption as a result of their illness (Cassidy et al., 1957). Self-neglect, the onset of stupor, and attempts at suicide all carry considerable risk to life and limb.

Neurotic depression

Otherwise termed as depressive neurosis or reactive depression, neurotic depression arises most typically in young adults of inadequate personality in response to stress. The depression of mood is similar in quality to normal unhappiness and tends to fluctuate as the patient can often be distracted from these feelings. Diurnal variation in mood is generally absent, or occasionally the reverse of that seen in psychotic depression. Anxiety, which may be phobic, is not uncommon. Unjustified ideas of guilt are rare as the patient tends to blame others for his predicament. Delusional ideas and hallucinations are not encountered. Bodily functioning is not markedly disturbed, and insomnia, if present, occurs in the early part of the night. Some psychiatrists do not accept the distinction between neurotic and psychotic depressions and regard the former as being a less severe form of the latter. Others view neurotic depression not as a disease entity but as an understandable response to what the patient sees as an intolerable and irremediable situation. From a clinical standpoint, however, the distress communicated by the patient and those around may equal or exceed that occasioned by psychotic depression.

Mania

The cardinal symptoms of mania are elation, pressure of speech, and physical hyperactivity. Classically the illness begins in adulthood in persons of cyclothymic temperament and pyknic physique. Carlson and Goodwin (1973) have recently described the manic episode as consisting of three stages. The first, hypomania, is characterized by increased speech and physical activity. The mood is laible but predominantly euphoric. Irritability occurs if demands are not met immediately. Grandiose, expansive ideas are obvious and may manifest themselves as overspending. Thought is coherent though at times tangential. An increased interest in sexual and religious matters may be evident. At this stage insight may be preserved, and the patient is not yet out of control. In the second phase, pressure of speech and action increases. The mood, though elated at times, becomes increasingly depressed at others. Irritability progresses to open anger and hostility. Definite flight of ideas occurs and speech becomes increasingly disorganized. Earlier preoccupations develop into frank delusions. During the final stage the patient engages in frenzied activity. Thought processes become incoherent; delusions become more bizarre, and hallucinations and ideas of reference may occur. Not all the patients reached this final stage. During recovery the patients passed through the earlier phases of the illness in reverse.

Biegel and Murphy (1971) analysed the item scores of 12 manics on their Manic-State Rating Scale. Core characteristics of mania included increased motor behaviour, increased verbal production, increased rapidity of thought processes, anger, poor judgement and increased social contact. In addition, their patients could be divided into those with higher elation–grandiosity scores and those with higher paranoia–destructiveness scores. The differences between their groups were independent of the degree of mania, age, sex, marital status, length of illness and the number of hospital admissions. An interesting finding was that 11 of their patients displayed observable degrees of depression.

Just as the introduction of more effective treatment stimulated interest in atypical forms of depression, so the advent of lithium therapy and prophylaxis has led to an improved awareness of the various manifestations of mania. Taylor and Abrams (1973) described 52 manics of whom on admission 48 had been diagnosed as schizophrenic and the remainder as suffering from other non-affective illnesses. Over 40% held delusions of persecution and over 10% exhibited first rank schizophrenic symptoms. The same authors investigated 55 patients with one or more catatonic features and found that 34 fulfilled diagnostic criteria for mania, whereas only four could be regarded as schizophrenic (Abrams and Taylor, 1976).

Special syndromes

Mixed states

The traditional view, at least amongst non-analysts, is that mania and psychotic depression represent opposite extremes of whatever process gives rise to the affective psychoses. This model, however, does not explain the not infrequent co-existence of manic and depressive symptoms (Kotin and Goodwin, 1972), nor the fact that a significant proportion of patients will pass directly from depression into mania, and vice versa, without any intervening period of euthymia. In addition, a number of psychological, neurophysiological and biochemical findings cast doubt on the validity of the bipolar model. Two alternatives are the triangular (Whybrow and Mendels, 1969) and continuum models (Court, 1972) (Fig. 1).

Atypical depression

The atypical or 'masked' depressions have assumed much importance in the light of recent advances in the treatment of depressive illness. They constitute those illnesses which present as either physical conditions or non-affective psychiatric disorders. Amongst the former are those depressions which present as pain, hypochondriasis, hysterical conversion symptoms, or psychosomatic disorders. Their true nature is usually revealed by the absence of any structural basis for the symptoms, a poor response to medical or surgical measures, and the presence of some depressive symptomatology (Lopez Ibor, 1972). The second group may present as anxiety states, dementia, or behavioural aberrations such as sexual misdemeanours in middle-aged men, shop-lifting in middle-aged women, and alcoholism.

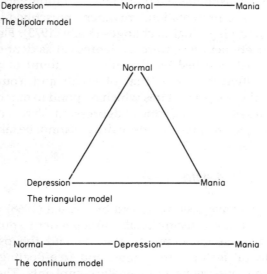

Fig. 1 Possible relationships between the normal state, depression and mania.

Bereavement reactions

Typical grief, following the loss of a close relative with whom there has been a significant amount of social interaction, can be divided into three phases. During the first the bereaved person's emotions are blunted and he behaves as though the loss had not occurred. After a period ranging from a few hours to two weeks attacks of yearning and distress occur against a background of unhappiness, apathy, and a sense of futility. Other features of this stage include anorexia, restlessness, irritability and a preoccupation with thoughts of the deceased, who may be thought of, or even perceived, as still being present. Those coming under psychiatric care tend to exhibit more self-blame and find acceptance of their loss more difficult. The final stage, of readjustment to life without the deceased, begins a few weeks after the onset of the second stage. Parkes (1965) has divided bereavement reactions into *typical grief* (outlined above), *chronic grief* in which resentment, guilt, identification symptoms and antisocial behaviour may be predominant, *inhibited grief*, which may not manifest itself for some years, and *nonspecific and mixed reactions.*

Anxiety states

A number of authors, notably Lewis (1966), have argued that anxiety states should be regarded as falling into the same category as the depressive disorders. More recent work has, however, shown that the two conditions can be distinguished on the basis of differences in premorbid personality, clinical presentation, treatment prescribed and responded to, prognosis and physiological changes (Kelly, 1973). Fleiss *et al.* (1971) found that anxiety neurotics were as depressed as depressive neurotics but could be distinguished by the greater amount of phobic anxiety displayed. A different view is that of Pollitt and Young (1971) who proposed that those anxiety states which respond to monoamine oxidase inhibitors represent atypical forms of depression. Tyrer (1976), however, suggests that a good response to these drugs cannot be taken as implying any particular diagnosis.

'Borderland states'

These conditions have been reviewed by Kessell (1968) who concludes that they represent a constitutionally independent entity lying in the borderland between the depressive states and the psychoneuroses. Prominent clinical features are phobic and free-floating anxiety along with depression, obsessions and somatic complaints. The onset is acute and usually follows a separation or physical illness. The patients are generally of obsessional personality and frequently give a history of previous separation anxiety.

Other special syndromes

Affective illness may occur in the mentally subnormal (Reid, 1972), in childhood and adolescence (Chapter 5) and old age (Chapter 14), and in association with pregnancy, physical illness and certain drug treatments.

Classification

In view of the plethora of aetiological hypotheses, it is hardly surprising that there is no universally accepted classification. Psychiatrists on the mainland of Europe have long accepted multiple-category systems; however, the main topic of contention amongst British and American psychiatrists has been whether depression is of one type or two. Other problems are the status of involutional melancholia and of those affective conditions bordering on schizophrenia and the neuroses. Most classification systems are based on the presenting symptomatology; others take into account previous illnesses, the family history, physiological and biochemical findings, or response to treatment.

Primary *vs* secondary affective disorder

This system classifies disturbances of affect according to whether they arise independently or as manifestations of other conditions. The classification proposed by Feighner *et al.* (1972) takes into account the duration of the illness, its phenomenology and the presence or absence of pre-existing medical or non-affective psychiatric illness, and avoids having to make the decision as to whether the affective disturbance is in keeping with the patient's background and circumstances. The primary affective disorders consist of primary depression and mania. The former is characterized by dysphoric mood and at least five of the following—appetite or weight loss, sleep disturbance, anergy, agitation or retardation, loss of interest or libido, self-reproach or guilt, poor concentration and suicidal thoughts. The patient must have been ill for at least one month with no history of pre-existing psychiatric disorder. Mania is defined as euphoria or irritability accompanied by five or all of the following—hyperactivity, increased flow of speech, flight of ideas, grandiosity, reduced sleep and distractability. The illness must have been of at least two weeks' duration and have arisen in the absence of pre-existing psychiatric disturbance. This classification does not acknowledge the dynamic concept of secondary mania, but describes two types of secondary depression, both phenomenologically identical to primary depression. The first is characterized by pre-existing non-affective psychiatric illness (which may or may not still be present) and the second by the concurrence of life-threatening or incapacitating medical illness.

Klein (1976) also advocates a primary versus secondary dichotomy but confines this to the depressive disorders and employs more sub-types to take into account the 'reactivity' of the illness and the nature of the pre-existing disorder. Primary depression consists of 'endogenomorphic depression' (phenomenologically similar to primary depression as defined above), reactive or situational dysphorias (which resemble neurotic depression) and schizoaffective itlness. The major subdivisions of the secondary forms are those associated with schizophrenia and schizoid states, personality disorder and neurosis, and with organic or toxic illness.

Unipolar *vs* bipolar affective disorder

Perris (1966) has defined bipolar patients as those who have experienced at least one episode of depression and one of mania (or hypomania), either separately or concurrently. Unipolars are those with a history of at least three separate episodes of psychotic depression with complete remission in between and no episodes of mania or hypomania. The usefulness of the occurrence of mania as a basis for categorizing affective illness has received much support (Perris, 1973). However, a major disadvantage of this system is that bipolar patients may be misclassified. Winokur and Morrison (1973) describe a patient who experienced eight depressive episodes before becoming manic 41 years after first becoming ill. A number of authors have suggested subdivisions of the bipolar–unipolar dichotomy. For example, Dunner *et al.* (1976a) have divided bipolar patients into types I and II according to whether the episodes of mania have been severe enough to warrant hospitalization (type I). A recent study of unipolar depressives suggests that they can be regarded as type T (tricyclic responders) or L (lithium responders). These differ in terms of premorbid personality, family history of mood swings, and the number of hospitalizations (Kupfer *et al.*, 1975). Finally, unipolar manics appear to differ from bipolar manics in age of onset and family history of affective illness and alcoholism (Abrams and Taylor, 1974). Such subclassifications as these can be regarded as no more than tentative. Time will tell whether they have any aetiological validity or therapeutic utility.

Depression spectrum disease *vs* pure depressive disease

On the basis of genetic studies Winokur (1971) has subdivided unipolar depressives into those with 'depression spectrum disease' and those with 'pure depressive disease'. The former occurs mainly in young females and is associated with a greater prevalence of depression among female than among male relatives; the difference is made up by sociopathy and alcoholism among male relatives. In contrast, pure depressive disease is commoner in men over 40, and male and female relatives show equal prevalence of depression.

Endogenous *vs* reactive depression

Proponents of this dichotomy claim that endogenous (psychotic) depression and reactive (neurotic) depression can be separated on the basis of precipitation, symptomatology, treatment and prognosis. The categorical system regards endogenous and reactive depression as distinct entities, the dimensional system as lying at opposite ends of a continuum. Intermediate forms should be rare if the former applies, commonplace if the dimensional view is correct. In spite of the simplicity of this proposition, statistical surveys have yielded conflicting results (Kendell, 1968).

Eysenck (1970) has criticized the statistical techniques so far employed and has proposed a binary dimensional system in which depressed patients are classified according to their scores on two separate and independent continua representing endogenous and reactive features. In a more recent discussion Foulds and Bedford (1976) consider the relationship between endogenous and reactive depression (employing the terms psychotic and neurotic respectively) in terms of the concept of classes of personal illness. The first, and lowest, consists of the dysthymic states, the second of neurotic symptoms, the third of integrated delusions (contrition, grandeur and persecution), and the fourth of delusions of disintegration. Higher classes take precedence over lower, but also involve the lower. Thus patients in class 3 exhibit symptoms of classes 2 and 1, but those in class 1 may not all exhibit symptoms of higher classes. They suggest the term 'state of depression' for neurotic depression, which they define as a profoundly painful dejection together with high self-blame in the absence of neurotic symptoms or delusions. Psychotic depression ('delusions of contrition') is in class 3 and consists of a preponderance of delusions of contrition over those of grandeur or persecution in the absence of delusions of disintegration. They add that psychotic depressives almost invariably suffer from neurotic symptoms and all experience anxiety, depression or both.

Winokur and Pitts (1964) are amongst those who doubt the existence of neurotic (reactive) depression as a distinct condition. They found that of 75 patients admitted with the diagnosis of reactive depression 63 were re-diagnosed on discharge (45 as endogenous depression). Unfortunately, the admission and discharge diagnoses were made by different psychiatrists; hence the findings could have been explained by differences in diagnostic practice and expertise.

Personal *vs* vital depression

This classification is similar to the endogenous *vs* reactive dichotomy but is based on whether the patient, not the doctor, can discern a connection between the depression and his circumstances (personal depression) (van Praag *et al.*, 1965).

Classification by symptom clusters

One way of attempting to categorize illnesses of unknown causation is to determine whether patients fall into statistically definable groups. Paykel (1971) subdivided depressed patients into four groups on the basis of cluster analysis. The *psychotic depressives* were the oldest and most severely depressed. Depressive delusions were encountered, along with guilt, retardation, anorexia and early waking. There was less evidence of preceding stresses and premorbid neuroticism. The *anxious depressives* tended to be middle-aged, moderately depressed, and exhibited anxiety and minor neurotic symptoms. They tended to have experienced previous similar episodes and displayed premorbid neuroticism. The *hostile depressives* were young, hostile and self-pitying. The remaining group consisted of *younger depressives with personality disorders* whose depression was generally mild but fluctuated with the environment. They had a high incidence of disturbed social relationships. Overall *et al.* (1965) employed factor analysis and were able to define three groups of depressed patients—*anxious-tense, hostile* and *retarded*. Both these systems proved to be of value in the prediction of response to drug therapy.

Similar studies have yielded comparable findings. In particular they tend to confirm the existence of a subgroup manifesting many features of psychotic depression.

Physiological classifications

Pollitt (1965) has divided depressive illness into type S and type J. In type S depressions there is a physiological shift (of the type described as occurring in psychotic depression) and no clear external cause for the mood change. Type J depressions, however, can be regarded as being justified and do not show the typical physiological dysfunctions.

Physiological measures, as opposed to symptoms, have proved disappointing in the investigation of any differences between psychotic and neurotic depressions. However, they suggest that to distinguish between agitated and retarded forms of the former might be of value. Retarded depressives have lower salivation rates, skin conductance levels and reactivity, forearm blood flow rates and pulse rates (Lader, 1973).

Pharmacogenetic classification

Pare *et al.* (1962), on the basis of responses to antidepressant medication amongst affected relatives, postulated the existence of two genetically determined types of depression—one responding to monoamine oxidase inhibitors, the other to tricyclics. However, their findings could be accounted for by inherited differences in drug metabolism (Alexanderson *et al.*, 1969; Johnstone and Marsh, 1973).

Biochemical classification

Biochemical studies of manic depressives have yielded conflicting findings, sometimes even when a clinically homogeneous population has been assessed by the same investigator. One possible explanation is that the studies undertaken were irrelevant; another is that affective disorders are best classified using biochemical, rather than clinical, criteria. The latter view, if substantiated, could have important implications for pharmacotherapy (Maas, 1975).

A pragmatic classification

Blinder (1966) has subdivided depressions according to the treatment they are most likely to respond to. He describes five types—depression with physiological retardation, depression with prolonged unresolved tension, depression characterized by profound ego disturbance, depression secondary to problems in living, and depression as the prodrome of organic illness.

A general scheme

The classification system adopted depends as much on where, and by whom, the psychiatrist was trained as on his orientation and experience. However, most accept the basic scheme set out in Fig. 2 as far as the unipolar–bipolar dichotomy. Beyond this point classification remains controversial.

Aetiology

Leaving aside ideological differences and methodological difficulties, there are a number of reasons why no generally accepted aetiological theory has emerged. Paramount are the assumptions that a uniform clinical presentation implies a single aetiology, and that phenomenological opposites have opposite causes. Further problems arise from the loose

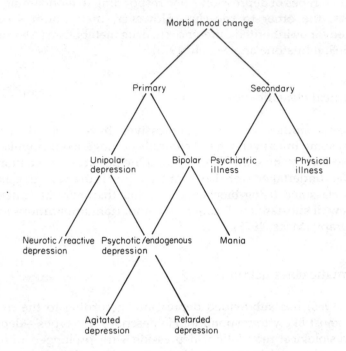

Fig. 2   The classification of affective disorders—a general scheme.

usage of the term depression, and from failures to distinguish between observation and inference, cause and effect, and predisposition and precipitation.

Genetic studies

The increased risk of manic depressive psychosis amongst the relatives of affected individuals (c.12%) and the higher concordance rates amongst monozygotic (68%) as opposed to dizygotic twins (23%), suggest that the predisposition toward the condition is inherited (Price, 1968). Both polygenic and monogenic transmissions have been proposed, and it has also been suggested that unipolar illness is inherited differently from bipolar (Perris, 1976). The view that predisposition to affective illness is determined by an X-linked dominant gene and that a second genetic factor mediates the appearance of mania (Winokur, 1971) has not received much support.

There have been few studies carried out on the inheritance of neurotic depression, but it appears that genetic factors are of less importance than in psychotic depression (Stenstedt, 1966).

Evolutionary hypotheses

In discussing why such a disadvantageous condition should be inherited, Price (1968) has compared depressive illness with two adaptive phenomena seen in lower animals— hibernation and behaviour following a decline in the dominance hierarchy. According to the latter model depressive behaviour has evolved from behavioural patterns which preserved group cohesiveness at times of change in social structure. The passive assumption of a submissive role, the avoidance of others, and an unwillingness to compete for food and sexual activity all resemble features of human depressive illness. Conversely, mania may represent atavistic behaviour evoked to consolidate a rise in dominance.

The possibility that some types of affective disorder may still be biologically advantageous was raised by a report of superior educational and occupational attainments among bipolar patients (Woodruff *et al.*, 1971). This study was carried out on white males admitted to a private hospital. The findings were not confirmed by a similar investigation on a public hospital sample which included negroes (Monnelly *et al.*, 1974).

Childhood environment

A number of studies have been carried out on the qualitative (e.g. rearing habits, parental attitudes) and quantitative (e.g. birth order, parental absence) aspects of the childhood of manic depressives. Cohen *et al.* (1954) described the mothers as being over-preoccupied with improving the family's social status, and as selecting the patient-to-be as the child most likely to achieve this. The fathers tended to be weak, dependent and self-deprecating, but lovable.

Granville-Grossman (1968) discussed the methodological issues involved in investigations of early parental loss, broken homes, parental age at birth, and birth order and concluded that there was no consistent evidence linking any of these factors to the development of affective illness. Subsequent studies, however, suggest that there may be a relationship between the early environment and depression. Hill (1969) found that females losing their fathers between the ages of 10 and 14 years were at greater risk of becoming depressed and committing suicide in later life. Munro and Griffiths (1969), however, reported that their sample of in-patient depressives showed an excess of maternal losses before the age of 15 years. It was suggested that early parental loss had its main effect on personality development and did not bear any relationship to specific mental illnesses. Birtchnell (1970a) found no differences between depressed and non-depressed psychiatric patients as to early parental loss, but the severely as opposed to the moderately depressed had a significant excess of maternal deaths during the first 20 years of life. Brown *et al.* (1975) found the loss of the mother by death or separation before the age of 11 as predisposing women toward depression. Brodie and Leff (1971) found no differences in number of siblings and birth order between unipolar and bipolar depressives. However, the latter showed more childhood parental losses. In contrast, Mayo (1970) found early parental losses to be evenly distributed between unipolars and bipolars. Brown *et al.* (1977) have claimed that the death of a parent predisposes toward a psychotic depression, whereas other causes of parental absence are more likely to be followed by neurotic depression.

To conclude, it now appears that there is a relationship between prolonged absence of a parent during early life and the subsequent development of a depressive illness. However, the nature of this relationship and whether it is confined to certain types of depressive illness remains obscure.

The depressive personality

Premorbid personality patterns may influence not only the symptomatology of manic depressive illness, but also its occurrence. Most of the studies of the personalities of those who become depressed have been superficial and impressionist and have suffered through being conducted during, rather than between, illnesses (Chodoff, 1972). Nevertheless, it appears that in general manic depressives tend to have cyclothymic temperaments or else fall into the normal range.

Kendell and Discipio (1970) using the Leyton inventory found that depressives had more obsessional personality traits than did normal controls. In an earlier study the same authors (Kendell and Discipio, 1968) showed that after recovery neurotic depressives were more neurotic and introverted than were normals and recovered psychotic depressives. Perris (1971) has claimed that bipolar depressives are less neurotic than unipolars.

Sociological viewpoints

At one extreme one can regard depression as a genetically determined disturbance of central neurotransmission which can produce symptoms at any time irrespective of the patient's circumstances. At the other, depression can be viewed as a reaction to an intolerable situation in which there is little prospect of support or guidance, and from which there seems no escape. Brown *et al.* (1975) have recently produced data to support the latter viewpoint. They found an excess of depression amongst working class women living in an inner London borough. They found also an excess of severely threatening events or major difficulties prior to the onset of the depression. The heightened reactions to such stresses amongst the working class women appeared to be related to a lack of support from their husbands, the loss of a mother before the age of 11, three or more children under the age of 15 living at home, and being unemployed.

Studies of life events prior to the onset of depression suffer from a number of potential drawbacks. Firstly, recollection may be affected by the illness. Lloyd and Lishman (1975) have demonstrated that depressives recall unpleasant memories more readily than pleasant ones. The attitude toward life events may also differ between depressives and normals, the former viewing them as more stressful (Schless *et al.*, 1974). Thirdly, the event may have been an early consequence of the illness (Cassidy *et al.*, 1957). Finally, problems may arise over the corroboration of the histories obtained and the selection of adequate control groups (Alarcon and Covi, 1972).

In a methodologically sound study carried out on an American population Paykel *et al.* (1969) found that depressed patients experienced more life events than did the general population, during the six months prior to their illness. Furthermore, these life events tended to be regarded as undesirable and involved losses or exits from the social field. Brodie and Leff (1971) found some degree of environmental stress preceded the first admissions of over 80% of their unipolar and bipolar patients. On subsequent admission, however, the rate for bipolar subjects fell to 54%. They discussed this finding in relation to the view that the first bipolar episode may be environmentally precipitated, but later episodes occur randomly.

Behavioural hypotheses

Depressive behaviour can be interpreted in terms of both classical and operant conditioning. Wolpe (1971) concentrated on the former in describing three types of reactive depression. The first, an exaggerated reaction to loss, can be regarded as having been conditioned by repeated losses in the past. Secondly, depression may arise in association with marked anxiety. In such cases desensitization to the cause of the latter may relieve the former. Finally, depression may result from a failure to control interpersonal relationships. Operant learning theory views depressive behaviour as a response to a sudden change in the pattern of social reinforcement of adaptive behaviour. Once precipitated, depression is maintained by attention and sympathy from others (Liberman and Raskin, 1971). Seligman (1972), however, has pointed out that the traditional approach of studying animals and men faced with rewards and punishments they can control does not apply to real life, where uncontrollable situations have to be faced. He has described a syndrome of 'learned helplessness' brought about by exposing animals to repeated uncontrollable trauma. This state bears a number of resemblances to depressive illness as seen in humans. In particular there is a reduction in voluntary activity, a difficulty in learning that their responses can be effective, lowered aggression, and losses of appetite, weight, libido and sociability.

Interactional hypotheses

In contrast to Liberman and Raskin (1971), Coyne (1976) regards depression as being maintained by the failure to evoke support and sympathy from others. Depression is viewed as a reaction to disruption of the social space in which the patient received support and validation of his experiences. The depressive repeatedly uses his symptoms to test the nature and security of his relationships. Unfortunately such constant questioning irritates those around. The patient therefore becomes further convinced of his rejection, displays more symptoms in order to maintain his increasingly uncertain sense of security, and thereby generates more hostility and rejection.

Psychoanalytic hypotheses

In his paper 'Mourning and Melancholia' Freud (1957) drew attention to the resemblances between grief and depression adding, however, that in the latter the loss may be symbolic rather than real, and that self-reproach and suicidal ideas are seen only in depression. He suggested that following a loss, the melancholic patient regresses to an emotional stage in which lost objects are dealt with by incorporation into the self, and in which sadistic feelings are more powerful than love. The incorporated object (and with it the self) is thus bitterly attacked. He later suggested the lost object is given up as being unworthy of love, incorporated into the ego by means of indentification, and then condemned by the superego. The view that internalized aggression is of relevance in the genesis of depression is supported by findings that depressive illness is less common in wartime, and that the rates of homicide and suicide tend to vary inversely (Kendell, 1973).

A number of authors have reformulated the classical concept of depression as arising from dammed up hostility. According to Bibring (1953) depression arises out of the helplessness felt by the ego on becoming aware of its inability to attain its ideals. Aggression is an inconstant and secondary response to those deemed responsible for causing or perpetuating the ego's helplessness and loss of esteem.

Freud regarded mania as occurring when the super ego relaxed its strictures and acted in harmony with the ego. Other psychodynamic views of mania include the concepts of the 'manic defence' and the 'flight into mania' as defences against, or reactions to, intolerable unhappiness and self-blame.

Cognitive hypotheses

Most clinicians regard the negativistic attitudes, beliefs and expectations of depressed patients as being secondary to their disturbed affect. However, it has been suggested that the affective change, whether neurotic or psychotic, arises out of a disturbance of cognition. Beck (1967) has delineated a 'depressive cognitive triad' consisting of negative evaluations of the environment, the self and the future. These views are acquired as the result of experience and lie dormant until mobilized following stress. Once the feelings of depression they engender become established further misconceptions are likely and the condition becomes self-perpetuating until interrupted by treatment.

Neurological hypotheses

The physiological symptoms of depressive illness resemble those seen following midbrain lesions. Kraines (1957) suggested manic depressive illness arises in the diencephalic-rhinencephalic-reticular system and that psychological features such as guilt and anxiety result from secondary involvement of the cerebral cortex. A more recent hypothesis implicates the limbic system—thought to contain the neuronal circuits whereby experiences are evaluated, stored and give rise to the appropriate affect. The amygdala appear to be concerned with the emotional aspects of this process, the hippocampi with the actual laying down of memories. Smythies (1970) has suggested that following a major disturbance of affect, changes occur at these sites so that the normal process whereby

412   S. Bhanji

experience and ideation give rise to affect is reversed. As a result false recollections and perceptions are generated to account for the emotion experienced. Both these views describe the pathways through which symptoms may be mediated, rather than the actual cause of manic depressive illness.

Reward/punishment systems

Animal self-stimulation experiments have demonstrated the existence of areas of the brain which appear to subserve sensations of pleasurable satisfaction or painful discontent. Wise *et al.* (1973) describe a reward/punishment system arising in the lower brain stem and ascending to the hypothalamus and limbic areas. Behaviour is potentiated by the noradrenergic components and suppressed by the serotonergic. They suggest that in depression a reduction in brain noradrenaline activity permits the serotonin system to predominate. An alternative view is that expressed by Crow (1973) who postulates the existence of two reward systems. One concerns reinforcement, but not changes in drive, and arises from cell bodies in the locus coeruleus which release noradrenaline from terminals distributed to the cortex. The second is concerned with incentive, motivation and changes in drive and motor responses. The cells are situated in the central mesencephalon and release dopamine from their endings in the corpus striatum and related nuclei. It is suggested that deficiency of central noradrenaline, such as may occur in depression, leads to a failure of the reinforcement system. In view of the difficulties inherent in extrapolating from animal neurophysiology to human psychopathology, both these hypotheses must be treated with caution. Nevertheless, they represent commendable attempts to integrate psychological, neurological and biochemical ideas regarding the causation and nature of the affective disorders.

Biochemical hypotheses

Biochemical investigations of affective illnesses have been concerned largely with water and electrolyte distribution, endocrine activity, and brain neurotransmitters. There have been several reports of intracellular sodium being increased in depression, and further increased in mania (Coppen, 1967). However, the significance of this and the role of other electrolytes such as calcium and magnesium await clarification. It has recently been proposed that some depressed patients have abnormal cell membrane electrolyte transport systems, and that these abnormalities may be genetically determined (Mendels and Frazer, 1974a). On the whole endocrinological studies have proved disappointing. A notable exception, however, is the finding of abnormal control of hydrocortisone secretion in some patients (Ettigi and Brown, 1977).

The most widely recognized hypothesis derives from the observations that reserpine causes brain monoamine depletion in animals and depression in man, and that drugs which increase the availability of monoamine neurotransmitters have antidepressant activity. The monoamine hypothesis postulates that depression is due to a deficiency of monoamine neurotransmitters at certain strategic sites in the brain, and the mania results from an excess. The monoamines most studied are the catecholeamines noradrenaline and dopamine, and the indoleamine serotonin.

Post mortem studies following suicide are bedevilled by methodological problems, but nevertheless appear to support the view that depression is associated with abnormal brain serotonin turnover. In the living the monoamine hypothesis can be investigated only by indirect means such as monitoring the levels of metabolites in the CSF and urine. The major metabolites of brain serotonin, noradrenaline, and dopamine are thought to be 5-hydroxyindoleacetic acid (5HIAA), 3-methoxy-4-hydroxy-phenylethyleneglycol (MHPG), and homovanillic acid (HVA) respectively (see Figs 3 and 4). Unfortunately, the site of origin of these metabolites is not known for certain. It has been suggested, for example, that 5HIAA in the lumbar CSF originates not in the brain but in the spinal cord, and that the urinary metabolites of noradrenaline reflect peripheral autonomic turnover. Furthermore, any changes observed may reflect transport from the CSF rather than metabolism, but this problem may be overcome by administering probenecid to block the active transport mechanism. Finally, diet, exercise and even simulating mania can affect the values obtained. In general, studies of CSF and urinary metabolites suggest that serotonin turnover is diminished in some cases of depression and may remain low in mania and on recovery. Noradrenaline turnover appears to be decreased in depression and increased immediately prior to and during mania. Finally, dopamine turnover is reduced in retarded depression.

A second indirect method of testing the monoamine hypothesis is to administer the appropriate antagonist or precursor. Reports of antimanic effects of the serotonin antagonist methysergide have not been confirmed in further studies (Coppen, 1972). Nor has the effectiveness of its precursor, tryptophan, in depression. L-dopa, a precursor of dopamine and noradrenaline, has been described as precipitating mania, but on the whole appears to be devoid of antidepressant effect (Mendels *et al.*, 1975).

The monoamine hypothesis has been further investigated by administering reserpine, the tyrosine hydroxylase inhibitor alpha-methylparatyrosine (see Fig. 3), and the tryptophan hydroxylase inhibitor parachlorophenylalanine (see Fig. 4). Mendels and Frazer (1974b) have

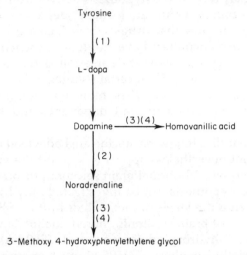

Fig. 3 The synthesis and metabolism of dopamine and noradrenaline. Enzymes mentioned: (1) tyrosine hydroxylase, (2) dopamine beta-hydroxylase, (3) monoamine oxidase, (4) catechol-ortho-methyl transferase.

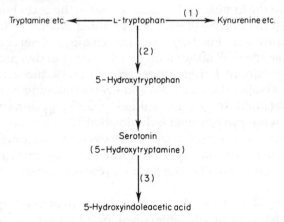

Fig. 4 The metabolism of L-tryptophan. Enzymes mentioned: (1) tryptophan pyrrolase, (2) tryptophan hydroxylase, (3) monoamine oxidase.

recently concluded that these compounds rarely, if ever, produce a true depressive syndrome in humans.

It seems likely that serum dopamine beta-hydroxylase activity in manics and depressives differs little, if at all, from that of normal subjects.

Meltzer *et al.* (1976), who divided their depressed patients according both to polarity and the presence of psychotic symptoms, found that only the psychotically depressed unipolars had activity levels significantly lower than in healthy subjects. Sack and Goodwin (1974) administered fusaric acid, which blocks dopamine beta-hydroxylase, to manic patients. The severely ill became worse: milder cases were unchanged or only slightly improved.

The enzyme trytophan pyrrolase (see Fig. 4) is of particular interest as claims have been made that its induction by steriod oral contraceptive agents may be responsible for the depression allegedly associated with the administration of such compounds. The possibility that endogenous depression is due to the metabolism of tryptophan being diverted away from the serotonin pathway was not supported by Frazer *et al.* (1973).

As can be seen from Figs 3 and 4, the monoamine neurotransmitters are degraded by monoamine oxidase (MAO) and Catechol-O-Methyl-Transferase (COMT). Sandler *et al.* (1975) have produced evidence consistent with increased MAO activity in depressive illness. Unfortunately no clinical details were given other than that their patients were selected on the basis of suitability for MAO inhibitor therapy. Nies *et al.* (1971) measured plasma and platelet MAO activity in normal subjects and hindbrain activity in autopsied patients. Monoamine oxidase activity was shown to increase with age and to be higher in females. This is in keeping with the age and sex incidence of psychotic depressive illness. Studies on red cell COMT activity have yielded conflicting results (Gershon and Jonas, 1975; Dunner *et al.*, 1971; White *et al.*, 1976).

As the evidence so far neither conclusively supports nor refutes the monoamine hypothesis a number of modifications have been proposed. One is that reduced serotonin activity is a constant feature of those prone to affective disorder. Illness occurs when a disturbance in catecholeamine activity supervenes (Prange *et al.*, 1974; Mendels and Frazer, 1975). A second possibility is that the affective psychoses are biochemically heterogeneous. Thus van Praag (1974) and Asberg *et al.* (1976) have divided psychotic depressives into those with reduced serotonin turnover and those without. Maas (1975) postulates the existence of two types of depression—type A in which there is a disturbance in noradrenaline metabolism or disposition, and type B in which serotonin is affected. A further view is that the disturbance lies not in the neurotransmitter availability but in receptor sensitivity (Prange *et al.*, 1972). The Medical Research Council (1972) have suggested that both factors are important and that more than one amine system may be implicated. Finally, it is possible that the biochemical changes are secondary to depressive symptomatology. Against this view is van Praag's finding that his biochemically distinct types of depression could not be differentiated clinically.

However, reduced dopamine turnover may be secondary to motor retardation (van Praag et al., 1975).

In his recent discussion of the monoamine hypothesis Baldessarini (1975) has stated that it does not take into account what is now known about the physiology of neurotransmitters and takes an over-simplified view of synaptic regulation. He concludes by stating that the monoamine hypothesis has stimulated much research, but has not led to a coherent biological view of abnormal behaviour, to an objective basis for differential diagnosis, or to the development of treatments more effective and safe than those obtained by empiricism and serendipity. Whilst not all would agree with these opinions, they do at least emphasize the inconsistent nature of the data and the need to revise the monoamine hypothesis as originally postulated.

The role of acetylcholine has been surprisingly little studied in view of reserpine's cholinomimetic effect, the anticholinergic actions of many antidepressants, and reports that physostigmine can relieve mania. One view is that affective disorder may result from an imbalance between central adrenergic (or serotonergic) and cholinergic receptors (Janowsky et al., 1972).

Cyclic adenosine monophosphate mediates the effects of a number of hormones and neurotransmitters. There have been several studies which demonstrate that urinary excretion of this substance is increased in mania and decreased in depression (e.g. Abdulla and Hamadah, 1970). The significance of these findings awaits clarification.

Enkephalin

A new development of possible promise is the identification of the polypeptide enkephalin as an endogenous morphine-like substance. Byck (1976) has postulated that enkephalin acts as the neurotransmitter subserving feelings of pleasure or indifference to aversive stimuli. A state of euphoria arises when there is increased binding of enkephalin to its receptor sites; dysphoria occurs with reduced binding.

Physical causes

Mood disturbances frequently accompany menstruation, parturition, physical illness and drug treatment, but in some instances exceed the normal reactions to discomfort and inconvenience or the successful outcome of treatment. The syndrome of premenstrual tension (Tonks, 1975) usually contains irritability, depression and anxiety, and has been described as the commonest form of endogenous depression. It is often assumed that hormonal changes preceding menstruation are responsible, but this has yet to be clearly established. Post-partum emotional disturbances (Pitt, 1975) range from tearfulness, dejection, anxiety, and minor cognitive impairment occurring transiently in about half of newly delivered women to severe affective psychosis following approximately one in every 500 deliveries. The prognosis of the post-partum affective psychosis is good, though the risk of recurrence following further pregnancies is about one in five. In view of their heterogeneous nature it is not surprising that there is more than one school of thought concerning the nature of puerperal affective illness. The first holds that the disorder is no different from nonpuerperal illness. The second regards pregnancy as being of prime aetiological significance and the psychosis as related to hormonal changes. Finally, post-partum illness has been explained in terms of conflict over pregnancy and motherhood.

Neurological disorders associated with mood changes resembling those encountered in the affective disorders include intracranial tumours, disseminated sclerosis, general paresis, subacute encephalitis, cerebral systemic lupus erythematosus, and Parkinsonism. Sufferers from the last condition are particularly prone to depression, though there is controversy over the reasons for this association. Mindham *et al.* (1976) found a high proportion of their patients become depressed during L-dopa therapy. The degree of depression was proportional to the degree of physical disability. Robins (1976), in contrast, found that his sample of Parkinsonian patients were significantly more depressed than age and sex matched chronically disabled controls with greater degrees of physical handicap. The complexity of the relationship between central nervous system illness and affect is further illustrated by multiple sclerosis. Surridge (1969) has suggested that depression seen in this condition is best regarded as a reaction to the illness, whereas the euphoria is a direct result of damage to the nervous system.

The endocrine disorders, Cushing's syndrome and Addison's disease, may each be associated with undue depression or elation. Persistent feelings of depression may figure prominently in the symptomatology of hyperparathyroidism and myxoedema.

The apathy and malaise of the anaemic may resemble that observed in depression, however the significance of low B12 and folate levels in some depressed patients awaits further exploration.

The occurrence of affective illness, usually depression, following viral infections is well recognized. It is usually assumed the illness acts as a non-specific stress. However, the suggestion has been made that the affective disorder results from a subclinical encephalitis. As regards surgical conditions, it appears thet hysterectomy is more often followed by depression than are other operations (Richards, 1974). Finally, it has been suggested (Kerr *et al.*, 1969), but not confirmed (Evans *et al.*, 1974), that depressive illness arising for the first time in middle-aged men may be the first manifestation of a malignancy.

The hypotensive drugs reserpine and alpha-methyl dopa have been claimed by some to produce depressive syndromes indistinguishable from psychotic depression. Adrenocorticotrophic hormone (ACTH) and steroid preparations may result in both depression or elation. The current consensus regarding oral contraceptives is that emotional side-effects are less common than first thought. Controversy still exists as to whether such effects are pharmacologically or psychologically mediated. Other drugs thought to occasionally give rise to a depressed affect include the phenothiazine tranquillizers. However, the impression that this applied to depot injections of fluphenazine (de Alarcon and Carney, 1969) was not supported by a larger study (Hirsch *et al.*, 1971). Finally, depression may follow sudden withdrawal of amphetamine-like compounds whether used hedonistically or as appetite suppressants.

Multifactorial approaches

A possible explanation for the diverse nature of the above theories is that the affective disorders are aetiologically heterogeneous conditions. it seems increasingly unlikely that for a given patient any single cause can be held responsible. The symptoms of affective illness appear to represent the final common pathway through which a number of factors exert their effect. Such factors include genetic predisposition, childhood experiences, environmental stress and internal change whether natural (e.g. the menopause) or pathological (e.g. glandular fever). Their effects may be modified by other variables such as social class and personality. The multifactorial approach to depression has been discussed by Blumenthal (1971) who argues that heterogeneity in symptomatology, heterogeniety in treatment response, and heterogeniety in aetiology are not necessarily related.

Treatment

The most important general decision in the management of affective disorder is whether to admit into hospital. Important clinical considerations in depressed patients are the risk of suicide (and rarely homicide or infanticide), the degree of self-neglect and the onset of stupor. Manics

require admission when their behaviour becomes intolerable or dangerous, or when they place their physical well-being in jeopardy through
lack of nutrition and sleep.

Psychosocial measures

In view of reports of impaired social functioning in depression (Weissman
et al., 1971) and the suggestion that adverse social circumstances can
cause, and not merely precipitate or perpetuate, depressive illness, it is
hardly surprising that *social manipulation* has been employed in the management of this condition. Such manoeuvres range from mundane matters such as writing letters recommending rehousing, to a restructuring
of intra-family relationships. A recent study, carried out on recovered
depressives receiving maintenance amitriptyline, placebo, or no drugs,
together with weekly psychotheapy or briefer monthly interviews, suggests that *psychotherapy* has little effect on depressive symptomatology
but is associated with improved social adjustment (Paykel *et al.*, 1975).
Behavioural approaches include desensitization to reduce anxiety, graded
systematic positive reinforcement to overcome feelings of inadequacy
and unworthiness, and assertive training (Wright and McDonald, 1974).

Physical measures

Chemotherapy

(a) *Antidepressant drugs*
Most depressives seen in hospital or clinic practice require a specific
antidepressant. The antidepressant drugs are thought to act by increasing
the availability of monoamine neurotransmitters at central receptor sites.

(i) *Tricyclics* are thought to act by blocking the neuronal re-uptake of
serotonin and noradrenaline. They also possess potent anticholinergic
properties, but these do not appear to be related to therapeutic efficacy.
Like the monoamine oxidase inhibitors (see below) they may take up to
two or three weeks to exert any therapeutic effect. During this time
side-effects tend to be at their height. Which drug is selected will depend
on a number of factors. For example, protriptyline has been claimed to
have the most rapid onset of action, dothiepin few side-effects, amitriptyline marked tranquillizing properties, and clorimipramine to be of
benefit in obsessional cases.

Approximately 30% of psychotic depressives fail to respond to a
tricyclic antidepressant. This finding cannot be entirely explained on the

basis of differences in sex, age and clinical symptomatology. One view is that such variations in drug response are due to genetically determined differences in drug pharmacokinetics. Unfortunately, studies on the relationship between plasma drug steady-state levels and clinical outcome have yielded conflicting results. Braithwaite *et al.* (1972) found a highly significant correlation between clinical outcome and plasma concentrations of amitriptyline and its active metabolite nortriptyline. In contrast, Burrows *et al.* (1972) detected no relationship between plasma nortriptyline levels and the therapeutic outcome. Asberg *et al.* (1971) reported that both low (below 50 ng/ml) and high levels (above 140 ng/ml) of nortriptyline were associated with a poor clinical response. However, the patients were studied for only two weeks, barely long enough for plasma steady-state levels to be reached, or for therapeutic response to be fully developed. Nevertheless, an upper therapeutic limit of plasma nortriptyline concentrations has been demonstrated in a better study (Kragh-Sorensen *et al.*, 1973). There have been fewer studies of imipramine levels, but it appears that low plasma concentrations are associated with poor outcome.

Methodological differences may account for the discrepant findings in studies of amitriptyline and nortriptyline levels; a further possibility is that differences in plasma drug-binding capacity were not taken into account (Glassman *et al.*, 1973).

(ii) *Monoamine oxidase inhibitors* act by retarding the intraneuronal breakdown of monoamines. They fall into two groups—the hydrazine derivatives (e.g. isocarboxid, phenelzine) and those related to amphetamine (e.g. tranylcypromine). The monoamine oxidase inhibitors (MAOIs) are used mainly in the treatment of neurotic depressive illness and can also be effective in phobic anxiety states. However, Tyrer (1976) has expressed the view that diagnosis is an unsatisfactory means of selection for MAOI therapy. Instead he advocates a target symptom approach. Primary symptoms most likely to respond are hypochondriasis, agoraphobia, social phobia, irritability, somatic anxiety and anergia. Primary depression, guilt, ideas of reference and personality disorders seldom respond.

Administration of the MAOIs is attended by two major hazards. The first is the risk of liver damage by hydrazine derivatives; the second derives from the interaction with drugs and foodstuffs which release or contain monoamines. In particular sympathomimetic amines, central depressants, some antihypertensives, tricyclic antidepressants and foods (such as matured cheese, yeast extracts, broad bean pods, banana skins and pickled herrings) containing dopamine or tyramine should be avoided during and for two weeks after treatment.

Three recent developments of theoretical and practical import concern the relationships between response to MAOI treatment and REM sleep suppression, acetylator status, and the degree of MAO inhibition. Akindele *et al.* (1970) demonstrated that the antidepressant affect of phenelzine coincided with the onset of pronounced REM suppression. This effect was dose related and appeared after a few days. Johnstone and Marsh (1973) compared the progress of slow and fast acetylators receiving phenelzine and placebo for neurotic depression. The slow acetylators responded to the active drug better than to placebo, whereas no drug–placebo difference was observed among the fast acetylators. Nies *et al.* (1974) reported that the chances of a favourable response to MAOIs were considerably greater if 80% inhibition of platelet MAO could be achieved. Where this did not occur, the response to phenelzine was no better than that to placebo.

(iii) *Monoamine precursors* such as *l*-tryptophan, whilst possessing some antidepressant activity, appear to be less effective than was first thought (Herrington *et al.*, 1974).

(b) *Lithium*

Lithium is now accepted as an effective anti-manic agent and is widely used in the prophylaxis of manic depressive illness (see below). Mendels (1976) has reviewed studies of the antidepressant effects of lithium used either alone, or in combination with ECT, tricyclics, or MAOIs. He concludes that there is convincing evidence to support the use of lithium as an antidepressant. Bipolar depression tends to respond better than unipolar and there is some evidence that a high red cell to plasma lithium ratio correlates with a favourable prognosis.

Electroconvulsive therapy

The Medical Research Council (1965) trial of antidepressant treatments demonstrated that 84% of those patients receiving ECT showed an improvement after four weeks. This compared favourably with the improvement rates achieved with imipramine (72%), phenelzine (38%) and placebo (45%). In general, male patients responded better than females to medication, but less well to ECT. Studies carried out on the predictive value of depressive symptomatology suggest that ECT is more effective in psychotic than in neurotic depression (Mendels, 1965). Of those patients who relapse following a course of ECT nearly all do so within three weeks. The use of ECT in mania has largely been superseded by the major tranquillizers and lithium.

The major side-effect of ECT is amnesia, which may persist for several weeks following treatment. Now that ECT is administered following general anaesthesia and muscle relaxants other ill-effects are rare, the death rate (usually due to cardiac arrest) being in the order of one per 25,000 treatments. Conditions in which ECT should be given with caution or witheld include severe myocardial or respiratory disease, marked osteoporosis or a major fracture, a recent cerebrovascular accident and peptic ulceration (see Chapter 20).

Flurothyl inhalation (under general anaesthesia and muscle relaxation) has been proposed, but not widely accepted, as an alternative method of inducing seizure activity. Post-seizure amnesia and confusion is reported as less than following ECT (Small *et al.*, 1968).

Other physical treatments

There is some evidence that *phenothiazine* compounds may possess anti-depressant effects. Overall *et al.* (1965) found thioridazine was more effective than imipramine in the treatment of anxious-tense depressives. Raskin and Crook (1976) reported that chlorpromazine could be helpful in the treatment of the older, more severely depressed patients with ideas of hopelessness and unworthiness. Young *et al.* (1976) have suggested that the thioxanthene derivative *flupenthixol* (1·5–4·5 mg/day) has an anti-depressant effect comparable to that of amitriptyline.

The observation that imipramine toxicity was more marked in thyro-toxics prompted investigations into the value of *triodothyronine, thyroid stimulating hormone* and *thyrotropin releasing factor (TRF)* as potentiators of the drug's antidepressant effects. This led to claims that TRF alone may alleviate depression. It appears, however, that its action is too transient and inconsistent to be of any value (van den Burg *et al.*, 1975).

Sleep deprivation therapy has been employed following the observation that some depressed patients improve following the loss of a night's sleep. Whilst it appears to be more effective for psychotic than neurotic or secondary depression, the value of sleep deprivation therapy has yet to be established under controlled conditions free of observer bias (Bhanji and Roy, 1975).

The management of resistant depression

Approximately 5–10% of psychotic depressives neither respond to stan-dard forms of treatment nor recover spontaneously. The first step in the management of such cases is a psychiatric, social and physical reappraisal, as it has been shown that a number of resistant psychotic depressives turn out to be misdiagnosed neurotic depressives, personal-ity disorders, or physical conditions. If the diagnosis is confirmed one is left with two simple choices—existing treatment can be enhanced, or new approaches attempted. As regards the former, it has been claimed that the effectiveness of the tricyclic drugs can be increased by the concurrent administration of chlorpromazine, which slows down drug hydroxylation, *l*-triodothyronine, which enhances the sensitivity of the noradrenergic receptors, or a monoamine oxidase inhibitor. The last two combinations should be prescribed with caution. There is some evidence that a combination of *l*-tryptophan and a monoamine oxidase inhibitor is more effective than either substance taken alone (Coppen *et al.*, 1963). Walinder *et al.* (1975) reported that *l*-tryptophan potentiated the antidepressant effect of clorimipramine, but Shaw *et al.* (1975) did not find this to be the case.

An experimental finding relevant to changes in therapy is that tricyclic antidepressants exert a differential effect on monoamine uptake (Maas, 1975). If this is the case a logical step following, for example, failure of a drug such as desipramine, which blocks mainly noradrenaline uptake, would be to prescribe clorimipramine, which blocks serotonin uptake. Other approaches are to employ such procedures as continuous narcosis, electro-narcosis, behaviour therapy and sleep deprivation therapy. However, the effectiveness of those forms of treatment is not generally accepted. When all else has failed psychosurgery may have to be considered (Schurr, 1973).

Anti-manic drugs

(a) *Phenothiazine and butyrophenone tranquillizers* are thought to exert their anti-manic effect by blockading central adrenergic receptors. Both types of drug may cause troublesome extrapyramidal side-effects. Treatment should be continued for several weeks after the episode has subsided.

(b) *Lithium salts* have been shown to have anti-manic effects in a number of clinical trials. The largest compared the effects of chlorpromazine (mean daily dose 1000 mg) and lithium carbonate (mean daily dose 1800 mg). For 'highly active' patients chlorpromazine was more effective, acted more quickly and had fewer side-effects, but there was a suggestion that lithium was superior for the 'mildly active' (Prien *et al.*, 1972). Because its effects may not be noticeable for some days most clinicians combine lithium with a neuroleptic.

Clinical course and prophylaxis

There have been many short-term, but few long-term studies of manic depressive illness. Those conducted before the introduction of modern treatment methods confirmed that both mania and depression remit spontaneously in the majority of cases but subsequent recurrence is the rule.

Murphy *et al.* (1974) have emphasized the variability in the course taken by the primary affective disorders. Their five-year follow-up of 37 patients showed that six were ill throughout this period, nine had no recurrences, and the remainder experienced from one to nine subsequent episodes of two weeks to one year's duration. Winokur and Morrison (1973) were able to follow up 213 out of 225 depressives admitted to hospital between 1934 and 1944. The length of the follow-up period ranged from one month to 20 years (mean approximately four years). They showed that depressed males were more likely to become chronically ill. A further finding was that less than 5 % became manic. Sainsbury (1968) has estimated that 15% of psychotic depressives will eventually kill themselves.

A recent multicentre retrospective study of over 1000 patients (Angst *et al.*, 1973) has revealed some differences between the courses of unipolar and bipolar psychoses. The median age of onset of the former was 30 years, of the latter 43 years. The lengths of the first cycle in unipolars, bipolars and involutionals were 45, 33 and 27 months respectively. Short cycles were more frequent amongst bipolar patients, long amongst the involutional cases. Less than 1% of the unipolar depressives experienced only one illness episode. The patients classified as bipolar included 5% with only a single attack of mania. Most of the episodes were of under three months duration and tended to be the same length for a given patient. As time progressed, however, the interval between episodes shortened. An interesting finding was that the median number of episodes per patient reached a limit (7–9 for bipolars, 4–6 for unipolars) i.e. recurrences appeared to be confined to the 20 years following the first episode.

Two recent developments have been the demonstration that continuation of antidepressant therapy beyond recovery reduces the probability of recurrence, and the acceptance of lithium salts as being of prophylactic value.

Mindham *et al.* (1973) conducted a double-blind trial on patients who had responded well to imipramine or amitriptyline and continued to receive smaller doses of the same drug or an identical placebo. During the six-month period of the trial there were significantly fewer relapses amongst those on active treatment (22% as opposed to 50%). Patients with residual symptoms derived more benefit from continuation therapy than those who had recovered completely. Paykel *et al.* (1975) assessed the effects of six forms of post-recovery care. Patients who had responded to amitriptyline received either regular psychotherapy or minimal contact, in addition to maintenance amitriptyline, an identical placebo, or no medication. Those on active medication fared best as regards depressive symptoms, whereas psychotherapy improved social adjustment.

Lithium prophylaxis is both safe and effective providing the plasma level is maintained between 0·6 and 1·5 mEq/l, and the drug is not given to patients with severe renal or cardiac disease. Abdominal pains, nausea, diarrhoea, tremor and thirst may occur early in treatment. Later on they may recur if the plasma level rises above the therapeutic range. More severe toxic effects include sleepiness which may proceed into coma. To ensure maximum effectiveness and safety the plasma levels should be monitored weekly during the early stages, and later at monthly intervals, if a relapse occurs, and when toxic effects are suspected. Minor toxicity can be relieved by stopping lithium and increasing sodium intake. Severe cases, however, may require haemodialysis. Long-term lithium may result in goitre and hypothyroidism, a nephrogenic diabetes insipidus, and excessive weight gain. An acute reversible dementia-like state has also been reported.

Quitkin *et al.* (1976) have recently discussed current opinion on lithium prophylaxis. They conclude that double-blind placebo controlled studies indicate that lithium can prevent episodes of mania, but its effect on depression is less clearly established. Prien *et al.* (1973) compared the prophylactic effects of lithium, imipramine and placebo. In bipolar patients lithium was significantly more effective than imipramine or placebo—the difference between the two active drugs being due largely to an excess of manic episodes in the imipramine-treated group. For unipolar depressives lithium and imipramine were equally effective, and both better than placebo. In contrast, Dunner *et al.* (1976b) found lithium to be significantly better than placebo in preventing recurrences of mania, but no more effective regarding depressive episodes. However, there was some indication that the depressive episodes were less severe in the lithium-treated patients.

Dunner and Fieve (1974) found that lithium failures contained a high proportion of rapid cyclers (more than four episodes per year) but did not differ from the successes in terms of age, sex, severity of manic episodes, or age of onset of illness. Dunner *et al.* (1976a) reported on 96 non-rapid cycling bipolars. The 44 who relapsed could not be distinguished in terms of sex, age, number of episodes in the previous two years, nature of previous episode, age of onset of first symptoms, age of first hospitalization, family history, and speed of onset of manic episodes. They did not confirm the view that lithium is more effective in patients with a history of mania in first degree relatives (Mendlewicz *et al.*, 1973) but employed a less accurate means of data collection. Finally, Prien and Caffey (1976) found that recurrent depressives were more likely to respond to lithium where the daily dose was above 1000 mg and plasma levels were maintained between 0·8 and 1·0 mEq/l.

The mechanism whereby lithium acts is not known. Possibilities in keeping with the biochemistry of affective illness are that it displaces intracellular sodium, reduces brain noradrenaline levels, and inhibits adenyl cyclase, the enzyme responsible for the formation of cyclic adenosine monophosphate.

Suicide

Topics of current interest to those concerned with the prediction and prevention of suicide include the nature of the act, the reliability of suicide statistics, and the differences between attempted and completed suicide.

Aetiological aspects

Theories as to causation of suicide range from those stressing external factors, such as the nature of society, to those which emphasize internal influences such as symptoms of illness. The classic sociological viewpoint is that of Emil Durkheim (1951) who suggested that suicide rates are low in societies which are well integrated and well regulated. *Egoistic* suicide occurs where there is lack of meaningful social interaction (poor integration). The *anomic* variety occurs when individual interests are not subordinated to those of society (poor regulation). Rarer forms are *altruistic* and *fatalistic* suicide. The former occurs as a self-sacrifice under conditions of excessive integration, the latter under excessive regulation as might occur in prison. Durkheim found that suicide rates were higher in older adults, males, Protestants as opposed to Catholics and Jews, the unmarried and divorced, the upper classes and the rich, soldiers as compared to civilians, and in the sane as opposed to the insane. As far as Western society is concerned Durkheim's views are still respected; however, they appear less applicable to cultures in which suicide is condoned, or even applauded, under certain circumstances. Most psychiatrists, while acknowledging social influences on suicide rates, regard mental illness as of equal, if not greater import. Thus Barraclough *et al*. (1975) were able to diagnose mental illness in 93 out of 100 cases of suicide. Of these 70 were depressed and 15 alcoholic. Murphy and Robins (1967) suggest that alcoholics kill themselves in response to a social disturbance, whereas depressives do so because of symptoms such as guilt and hopelessness. Arguments against a strictly medical view of suicide include the possibility that mental illness may itself be a reaction to society, and the likelihood that accidental deaths in persons known or thought to be depressed will be misclassified as suicide. An intermediate proposal is that of Henry and Short (1954) who see suicide as the result of interaction between external and internal restraint. The former derives both from the individual's position in the social hierarchy (vertical restraint) and from his relationships with others (horizontal restraint). Internal restraint determines the degree to which aggression is internalized when frustrated. Suicide occurs in a situation of high internal and low external restraint.

Epidemiology

The World Health Organization estimates that every day at least 1000 people will kill themselves. The actual rates vary considerably from country to country. For example the male suicide rate for Hungary during 1969 was 48·3 per 100,000 and the rate for females 18·9 per 100,000. Malta's male rate was 1·9 per 100,000 and negligible for females (WHO Working Group, 1974). Such differences may reflect real variations in suicide rates which, if their source could be traced, would throw much light on the causation and precipitation of suicidal behaviour. On the other hand, they may derive from international differences in the procedures for assessing, classifying and recording deaths not due to natural causes. Brooke and Atkinson (1974) have analysed the responses to questionnaires returned to the WHO by 24 countries. They conclude that there is a general lack of uniformity and go on to add that as long as suicide attracts a stigma people will find a verdict of accidental or undetermined death more acceptable. Their view that the differences in suicide rates are likely to be artifactual was supported by their data from 21 assessors (from eight countries) asked for their opinion on 40 possible suicides. Complete agreement as to cause of death was obtained in only seven of the cases. The number of suicide verdicts ranged from 16 by a Norwegian to 32 by a Dane and a Nigerian. The main source of variance seemed due to a choice between recording an open verdict and one of suicide.

In spite of misgivings as to the reliability of the available data a number of general conclusions are possible. The incidence of suicide appears to be lower in smell non-industrial communities and in rural areas. Rates are also lower in those who remain in their country of origin. Males are more likely to kill themselves than are females. Suicide rates are higher amongst the old and upper classes. Living alone and being unmarried are also associated with a greater likelihood of suicide. However, the view that a majority of suicides are committed by the mentally ill is by no means universally accepted. Nevertheless, the seasonal incidence of suicide closely parallels that of psychotic depression.

Method employed

The preferred method of suicide varies from country to country and in many cultures depends on the sex of the subject. In Europe drug over-dosage appears to be the commonest means of suicide; amongst those using other methods there is a male preference for the more violent means of suicide.

The precursors of suicide

There is some evidence that loss of a parent during childhood increases the risk of suicide in later life. Hill (1969) suggested that the loss of their fathers between the ages of 10 and 14 years predisposed girls toward suicidal depression later in life. Paffenbarger and Asnes (1966) examined the college records of 10,000 male former students and compared those of the 225 who had committed suicide with those of living classmates chosen at random. The suicide group were more likely to be the sons of college-trained parents who had separated. There was also an excess of paternal deaths. As students they had tended not to participate in extracurricular activities (but nevertheless failed to graduate) and had assessed themselves as prone to insomnia, worry, self-consciousness, feelings of persecution, a secretive-seclusive nature, and feelings of anxiety and depression.

More immediate precursors of suicide include the recent death of a parent (Birtchnell, 1970b), disruption of a social relationship (Murphy and Robins, 1967) and a previous suicide attempt (Kessel and McCulloch, 1966). A number of investigations have found a premenstrual excess of attempted and completed suicides.

A majority of suicides are preceded by some warning or intimation from the subject. Robins et al. (1959) interviewed relatives and close friends of the deceased and found that 69% had communicated their suicidal intentions—41% by a direct explicit statement usually to more than one person.

Suicide in psychotic depression

Approximately 15% of psychotic depressives will kill themselves. Sains-bury (1968) has listed the following factors as being associated with an increased risk of suicide; an age of over 40 years (particularly if the first episode); male sex; recent widowhood or divorce; a family history of suicide; a previous history of suicide attempts (psychotic depressives are less likely to repeat attempts, but more likely to succeed if they do); the onset and end of the illness; the presence of agitation, insomnia, guilt and feelings of inadequacy; the co-existence of alcoholism or psychopathic traits; and the menopause or the presence of physical illness.

Attempted suicide

For every person who kills himself at least 10 will attempt the act but survive. One of the major developments in the study of suicide has been the drawing of a distinction between suicide and attempted suicide (parasuicide). In the latter it is the act itself, rather than the ending of life, which is important. The differences between these phenomena are summarized in Table I.

Table I

	Attempted suicide	Suicide
Incidence	Rising	Declining
Sex	Female	Male
Age	Young	Late middle-age
Social class	Lower	Upper
Childhood	Broken home	Bereavement
Physical health	Good	May have terminal illness or be handicapped
Personality	'Antisocial'	Well-adjusted
Diagnosis	Situational reaction Personality disorder Psychotic depression (only 10%)	Psychotic depression (75%) Alcoholism
Precipitant	Acute personal crisis	Guilt, hopelessness Social stress in alcoholism Painful or disabling physical illness
Setting	Impulsive, though with forewarning and in presence of others	Carefully premeditated, most give warning. Act carried out when alone

Some 40% of those who attempt suicide have a previous history of such acts and approximately 20% will make further attempts within a year (one in 10 with fatal outcome) (Kessel and McCulloch, 1966). Suggested motives include the testing out of others' feelings, the arousal of guilt, and removal from the scene of conflict.

Suicidal thoughts

A number of attempts have been made to classify self-destructive behaviour. Most contain categories corresponding to completed and

attempted suicide—some also include suicidal thoughts. Paykel *et al.*
(1974) interviewed 720 subjects in a general population survey carried out
in Connecticut. Almost 9% reported feeling suicidal in the previous year.
These included 3·5% who felt life was no longer worthwhile, 2·8% who
wished themselves dead, 1·0% who had thought of ending their lives,
1·0% who had seriously contemplated suicide, and 0·6% who had actually
made an attempt.

Suicide prevention schemes

A number of suicide prevention agencies have come into operation in
recent years. Most provide a 24-hour telephone service manned by
trained volunteers. Their evaluation is difficult owing to problems in
obtaining adequate control groups to allow for regional variations in the
frequency of attempted suicide, the tendency for rates to increase, and
coincidental factors such as the change from coal gas to non-toxic natural
gas. Nevertheless most psychiatrists have welcomed their advent,
though some regard them more as crisis intervention services than as
preventers of attempted or completed suicide.

References

Abdulla, Y. H. and Hamadah, K. (1970). 3', 5' cyclic adenosine monophosphate in
  depression and mania. *Lancet* 1, 378–381.
Abrams, R. and Taylor, M. A. (1974). Unipolar mania: A preliminary report. *Arch.
  Gen. Psychiat.* 30, 441–443.
Abrams, R. and Taylor, M. A. (1976). Catatonia: A prospective clinical study.
  Arch. Gen. Psychiat. 33, 579–581.
Akindele, M. O., Evans, J. I. and Oswald, I. (1970). Mono-amine oxidase
  inhibitors, sleep and mood. *Electroenceph. Clin. Neurophysiol.* 29, 47–56.
Alarcon, R. D. and Covi, L. (1972). The precipitating event in depression: Some
  methodological considerations. *J. Nerv. Ment. Dis.* 155, 379–391.
Alexanderson, B., Price Evans, D. and Sjoqvist, F. (1969). Steady-state plasma
  levels of Nortriptyline in twins: Influence of genetic factors and drug therapy.
  Br. Med. J. 4, 764–768.
Angst, J., Baastrup, P., Grof, P., Hippius, H., Poldinger, W. and Weis, P. (1973).
  The course of monopolar depression and bipolar psychoses. *Psychiat. Neurol.
  Neurochir.* 76, 489–500.
Asberg, M., Cronholm, B., Sjoqvist, F. and Tuck, D. (1971). Relationship between
  plasma level and therapeutic effect of Nortriptyline. *Br. Med. J.* 3, 331–334.
Asberg, M., Thoren, P., Traskman, L., Bertilsson, L. and Ringberger, V. (1976).
  'Serotonin Depression'—A biochemical subgroup within the affective dis-
  orders? *Science* 191, 478–480.

Bagley, C. (1973). Occupational class and symptoms of depression. *Soc. Sci. Med.* **7**, 327–340.

Baldessarini, R. J. (1975). The basis for amine hypotheses in affective disorders: A critical evaluation. *Arch. Gen. Psychiat.* **32**, 1087–1093.

Barraclough, B., Bunch, J., Nelson, B. and Sainsbury, P. (1975). A hundred cases of suicide: Clinical aspects. *Br. J. Psychiat.* **123**, 355–373.

Beck, A. T. (1967). 'Depression: Clinical, Experimental, and Theoretical Aspects'. Harper and Row, New York.

Bhanji, S. and Roy, G. A. (1975). The treatment of psychotic depression by sleep deprivation: A replication study. *Br. J. Psychiat.* **127**, 222–226.

Bibring, E. (1953). The mechanism of depression. *In* 'Affective disorders' (Ed. P. Greenacre), pp. 13–48. International University Press, New York.

Biegel, A. and Murphy, D. L. (1971). Assessing clinical characteristics of the manic state. *Am. J. Psychiat.* **128**, 688–694.

Birtchnell, J. (1970a). Depression in relation to early and recent parent death. *Br. J. Psychiat.* **116**, 299–306.

Birtchnell, J. (1970b). The relationship between attempted suicide, depression and parent death. *Br. J. Psychiat.* **116**, 307–313.

Blinder, M. G. (1966). The pragmatic classification of depression. *Am. J. Psychiat.* **123**, 259–269.

Blumenthal, M. D. (1971). Heterogeneity and research on depressive disorders. *Arch. Gen. Psychiat.* **24**, 524–531.

Braithwaite, R. A., Goulding, R., Theano, G., Bailey, J. and Coppen, A. (1972). Plasma concentration of Amitriptyline and clinical response. *Lancet* **1**, 1297–1300.

Brodie, H. K. H. and Leff, M. J. (1971). Bipolar depression—a comparative study of patient characteristics. *Am. J. Psychiat.* **127**, 1086–1090.

Brooke, E. M. and Atkinson, M. (1974). *In* 'Suicide and Attempted Suicide' (Ed. E. M. Brooke), pp. 15–70. WHO, Geneva.

Brown, G. W., Bhrolchain, M. N. and Harris, T. (1975). Social class and psychiatric disturbance among women in an urban population. *Sociology* **9**, 225–254.

Brown, G. W., Harris, T. and Copeland, J. R. (1977). Depression and loss. *Br. J. Psychiat.* **130**, 1–18.

Burrows, G. D., Davies, B. and Scoggins, B. A. (1972). Plasma concentration of Nortriptyline and clinical response in depressive illness. *Lancet* **2**, 619–623.

Byck, R. (1976). Peptide transmitters: A unifying hypothesis for euphoria, respiration, sleep, and the action of lithium. *Lancet* **3**, 72–73.

Carlson, G. A. and Goodwin, F. K. (1973). The stages of mania: A longitudinal analysis of the manic episode. *Arch. Gen. Psychiat.* **28**, 221–228.

Cassidy, W. L., Flanagan, M. B., Spellman, M. and Cohen, M. E. (1957). Clinical observations in manic-depressive disease. A quantitative study of one hundred manic-depressive patients and fifty medically sick controls. *J. Am. Med. Ass.* **164**, 1535–1546.

Chodoff, P. (1972). The depressive personality: A critical review. *Arch. Gen. Psychiat.* **27**, 666–673.

Cohen, M. B., Baker, G., Cohen, R. A., Fromm-Reichmann, F. and Weigert, E. V. (1954). An intensive study of twelve cases of manic-depressive psychosis. *Psychiatry* **17**, 103–138.

Cooper, J. E., Kendell, R. E., Gurland, B. J., Sharpe, L., Copeland, J. R. M. and

Simon, R. (1972). 'Psychiatric Diagnosis in New York and London'. Oxford University Press, Oxford.

Coppen, A. (1967). The biochemistry of affective disorders. Br. J. Psychiat. 113, 1237–1264.

Coppen, A. (1972). Indoleamines and affective disorders. J. Psychiat. Res. 9, 163–171.

Coppen, A., Shaw, D. M. and Farrell, J. P. (1963). Potentiation of the antidepressive effect of a monoamine-oxidase inhibitor by Tryptohan. Lancet 1, 79–81.

Court, J. H. (1972). The continuum model as a resolution of paradoxes in manic-depressive psychosis. Br. J. Psychiat. 120, 133–141.

Coyne, J. C. (1976). Toward an interactional description of depression. Psychiatry 39, 28–40.

Crow, T. (1973). Catecholamine-containing neurones and electrical self-stimulation: 2.A theoretical interpretation and some psychiatric implications. Psychol. Med. 3, 66–73.

de Alarcon, R. and Carney, M. W. P. (1969). Severe depressive mood changes following slow-release intramuscular fluphenazine injection. Br. Med. J. 3, 564–567.

Dunner, D. L., Cohn, C. K., Gershon, E. S. and Goodwin, F. K. (1971). Differential catechol-o-methyl-transferase activity in unipolar and bipolar affective illness. Arch. Gen. Psychiat. 25, 348–353.

Dunner, D. L. and Fieve, R. R. (1974). Clinical factors in lithium carbonate prophylaxis failure. Arch. Gen. Psychiat. 30, 229–233.

Dunner, D. L., Fleiss, J. L. and Fieve, R. R. (1976a). Lithium carbonate prophylaxis failure. Br. J. Psychiat. 129, 40–44.

Dunner, D. L., Stallone, F. and Fieve, R. R. (1976b). Lithium carbonate and affective disorders: V. A double-blind study of prophylaxis of depression in bipolar illness. Arch. Gen. Psychiat. 33, 117–120.

Durkheim, E. (1951). 'Suicide'. Free Press, Glencoe, Illinois.

Essen-Moller, E. and Haguell, O. (1961). The frequency and risk of depression within a rural population group in Scandinavia. Acta. Psychiat. Scand., Suppl. 162, 28–32.

Ettigi, P. G. and Brown, G. M. (1977). Psychoneuroendocrinology of affective disorder: An overview. Am J. Psychiat. 134, 493–501.

Evans, bn. J. R., Baldwin, J. A. and Gath, D. (1974). The innidence of cancer among in-patients with affective disorders. Br. J. Psychiat. 124, 518–525.

Eysenck, H. J. (1970). The classification of depressive illness. Br. J. Psychiat. 117, 241–250.

Feighner, J. P., Robins, E., Guze, S. B., Woodruff, R. A., Winokur, G. and Munoz, R. (1972). Diagnostic criteria for use in psychiatric research. Arch. Gen. Psychiat. 26, 57–63.

Fleiss, J. L., Gurland, B. J. and Cooper, J. E. (1971). Some contributions to the measurement of psychopathology. Br. J. Psychiat. 119, 647–656.

Foulds, G. A. and Bedford, A. (1976). Classification of depressive illness. Psychol. Med. 6, 15–19.

Frazer, A., Pandey, G. N. and Mendels, J. (1973). Metabolism of tryptophan in depressive disease. Arch. Gen. Psychiat. 29, 528–535.

Freud, S. (1957). 'Mourning and Melancholia'. Hogarth Press. London.

Gershon, E. S. and Jonas, W. Z. (1975). Erythrocyte soluble catechol-o-methyl transferase activity in primary affective disorder: A clinical and genetic study. Arch. Gen. Psychiat. 32, 1351–1356.

Gittleson, N. L. (1966). Depressive psychosis in the obsessional neurotic. *Br. J. Psychiat.* **112**, 883–887.

Glassman, A. H., Hurwic, M. J. and Perel J. M. (1973). Plasma binding of imipramine and clinical outcome. *Am. J. Psychiat.* **130**, 1367–1369.

Granville-Grossman, K. L. (1968). The early environment in affective disorder. *In* 'Recent Developments in Affectime Disorders' (Eds A. Coppen and A. Walk), pp. 65–79. Headley Bros, Ashford, Kent.

Hare, E., Price, J. S. and Slater, E. (1972). Parental social class in psychiatric patients. *Br. J. Psychiat.* **121**, 515–524.

Hashmi, F. (1970). Immigrants and emotional stress. *Proc. Roy. Soc. Med.* **63**, 631–632.

Hemsi, L. K. (1967). Psychiatric morbidity of West Indians. *Social Psychiat.* **3**, 133–135.

Henry, A. F. and Short, J. F. (1954). 'Suicide and Homicide'. MacMillan, The Free Press of Glencoe, New York.

Herrington, R. N., Bruce, A., Johnstone, E. C. and Lader, M. H. (1974). Comparative trial of L-Trytophan and E.C.T. in severe depressive illness. *Lancet* **2**, 731–734.

Hill, O. W. (1969). The association of childhood bereavement with suicidal attempt in depressive illness. *Br. J. Psychiat.* **115**, 301–304.

Hirsch, S. R., Gaind, R., Rohde, P. D., Stevens, B. C. and Wing, J. K. (1973). Out-patient maintenance of chronic schizophrenic patients with long-acting fluphenazine. *Br. Med. J.* **1**, 633–637.

Janowsky, D. S., el Gousef, M. K., Dais, J. M. and Sekerke, M. J. (1972). A cholinergic-adrenergic hypothesis of mania and depression. *Lancet* **2**, 632–635.

Johnstone, E. C. and Marsh, W. (1973). The relationship between response to phenelzine and acetylator status in depressed patients. *Proc. Roy. Soc. Med.* **66**, 947–949.

Kelly, D. (1973). The inter-relationship of depression and anxiety. *In* 'Aspects of Depression' (Eds M. Lader and R. Garcia), pp. 13–20. World Psychiatric Association, Madrid.

Kendell, R. E. (1968). The problem of classification. *In* 'Recent Advances in Affective Disorders' (Eds A. Coppen and A. Walk), pp. 15–26. Headley Bros, Ashford, Kent.

Kendell, R. E. (1973). The relationship between aggression and depression. *In* 'Aspects of Depression' (Eds M. Lader and R. Garcia), pp. 39–49. World Psychiatric Association, Madrid.

Kendell, R. E. (1976). The classification of depressions: A review of contemporary confusion. *Br. J. Psychiat.* **129**, 15–28.

Kendell, R. E. and Discipio, W. J. (1968). Eysenck personality inventory scores of patients with depressive illnesses. *Br. J. Psychiat.* **114**, 767–770.

Kendell, R. E. and Discipio, W. J. (1970). Obsessional symptoms and obsessional personality traits in patients with depressive illnesses. *Psychol. Med.* **1**, 65–72.

Kerr, T. A., Schapira, K. and Roth, M. (1969). The relationship between premature death and affective disorders. *Br. J. Psychiat.* **115**, 1277–1282.

Kessel, N. and McCulloch, W. (1966). Repeated ants of self-poisoning amd self-injury. *Proc. Roy. Soc. Med.* **59**, 89–92.

Kessell, A. (1968). The borderlands of the depressive states. *Br. J. Psychiat.* **114**, 1135–1140.

Klein, D. F. (1976). Differential diagnosis and treatment of the dysphorias. *In* 'Depression: Behavioural, Biochemical, Diagnostic and Treatment Concepts'

(Eds D. M. Gallant and G. M. Simpson), pp. 127–142. Spectrum, New York.

Kotin, J. and Goodwin, F. K. (1972). Depression during mania: Clinical observations and theoretical implications. *Am. J. Psychiat.* **129**, 679–686.

Kragh-Sorensen, P., Asberg, M. and Eggert-Hansen, C. (1973). Plasmanortriptyline levels in endogenous depression. *Lancet* **1**, 113–115.

Kraines, S. H. (1957). The physiologic basis of the manic-depressive illness: a theory. *Am. J. Psychiat.* **114**, 206–211.

Kreitman, N., Sainsbury, P., Pearce, K. and Costain, W. R. (1965). Hypochondriasis and depression in out-patients at a general hospital. *Br. J. Psychiat.* **111**, 607–615.

Kupfer, D. J., Pickar, D., Himmelhoch, J. M. and Detre, T. P. (1975). Are there two types of unipolar depression? *Arch. Gen. Psychiat.* **22**, 866–871.

Lader, M. (1973). Psychophysiology of depression. *In* 'Aspects of Depression' (Eds M. Lader and R. Garcia), pp. 179–187. World Psychiatric Association, Madrid.

Lazare, A. and Klerman, G. L. (1968). Hysteria and depression: The frequency and significance of hysterical personality features in hospitalized depressed women. *Am. J. Psychiat.* **124**, May Suppl. 48–56.

Leff, J. P., Fischer, M. and Bertelsen, A. (1976). A cross-national epidemiological study of mania. *Br. J. Psychiat.* **129**, 428–437.

Lehmann, H. E. (1971). Epidemiology of depressive disorders. *In* 'Depression in the 1970's' (Ed. R. R. Fieve), pp. 21–30. Excerpta Medica, Amsterdam.

Lewis, A. J. (1934). Melancholia: A clinical survey of depressive states. *J. Ment. Sci.* **80**, 277–378.

Lewis, A. J. (1966). Affective disorder. *In* 'Price's Textbook of the Practice of Medicine' (Ed. R. Bodley Scott), pp. 1177–1185. Oxford University Press, Oxford.

Liberman, R. P. and Raskin, D. E. (1971). Depression: A behavioural formulation. *Arch. Gen. Psychiat.* **24**, 515–523.

Lloyd, G. G. and Lishman, W. A. (1975). Effect of depression on the speed of recall of pleasant and unpleasant experiences. *Psychol. Med.* **5**, 173–180.

Lopez Ibor, J. J. (1972). Masked depressions. *Br. J. Psychiat.* **120**, 245–258.

Lyons, H. A. (1971). Psychiatric sequelae of the Belfast riots. *Br. J. Psychiat.* **118**, 265–273.

Maas, J. W. (1975). Biogenic amines and depression: Biochemical and pharmacological separation of two types of depression. *Arch. Gen. Psychiat.* **32**, 1357–1361.

Madden, J. L., Luhan, J. A., Kaplan, L. A. and Manfredi, H. M. (1952). Non-dementing psychoses in older persons. *J. Am. Med. Ass.* **150**, 1567–1570.

Mayo, J. A. (1970). Psychosocial profiles of patients on Lithium treatment. *Int. Pharmacopsychiat.* **5**, 190–202.

Medical Research Council (1965). Clinical trial of the treatment of depressive illness. *Br. Med. J.* **1**, 881–886.

Medical Research Council Brain Metabolism Unit (1972). Modified amine hypothesis for the aetiology of affective illness. *Lancet* **2**, 573–577.

Meltzer, H. Y., Hyong, W. C., Carroll, B. J. and Russo, P. (1976). Serum dopamine-B-hydroxylase activity in the affective psychoses and schizophrenia: Decreased activity in unipolar psychotically depressed patients. *Arch. Gen. Psychiat.* **33**, 585–591.

Mendels, J. (1965). Electroconvulsive therapy and depression: III A method for prognosis. *Br. J. Psychiat.* **111**, 687–690.

Mendels, J. (1976). Lithium in the treatment of depression. *Am. J. Psychiat.* **133**, 373–378.

Mendels, J. and Frazer, A. (1974a). Alterations in cell membrane activity in depression. *Am. J. Psychiat.* **131**, 1240–1246.

Mendels, J. and Frazer, A. (1974b). Brain biogenic amine depletion and mood. *Arch. Gen. Psychiat.* **30**, 447–451.

Mendels, J. and Frazer, A. (1975). Reduced central serotonergic activity in mania: Implications for the relationship between depression and mania. *Br. J. Psychiat.* **126**, 241–248.

Mendels, J., Stinnett, J. L., Burns, D. and Frazer, A. (1975). Amine precursors and depression. *Arch. Gen. Psychiat.* **32**, 22–30.

Mendlewicz, J., Fieve, R. R. and Stallone, F. (1973). Relationship between the effectiveness of lithium therapy and family history. *Am. J. Psychiat.* **130**, 1011–1013.

Miller, W. R. (1975). Psychological deficit in depression. *Psychol. Bull.* **82**, 238–260.

Mindham, R. H. S., Howland, C. and Shepherd, M. (1973). An evaluation of continuation therapy with tricyclic antidepressants in depressive illness. *Psychol. Med.* **3**, 5–17.

Mindham, R. H. S., Marsden, C. D. and Parkes, J. D. (1976). Psychiatric symptoms during L-dopa therapy for Parkinson's disease and their relationship to physical disability. *Psychol. Med.* **6**, 23–33.

Monnelly, E. P., Woodruff, R. A. and Robins, L. N. (1974). Manic-depressive illness and social achievement in a public hospital sample. *Acta Psychiat. Scand.* **50**, 318–325.

Munro, A. and Griffiths, A. B. (1969). Some psychiatric non-sequelae of childhood bereavement. *Br. J. Psychiat.* **115**, 305–311.

Murphy, G. E. and Robins, E. (1967). Social factors in suicide. *J. Am. Med. Ass.* **199**, 303–308.

Murphy, G. E., Woodruff, R. A., Herjanic, M. and Super, G. (1974). Variability of the clinical course of primary affective disorder. *Arch. Gen. Psychiat.* **30**, 757–761.

Nies, A., Ravaris, O. L. and Sylwester, D. (1971). Relation of sex and ageing to monoamine oxidase activity of human brain, plasma, and platelets. *Arch. Gen. Psychiat.* **24**, 536–539.

Nies, A., Robinson, D. S., Lamborn, K. R., Ravaris, C. L. and Ives, J. O. (1974). The efficacy of the MAO inhibitor, Phenelzine. *In* 'Present Status in Research and Clinical Use of MAO Inhibitors'. IX Cong. Collegium Internationale Neuropsychopharmacologicum, Symposium No. 11. Paris.

Nystrom, S. and Lindegard, B. (1975). Depression: Predisposing factors. *Acta Psychiat. Scand.* **51**, 77–87.

Odegaard, O. (1961). The epidemiology of depressive psychoses. *Acta. Psychiat. Scand., Suppl.* **162**, 33–38.

Overall, J. E., Hollister, L. E., Johnson, M. and Pennington, V. (1965). Computer classifications of depressions and different al effect of antidepressants. *J. Am. Med. Ass.* **192**, 561.

Paffenbarger, R. S. and Asnes, D. P. (1966). Chronic disease in former college students: III. Precursors of suicide in early and middle life. *Am. J. Publ. Hlth* **56**, 1026–1036.

Pare, C. M. B., Rees, L. and Sainsbury, M. J. (1962). Differentiation of two genetically specific types of depression by the response to anti-depressants. *Lancet* **2**, 1340–1343.

Parkes, C. M. (1965). Bereavement and mental illness. *Br. J. Med. Psychol.* **38**, 1–26.

Paykel, E. S. (1971). Classification of depressed patients: A cluster analysis derived grouping. *Br. J. Psychiat.* **118**, 275–288.

Paykel, E. S., Myers, J. K., Dienelt, M. N., Klerman, G. L. Lindenthal, J. J. and Pepper, M. P. (1969). Life events and depression. *Arch. Gen. Psychiat.* **21**, 753–760.

Paykel, E. S., Myers, J. K., Lindenthal, J. J. and Tanner, J. (1974). Suicidal feelings in the general population: A prevalence study. *Br. J. Psychiat.* **124**, 460–469.

Paykel, E. S., Dimascio, A., Haskell, D. and Prusoff, B. A. (1975). Effects of maintenance amitriptyline and psychotherapy on symptoms of depression. *Psychol. Med.* **5**, 67–77.

Perris, C. (1966). A study of bipolar (manic-depressive) and unipolar recurrent depressive psychoses. *Acta. Psychiat. Scand., Suppl.* **194**, 1–188.

Perris, C. (1971). Personality patterns in patients with affective disorders. *Acta. Psychiat. Scand., Suppl.* **221**, 43–51.

Perris, C. (1973). New approaches to the classification of affective disorders. *In* 'Aspects of Depression' (Eds M. Lader and R. Garcia), pp. 95–107. World Psychiatric Association, Madrid.

Perris, C. (1976) Frequency and hereditary aspects of depression. *In* 'Depression: behavioural, biochemical, diagnostic and treatment concepts' (Eds D. M. Gallant and G. M. Simpson), pp. 75–95. Spectrum, New York.

Pitt, B. (1975). Psychiatric illness following childbirth. *In* 'Contemporary Psychiatry' (Eds T. Silverstone and B. Barraclough), pp. 409–415. Headley Bros, Ashford, Kent.

Pollitt, J. and Young, J. (1971). Anxiety state or masked depression? A study based on the action of monoamine oxidase inhibitors. *Br. J. Psychiat.* **119**, 143–150.

Pollitt, J. D. (1965). Suggestions for a physiological classification of depression. *Br. J. Psychiat.* **111**, 489–495.

Prange, A. J., Wilson, I. C., Knox, A. E., McClane, T. K., Breese, G. R., Martin, B. R., Alltop, L. B. and Lipton, M. A. (1972). Thyroid-imipramine clinical and chemical interaction: Evidence for a receptor deficit in depression. *J. Psychiat. Res.* **9**, 187–195.

Prange, A. J., Wilson, I. C., Lynn, C. W., Alltop, L. B. and Stikeleather, R. A. (1974). L-Tryptophan in mania: Contribution to a permissive hypothesis of affective disorders. *Arch. Gen. Psychiat.* **30**, 56–62.

Price, J. (1968). The genetics of depressive behaviour. *In* 'Recent Developments in Affective Disorders' (Eds A. Coppen and A. Walk), pp. 37–54. Headley Bros, Ashford, Kent.

Prien, R. F. and Caffey, E. M. (1976). Relationship between dosage and response to lithium prophylaxis in recurrent depression. *Am. J. Psychiat.* **133**, 567–570.

Prien, R. F., Caffey, E. M. and Klett, C. J. (1972). Comparison of lithium carbonate and chlorpromazine in the treatment of mania: Report of the Veterans Administration and National Institute of Mental Health collaborative study group. *Arch. Gen. Psychiat.* **26**, 146–153.

Prien, R. F., Klett, C. J. and Caffey, E. M. (1973). Lithium carbonate and imipramine in prevention of affective episodes: A comparison in recurrent affective illness. *Arch. Gen. Psychiat.* **29**, 420–425.

Quitkin, F., Rifkin, A. and Klein, D. F. (1976). Prophylaxis of affective disorders: Current status of knowledge. *Arch. Gen. Psychiat.* **33**, 337–341.

Rao, A. V. (1970). A study of depression as prevalent in South India. *Transcult. Psychiat. Res. Rev.* **7**, 166–167.

Raskin, A. and Crook, T. H. (1976). The endogenous-neurotic distinction as a predictor of response to antidepressant drugs. *Psychol. Med.* 6, 59–70.

Reid, A. H. (1972). Psychoses in adult mental defectives: I. Manic depressive psychosis. *Br. J. Psychiat.* 120, 205–212.

Richards, D. H. (1974). A post-hysterectomy syndrome. *Lancet* 2, 983–985.

Robins, A. H. (1976). Depression in patients with Parkinsonism. *Br. J. Psychiat.* 128, 141–145.

Robins, E., Gassner, S., Kayes, J., Wilkinson, R. H. and Murphy, G. E. (1959). The communication of suicidal intent: A study of 134 consecutive cases of suicide. *Am. J. Psychiat.* 115, 724–733.

Seck, R. L. and Goodwin, F. K. (1974). Inhibition of dopamine-β-hydroxylase in manic patients: A clinical trial with fusaric acid. *Arch. Gen. Psychiat.* 31, 649–654.

Sainsbury, P. (1968). Suicide and depression. *In* 'Recent Developments in Affective Disorders' (Eds A. Coppen and A. Walk), pp. 1–13. Headley Bros, Ashford, Kent.

Sandler, M., Bonham Carter, S., Cuthbert, M. F. and Pare, C. M. B. (1975). Is there an increase in monoamine-oxidase activity in depressive illness? *Lancet* 1, 1045–1048.

Schless, A. P., Schwartz, L., Goetz, C. and Mendels, J. (1974). How depressives view the significance of life events. *Br. J. Psychiat.* 125, 406–410.

Schurr, P. H. (1973). Psychosurgery. *Br. J. Hosp. Med.* 10, 53–60.

Schwab, J. J., Bialow, M., Holzer, C. E., Brown, J. M. and Stevenson, B. E. (1967a). Sociocultural aspects of depression in medical inpatients: I. Frequency and social variables. *Arch. Gen. Psychiat.* 17, 533–538.

Schwab, J. J., Bialow, M. R., Brown, J. M., Holzer, C. E. and Stevenson, B. E. (1967b). Sociocultural aspects of depression in medical inpatients: II. Symptomatology and class. *Arch. Gen. Psychiat.* 17, 539–543.

Seligman, M. E. P. (1972). Learned helplessness. *Ann. Rev. Med.* 23, 407–412.

Shaw, D. M., Macsweeney, D. A., Hewland, R. and Johnson, A. L. (1975). Tricyclic antidepressants and tryptophan in unipolar depression. *Psychol. Med.* 5, 276–278.

Small, J. G., Small, I. F., Sharpley, P. and Moore, D. F. (1968). A double-blind comparative evaluation of flurothyl and E.C.T. *Arch. Gen. Psychiat.* 19, 79–86.

Smythies, J. R. (1970). 'Brain Mechanisms and Behaviour'. Blackwell, Oxford and Edinburgh.

Spicer, C. L., Hare, E. H. and Slater, E. (1973). Neurotic and psychotic forms of depressive illness: Evidence from age-incidence in a national sample. *Br. J. Psychiat.* 123, 535–541.

Stallone, F., Huba, G. J., Lawlor, W. G. and Fieve, R. R. (1973). Longitudinal studies of diurnal variations in depression: A sample of 643 patient days. *Br. J. Psychiat.* 123, 311–318.

Stenstedt, A. (1959). Involutional melancholia: An etiologic, clinical and social study of endogenous depression in late life, with special reference to genetic factors. *Acta Psychiat. Scand., Suppl.* 127.

Stenstedt, A. (1966). Genetics of neurotic depression. *Acta Psychiet. Scand.* 42, 392–409.

Surridge, D. (1969). An investigation into some psychiatric aspects of multiple sclerosis. *Br. J. Psychiat.* 115, 749–764.

Taylor, M. A. and Abrams, R. (1973). The phenomenology of mania: A new look at some old patients. *Arch. Gen. Psychiat.* 29, 520–522.

Teja, J. S., Narang, R. L. and Aggarwal, A. K. (1971). Depression across cultures. *Br. J. Psychiat.* **119**, 253–260.

Tonks, C. M. (1975). Premenstrual tension. *In* 'Contemporary Psychiatry' (Eds T. Silverstone and B. Barraclough), pp. 399–408. Headley Bros, Ashford, Kent.

Tonks, C. M., Paykel, E. S. and Klerman, G. L. (1970). Clinical depression amongst negroes. *Am. J. Psychiat.* **127**, 329–335.

Tyrer, P. J. (1976). Towards a rational therapy with monoamine oxidase inhibitors. *Br. J. Psychiat.* **128**, 345–360.

van den Burg, W., van Praag, H. M., Bos, E. R. H., Piers, D. A., van Zanten, A. K. and Doorenbos, H. (1975). TRH as a possible quick-acting but short-lasting antidepressant. *Psychol. Med.* **5**, 404–412.

van Praag, H. M. (1974). Toward a biochemical classification of depression. *In* 'Advances in Biochemical Psychopharmacology' (Eds E. Costa, G. L. Gessa and M. Sandler), Vol. 2, pp. 357–368. Raven Press, New York.

van Praag, H. M., Uleman, A. M. and Spitz, J. C. (1965). The vital syndrome interview. *Psychiat. Neurol. Neurochir.* **68**, 329–246.

van Praag, H. M., Korf, J., Lakke, J. P. W. F. and Schut, T. (1975). Dopamine metabolism in depressions, psychoses, and Parkinson's Disease: The problem of the specificity of biological variables in behaviour disorders. *Psychol. Med.* **5**, 138–146.

Videbech, T. (1975). The psychopathology of anancastic endogenous depression. *Acta Psychiat. Scand.* **52**, 336–373.

Walinder, J., Skott, A., Nagy, A., Carlsson, A. and Bjorn-Crik, E. (1975). Potentiation of antidepressant action of clomipramine by tryptophan. *Lancet* **1**, 984.

Weissman, M. M., Paykel, E. S., Siegel, R. and Klerman, G. L. (1971). The social role performance of depressed women: Comparisons with a normal group. *Am. J. Orthopsychiat.* **41**, 390–405.

White, H. L., McLeod, M. N. and Davidson, J. R. T. (1976). Catechol O-methyltransferase in red blood cells of schizophrenic, depressed and normal human subjects. *Br. J. Psychiat.* **128**, 184–187.

Whybrow, P. C., and Mendels, J. (1969). Toward a biology of depression: Some suggestions from neurophysiology. *Am. J. Psychiat.* **125**, 1491–1500.

Winokur, G. (1971). The genetics of manic-depressive illness. *In* 'Depression in the 1970s' (Ed. R. R. Fieve), pp. 47–53. Excerpta Medica, Amsterdam.

Winokur, G. and Morrison, J. (1973). The Iowa 500: Follow-up of 225 depressives. *Br. J. Psychiat.* **123**, 543–548.

Winokur, G. and Pitts, F. N. (1964). Affective disorder: I. Is reactive depression an entity? *J. Nerv. Ment. Dis.* **138**, 541–547.

Wise, C. D., Berger, B. D. and Stein, L. (1973). Evidence of noradrenergic reward receptors and serotonergic punishment receptors in the rat brain. *Biol. Psychiat.* **6**, 3–21.

Wolpe, J. (1971). Neurotic depression: Experimental analog, clinical syndromes and treatment. *Am. J. Psychother.* **25**, 362–368.

Woodruff, R. A., Robins, L. N., Winokur, G. and Reich, T. (1971). Manic depressive illness and social achievement. *Acta Psychiat. Scand.* **47**, 237–249.

World Health Organization Working Group (1974). *In* 'Suicide and Attempted Suicide' (Ed. E. M. Brooke), pp. 71–106. WHO, Geneva.

Wright, S. and McDonald, C. (1974). Review of behavioral treatment of depression. *Psychol. Rep.* **34**, 1335–1341.

Young, J. P. R., Hughes, W. C. and Lader, M. H. (1976). A controlled comparison of flupenthixol and amitriptyline in depressed outpatients. *Br. Med. J.* **1**, 1116–1118.

Zung, W. (1973). From art to science: The diagnosis and treatment of depression. *Arch. Gen. Psychiat.* **29**, 328–337.

13 Psychiatric manifestations of organic illness

Roy McClelland

Introduction

The elucidation of neuropsychiatric symptoms evoked by cerebral and systemic disease and their differentiation from mental states unrelated to such processes are important parts of psychiatric practice (Bleuler, 1951). Often accompanying neurological signs leave no doubt as to the presence of underlying organic disease and the psychiatric symptoms are of secondary importance. However, in the prodromal stages of many physical illnesses, especially in the elderly, disturbances in the patient's mental life may be the only clues to the presence of illness, e.g. mild congestive cardiac failure or bronchial pneumonia. Some intracranial pathologies such as a frontal meningioma may cause major changes in the patient's mental state for long periods before significant neurological signs develop.

The role assigned to organic disease in causing mental symptoms has changed over the past hundred years, since Jackson stated, 'I do not believe that there is such a thing as loss or deficit of function of any nervous elements without a proportionate material alteration of their structure and nutrition'. Although the debate continues as to the biological or other bases of some psychological syndromes, there is now sound evidence that those recognized organic pathologies which effect the nervous system often produce a reaction pattern whose symptomatology is distinguishable from othe types of mental disorder. The importance of this diagnostic issue is heightened by the size of the problem. Several epidemiological studies of those over 65 years old concur that about 10% suffer from organic mental disorder (Kay *et al.*, 1964). About half of the elderly in psychiatric hospitals receive a diagnosis of 'dementia'.

Misdiagnosis is not uncommon in the early stages of organic mental disorder. In one study of consecutive admissions originally given a 'functional' diagnosis, independent inquiry established physical disease as making a significant contribution in over 20% (Herridge, 1960). The most common early misdiagnoses appear to be schizophrenia and neurotic reactions, non-specific 'dementia' in the elderly, and Korsakoff syndrome in patients with a history of alcohol abuse. Shulman (1967) on screening a group of psychiatric in-patients detected Vitamin B12 deficiency in 8% and in at least half of these it was probably a significant causal factor in their illness. A higher than expected incidence of tumours has been reported from post mortem studies of psychiatric in-patients. Part of the problem relates to difficulties in assessing functional disturbance of the nervous system which increase sharply as one moves from basic sensory and motor processes to higher functions. Mental phenomena are further complicated by their multiple dependence on personality and environment as well as the disease process itself. In spite of this individual colouring several consistent reaction patterns can be identified with reasonable reliability. Although the type of reaction is usually not a function of the specific pathology, it often gives important clues to both the location and the behaviour of the disease process (Lishmann, 1978). The subject of mental reactions to general physical disorder is also considered in Chapter 18.

Clinical syndromes

The acute organic reaction (acute confusional state)

The central and most constant feature in the acute organic reaction, is impairment of consciousness ranging from minimal diminution in alertness to coma. The degree of impairment is most meaningfully assessed by establishing the minimal stimulus which elicits a response and the quality of the response obtained. Mild impairment of conscious awareness manifests itself in difficulties obtaining and holding attention and concentration, with for example a tendency to wander off the theme of a conversation or mild drowsiness. Paralleling these disturbances are impairment of recent memory causing defective registration of new experiences, and impairment of intellect, leading to defective reasoning. Time sense depends on state of awareness, intellectual grasp, and recent memory and is therefore a sensitive measure of minimal clouding (e.g. time of day, duration of interview).

Perceptual distortions, emotional disturbances, and general psychomotor activity are less constant features although they can dominate the clinical picture. In delirium, illusions and hallucinations usually of a visual nature are prominent and the patient is often excited, frightened and over-active. In some toxic states a characteristic hallucinatory pattern is often found (e.g. alcohol withdrawal, LSD, or cocaine abuse) while disturbance within a particular sensory modality is also a function of those environmental conditions which make the greatest demands on the related perceptual skills. For instance, increased visual misinterpretation usually occurs under poor lighting conditions (Wolff and Curran, 1935).

Temporal patterns are useful in differentiating the acute organic reaction from the chronic reaction. In the former the onset is characteristically sudden, there is usually considerable variation with time, and the patient usually recovers completely once the underlying process has been removed. Although the acute organic reaction is characterized by diffuse impairment of cerebral function impairment of consciousness has a central position and it seems probable that the site of primary dysfunction is in the brain stem reticular formation (Brain, 1962). Hence a discrete brain stem lesion may produce the acute organic reaction, although it is more commonly seen in association with diffuse cerebral pathology.

The chronic organic reaction (dementia)

This may be defined as an acquired, global, impairment of intellect, memory and personality without impairment of consciousness. By definition it excludes mental retardation and focal dysfunction, but it does not imply progressiveness or ireversibility of the condition. Intellectual deterioration is the hallmark, but in the early stages this may only be manifest in loss of interest and initiative, or in a slight lowering of work performance and only later progress to more marked impairment of grasp, abstract sense and judgement. Memory impairment is a second characteristic feature with early difficulties in recounting recent personal events and current affairs. In the more severely affected this may lead to disorientation for time, and ultimately to loss of remote memory and disorientation for persons and places. Perseveration is common in established cases and often accompanied by purposeless overactivity or compensatory over-orderliness (Goldstein, 1952).

Several trends are discernible in personality deterioration. In the early stages emotional disturbance such as anxiety and depressive reactions, irritability, emotional explosiveness, perplexity and suspiciousness probably reflect the individuals premorbid personality, attempting to cope in the face of failing abilities. In the later stages emotional lability and blunting are more typical, while coarsening of personality and loss of social control usually result from extensive frontal lobe involvement (Roth and Myers, 1969).

There is often considerable variation in the relative degree of impairment in each of these areas of psychic function. In the initial stages some patients may show deficit in only one sector while others are more diffusely affected and may also have such focal deficits as dysphasia, and dyspraxia. It should be stressed that the concept of dementia employed here is not a pathological or aetiological diagnosis but a state of diffuse cerebral dysfunction, and although the causative pathology has usually a widespread distribution there are important exceptions, notably lesions involving the frontal or temporal lobes, and the diencephalon.

Dysfunction suggestive of focal cerebral lesions

As already indicated, both the acute and chronic organic reactions may be produced by focal lesions but usually there is additional evidence for such a process. In this respect neurological deficit, especially a focal fit, cranial nerve palsies, or hemisyndromes are more reliable. However, if only cortical association areas are involved delineation of focal cognitive deficit assumes great clinical importance.

Amnesia

Focal amnesia may result from bilateral hippocampal gyrus lesions or bilateral damage to other cell stations in the Papez circuit, notably anterior thalamus, structures surrounding the third ventricle, posterior hypothalamus and the mammillary bodies (Brierley, 1966). There is a characteristic deficit of recent memory while registration is quite normal (e.g. impaired recall of name and address after five minutes). Disturbance of time sense including the temporal order of recent past events is characteristic while remote memory is unaffected, and other cognitive functions usually remain intact. Confabulation (falsification of memory in clear consciousness) is sometimes a feature especially with diencephalic lesions, and in the Korsakoff states there is usually associated attitudinal changes and lethargy. In contrast memory impairment associated with diffuse cerebral disease usually involves remote events, and other cognitive deficits can often be found.

Aphasia

Impairment of language is a prominent feature with lesions involving the dominant hemisphere and nomial aphasia a characteristic but non-localizing finding (Butler and Benson, 1974).

Posterior aphasias (high output, jargon, sensory or Wernicke's aphasia). A failure to understand verbal communications associated with an *excessive* output of paraphasic contaminated language is most commonly associated with lesions in the posterior aspect of the dominant superior temporal gyrus. Patients with lesions more peripheral to the sylvian fissure in the border zone between the temporal and parietal lobes have similar deficits but no jargon, are able to repeat and may also show echolalia (Transcortical Sensory Aphasia). The association of nominal aphasia with dyslexia, dysgraphia, dyscalculia, right–left disorientation and finger agnosia (Guerstmann's syndrome) is found with lesions of the dominant angular gyrus. Fluency of speech is common to all of the posterior aphasias.

Anterior aphasias (low output, motor, Broca's aphasia). Lesions of the inferior frontal gyrus frequently cause *loss* of fluency associated with multiple grammatical errors and indistinct productions of both correct and incorrect phonemes. Again more peripheral lesions affecting the antero-superior border of the pre-motor area produce deficits which show a marked improvement with practice (Transcortical Motor Aphasia).

Agnosia

Central to all agnosias is a high order perceptual defect often associated with related spatial and language difficulties (Warrington, 1974). The right parietal region appears to be critical for the processing of visual and other sensory data. In visuo-spatial agnosia there is defective appreciation of spatial relationships and impaired execution of simple constructional tasks, often associated with neglect of left visual space. Curious left-sided body image disturbances such as neglect or denial of ownership of a limb (anosagnosia) and failure to recognize familiar faces (prosopagnosia) may also accompany right hemisphere lesions. The dominant parietal lobe is essential for the encoding of visual information in terms of linkages with verbal symbols. Typical deficits include bilateral tactile agnosia and visual object agnosia (inability to name and use common objects).

Apraxia

The parietal lobes are also involved in higher order executive functions. Typical deficits with non-dominant lesions include dressing apraxia and contralateral motor apraxia, while dominant hemisphere lesions are associated with bilateral motor apraxia (e.g. copying a complex task like striking a match) and ideational apraxia (e.g. executing a complex instruction like 'light this cigarette').

Other psychiatric manifestations of organic disease

It should be appreciated that the correlation between intracerebral pathology and these organic reactions is not perfect. On the one hand, lesions may sometimes evoke major disturbances of psychological function, while on the other hand primary functional disturbances may simulate one of the organic reactions. Although *schizophreniform reactions* may be precipitated by a wide range of non-specific triggers including organic illness in the constitutionally vulnerable (Bleuler, 1951), they appear to be more commonly associated with lesions of the temporal lobe (Davison and Bagley, 1969). In such circumstances the clinical picture may be atypical with no family history, stable premorbid personality, late onset or the prominence of visual as opposed to auditory hallucinations. Ultimately it may be the atypical response to treatment which alerts suspicions of an organic basis.

Pathoplastic factors, especially premorbid emotional stability and habitual reaction patterns may contribute in the early stages to a *neurotic reaction* which dominates the clinical picture. Thus depressive, anxiety and obsessional and states of late onset occurring in the absence of obvious environmental stress should raise suspicions of a possible organic basis. On the other hand, symptoms suggestive of a dementia may be found in some patients who are ultimately found to be suffering from a depressive illness. Hysterical simulation of an organic reaction such as dull behaviour, amnesia or Ganser symptoms (approximate answers) usually occur in the young or unintelligent and a clear motive can often be found. Behaviour usually proves to be inconsistent, while with hysterical amnesia there is characteristically either a sudden and often inconsistent loss of specific and appropriate themes or else a dense global amnesia which is not seen in organic states in the absence of a period of unconsciousness or gross cognitive deficit. But even in such cases a previous history of organic impairment or epilepsy will often be found probably providing the essential learning experience of the rewards of illness behaviour (Kendell, 1974).

Hypokinesis, somnolence, mutuism, stupor and catatonic symptoms although often part of some functional illness may arise with lesions of the cingulate regions, diencephalon or brain stem.

Complex epileptic phenomena

Epileptic seizures can be classified into two main groups. Firstly there is generalized epilepsy probably arising from centrencephalic structures and associated with inter-ictal EEG features of bilateral, synchronized discharges usually of spike and wave form. Fits are generalized from the outset the most typical being classical *petit mal* attacks and non-localized *grand mal* convulsions in both of which consciousness is lost from the outset. Local cerebral pathology is rarely found. Secondly, there are focal, partial or secondary generalized seizures in which the epileptic discharges commence in an area of cortical or sub-cortical grey matter. Because the initial events do not involve centres which control consciousness they may be experienced by the patient (an aura). Local pathology is common. Fits occurring for the first time in individuals over 30 years of age are virtually always a symptom of underlying cerebral pathology or systemic disorder.

A typical *grand mal* fit is easily recognized leaving no doubt as to the nature of the attack. Need for further investigation is obvious, although due consideration should be given to a history of alcoholism or drug abuse. However, the majority of focal fits arise from temporal lobe structures and as many as half of patients so affected may not have experienced a *grand mal* fit (Currie *et al.*, 1971). Some form of psychomotor seizure is quite common and the associated complex symptomatology and behaviour disturbance can lead to confusion with functional psychiatric disorders.

In the absence of the diagnostic features of a *grand mal* fit, namely tonic and clonic movements followed by a period of confusion, other ictal symptoms need to be clarified. The cluster of sudden, usually brief episodes, heralded by an aura and followed by a period of confusion form the lowest common denominator of most fits. The most common auras reported in one study of temporal lobe epilepsy were cephalic or abdominal sensations, perceptual disturbances especially visual and simply auditory hallucinations, *déjà vu* experiences and emotional disturbances, such as anxiety and depression (Currie *et al.*, 1971). Anxiety symptoms often have a prominent epigastric component; olfactory hallucinations usually point to lesions of the uncinate lobe. Important motor symptoms include adversion, focal tonic or clonic movements and more complex activities which are usually stereotyped and inappropriate (e.g. plucking, muttering, undressing). Autonomic accompaniments include pallor and sweating and the patient may be incontinent.

Clinical features of common intracerebral pathologies

The degenerations (primary dementias)

Senile dementia. By definition senile dementia occurs in those over 65 years of age, is much more common in women than men and together with arterio-sclerotic dementia accounts for over half of the major psychiatric disorders in this age group (Kay *et al.*, 1964). The clinical course is usually slow and insidious beginning with a slight accentuation of personality characteristics or an exacerbation of premorbid neurotic traits, and as a consequence depressive and paranoid reactions are quite common. Memory and intellectual impairment gradually emerge while personality and behavioural changes at this stage are often characterized by restlessness, blunting of emotions, anger outbursts or deterioration in personal habits. As the condition progresses focal cognitive deficits such as aphasia or apraxia and neurological signs become increasingly common. Hospitalization is often necessary in the later stages, especially if there is a lack of support at home, and is often precipitated by some relatively mild acute illness which has led to decompensation.

The underlying pathology is a diffuse cerebral atrophy associated with a loss of neurones, gliosis, senile plaque formation and neuro-fibrillary degeneration. The process appears to be genetically and pathologically distinct from normal senescence and arterio-sclerotic degeneration (Roth, 1971). The distinction between senile degeneration and Alzheimer's disease is less clear-cut.

Alzheimer's disease is the commonest cerebral degeneration in the pre-senium and again females outnumber males in the ratio 2:1. The clinical course although slow at first soon gathers speed and death usually occurs within two to three years (Wolstenholme and O'Connor, 1970). Early memory impairment is a characteristic feature while in the later stages personality changes, emotional blunting and irritability become more prominent. Eventually parietal lobe signs such as agnosia and apraxia appear, frequently accompanied by long tract signs or epilepsy. The underlying pathological changes are characterized by *diffuse* atrophy often more marked in the frontal and temporal regions; with typical plaque formation and neuro-fibrillary tangles in the grey areas of the cortex (Corsellis, 1969).

Pick's disease is an uncommon degenerative condition with a similar female/male ratio to Alzheimer's disease. Onset is usually in the fifties and sixties and it has a slow insidious course. Earliest manifestations are usually in personality with for example a loss of social restraint, changes in character or drive, increasing fatuousness or apathy. Loss of insight, dysphasia and incontinence also occur in the early stages before severe memory and intellectual impairment have become obvious. Underlying pathological changes usually consist of a *patchy* atrophy especially within the frontal and temporal lobes without the characteristic plaque and neuro-fibrillary changes found in Alzheimer's and senile dementia (Sim and Sussman, 1962).

Huntington's chorea is a rare condition characterized by the association of pre-senile dementia and choreaform movements beginning in middle life. The earliest mental changes are usually in personality often with increasing irritability, apathy and neglect and the development of paranoid ideas (Oliver, 1970). At this stage it may be misdiagnosed as personality disorder, affective illness or schizophrenia. Unsteadiness and clumsiness are also common early signs, while choreaform movements become gradually more prominent and widespread. Dementia is very insidious and distractability a characteristic feature. The condition occasionally begins in childhood when intellectual deterioration is much more fulminant and epilepsy exceedingly common. Unaffected family members show a marked excess of both social and psychopathology including schizophrenia and suicide.

The characteristic underlying pathology is a marked atrophy of the frontal lobes and caudate nucleus although other sub-cortical nuclear groups may be involved. The condition has a clear autosomal dominant inheritance with full penetrance, and has recently been associated with reduced glutamic-acid-decarboxylase activity and hence a reduction in the activity of gamma-aminobutyric acid (GABA) containing neurones in the basal ganglia (Bird *et al.*, 1973).

Creutzfeldt-Jakob disease is an uncommon disorder beginning in middle life and affecting both sexes in the same way. It causes a rapidly progressive dementia with neurological deficits especially impairment of speech, vision and various motor signs including cerebellar ataxia, spasticity, rigidity, tremor and chorea. Myoclonic jerks are common and if anterior horn cells are affected associated muscle atrophy appears. Death usually occurs within a year although in some more fulminant forms of the disease in which acute confusion, marked cortical blindness and myoclonic jerks are prominent, death may ensue within three to six months.

Widespread spongiform atrophy occurs throughout the cortex and sub-cortical nuclear groups and often the cerebellum, brain stem and spinal cord are involved. There is increasing evidence that the condition may be due to a slow virus transmissible to other primates (Gibbs and Gajdusek, 1969).

Arterio-sclerotic dementia

Vascular disease of the nervous system is slightly more common in men than women and usually occurs in the late sixties and seventies, but may commence in the presenium when it is usually associated with evidence of more widespread vascular disease, especially hypertension. The condition has a step-wise course often heralded by sudden strokes of varying severity and progressing to severe coma, hemiparesis or dysphasia. Variable patchy neurological and cognitive deficits are left in the wake of such acute ischaemic episodes or infarctions, while between the more dramatic strokes transient clouding and fluctuating cognitive impairment are common together with such somatic symptoms as headache, dizziness, syncope and epilepsy (Birkett, 1972). Death in most cases is due to renal failure, ischaemic heart disease or a major cerebro-vascular accident.

Tumours

Mental symptoms usually occur at some stage in the history of a cerebral tumour and in a number they may be the first clinical signs. These symptoms, however, are usually of little diagnostic or localizing value and the diagnosis ultimately rests on evidence of raised intracranial pressure, focal neurological signs or focal epilepsy.

A wide range of psychiatric symptoms may occur but the most common syndrome is the acute organic reaction. Focal syndromes are also common and less often a global dementia may be found. Isolated hallucinatory disturbances may be experienced, more commonly with tumours of the temporal and frontal lobes. Affective and neurotic symptoms especially dullness, euphoria, depression and anxiety are usually accompanied by other evidence of organic impairment, although they are in part determined by premorbid traits and constitution.

Mental symptoms and their severity are to some extent a function of the type of tumour, both its rate of growth and invasiveness, and therefore are most frequently found with astrocytomas, less with gliomas, and least with meningiomas. The more rapidly growing tend to produce acute impairment of consciousness while the more slowly expanding often manifest themselves in personality change or intellectual impairment. In addition raised intracranial pressure may affect brain stem function and so lead to impairment of consciousness.

The location of the tumour is also a factor determining the frequency and intensity of mental symptoms (Hecan and Ajuriaguerra, 1956). Tumours of the frontal lobe frequently cause either impairment of consciousness or dementia especially if bilateral. The dementia is often accompanied by apathy, loss of spontaneity or affective disturbances especially euphoria and irritability. There may also be isolated behavioural disturbances and loss of social control. Tumours of the corpus callosum usually produce severe mental disturbances probably because of ready spread to neighbouring hemispheres. Those of the anterior corpus callosum tend to cause a typical 'frontal lobe' type picture although they may produce a florid schizophreniform syndrome.

Tumours of the temporal lobe may cause fits often with complex symptomatolgy. Affective symptoms, including depression, anxiety, and irritability, and schizophreniform states are more commonly associated with tumours in this region while aphasia may be caused by neoplasms arising in the dominant hemisphere.

In parietal lobe tumours focal cognitive deficit may be evident with, for example, dysphasia or elements of Gerstmann's syndrome accompanying tumours of the left hemisphere and agnosia with those arising in the right. Neurological signs are also very frequent.

Although tumours of the diencephalon and around the third ventricle only infrequently produce psychiatric symptoms these are usually quite characteristic, namely an amnesic syndrome, severe dementia, excessive somnolence or akinetic mutism.

Normal pressure hydrocephalus

Brief mention must be made of this unusual but treatable cause of dementia. The pathophysiological process is often quite obscure although in some, obstruction to the flow of CSF from the base of the brain through to the arachnoid villi has resulted from earlier sub-arachnoid haemorrhage, meningitis or head injury with adhesion formation (Adams *et al.*, 1965). There are usually no diagnostic symptoms or signs although dementia is often rapid and ataxia and incontinence of urine are common clinical features. The presence of 'normal pressure hydrocephalus' should always be considered especially in cases of pre-senile dementia, when the diagnosis can readily be made with the use of either radio-iodinated-albumen-cisterography or air-encephalography. These demonstrate the presence of enlarged ventricles and the failure of air passage over the surface of the cerebral hemispheres which show no evidence of atrophy. The shunting of CSF will halt the process and in some lead to clinical improvement (Rice and Gendelman, 1973).

Infections of the central nervous system

Virus encephalitis

Most virus infections of the central nervous system have a dramatic acute phase characterized by pyrexia, focal neurological signs, seizures, vomiting and photophobia. Impairment of consciousness usually progresses rapidly to coma often through a stage of delirium. The final outcome is partly a function of age, and in childhood is associated with a high mortality and severe neurological, cognitive and behavioural deficits (Whitty *et al.*, 1969).

Epidemic encephalitis is mainly a problem in southern and eastern European countries and in the southern states of America. They are usually arthropod borne and the very young and old are most at risk. Mortality is high in the acute phase and among children who survive, deficits such as mental handicap and spastic paralysis are common. Adults are generally less severely affected usually with little more than protracted feelings of malaise and lethargy.

Herpes simplex is a common cause of severe sporadic encephalitis especially in Great Britain. In the early stages meningeal irritation and focal neurological signs are common and complex hallucinatory experiences and other psychiatric symptomatology frequently accompany a rapidly evolving acute organic reaction. There is often major involvement of the temporal lobes and orbital frontal structures, and the clinical features may simulate the presence of a tumour in this region (Potter, 1969). Mortality in such severe cases is high (about 40%) and chronic sequelae are common among survivors. In the young this either takes the form of mental retardation, epilepsy or focal neurological deficit, while in adults dementia is prominent.

Encephalitis may also follow in the wake of systemic virus infections such as influenza, acute exanthemata (measles, rubella, chicken pox, scarlet fever) or after vaccination. In the mild cases recovery usually occurs after two to three weeks while the severely affected either succumb or ultimately progress to complete recovery.

Sub-acute sclerosing pan-encephalitis is an uncommon but severe insidious progressive disorder chiefly affecting children and adolescents. Most cases are probably due to measles virus although others such as the paramyxo virus may be involved. The characteristic clinical feature is a sudden cessation of cognitive development followed by a progressive deterioration of intellectual skills and increasing behaviour disorder. A low grade pyrexia is common and neurological signs soon emerge, especially myoclonic jerks, extrapyramidal rigidity and athetoid movements. In the later stages epilepsy and spastic paresis often develop. In some children psychiatric symptomatology including bizarre behaviour and psychotic features may be prominent possibly reflecting the degree of temporal lobe involvement.

Syphilis

The incidence of syphilitic infection of the nervous system has decreased considerably throughout this century. Chronic meningo-vascular syphilis usually occurs in the first five years after primary infection and the associated gumma may produce a gradually progressive dementia or cloudy state. Focal neurological deficit such as cranial nerve lesions with basal meningeal involvement, fits, aphasia, hemiparesis with convexity lesions or strokes of varying severity resulting from vascular involvement are usually evident.

General paralysis of the insane is the result of direct spirochaetal involvement of the nervous system. The essential feature is a progressive dementia and in the classical form, which is now rarely seen, personality and affective changes are prominent. Typical dementia or depressive psychosis are now more common although virtually any psychiatric syndrome may be found in the early stages (Dewhurst, 1969). Again neurological signs are prominent, the most common being pupillary abnormalities, especially impaired light reaction, coarse tremor usually of facial musculature dysarthria, long tract signs and epilepsy. When tabo-paresis co-exists posterior column signs can usually also be found.

Cerebral abscess

In the early stages of some abscesses there may be few clear diagnostic signs and the diagnosis should therefore be considered in cases of mild confusion or change of temperament associated with general ill-health and mild pyrexia. Vague headache, general malaise, pyrexia and mild confusion are common and there is usually evidence of raised intracranial pressure, focal neurological signs, focal epilepsy and meningeal irritation.

Psychiatric aspects of head injury

The chronic sequelae of head injury, mainly the results of road traffic accidents have increased dramatically in recent years and currently adds approximately 1000 persons each year to the severely disabled (Lewin, 1968). The majority of long-term problems are psychiatric and among the severely head-injured up to half may have chronic psychiatric problems (Fahey *et al.*, 1967). Epilepsy develops in about 5% of those with closed head injuries and rise to about 30% following an open head injury; most seizures are within five years of the injury (Paillas *et al.*, 1972). Long-term neurological problems are relatively uncommon and usually consist of cranial nerve deficits especially anosmia or visual or auditory impairment.

The degree of brain damage following a closed head injury is a function of both *decelerating forces* producing shearing stresses throughout cortical and subcortical structures and the *direct impact damage* occurring at either the site of contract or contra coup. To these may be added the effects of oedema, anoxia and haemorrhage (both intracerebral and subdural). Following open head injury direct local damage is usually more marked than the effects of shearing stresses and infection is often a complication (Jennett, 1975). Common to most head injuries is a period of concussion characterized by a variable degree of paralysis of many cerebral functions including consciousness, respiration and vasomotor tone. Dysfunction of brain stem structures due to shearing stresses appears to be the central mechanism. Concussion is usually followed by an interval of impaired consciousness throughout which there is a defective registration of ongoing events and for which there is subsequent amnesia.

The duration of post-traumatic amnesia is a useful measure of the severity of the underlying brain damage especially in closed head injury and, together with more direct measures of brain damage such as depth and amount of tissue destruction, shows a positive correlation with the severity of long-term sequelae. In addition psychiatric complications more commonly follow lesions of the left hemisphere and especially those involving the temporal lobe (Lishman, 1968). Other physical factors which contribute to the long-term outcome include the development of normal pressure hydrocephalus, subdural haematoma and epilepsy. In many situations the emotional impact of the brain injury or subsequent intellectual impairment may be sufficiently stressful to cause neurotic decompensation especially in those whose premorbid personalities were more vulnerable. The presence of a compensation issue also substantially increases the likelihood of long-term sequelae (Miller, 1961). The relative contribution of each of these factors varies considerably from patient to patient and for convenience the more common psychiatric syndromes following head injury are considered separately.

Organic reactions

Following severe injury intellectual impairment, memory defects and personality changes, especially blunting, coarsening and loss of affective control, have been found in a substantial proportion (10–50%). The degree of dementia bears a close relationship to measures of the severity of the head injury and long-term prognosis is usually much worse following an open head injury or a period of post-traumatic amnesia greater than 24 hours. Personality change is more often observed with left hemisphere lesions especially those affecting frontal and temporal lobe structures (Lishman, 1968). Where the deficit appears to be disproportionately large compared with severity of the injury then complications should be considered especially normal pressure hydrocephalus or a subdural haematoma.

There is, however, commonly a gradual improvement often over many months and even years provided suitable rehabilitative measures are taken. This may in part be the consequence of re-education of intact brain tissue but it is probable that motivational disturbances and emotional responses to the injury and impairment make substantial contributions to the overall disability in the early stages (Lishman, 1973). The potential effects of these factors make assessment of mild degrees of intellectual impairment very difficult and serial psychometric testing may be necessary.

Psychosis

Psychotic reactions have been observed more commonly than expected in the late post-traumatic period. In part these may be the result of non-specific effects of stress precipitating specific reactions in those individuals who are constitutionally vulnerable. However, there does appear to be a group who develop schizophreniform reactions in the absence of constitutional loading and in whom damage to temporal lobe structure has been noted (Davison and Bagley, 1969).

Neurotic disorders

Post-traumatic neuroses form the largest group of complications and consist of the full range of neurotic symptoms including depression anxiety and obsessional reactions, impaired concentration, and a prominence of somatic complaints especially headache, giddiness and fatiguability. Psychogenic factors either predating or relating to the situation of the head injury are often of major significance while frequently there is a history of premorbid personality difficulties (Fahey *et al.*, 1967). There is usually little evidence of severe head injury especially in those whose symptoms are of long standing.

It is perhaps presumptive to include within this category the clearly recognized 'post-traumatic syndrome'. However, many of the symptoms occur with notable excess in association with compensation issues, and usually follow milder degrees of head injury (Miller, 1961). The clinical features consist of dizziness, intolerance of noise, impaired concentration and irritability. It is possible that in the early post-traumatic period many of the symptoms do have an organic basis but these persist in those individuals whose personalities are more vulnerable and perhaps condition readily to the rewards of illness (Lishman, 1973; Rutherford *et al.*, 1977).

Psychiatric aspects of epilepsy

The prevalence of epilepsy among psychiatric patients is much higher than that found in the normal population (0·6%) and in different countries between 3–10% of all psychiatric admissions have epilepsy (Slater and Roth, 1969). This association appears to be due to one of two mechanisms. In some patients both the mental disturbance and epilepsy are derived from a common underlying pathology such as neuronal degeneration or a tumour, and among the severely mentally handicapped, where the prevalence of epilepsy is approximately 20%, this is the principal relationship. In a second group the fits themselves may either directly or indirectly be the cause of mental disturbance and thus contribute to the higher rate of mental illness found in patients with epilepsy (Pond and Bidwell, 1960). However, epilepsy rarely occurs as an isolated problem and therefore the effects of other variables need to be taken into consideration before concluding that seizures are a direct cause of mental disturbance. Important variables related to epilepsy are the presence of underlying brain damage and current anticonvulsant therapy while more independent factors include the constitutional predisposition and underlying personality of the affected individual, together with complex psychosocial interactions. Most early studies failed to make proper allowance for these issues, giving rise to such erroneous concepts as 'the epileptic personality', a stereotype for those suffering from epilepsy (Tizard, 1962). For example, in a child population study Rutter *et al.* (1970) observed a high incidence of social rejection and broken homes among children with epilepsy and there was also a significantly higher incidence of physical handicaps, intellectual and language impairment. Nevertheless, the presence of epilepsy does appear to render the affected individual more vulnerable to psychological stress and deprivation. In addition there are a few direct associations between certain psychiatric syndromes and some epileptic features. These relationships can conveniently be considered first for problems related to the seizure itself and occurring in the peri-ictal period, and for problems arising in the inter-ictal period and not directly related to any seizure.

Peri-ictal problems

Focal epilepsy, especially those arising from deep temporal and frontal lobe structures often give rise to complex symptomatology which although possibly of important localizing value may, in the absence of true *grand mal* features, lead to diagnostic confusion with abnormal emotional states, psychoses and behaviour disorder. The spontaneous and episodic nature of the attacks and the presence of associated confusion should help differentiate psychomotor seizures from other clinical states. Individual symptoms have been discussed earlier. Among children brief absences may be misinterpreted as day-dreaming or inattentiveness while others having frequent paroxysmal discharges may show impairment of cognitive performance. Falling down attacks can give rise to diagnostic difficulties between hysterical dissociation states and akinetic seizures, but the latter are usually associated with other types of seizure disorder especially *grand mal* epilepsy. Such attacks also need to be differentiated from vertebro-basilar ischaemia in older adults, faints, and more rarely hypoglycaemia. Behavioural automatisms consisting of apparently purposeful but inappropriate behaviour, for example, searching or undressing, may occur as a feature of some focal seizures usually of temporal or frontal lobe origin, and also as part of any post-ictal confusional state (Fenton, 1972). Both the complexity of such behaviour and the fact that it can persist for several minutes has led to much speculation as to the possible epileptic basis of episodic behaviour disturbances including outbursts of violence or temper ('epileptic equivalents'). Nevertheless, violent behaviour in relation to seizures appears to be very rare indeed, and in a national study of 190 patients with epilepsy in prisons and borstals only two showed any convincing evidence of automatic behaviour that might have been responsible for their crime (Gunn and Fenton, 1971). In the great majority of episodic behaviour disturbances no convincing evidence of epilepsy is usually to be found while a careful psychosocial appraisal generally provides a reasonable explanation. Both true fits and hysterical attacks may co-exist especially in the young and those with emotional or interpersonal difficulties.

The inter-ictal period

The effect of epileptic attacks on intellect is generally much less than constitutional endowment or underlying brain damage, but in some individuals it may contribute together with the effects of anticonvulsant medication (Pond, 1974). Although uncomplicated epilepsy usually does not cause any obvious impairment of intellect (Rutter *et al.*, 1970), more severe forms including status epilepticus and hypsarrhythmia, especially in the first two years of life, have been reported as principal causes of severe mental retardation in about 4% of severely handicapped children, and Chaudhry and Pond (1961) observed cognitive deterioration among brain-damaged children who had frequent seizures. Epilepsy in the severely mentally handicapped is also highly correlated with hyper-kinesis and behavioural disturbances, and is a major reason for hospital-ization rather than alternative forms of long-term care.

The hyperkinetic syndrome and rage reactions appear to occur more commonly in patients with epilepsy (8%) compared with the normal population, and are especially associated with temporal lobe epilepsy (Ounsted et al., 1966). Both may ultimately be derived from the same common source of severe childhood status or brain damage leading to impairment of temporal lobe functions while secondary intellectual impairment may also play a significant part in these behaviour disorders (Werry, 1968).

The classical description of the epileptic personality as 'languid, spirit-less, slow and sticky' has not stood the test of more careful and systematic enquiry. However, there is some evidence that the incidence of personal-ity disturbances may be higher among patients with epilepsy (Tizard, 1962), with possible relationships existing between the type of epilepsy and the form of personality disturbance. Aggressiveness appears to be over-represented in patients with focal temporal lobe epilepsy while generalized spike and wave discharges have been observed more com-monly in association with neurotic disorder (Serafetinides, 1965). Again other variables, such as age of onset of seizures, may be critical for in a study of patients with temporal lobe epilepsy in which no excess of mental disturbances was observed, the mean age of onset was consider-ably higher than in studies in which psychiatric problems have been reported (Currie et al., 1971). Parental reactions to fits including rejection and overprotection, the effects of poorly controlled seizures on schooling, and the wider social response of the community may ultimately create an unsatisfactory psychological environment for normal personality development. When seizures are severe enough to cause educational problems the prognosis is usually not good, with many so affected con-tributing to the hard-core of young adults with a poor employment record and mental disorder (Pond and Bidwell, 1960).

There is an association between epilepsy and psychotic disturbances usually of a schizophreniform type especially in those with temporal lobe epilepsy. These psychoses generally lack the usual features of constitu-tional loading such as a positive family history and schizoid personality, and usually occur several years after the onset of epilepsy (Slater et al., 1963). There is additional evidence that the reactions are more commonly associated with epileptic discharges arising from the dominant hemisphere. These features suggest a common origin for the epilepsy and behaviour disturbances in a damaged temporal lobe. However, a more complex interaction may exist for an inverse relationship between the frequency of seizures and the presence of psychotic behaviour has been reported (Flor-Henry, 1976).

Clinical evaluation of organic mental states

Initial assessment

Although the clinical problem will vary considerably from patient to patient several clear stages or levels of evaluation are common to most. The first is the differentiation between functional and organic conditions and if the latter is suspected then one's ultimate goal is the pursuit of the underlying pathology. As initial psychiatric assessment involves the acquisition of much information from many aspects of the patient's current life situation and mental state, there is therefore a great need for simple reliable and rapid screening procedure for 'organicity'. Certain features should heighten one's suspicions of underlying physical pathology and in particular cognitive skills (coping ability, attention, orientation, memory, grasp) should be routinely assessed in all cases as it is in this area of mental functioning that differentiation between organic and functional states can be made.

Deterioration in the patient's coping skills at work or in his social competence, while not being specific to organic states, will nevertheless often provide early clues to impaired cognitive function. The patient's attention, how it has to be elicited and how distractable he is, will be evident from the general tone of the interview. Concentration can be assessed more formally by simple tasks such as the months of the year in reverse order or serial computation of numbers, due allowance being made for the patient's native intelligence. Reasons for any difficulties, manifested as delays or errors, should be sought. The patient's sense of time is a very sensitive parameter of organic disease with its dependence upon intact memory, grasp and consciousness, while disorientation for persons and places can usually be found in established dementia. Systematic enquiry should be made for recent memory difficulties, for example need to keep notes as reminders, and recent memory can usefully be assessed by giving the patient a small amount of data to remember, such as a name and address. Once the data has been acquired (tested by immediate recall) the number of errors found after delayed recall (three to five minutes of intervening questioning), gives a crude measure of impairment. Deterioration of grasp and intellect may be evident from alteration in work performance or discrepancies between usual work level and present grasp of current affairs, general knowledge, or in the definition of some proverbs. A more thorough assessment can be obtained from the Mill Hill and Progressive Matrices which can be administered by a nurse.

Other features while not specific to organic disease should nevertheless alert one to the possibility of an underlying physical basis. They can be usefully considered under the global heading of personality change. The patient may present with complaints of difficulty in concentration at work or a relative or spouse may report some alteration in behaviour or personality. During interview, slowness and perseveration may be manifest while affective changes more commonly found in association with organic disease are fluctuations in mood and fearfulness (associated in particular with acute organic reactions), lability, euphoria, shallowness, blunting, apathy and a tendency to over-react with aggression, irritability or anxiety (especially in the chronic organic reactions). Disturbances in interest and drive are much more difficult to assess but nevertheless those more frequently found in organically induced states include impulsiveness, indifference, apathy, loss of spontaneity, aimlessness, fatigue, restlessness or a reversal of sleep pattern with restlessness at night and somnolence during the day. There may be loss of social control with disinhibition or a loss of sensitivity. Paranoid ideas, ideas of reference, hallucinations especially of a visual modality are also common in organic states. Neurotic and psychotic symptoms arising *de novo* in late adult life and in the absence of obvious stresses should also lower one's threshold to a search for physical pathology.

Definitive evaluation

If some of the foregoing symptoms are elicited in the course of initial psychiatric assessment then there is a need for a thorough search for organic factors as potential major contributors to the presenting problems. The next level of investigation is therefore addressed to the questions 'Is there major cerebral dysfunction indicative of physical pathology?', 'Is the dysfunction of a diffuse or focal nature?'. These questions can best be answered by three parallel lines of investigation, namely detailed clinical evaluation, psychometric evaluation and electroencephalography.

Clinical assessment

Clinical assessment of cognitive function should include, in addition to the general parameters (coping skills, concentration, memory and grasp) outlined above, a careful scrutiny for evidence of focal deficit, namely amnesia, aphasia, agnosia, apraxia. It is also usually convenient at this stage for the clinician to attune his perceptual set to the third level of enquiry, the search for specific pathology.

The rate of onset of an organic state differentiates several groups, with a slow insidious onset characteristic of most of the degenerations especially senile dementia and a more rapid onset typical of tumours. An abrupt onset and stepwise course is characteristic of cardio-vascular disease while a fluctuating course is found with many systemic disorders producing an acute organic reaction. Brief transient acute episodes suggest either epilepsy, cardio-vascular disease, hypoglycaemia or drug abuse.

Thorough physical assessment is essential in all cases. A family history of dementia, Huntington's chorea or epilepsy may be relevant. In the past medical history, head injury, alcoholism or arterio-sclerosis may be important in themselves or point to a subsequent subdural haematoma, while normal pressure hydrocephalus may result from earlier meningitis, subarachnoid haemorrhage or previous head injury. In recent history, falls or blackouts may point to epilepsy, cerebro-vascular disease, syncope, or hypoglycaemia. General health also needs to be evaluated and such non-specific changes as malaise, weight loss or anorexia may indicate underlying anaemia, uraemia, neoplastic disease, metabolic disorder or infection such as cystitis or pneumonia. Dietary indiscretions and current medication may all have a bearing on the present problems. On physical examination the presence of raised intracranial pressure with headache, visual disturbance and vomiting, suggest a space occupying lesion while focal lesions generally produce focal neurological deficit or focal fits. The pupillary abnormalities of GPI, nystagmus of drug intoxication and the extra-ocular palsies of Wernicke's encephalopathy provide important diagnostic clues. Other common neurological signs of intracerebral disease among psychiatric patients include choreaform movements, incoordination, dysarthria or ataxia, evidence of peripheral neuropathy and incontinence of urine. Low grade pyrexia is suggestive of sub-acute encephalitis, a cerebral abscess or possibly an embolus from a sub-acute bacterial entercarditis. Cardio-respiratory status and liver function need to be carefully assessed, and evidence of carcinoma sought from examination of breasts, axilla, rectum and vagina.

Psychological testing

Psychologists have long been concerned with mental illness and have regarded psychiatric diagnostic labels as fundamentally important to the scientific analysis of both mental abnormality and intellectual ability. In particular, brain damage and intellectual functioning have been inextricably bound up with assessment problems in clinical psychology. In interpreting results of psychological tests one must guard against the assumption that intellectual impairment is a unique feature of brain damage for cognitive impairment is common to several mental conditions (Savage, 1974). This has been compounded by the difficulties of providing satisfactory external criteria of brain damage, the instability of psychiatric diagnosis and the lack of suitable age–sex matched normative data for the many specific tests. The Wechsler Deterioration Indices are perhaps the most widely used measures of organic impairment. 'In general, the gradual falling off of ability in later age may be considered as an indication of normal decline; a marked and disabling loss, at any age, as a sign of definite impairment' (Wechsler, 1958). One major problem, however, is the assessment of *previous* cognitive level. It was noted that the age curves of the subtests in the Weschler Adult Intelligence Scale (WAIS) decline at different rates so that deterioration could be assessed by comparing 'slowly' declining abilities using Hold Tests (information, vocabulary, object assembly and picture completion) with abilities which declined 'quickly' using Don't Hold Tests (Digit Span, Similarities, Digit Symbol and Block Design). Experience with the WAIS suggests that verbal abilities are more resistant to impairment than performance and that a discrepancy of greater than 20 points between the two scales is a statistically significant indication of organic impairment. Nevertheless results should be interpreted in conjunction with other psychological measures of brain damage.

Available evidence suggests that performance on verbal-learning tests is significantly impaired by brain damage. Two useful and frequently used tests are The Modified Word Learning Test and The Paired Associate Learning Test. Perceptual and motor-perceptual assessment techniques have also been used to diagnose organic disorders. Among the most useful and best standardized are The Minnesota Percepto-Diagnostic Test, The Benton Visual Retention Test, Graham-Kendall Memory for Designs Test, The Trail Making Test, and the Halstead Category Test (see Savage, 1974, for review of recent evaluations of these tests).

As some intellectual functions appear to be localized within one of the cerebral hemispheres, use has been made of the fact that some psychological tests focus on these specific skills to localize aeas of brain damage. In general verbal capacity is better than performance in patients with right hemisphere lesions and it is generally assumed that marked discrepancies between verbal and performance on the WAIS in favour of verbal capacity is not only characteristic of diffuse cerebral pathology but may also be indicative of pathology in the right hemisphere. The reverse pattern (Performance IQ greater than Variable IQ) differentially characterizes left hemisphere disturbance. The Halstead Category Test, in which the subject is presented with a series of pictures projected on to a screen and asked to press one of four possible levers according to four possible concepts linking the pictures (colour, shape, etc.), is thought to be particularly sensitive to frontal lobe dysfunction. The Rey-Osterreth Test which involves copying and recall of a design is differentially sensitive to right temporal lesions while tests such as visual naming and word fluency assess dominant (usually left) fronto-temporal function. Psychological tests are usually inappropriate if there is any significant element of impairment of consciousness.

Electroencephalography

Clinical electroencephalography can be of considerable value in the investigation of patients presenting with mental illness of suspected organic origin, and usually helps to answer the following questions:

Is there supportive evidence for an organic basis for the patient's symptoms?

Is the observed organic function diffuse or localized?

What pathology is most likely to account for these dangers?

Is there supportive evidence for a diagnosis of epilepsy?

However, in considering such problems it is necessary to remember that the EEG itself does not demonstrate cerebral anatomy or pathology; it is at best a reflection of brain function or dysfunction and the answers to clinical questions must be sought from an interpretation of the distortions of normal activities or super-added features (McClelland and Binnie, 1977). To make sense of the information provided by an EEG analysis therefore it is necessary to be familiar with the range of normal features. Since Berger's original description (Berger, 1929) it has generally been assumed that the EEG signals arise from the electrical activity of cells in the cerebral cortex and the consensus of evidence to date would suggest its origin from the averaged effect of numerous post-synaptic potentials recurring on the dendrites of the large superficial pyramidal cells of the cerebral cortex. Several cortical isolation experiments have demonstrated that synchronization of these cells depends upon input from sub-cortical sources. So the scalp-recorded EEG is a function of both superficial pyramidal cells and these distant, principally mid-line, nuclear groups.

By the age of 20–25 years the characteristics of an individual's EEG have become more or less stable and will remain so in health until old age. At this time the only activity of prominence in the resting but awake state is rhythmic and continuous, occupying a frequency band of 0·5–60 Hz, and of 10–100 microvolts (mV) peak to peak in amplitude. In the majority of adult EEGs the most prominent rhythm occurs mainly over the posterior half of the scalp, especially in the parieto-occipital region at 8–13 Hz. This 'alpha rhythm' is usually present when the eyes are closed and is attenuated during attention especially on opening the eyes. In most subjects the alpha rhythm remains fairly stable varying at most by ± 0·5 Hz. Fast activity (beta), above 13·5 Hz is sometimes found distributed in the precentral regions while small amounts of slower activity (theta) at 4–7·5 Hz, and 'delta' below 4 Hz are occasionally seen in the alert state.

Two physiological variables, age of subject and state of awareness, have a profound effect on the features of the EEG. When an adult becomes drowsy the first indication in the EEG is usually of a reduction of muscle potentials accompanied by an increase in slow undulating movements of the eyeballs which produce slow fluctuating potentials seen in the frontal electrodes. Associated with this the alpha rhythm usually becomes less continuous and as light sleep is entered this rhythm diminishes rapidly to be replaced by mixed frequency activity in the 2–7 Hz range. At this stage sensory stimulation evokes monophasic electronegative discharges mainly seen at the vertex. As the sleep state deepens bursts of 12–14 Hz spindle activity appear bilaterally usually in the fronto-central region and stimulation usually evokes complex high amplitude bi-or triphasic slow waves, again in the fronto-central region. In deep sleep, slow wave activity is prominent and often of large amplitude (over 70 mV). During continuous recording of natural sleep a further stage can be identified; paradoxically while the patient is in deep sleep, the EEG becomes typical of light sleep and there are associated rapid eye movements (REM sleep). Many EEG phenomena which may be of clinical diagnostic importance are influenced by state of awareness so that EEGs are therefore often recorded under conditions of natural or drug induced sleep.

The second physiological parameter which must be considered is the age of the subject. From birth to adult life there are characteristic changes in the frequency of dominant rhythm, although there is a great variability both within and between subjects, a variability which itself decreases with a maturation. In the neonate two main EEG patterns have been recognized, the first is seen mainly in light sleep and the awake state when the record is of low voltage of variable frequencies less than 7 Hz and having a fairly diffuse distribution (activité moyenne). During deeper sleep characteristic bursts of 1–3 Hz activity and of large voltage (50–100 mV) are seen (activité alternans). In the 3–12 month period more monorhythmic activity appears first in the central region at 5–8 Hz and by 5 months occipital activity appears first at about 3–4 Hz and of about 50 mV in amplitude. This posteriorly distributed rhythm gradually increases in frequency with age to become the adult alpha rhythm reaching a maximum amplitude around 10–12 years of age. Subsequent maturational changes include a slight diminution in the power and variability of the record and in the amount of activity outside the alpha band. From about the age of 60, there is often a slight slowing of the alpha rhythm or a reduction in its amplitude, and slow wave forms often appear.

In view of the nature of the EEG it is perhaps not surprising that the features seen in association with organic disease are more a reflection of the location, distribution and rate of development of pathology and less as characteristics or unique features of specific pathologies.

As mentioned above conditions causing an acute organic reaction in the main have a widespread effect on cerebral function, although perhaps the central pathophysiological mechanism lies on a common alteration of function within midline structures. Changes shown in the EEG are quite characteristic and may even precede the onset of clinically detectable confusion. In general there is first a decrease in the frequency and responsiveness of the alpha rhythm which may progress to more severe disturbances including increased amounts of activity at slower frequencies in both the theta and delta ranges. Changes are usually quite diffuse and symmetrical throughout the EEG especially when the causes are extracerebral, for example metabolic or toxic disorders. Primary intracerebral pathologies usually produce additional features at some stage and these will depend on the distribution (focal or diffuse), location if focal, and to some extent on the nature of the underlying pathology. Again widespread EEG abnormalities are characteristic of diffuse cerebral disease, for example encephalitis such as sub-acute sclerosing panencephalitis in which one pathognomonic feature includes bilaterally synchronous paroxysmal discharges (period ranging from 1 to 13 seconds).

In the senile and pre-senile dementias the pathology underlying is again usually of a diffuse nature and consequently the EEG changes are also diffuse. There is usually a slowing of the alpha rhythm which may be reduced in amplitude, while diffuse beta activity sometimes with slow components may become prominent. In more severe cases the alpha rhythm may disappear entirely with the dominant activity falling within the theta range. However, the EEG may be surprisingly normal even in the presence of clinically evident dementia (Levy, 1969). Again some pathognomonic features may be seen, e.g. the marked absence of all rhythmic activity in Huntington's chorea or periodic complexes at 1–2 Hz seen in Creutzfeldt-Jacob Disease.

As mentioned earlier, the full spectrum of psychiatric symptoms and especially organic personality change, the acute or chronic organic reactions or a focal syndrome may be produced by a strategically placed focal intracerebral lesion, the most common being of neoplastic or vascular origin. A normal EEG is relatively uncommon with discrete cerebral pathology causing symptoms although again this picture will depend on the location of the abnormality and its time course, the scalp-recorded EEG being less commonly affected by lesions of the posterior fossa or with chronic minor or non-progressive pathology. In the case of a space occupying mass the presence of localized delta accompanied by depression of normal background activities at the same site usually provide the best localizing signs. Alterations of background activity in isolation, while less reliable as localizing signs, may provide vital clues to the presence of primary intracerebral pathology. These include asymmetries both of the amplitude and the frequency of background rhythm (Driver, 1970). Although the brain often reacts with similar responses to different influences, occasionally differentiation between pathologies can be made. For example, it has been observed that ischaemic disorders affecting the territory of the middle cerebral artery tend to produce more strictly unilateral EEG changes than space occupying lesions in this region (Van der Drift and Magnus, 1961). Temporal changes from serial EEGs provide a further help in the differientiation of pathologies, for example, gradual improvement following a cerebral vascular accident contrasting with the deteriorating changes associated with progressive cerebral disease such as a tumour.

The EEG has probably been found to be of greatest value in the study of the many and varied manifestations of epilepsy. Though no EEG feature alone is sufficient to make a diagnosis in the absence of clinical seizures, 'paroxysmal high voltage electrical potentials of almost any form or frequency may be considered epileptic from the EEG point of view' (Penfield and Jasper, 1954), the most important from the diagnostic point of view being sharp waves, spikes and spike and wave complexes. The EEG can be of great value in the analysis of complex symptomatology such as episodic posturing or hallucinatory phenomena compatible with alternative psychiatric diagnosis.

Characteristic EEG phenomena occur during fits and in the inter-seizure period and for this reason the classification of the epilepsy has increasingly become an electro-clinical classification (Gastaut, 1970). One major sub-category of the epilepsies are the primary generalized seizures in which some form of bilaterally synchronous rhythmic activity in the form of spikes or spike and wave complexes are seen in the EEG (*petit mal*, primary, generalized epilepsy). The second major sub-category are the focal epilepsies in which there is either clinical or neurophysiological evidence of focal onset. Important EEG features include the inter-ictal spike focus and the ictal focal spike or slow wave rhythm which may be of diagnostic value in localizing the lesion responsible for the epilepsy (Driver, 1970).

Special investigations

Although the many disease processes (see Table I) which may alter behaviour and mental life often have a few distinctive features such as the temporal pattern or specific accompanying neurological or physical signs, the final diagnosis can often only be reached after some physical or biochemical investigation. Primary intracerebral pathology may be

Table I   *Causes of organic reactions*

Intracerebral

Epilepsy

Degenerations:	Senile degeneration
	Alzheimer's disease
	Pick's disease
	Huntington's chorea
	Creutzfeldt-Jakob disease

Neoplasms:	Primary growths
	Secondaries
Infections:	Encephalitis
	Abscess
	Syphilis
	Parasites

Physical:	Trauma
	Space occupying lesions:
	neoplasm, abscess, subdural haematoma, intracerebral haematoma, parasites, hydrocephalus.

| Vascular: | Ischaemia, infarction, haemorrhage; causes: atherosclerosis, hypertension, embolism, SLE. |

Extracerebral

| Anoxic | Hypotension, heart failure, cardiac arrhythmias, anaemia, CO poisoning, respiratory failure. |

Nutritional and Metabolic:	Vit. B group deficiencies, vit. B12 and folic acid deficiencies.
	Diabetes, hypoglycaemia, hypothyroidism, hypo- and hyper-parathyroidism, steroid excess or deficiencies.
	Electrolyte imbalance, porphyria.
	Renal failure, liver failure.

Toxic:	Alcohol and drugs—intoxication and withdrawal.
	Metal poisoning, and other chemicals inorganic and organic.
	Systemic infections.

confirmed by the presence of an abnormal skull X-ray with pineal shift or bony erosion, while the ESR, haematology, Wasserman Reaction (or VDRL) and chest X-ray provide an important screen for systemic disorder.

Acute organic reactions and focal syndromes in all age groups and chronic reactions especially in younger people may require a more thorough search for remediable causes. Metabolic tests include assessment of plasma proteins, liver and renal function tests, urea, electrolytes, (including calcium, phosphate, bicarbonate), blood sugar, vitamin B12 and folic acid, thyroid function and evidence of porphyria. Drug abuse may be a problem in younger people and urinary estimations of the more common varieties especially barbiturates may be carried out. An ECG should also be considered. If a primary intracerebral lesion is still under suspicion, lumbar puncture may be of help when CSF, WR and Lange curve should be carried out together with protein and electrolyte estimation; cell culture may provide evidence of infection, degeneration or tumour. A gamma scan is a useful non-invasive test but ultimately cerebral angiography is essential for diagnosing and localizing a cerebral tumour or subdural haematoma. It is also the most direct way of demonstrating disease of the cerebral blood vessels. Airencephalography may provide evidence of normal pressure hydrocephalus, a focal space occupying lesion or confirm, in a younger person, that a dementia is in fact due to some diffuse degenerative process.

Computer assisted tomography (EMI scanner) promises to be a most useful aid in the investigation of suspected intracerebral pathology. The unique power of this scanner resides in a fine collimated X-ray beam and a system of crystal detectors which permit the resolution of serial sections of tissue into a fine matrix on the basis of relative absorption of photons. Recent evidence suggests that the EMI scanner as a single test provides accuracy of localization comparable with the sum total of conventional contrast radiographic procedures while having the added advantage of being essentially non-invasive. To date the majority of reliability studies have been based on the investigation of cases with well established pathology so its role in the prodromal stages of primary intracerebral disease remains to be seen. However, in established organic states the technique has been used successfully to differentiate between diffuse intracerebral pathology such as Alzheimer's disease, hydrocephalus, vascular disease, intracerebral haemorrhage and neoplasms (Ambrose et al., 1975).

Finally, in this search for remediable or treatable factors the multifactorial nature of many of the 'organic' states should be considered especially in the elderly who form an increasing proportion of clinical practice. Confusion in an old person may not be the result of any single major cause but may be partly due to some specific illness and the interaction of several minor systemic problems such as pressure sores, mild congestive cardiac failure, anaemia and the like. In the dementing elderly, major psychological or social disturbances such as removal from familiar surroundings may precipitate an acute confusional state. In general, the more severe the underlying dementia the more readily will such a confusional episode arise and the less specific and obvious the precipitant (Arie, 1973).

References

Adams, R. D., Fisher, C. M., Hakim, S., Oiemann, R. G. and Sweet, W. H. (1965). Symptomatic occult hydrocephalus with 'normal' C.S.F. pressure. *New Eng. J. Med.* **273**, 117–126.

Ambrose, J., Gooding, M. R. and Richardson, A. E. (1975). An assessment of the accuracy of computerized transverse axial scanning (EMI Scanner) in the diagnosis of intra-cranial tumour. *Brain* **98**, 569–582.

Arie, T. (1973). Dementia in the elderly: management. *Br. Med. J.* **4**, 602–604.

Berger, H. (1929). Uber das Elektrenkephalogramm des Menschen. *Arch. Psychiat. Nerv Krankh.* **87**, 527.

Bird, E. D., Mackay, A. V. P., Rayner, C. N. and Iversen, L. L. (1973). Reduced glutamic acid decarboxylase activity of post mortem brain in Huntington's Chorea. *Lancet* **1**, 1090.

Birkett, D. P. (1972). The psychiatric differentiation of senility and arteriosclerosis. *Br. J. Psychiat.* **120**, 321–325.

Bleuler, M. (1951). Psychiatry of cerebral diseases. *Br. Med. J.* **2**, 1233–1238.

Brain, Lord (1962). 'Diseases of the Nervous System', p. 816. Oxford University Press, Oxford.

Brierley, J. (1966). The neuropathology of amnesia states *In* 'Amnesia' (Eds C. W. M. Whitty and O. L. Zangwill). Butterworth, London.

Butler, R. B. and Benson, D. F. (1974). Aphasia: a clinical—anatomical correlation. *Br. J. Hosp. Med.* **12**, 211–217.

Chaudhry, M. R. and Pond, D. A. (1961). Mental deterioration in epileptic children. *J. Neurol. Neurosurg. Psychiat.* **24**, 213–219

Corsellis, J. A. N. (1969). The pathology of dementia. *Br. J. Hosp. Med.* **2**, 695–703.

Curr e, S., Heathfield, K. W. G., Henson, R. A. and Scott, D. F. (1971) Clinical causes and prognosis of temporal lobe epilepsy. *Brain* **94**, 173–190.

Davison, K. and Bagley, C. (1969). Schizophrenia-like psychoses associated with organic disorders. *In* 'Current Problems in Neuropsychiatry' (Ed. R. W. Herrington). Headley Bros, Ashford, Kent.

Dewhurst, K. (1969). The neurosyphilitic psychosis today. *Br. J. Psychiat.* **115**, 31–39.

Driver, M. V. R. (1970). *In* 'Seminars on Electroencephalography' (Eds M. V. Driver, G. W. Fenton and R. Harris). Reprinted from *Proc. J. Electro-physiol. Technol. Ass.* **17**. Nos 2 and 4.

Fahey, T. J., Irving, R. H. and Millac, P. (1967). Severe head injury. *Lancet* **2**, 475–479.

Fenton, G. W. (1972). Epilepsy and automatism. *Br. J. Hosp. Med.* **7**, 57–64.

Flor-Henry, P. (1976). Epilepsy and psychopathology. In 'Recent Advances in Clinical Psychiatry' (Ed. K. Granville-Grossman). Churchill Livingstone, Edinburgh.

Gastaut, H. (1970). Clinical and EEG classification of epileptic seizures. Epilepsia 11, 102–113, 114–119.

Gibbs, C. J., Jnr., and Gajdusek, D. C. (1969). Infection as the etiology of spongiform encephalopathy. Science 165, 1023–1025.

Goldstein, K. (1952). The effect of brain damage on personality. Psychiatry 15, 245–260.

Gunn, J. and Fenton, G. (1971). Epilepsy, automatism and crime. Lancet 1, 1173–1176.

Hecan, H. and Ajuriaguerra, J. de. (1956). 'Troubles Mentaux Cours des Tumeurs Intracraniennes'. Massen, Paris.

Herr dge, C. F. (1960). Physical disorders in psychiatric illness. Lancet 2, 949–951.

Jennett, B. (1975). Head injuries. Medicine 32, 1873–1884.

Kay, D. W., Beamish, P. and Roth, M. (1964). Old age mental disorders in Newcastle-upon-Tyne. Br. J. Psychiat. 110, 146–158.

Kendell, R. E. (1974). A new look at hysteria. Medicine 11, 1780–1782.

Levy, R. (1969). The neurophysiology of dementia. Br. J. Hosp. Med. 2, 688–690.

Lewin, W. (1968). Rehabilitation after head-injury. Br. Med. J. 1, 465–470.

Lishman, W. A. (1968). Brain damage in relation to psychiatric disability after head injury. Br. J. Psychiat. 113, 373–410.

Lishman, W. A. (1973). The psychiatric sequelae of head injury. Psychol. Med. 3, 304–318.

Lishman, W. A. (1978). 'Organic Psychiatry'. Blackwell, Oxford.

McClelland, R. J. and Binnie, C. D. (1977). Techniques and instrumentation in clinical neurophysiology. In 'Physical Techniques in Medicine' (Ed. J. McMullan) Vol. I. Wiley, Chichester.

Miller, H. (1961). Accident neurosis. Br. Med. J. 1, 919–925, 992–998.

Oliver, J. E. (1970). Huntington's Chorea in Northamptonshire. Br. J. Psychiat. 116, 241–253.

Ounsted, C., Lindasy, J. and Norman, R. (1966). 'Biological Factors in Temporal Lobe Epilepsy'. Clinics in Developmental Medicine No. 22. Heinemann, London.

Paillas, J. E., Paillas, N. and Bureau, M. (1972). Post-traumatic epilepsy. Epilepsia 11, 5–15.

Penfield,W. and Jasper, H. (1954). 'Epilepsy and the Functional Anatomy of the Human Brain'. J. and A. Churchill, London.

Pond, D. A. (1974). Children with epilepsy. Teach-In, 416–420.

Pond, D. A. and Bidwell, B. H. (1960). A survey of epilepsy in 14 general practices. Epilepsia 1, 285–299.

Potter, J. M. (1969). Herpes simplex encephalitis—clinical aspects. In 'Virus Diseases and the Nervous System' (Eds C. W. N. Whitty, J. J. Hughes and F. O. MacCallum). Blackwell, Oxford.

Rice, E. and Gendelman, S. (1973). Psychiatric aspects of normal pressure hydrocephalus. J. Am. Med. Ass. 233, 409–412.

Roth, M. (1971). Classification and aetiology in mental disorder of old age. In 'Recent Developments in Psychogeriatrics' (Eds D. W. K. Kay and A. Walk). Br. J. Psychiat. Special Publication No. 6.

Roth, M. and Myers, D. H. (1969). The diagnosis of dementia. Br. J. Hosp. Med.2, 705–717.

Rutherford, W. H., Merrett, J. D. and McDonald, J. R. (1977). Sequelae of concussion caused by minor head injuries. *Lancet* i, 1–4.

Rutter, M., Graham, P. and Yule, W. (1970). 'A Neuropsychiatric Study in Childhood'. Clinics in Developmental Medicine Nos 35/36. Heinemann, London.

Savage, R. D. (1974). Intellectual assessment. *In* 'The Psychological Assessment of Mental and Physical Handicaps' (Ed. P. Mittler). Tavistock, London.

Serafetinides, E. A. (1965). Aggressiveness in temporal lobe epileptics and its relation to cerebral dysfunction and environmental factors. *Epilepsia* 6, 33–42.

Shulman, R. (1967). A survey of vitamin B 12 deficiency in an elderly psychiatric population. *Br. J. Psychiat.* 113, 241–256.

Sim, M. and Sussman, I. (1962). Alzheimer's Disease: its natural history and differential diagnosis. *J. Nerv. Ment. Dis.* 135, 489–499.

Slater, E. and Roth, M. (1969). 'Clinical Psychiatry', p. 450. Bailliere, Tindall and Cassell, London.

Slater, E., Beard, A. and Glithero, E. (1963). Schizophrenia-like psychoses of epilepsy. *Br. J. Psychiat.* 109, 95–150.

Tizard, B. (1962). The personality of epileptics: a discussion of the evidence. *Psychol. Bull.* 59, 196–210.

Van der Drift, J. H. A., and Magnus, O. (1961). bintra-cranial haemorrhage. *In* 'Electro-encephalography and Cerebral Tumours' (Eds O. Magnus, W. Strom Van Leeuwen and W. A. Cobb), pp. 141–159. Elsevier, Amsterdam.

Warrington, E. K. (1974). Neurological deficits. *In* 'The Psychological Assessment of Mental and Physical Handicaps' (Ed. P. Mittler). Tavistock, London.

Wechsler, D. (1958). 'The Measurement and Appraisal of Adult Intelligence' (4th edn). Williams and Wilkins, Baltimore.

Werry, J. (1968). Developmental hyperactivity. *Paediat. Clin. N. America.* 15, 581–599.

Whitty, C. W. M., Hughes, J. T. and MacCallum, F. O. (Eds). (1969). 'Virus Diseases and the Nervous System'. Blackwell, Oxford.

Wolff, H. G. and Curran, D. (1935). The nature of delirium, and allied states. *Archs Neurol. Psychiat.* 33, 1175–1215.

Wolstenholme, G. E. W. and O'Connor, M. (Eds) (1970) 'Alzheimer's Disease and Related Conditions', Ciba Foundation Symposium. Churchill, London.

14 The psychiatry of old age
I General principles and functional disorders

Peter M. Jefferys, Robin Jacoby and Robin Murray

Over the past twenty years several distinguished British psychiatrists, of whom Felix Post and Martin Roth are the best known, have maintained a major interest in the psychiatric illnesses of the elderly. Their interest and enthusiasm has provided a substantial framework of clinical and epidemiological findings concerning the psychiatry of old age (Roth, 1955; Roth *et al.*, 1967; Post, 1962, 1965). Nosological issues have been clarified, the organic psychoses better understood, and links with the psychiatry of younger age groups established. Workers from a variety of disciplines including neuropathologists (Corsellis, 1962), geriatricians (Isaacs, 1971), behavioural scientists and social workers (Goldberg *et al.*, 1970) have shared in the progress and Health Service planners have become more aware of the needs of the elderly with psychiatric illness (Brothwood, 1971).

There has been an unfortunate lack of agreement about the meaning of the term *psychogeriatrics*. Although most psychiatrists working in this area use the word to refer to the assessment, treatment and management of elderly people suffering all kinds of mental disorders, some use the term only in reference to confused old people, and others where mental and physical disease occur simultaneously. Because of the potential for misunderstanding we prefer the term 'the psychiatry of old age'.

The size of the problem. The number of elderly people in developed countries has increased substantially in recent years, and in Western Europe approximately 13% to 16% of the population are now aged 65 and over. In the United Kingdom there are more than $7\frac{1}{2}$ million people at least 65 years old, a third of them 75 years and over, and further large increases are projected. The elderly show high physical, social and psychiatric morbidity and consequently have heavy demands on health and social services (Roth, 1973).

In Britain this is reflected in the increase with age of mental hospital admission rates. The number and proportion of chronic confused elderly cared for in psychiatric hospitals, geriatric hospitals and local authority homes increases each year (Isaacs, 1971; Kay *et al.*, 1962). To obtain a true picture of the extent of psychiatric disorder within the community, surveys have been done in several European countries with impressively similar findings (Kay *et al.*, 1964). In summary, it may be said that approximately 5% of the elderly have severe psychosyndromes, 5% mild or early psychosyndromes, 3% have major functional psychoses, and 10% have neurotic and character disorders.

Perhaps surprisingly only 5% of the total elderly are in institutions. In their survey Kay *et al.* (1964) found that half of all the cases of dementia had progressed to a severity equal to that found in demented hospital patients, yet fewer than one-fifth were in hospital; and of the cases of depressive illness, the majority were not receiving any form of psychiatric treatment. The latter finding emphasizes the scope that exists for improving recognition of undisclosed mental illness among this age group.

Psychiatric services for the elderly

As the number of old people with psychiatric problems has increased, so has their need for specialized services (Brothwood, 1971). In Britain a number of psychiatrists have been appointed with a special interest in or responsibility for the elderly, and have organized or developed psychiatric services for the elderly in their districts. The patterns of services in different areas show considerable variety (Donovan *et al.*, 1971), reflecting variations both in demand and resources as well as contrasting strategies (Kushlik and Blunden, 1974; Baker and Byrne, 1977). Arie (1970), however, has proposed some sound and sensible guidelines which are as follows: Availability, Flexibility, Assessment, Good Communications and Responsibility. These are largely self-explanatory and need only slight amplification.

'Availability' is essential for the not uncommon crises, and means not only coping with the crisis on hand, but also preventing others by foresight and early intervention. 'Flexibility' reflects the need for doctors to co-operate with other disciplines including the social, community and nursing services. Indeed, the psychiatrist who wants to provide a high quality of care for the elderly is very dependent on the skills, resources and goodwill of such agencies. From this follows 'Good Communication'. Many paramedical personnel (nurses, social workers, occupational therapists and home wardens) can feel very isolated and overburdened, especially when coping with demanding, elderly sick people. If they are given the opportunity to provide information for and accept information and guidance from others in the service, they will clearly cope better. Conversely, poor communication leads to resentment and inefficiency. 'Responsibility' implies a commitment to the community, and a need for the service to constantly re-examine and if necessary alter its approaches in the light of experience.

The facilities for a comprehensive service will now be reviewed. The principle of flexibility should, however, be borne constantly in mind; elderly patients should be cared for in the place most suitable for each individual. Thus, some patients may be treated at home with the help of social agencies and community nursing services as well as by the medical profession. A patient able to live at home may benefit from attendance at a local day centre or day hospital. In-patient care may benefit not only the patient, but can be used to provide holiday relief for hard-pressed relatives.

1 *In-patient facilities*. Acute admission and assessment beds are required for the elderly with functional disorders and with confusional illnesses. Current guidelines from the Department of Health (1975) suggest that a district of 200,000 population should have up to 20 beds for the elderly with functional illness, and 10–14 assessment beds for the acutely confused under geriatric and psychiatric supervision. There is continuing debate about the merits of segregating the elderly from the younger mentally ill (Jolly and Arie, 1976), and local geography and ward design can be crucially important.

The elderly with severe dementia requiring long-term psychiatric hospital care because of behaviour disturbance in the absence of significant physical disability are mostly placed in mental hospitals at present. The Department of Health suggests 60–80 beds for a district of 200,000 people. However, the actual number of beds needed for severely demented patients depends not only on demand, but also on the availability of alternative resources such as day and residential care, geriatric provision and sheltered housing. Whatever the total, the psychiatrist responsible for elderly patients on long stay wards must recognize the crucial importance of nursing and remedial staff morale in providing humane care.

2 *Day hospitals*. Over the past decade there have been dramatic increases

in the numbers of people living at home and attending psychiatric and geriatric day centres. Day care is particularly relevant to the elderly with functional disorders, but can also provide invaluable support for families caring for a severely demented relative. The Department of Health suggest 130 day places for those with functional disorders, and 50 to 80 places for the severely mentally infirm for a population of 200,000.

3 *Primary care.* General practitioners with the support of community based nurses (health visitors and district nurses) deal with most psychiatric morbidity in the elderly living at home. Indeed, the psychiatric services would be overwhelmed if GPs referred a higher proportion of the elderly. In good practices the 'at risk' elderly are visited regularly by the doctor or a community based nurse, and the psychiatrist is available to give specialist advice to patients, relatives or members of the primary team.

4 *Local authority provision.* Local authorities have a statutory responsibility to help the elderly in a variety of ways. They provide residential homes ('part 3 accommodation') and in some areas have developed sheltered housing for the elderly. The proportion of elderly residents in local authority houses who have psychiatric problems, particularly confusion, appears to have been increasing (Kay *et al.*, 1970), thus presenting substantial difficulties to other residents and a largely untrained staff. In some places designated homes for the 'elderly mentally infirm' have been set up, but controversy exists about the value of segregating the confused (Meacher, 1972).

Social services can play an essential role in maintaining the mentally ill old person in the community. Meals on wheels and home helps are the two most available, but in some areas laundry services, regular visiting by paid or voluntary workers, and day centres are also available.

5 *Geriatric medicine.* The elderly patient under the care of a geriatrician commonly possesses multiple handicaps or disabilities, with affective disorder and confusion being particularly common (Kay *et al.*, 1970; Copeland *et al.*, 1975). Close links are, therefore, required between geriatric and psychiatric services. Some authorities have suggested the establishment of shared units known as 'Psychogeriatric Assessment Units'. Recent research (Copeland *et al.*, 1975) suggests that this is unnecessary provided that pre-admission assessment, liaison and joint consultation between the two disciplines are good. This co-operation is greatly facilitated if geriatrician and psychiatrist work in the same hospital and assessment facilities are good, with easy transfer of patients from one service to the other. The two services have to share responsibility for

severely demented people who need hospital care. Psychiatrists generally take responsibility for those with severe dementia, but not other significant physical disease (except incontinence), while geriatricians often care for the demented with other significant physical illness.

The principles of care

Assessment

The importance of careful assessment including attention to physical illness and social factors cannot be over-emphasized. Arie (1970, 1973) believes that wherever possible the initial assessment should take place in the patient's own home. While there are important benefits from this it is not always feasible. Hospital facilities are required for those too ill or disturbed to be adequately assessed at home or as out-patients. High quality assessment can often be provided in a designated admission ward where investigation facilities are concentrated, and psychiatrist, geriatrician and other staff can co-operate.

Wherever assessment is carried out an adequate history must be obtained. Since the elderly mentally ill are often unable to give a lucid history, it is vital to seek out other informants such as relatives and neighbours. This may, for instance, be the only way to distinguish between depressive pseudodementia and true dementia. Post (1971) considers that ascertaining the temporal course of the illness is of great diagnostic value:

(a) *Acute onset*. If psychiatric disorder develops within a week or two in an elderly person who until then had been living a well-adjusted existence then three conditions should be considered: acute confusional state; acute affective disorder; acute paranoid state. A diagnosis of acute confusional state is favoured by the presence of visual hallucinations, recent physical illness—even seemingly trivial chest, urinary or skin infection—and is frequently precipitated by drugs.

(b) *Indefinite onset*. When a patient presents a variety of complaints whose onset cannot be clearly defined, and which are not markedly different from his normal state, then there are two possibilities; chronic neurosis or slowly developing depression in a neurotic personality.

(c) *Gradual development*. Most elderly persons referred to a psychiatrist have a history of deteriorating mental health over the course of a few months to a couple of years. Where mood disorders or paranoid allegations were preceded by a decline in cognitive functions then a slowly developing organic-cerebral disorder is most likely. Of special diagnostic value are disorientation first noted in unaccustomed surroundings, and difficulties in daily living. Nocturnal confusion, occupational delirium, incontinence and micturition in the wrong place are almost pathognomonic of cerebral disease. On the other hand, where depressive symptoms precede a history of memory difficulty, lack of concentration and disorientation, then primary affective disorder is more likely.

Drug treatment

The use of psychotropic drugs in the elderly poses a number of special problems (Van Praag, 1977). Firstly, abnormally high blood levels may develop because of reduced degradation (due to delayed enzyme induction) and diminished excretion (due to impaired renal function). Secondly, many elderly patients suffer from somatic diseases which may make the prescription of psychotropic drugs more hazardous, e.g. barbiturates may suppress respiratory drive in the chronic bronchitic or enhance the degradation of anticoagulants, thus reducing their effect. Thirdly, paradoxical reactions are more common among the elderly, e.g. agitation caused by barbiturates, aggressiveness by benzodiazepines. As a result more side-effects can be expected in the elderly. Indeed, Learoyd (1972) found no less than 16% of patients admitted to a psychogeriatric ward had more or less serious side-effects of psychotropic medication. Side-effects are not only more frequent, but also more severe. Drugs which produce hypotension or constipation in the young may lead to a cerebrovascular accident or paralitic ileus in the elderly. For all these reasons the following rules should be observed: (a) the initial dose should be small and increased gradually on the basis of the ratio between therapeutic and unwanted effects; (b) the minimum effective dose should be established, and regular efforts should be made to ascertain whether one could do with less or even without drugs at all; (c) regular drug monitoring is imperative; (d) combined pharmacotherapy should be avoided if at all possible.

Prescribing for confused and disturbed patients can be particularly difficult, and may lead to greater disturbance, sometimes even stupor or coma. Acute delirium secondary to pneumonia is unlikely to be improved by large doses of neuroleptics which render the patient semi-stuporose and unable to cough. Sympathetic nursing care may achieve as much as drugs, but when the medication is necessary small oral doses of thioridazine, chlormethiazole or promazine are useful. Intramuscular tranquillizers should be avoided if possible as they may be perceived as an assault thus exacerbating disturbance.

Psychotherapy

As a general rule psychotherapy with the elderly is conducted on a simpler basis than with younger patients. Complex interpretations of childhood events are unacceptable to most elderly patients, and interpretative approaches usually have a much smaller role to play. However, a relationship based on genuineness, empathy and warmth remains the basis of treatment, and psychotherapy of a simple and immediately relevant nature can be useful and effective.

Occupational therapy

The prime task of the occupational therapist with the elderly is to maintain functions which younger people often take for granted, e.g. dressing, self-care, and the ability to handle personal affairs. Some elderly people living alone and thought capable of looking after themselves may not, in fact, have been doing so for a considerable time. Thus, a detailed assessment should be made of every patient's functional abilities as soon as the clinical state permits. It is not only the dementing patient who is liable to suffer from loss of function; many elderly people who have spent months in hospital receiving total care may need retraining to look after themselves at home. It is often preferable not to keep such patients in hospital until they are considered absolutely fit and then precipitously discharge them. It is better for the patient to undergo a series of graded 'home trials', perhaps initially under supervision; such a plan may prevent relapse and re-admission of a patient who has become institutionalized.

Social measures

A rigidly biological approach to mental illness is as limiting in the elderly as it is in the rest of psychiatry. Social isolation may be treated by involving neighbours and community services and by encouragement to attend clubs and day centres. Help in re-modelling family and other social relationships can be used alongside physical and psychological treatments.

Attention to physical disorder

The elderly are particularly prone to physical disorders, and almost 40% of the physically impaired in the community show evidence of mental disorder (Harwin, 1973); psychiatric illness can, of course, co-exist with as well as be caused by physical illness. All patients should undergo physical examination whether in domiciliary or hospital practice. For patients in hospital, laboratory tests including chest X-ray, basic haematology and biochemistry, and urine culture should be routine. Thyroid function tests, ECG and treponemal serology may also be indicated, and the clinician's threshold for suspicion of B12 and folate deficiencies should be low (Sneath *et al.*, 1973). Deafness deserves particular attention, since it is common in the elderly, leads to marked social isolation even within family boundaries, and may predispose to paranoid illness (Cooper *et al.*, 1974).

Affective disorders

The greater incidence and prevalence of affective illness in the elderly is an indication of the seriousness of the problem. First admission rates for depressive illness rise in middle life to peak in the sixth and seventh decades (Spicer *et al.*, 1973). Suicide rates begin to increase in the fifth decade and remain high in late life (Sainsbury, 1962), the rate for men exceeding that for women. Sainsbury (1962) also found that depressive illness more frequently heralded attempted or successful suicide in the elderly than it did in younger people.

The incidence of manic illness does not rise in late life like that of depression. Indeed for women the incidence as judged by first admission does not rise at all and for men the rise is insignificant. Post (1965) states that only 5–10% of elderly patients referred for treatment of affective illness show manic features. Thus, it is depressive illness which is more common in late life, and this ranges from the sub-clinical to the severe and life-threatening.

Depressive illness

Aetiology

Common sense observes that old age is a period of loss; loss of social position, loss of physical capacity, both leading to loss of self-esteem, and above all loss of close friends and relatives through bereavement. It is interesting that these factors, which amount to emotional and social isolation, are also closely associated with suicide. This cannot, however, be the exclusive reason for the greater incidence of depression in old age, since these specific precipitating factors are not found significantly more often in elderly as compared with younger depressives (Post, 1976).

Late onset depression is not characterized genetically, in fact the converse is true, a family history of affective illness being more common in patients with illnesses of early onset (Stenstedt, 1959; Angst, 1966; Hopkinson and Ley, 1969). Also, elderly patients have not been found to have a weaker premorbid personality structure.(Post, 1976).

Many earlier authorities considered senile depression to be causally linked to structural brain disease, either arterio-sclerotic or parenchymatous. The evidence has not borne this out. In a longitudinal study of 100 patients, Post (1962) found a somewhat higher prevalence of focal cerebral disease in the patients on admission to hospital for affective disorder, but he concluded that the association was of the structural disorder acting as a precipitant of the functional illness. This conclusion was made on the grounds that the presence of focal cerebral disease, which could not be treated, did not preclude successful treatment of the depression, that cerebral episodes could precede or coincide with depression, and that the incidence of fresh cerebral disease in the (prolonged) follow-up period was no greater than in the population as a whole. As to senile dementia, this is a common disease like depression, and the two may certainly coincide, but there is no good evidence that senile depression announces the onset of senile dementia.

No firm conclusions can be drawn to explain the greater frequency of depression in old age, especially since the more obvious factors of loss, which cannot be ignored, would require the crime of Procrustes to make them a sufficient explanation. This has led some workers to suggest that the ageing process itself in some way predisposes the elderly to depressive breakdown, either through alterations in rate-limiting factors of monoamine metabolism, or by changes in cerebral arousal (reviewed by Post, 1975).

Clinical manifestations

Earlier writers sought to differentiate several types of depressive illness on the basis of the clinical picture. Post (1965) described seven types (organic, depressive pseudodementia, senile melancholia, agitated, reactive, neurotic and masked), although he was careful to point out that these catergories were not rigid, nor to be expected in pure culture. Classification along these and other lines has been of limited value in studies of prognosis, but of no use in the management of individual cases.

In most patients the diagnosis is not difficult and is made on the basis of typical history, appearance, behaviour and thought content. Retardation is less common than agitation with its psychological component of

2 P. M. Jefferys et al.

anxiety. Indeed, in so far as one may refer to specific types at all, agitated depression is most frequently seen with characteristic importuning and reiterative pleas for reassurance. Post (1965) has suggested that senile melancholia with psychotic gait and other, often bizarre and nihilistic delusional preoccupations is an extreme form of agitated depression.

Diagnostic difficulties may arise in differentiating depression from a dementing process, from schizophrenia, or when there are no obvious depressive symptoms (so called masked depression). As already mentioned the problem of *depressive pseudodementia* requires an adequate history from a reliable informant, who may be able to state that decline in cognitive ability coincided with the onset of depressive symptoms. Since dementia can co-exist with depression no harm is done by treating the former as the latter. Kendell (1974) demonstrated only a slight tendency to misdiagnose dementia for depression in a survey of a large sample, which suggests that, in Britain at least, psychiatrists are not unduly misled by depressive pseudodementia.

Difficulty in differentiation from late paraphrenia occurs in a setting of paranoid ideation which is neither clearly schizophrenic, i.e. in association with first rank symptoms, nor clearly depressive, i.e. where the persecution is felt to be a justifiable punishment. In such cases it may be impossible to make a firm diagnosis, and a trial of treatment for one of the conditions only must be started. If this fails it may well be that the other condition has become more clearly manifest as time has progressed. Such cases are distinct from schizo-affective reactions in the elderly, a difficult entity to define which appears to occupy an intermediate position between depression and schizophrenia (Post, 1971).

Masked depression is controversial since it is open to the objection that a diagnosis of depression without evident depression is suspect. None the less it has found favour with clinicians. The story is usually one of longstanding neurotic symptoms most often hypochondriacal, in which there occurs a definite, but not always recognized exacerbation. There may be appetite disturbance with weight loss, a falling off in daily functional ability and changes in sleep pattern, which can be difficult to detect because of longstanding sleep disturbance. Although an elusive diagnosis, the proof of the pudding is in the eating, and the response of these patients to treatment is gratifying.

Management

Many of the principles of management of depressive illness in the elderly are applicable at any age. Drugs have shifted the emphasis towards the general practitioner's surgery, such that it is now the more severely ill who are admitted to psychiatric facilities (Post, 1972). Tricyclic antidepressants are the drugs of choice, and there is no evidence of the superiority of one preparation over another. The elderly are extremely sensitive to tricyclics and the initial, and usually the maintenance, doses should be lower than for younger adults. Amitriptyline, imipramine or nortriptyline, for instance, should be commenced at 20–30 mg daily, increasing gradually over about 14 days to therapeutic maximum. The dose may be weighted towards a larger dose at night as prolonged half-life gives sustained release preparations no advantage over standard ones (Ziegler *et al.*, 1977). However, divided dosage may be desirable to avoid toxicity, which can be severe with quite small amounts of drug.

Provided rapid deterioration does not necessitate it, no change of treatment should be made until an adequate trial of the tricyclic has been completed (at least three to four weeks). It is probably wise to continue for about three to six months after recovery from a first illness. After subsequent illnesses, especially those separated by relatively short intervals, the drug should be continued for longer, and for some recurrent cases small to moderate doses may be continued indefinitely. Although no studies have been carried out specifically in the elderly Mindham *et al.* (1972) demonstrated an advantage of maintenance tricyclics over placebo in patients recovered from depression.

The use of monoamine oxidase inhibitors (MAOIs) is much less common because they are considered by many to be ineffective and by others to be too dangerous. Tyrer (1976) claims that MAOIs are of no use in serious depression, but suggests that symptoms such as hypochondriasis, somatic anxiety, irritability, agoraphobia, social phobias and anergia respond to MAOIs, which are in effect 'delayed psychostimulants'. Clinical experience favours the infrequent use of MAOIs in the elderly as a second choice in depression.

Treatment adherence (drug compliance) is as much a problem in the elderly as in other groups (Blackwell, 1976), but the problem is augmented by forgetfulness, which may fall short of pathological memory impairment. This can lead to missed or to extra doses. It is not a problem in hospital, but at home sensible and unobtrusive supervision by a suitable relative or friend may help to avoid trouble.

Electroconvulsive therapy is still a vexed treatment because it is distasteful to most patients and to many psychiatrists. However, as Post (1976) has pointed out, ECT is most likely to rapidly relieve 'potentially dangerous psychotic states'. The severely suicidal patient is a case in point. Others responding to ECT are those in whom tricyclics have failed, especially those presenting an 'endogenous' picture, but Post (1972) found that even patients whose symptomatology was primarily 'neurotic' sometimes required ECT to effect discharge from hospital. A peculiar and interesting case is that of the life-long hypochondriac, whose essentially neurotic symptoms may effloresce into a state of severe and sometimes psychotic hypochondriasis. This form of masked depression frequently responds to antidepressants and/or ECT.

Prognosis

The prognosis of depression in the elderly has altered for the better. In 1934/1936 before the first specific treatment (ECT) only just over 30% of patients in one survey, who were admitted for affective disorder, were discharged within six months, but by 1948/1949 the figure had risen to almost 60% (Roth, 1955). At another hospital around 1955 about 80% of affective patients were discharged within six months (Post, 1965). The figure now is probably even higher.

Long-term follow-up studies do not give such a rosy picture, for continuing morbidity of one kind or another is great. Of Post's (1962) group of 100 only 28% remained symptom-free over the follow-up period; 14% never recovered. Those factors associated with good prognosis are onset of illness before the age of 70, a family history of affective disorder, recovery from earlier attacks before the age of 50, an extroverted personality with good social adjustment and an euthymic temperament. Factors favouring a bad prognosis are first onset of illness after 70, pathological changes in the brain and serious physical illness elsewhere, a senile habitus (especially in women over 70) and uninterrupted illness for two years or more when recovery is rare.

Manic illness

In essence manic illnesses are the same as in younger patients, but Post (1965) has claimed that mixed affective states are more common and that manic illness nearly always shows depressive admixture. Management is also similar to that of younger patients, but special regard should be paid to actual or potential frailty which can hazard the elderly, hyperactive patient. Particular attention must be given to maintenance of bodily functions and fluid balance, and close supervision is mandatory to avoid injury; the elderly hyperactive patient may, for example, easily trip and sustain a fractured neck or femur. For this reason all but the mildest cases are best managed in hospital.

Lithium is found by many clinicians to be as useful in the elderly as in younger patients. The indications for use are much the same, but potential toxicity requires attention since factors which reduce renal excretion are common in later life. These are heart and kidney disease, low sodium and fluid intake, thiazide diuretics and even old age itself. Thus lithium therapy should not be lightly undertaken, and the serum level should be maintained at the lower end of the therapeutic range (Post, 1976). Thyroid function should be carefully observed, lest lithium induced myxoedema go undetected.

Schizophrenia-like states

Although schizophrenia is generally considered a disease of young adults, some 4% of all schizophrenia-like illness in men and 14% in women arise after the age of 65 years. Kay (1972) claims that such illnesses account for about 5% of psychiatric first admissions after this age. There has been considerable dispute over the aetiology, prognosis and even most appropriate nomenclature for these conditions. Kay and Roth (1961) coined the term 'late paraphrenia' for

> all cases with a paranoid symptom complex in which signs of organic demen-
> tia or sustained confusion were absent and in which the condition was
> judged from the content of the delusional and hallucinatory symptoms not to
> be due to a primary affective disorder.

Thus, the term 'late paraphrenia' emphasizes that in the elderly illnesses occur with a more or less organized delusional system in the setting of well preserved personality and intellect which are quite distinct from dementia and affective disorder. In his monograph on persecutory states in the elderly, Post (1966) described 93 cases collected over ten years. Thirty-four patients exhibited Schneiderian first rank symptoms and were regarded as 'schizophrenic'. A second group of 37 'schizo-phreniform' patients had more understandable delusional preoccupa-tions. The final group of 22 patients was characterized by hallucinations (usually auditory) and persecutory beliefs secondary to these hallucina-tions; this was termed the 'paranoid hallucinosis' syndrome. Post tried to separate the three groups on the basis of aetiology, clinical characteristics and outcome, but could not. He concluded that together they represented a continuum.

Predisposing factors

When a schizophrenic illness starts late in life the risk among relatives is lower than in schizophrenia as a whole, but higher than in the general population (Kay, 1972). There may in some cases be evidence of long-standing personality disorder, and like schizophrenics in general these patients are often unmarried or separated. Social isolation has often resulted from life-long personality traits, but may be aggravated in old

486 P. M. Jefferys et al.

age by the death of relatives. While habitual self-seclusion may have been tolerable in earlier life, it can become more troubling with advancing years.

Impaired hearing has been consistently found in 30% or more of elderly people with schizophrenia-like states. Cooper *et al.* (1974) for instance, reported that deafness predating psychosis was not only more common in elderly schizophrenics than in depressed persons of the same age, but it was also more severe and of longer duration. Visual defects too, are more frequent than expected (Kay, 1972). Schizophrenia in the elderly is also not infrequently symptomatic of focal brain disease; 7·5% of Post's (1966) cases had cerebrovascular disease, and a further 9·5% had GPI, epilepsy or dementia.

Management

The first step in management is to be sure that the symptoms are not secondary to some other disorder. In affective disorder paranoid symptoms are associated with ideas of guilt and retribution, and disappear when the mood returns to normal. Paranoid ideas may also colour organic brain syndromes, but they are usually transient or fragmentary and visual hallucinations are common.

Some paraphrenics can be managed as out-patients or on the basis of day care. The decision to admit to hospital is influenced both by the severity of illness and by social factors. Clearly, the lady who is driven on to the street in her night attire because she hears the neighbours plotting against her needs in-patient treatment. But it may also be desirable to admit the quietly isolated patient who is deteriorating unobserved in a bedsitter, or a patient whose family have turned against him through long exposure to even quite mild symptoms.

Hospital admission itself may sometimes be followed by remission of symptoms. Other patients benefit from antipsychotic medication. Post (1966) demonstrated the value of these drugs and the likelihood of relapse in patients who failed to take this medication after discharge. Selection of the appropriate antipsychotic should be empirical. One should delineate the target symptoms and also the side-effects to be avoided. For example, haloperidol may be the drug of choice in a patient in whom low blood pressure would be hazardous, while a patient who developed severe extrapyramidal symptoms should be switched to thioridazine. The dosage should usually be 30–50% of the usual adult dose, e.g. 50–300 mg of chlorpromazine or 1–8 mg haloperidol daily. Anticholinergics should not be prescribed automatically as they are not invariably necessary and may themselves cause side-effects. A more detailed exposition of the indications for and against various drugs in the treatment of the elderly psychotic is provided by Gullevich (1977).

Although the majority of patients receiving adequate antipsychotic medication undergo remission there are some who do not respond. If a full trial of drug therapy is unsuccessful it is better not to add to the patient's burden with prolonged treatment by strong ineffective medication.

Outcome

Patients with late paraphrenia have a virtually normal expectation of life. Roth (1955) found that two years after admission to hospital only 20% of paraphrenics had died compared with 80% of those with senile dementia. However, before the neuroleptics were introduced the course of the illness was nearly always chronic, and psychotic symptoms would persist for many years with only minor fluctuations in intensity. Thus, in the past many of these patients spent the remainder of their lives in mental hospitals.

However, the progress is now much better. As Post (1966) pointed out a favourable response can be sustained with long-term medication both in the classical schizophrenic and in the less typical paranoid syndromes. However, since there is little hope of changing their personalities or the pattern of their lives in old age, careful follow-up and painstaking social work are of great value.

References

Angst, J. (1966). 'Zur Atiologie und Nosologie Endogener Depressiver Psychosen'. Springer, Berlin.

Arie, T. (1970). The first year of the Goodmayes psychiatric service for old people. *Lancet* **2**, 1179–1182.

Arie, T. (1973). Dementia in the elderly; diagnosis and assessment. *Br. Med. J.* **4**, 540–543.

Baker, A. A. and Byrne, R. J. J. (1977). Another style of psychogeriatric service. *Br. J. Psychiat.* **130**, 123–126.

Blackwell, B. (1976). Treatment adherence. *Br. J. Psychiat.* **129**, 513–531.

Brothwood J. (1971). The organisation and development of services for the aged with special reference to the mentally ill. *In* 'Recent Developments in Psychogeriatrics' (Eds D. W. K. Kay and A. Walk). *Br. J. Psychiat.* Special Publication No. 6.

Cooper, A. F., Curry, A. R., Kay, D. W. K., Garside, R. F. and Roth, M. (1974). Hearing loss in paranoid and affective psychosis of the elderly. *Lancet* **2**, 851–854.

Copeland, J. R. M., Kelleher, M. J., Barron, G., Cowan, D. W. and Gourlay, A. J. (1975). Evaluation of a psychogeriatric service: the distinction between psychogeriatric and geriatric patients. *Br. J. Psychiat.* **126**, 21–29.

Corsellis, J. A. N. (1962). 'Mental Illness and the Ageing Brain'. Maudsley Monograph No. 9. Oxford University Press, Oxford.

Department of Health and Social Security (1975). Better Services for the Mentally Ill. Cmnd 6233. HMSO, London.

Donovan, J. F., Williams, I. E. and Wilson, T. S. (1971). A fully integrated psychogeriatric service. *In* 'Recent Developments in Psychogeriatrics' (Eds D. W. K. Kay and A. Walk). *Br. J. Psychiat.* Publication No. 6.

Goldberg, E. M., Mothery, A. and Williams B. T. (1970). 'Helping the Aged: A Field Experiment in Social Work'. London, Allen and Unwin.

Gullevich, G. D. (1977). Psychopharmacological treatment of the aged. *In* 'Psychopharmacology, From Theory to Practice' (Eds J. Barchas *et al*). Oxford University Press, New York.

Harwin, B. (1973). Psychiatric morbidity among the physically impaired elderly in the community. *In* 'Roots of Evaluation' (Eds J. K. Wing and H. Hafner). Nuffield Provincial Trust, Oxford University Press, Oxford.

Hopkinson, G. and Ley, P. (1969). A genetic study of affective disorder. *Br. J. Psychiat.* **115**, 917–922.

Isaacs, B. (1971). Studies of Illness and Death in the Elderly in Glasgow. Scottish Health Service Studies No. 17. Scottish Home and Health Department, Edinburgh.

Jolley, D. J. and Arie, T. (1976). Psychiatric service for the elderly. How many beds? *Br. J. Psychiat.* **129**, 418–423.

Kay, D. W. K. (1972). Schizophrenia and schizophrenia-like states in the elderly. *Br. J. Hosp. Med.* October, 369–376.

Kay, D. W. K., Beamish, P. and Roth, M. (1962). Some medical and social characteristics of elderly people under state care. *In* 'The Sociological Review Monograph' (Ed. P. Halmos), No. 5, pp. 173–93. University of Keele.

Kay, D. W. K., Beamish, P. and Roth, M. (1964). Old age mental disorders in Newcastle-upon-Tyne. Part 1: a study of prevalence. *Br. J. Psychiat.* **110**, 146–158.

Kay, D. W. K., Bergmann., K., Foster, E. M., McKechnie, A. A. and Roth, M. (1970). Mental illness and hospital usage in the elderly. *Comp. Psychiat.* **2**, 26–35.

Kendell, R. E. (1974). The stability of psychiatric diagnoses. *Br. J. Psychiat.* **124**, 352–356.

Kushlik, A. and Blunden, R. (1974). Proposals for the Setting Up and Evaluation of an Experimental Service for the Elderly. A Document for Discussion. Health Care Evaluation Research Team. Research Report No. 107.

Learoyd, B. M. (1972). Psychotropic drugs and the elderly patient. *Med. J. Aust*, **1**, 1131–1132.

Meacher M. (1972). 'Taken for a Ride. Special Residential Homes for Confused Old People. A Study of Separatism in Social Policy'. Longman, London.

Mindham, R. H. S., Howland, C. and Shepherd, M. (1972). Continuation therapy with tricyclic antidepressants in depressive illness. *Lancet* **2**, 854–855.

Post, F. (1962). 'The Significance of Affective Symptoms in Old Age'. Maudsley Monograph No. 10. Oxford University Press, Oxford.

Post, F. (1965). 'The Clinical Psychiatry of Late Life'. Pergamon, Oxford.

Post, F. (1966). 'Persistent Persecutory States of the Elderly'. Pergamon, Oxford.

Post, F. (1971). Schizo-affective symptomatology in late life. *Br. J. Psychiat.* **118**, 437–445.

Post, F. (1971). The diagnostic process. *In* 'Recent Developments in Psychogeriatrics' (Eds D. W. Kay and A. Walk). *Br. J. Psychiat.* Special Publication No. 6.

Post, F. (1972). The management and nature of depressive illness in late life: a follow-through study. *Br. J. Psychiat.* **121**, 393–404.

Post, F. (1975). Dementia, depression and pseudodementia. *In* 'Psychiatric Aspects of Neurological Disease' (Eds D. F. Benson and D. F. Blumer). Grune and Stratton, New York.

Post, F. (1976). Geriatric depression. 'Depression' (Eds D. H. Gallant and G. M. Simpson). Spectrum, New York.

Prien, R. F. and Caffey, E. M. (1976). Relationship between dosage and response to lithium prophylaxis in recurrent depression. *Am. J. Psychiat.* **133**, 567–570.

Roth, M. (1955). The natural history of mental disorders in the senium. *J. Ment. Sci.* 281–301.

Roth, M., Tomlinson, B. E. and Blessed, G. (1967). The relationship between measures of dementia and degenerative changes in the cerebral grey matter of elderly subjects. *Proc. Roy. Soc. Med.* **60**, 254–259.

Roth, M. (1973). The principles of providing a service for psychogeriatric patients. *In* 'Roots of Evaluation' (Eds J. K. Wing and H. Hafner). Nuffield Provincial Hospitals Trust, Oxford University Press, Oxford.

Sainsbury, P. (1962). Suicide in later life. *Geront. Clin.* **4**, 161–170.

Sneath, P., Chanarin, I., Hodkinson, H. M., McPherson, C. K. and Reynolds, E. H. (1973). Folate status in a geriatric population and its relation to dementia. *Age and Ageing* **2**, 177–182.

Spicer, C. C., Hare, E. H. and Slater, E. (1973). Neurotic and psychotic forms of depressive illness. *Br. J. Psychiat.* **123**, 535–541.

Stenstedt A. (1959) Involuntional melancholia. *Acta. Psychiat. Scand., Suppl.* 127.

Tyrer, P. (1976). Towards rational therapy with monoamine oxidase inhibitors. *Br. J. Psychiat.* **128**, 354–360.

Van Praag, H. M. (1977). Psychotropic drugs in the aged. *Comp. Psychiat.* **18**, 429–442.

Ziegler, V. E., Meyer, D. A., Rosen, S. H., Knesevich, J. W. and Biggs, J. T. (1977). Amitriptyline dosage schedule , sampling time and tricyclic plasma levels. *Br. J. Psychiat.* **131**, 168–171.

14 The psychiatry of old age
II Aspects of dementia

Maria Ron

Some aspects of dementia

A broad outline of the clinical features of dementia and its various aetiologies has already been given in Chapter 13. Here some specific problems of dementia, its relationship to normal senescence and the differential diagnosis from other psychiatric conditions will be discussed.

The magnitude of the problem

As a result of enhanced life expectancy the numbers of elderly people living in the community have increased in the last few decades, leading inevitably to a higher incidence of dementia. Kay *et al.* (1964) found that 4·9% of people over 65 living in the Newcastle area suffered from severe dementia, and another 5·2% were mildly demented. Bollerup (1975), reviewing studies from other countries, has found a similar incidence.

Dementia in the presenium is less common. Sjögren *et al.* (1952) calculated the joint incidence of Alzheimer's and Pick's diseases to be 0·1% for the general population. Other dementing illnesses such as Huntington's chorea are far less common—5·2 per 100,000 for the West of Scotland (Bolt, 1970).

By 1981 it is to be expected that in England and Wales those over 65 will constitute 16·2% of the total population (over 8 million) (Brothwood, 1971). If this prediction proves to be correct, nearly half a million people over 65 will be suffering from severe dementia and the subsequent demands that such numbers will make upon hospitals and ancillary services will be considerable.

The relationship between dementia and ageing

The similarities between the lesions found in the brains of normal elderly people and those found in pre-senile and senile dementia have been recognized for a long time. This, coupled with the observation that 'forgetfulness' is part of the normal process of ageing, has led some to consider dementia as an extreme form of senescence (Newton, 1948). More recently this view has come under attack.

The fact that senile dementia occurs four times more often in first degree relatives (Larsson et al., 1963) is perhaps the best argument against considering it solely as an accelerated form of ageing. Although the pathological lesions of senile dementia and ageing appear qualitatively identical, recent quantitative studies have demonstrated important differences. Tomlinson et al. (1968) and Dayan (1970) found these lesions to be extremely rare in normals under the age of 60. Furthermore, in dementia the lesions spread to all cortical layers and the neuro-fibrillary tangles were particularly frequent in Ammon's horn; neither of these features is seen in non-demented old people. Animal studies (Dayan, 1971) have also contributed to dispel the belief that senile plaques and tangles are a constant feature of ageing. However, the role of the senile plaques and neuro-fibrillary tangles in the production of the clinical signs of dementia is debatable, and the loss of neurones is likely to be the crucial lesion, other changes being secondary to it. To date quantitative estimates of neuronal loss are few and comparison between normality and disease states is not yet possible, but the scanty available evidence suggests that age related neuronal loss is not a universal feature in all species and that constancy over time of neuronal populations has been established for certain discrete nuclei in men and animals (Hanley, 1974).

Miller (1974), reviewing the psychological aspects of the problem, describes some relevant differences between dementia and normal ageing, e.g. qualitative differences in performance of tasks of psychomotor speed, although in this field the arguments remain inconclusive.

Recent biochemical evidence favours the difference between ageing and dementia. White et al. (1977) studied choline acetyl transferase (CAT) activity, a potential marker of the presynaptic cholinergic system and perhaps related to the formation of neuro-fibrillary tangles, in the brains of normal and demented elderly patients. In patients suffering from senile dementia of the Alzheimer's type CAT was selectively reduced.

In summary, the evidence so far is strong enough to consider dementia as being different from accelerated ageing, although the similarities between the two are important. Roth (1971) suggested that a certain threshold needs to be reached for pathological lesions to produce clinical signs of dementia and that for this to occur the presence of a certain genetic factor is necessary. So far this model appears to fit best the known facts.

The relationship between Alzheimer's disease and senile dementia

The similarities between the pathological lesions found in these two conditions have been recognized for a long time. On the other hand, clinical features such as focal cortical signs (e.g. aphasia, apraxia, agnosia, etc.), extrapyramidal signs, epilepsy and lack of spontaneity have been held to be specific to Alzheimer's disease. These differences have led some to make a distinction between Alzheimer's disease and 'simple' senile dementia characterized by a global impairment of memory but in which aphasia, apraxia and agnosia are conspicuously absent even in the advanced stages of the illness (Delay and Brion, 1962).

Pilleri (1966) described in man a clinical picture equivalent to the Klüver-Bucy syndrome found in primates after bilateral temporal lobectomy. The main features in man are visual agnosia, apathy, blunting of affect, a tendency to handle any object in sight and to put it inside the mouth in a similar way to the oral exploratory behaviour encountered in young children (hypermetamorphosis). Disinhibited sexual behaviour and bulimia are sometimes present. The syndrome is produced by bilateral lesions in the inferomedial areas of the temporal lobes and it appears that widespread brain pathology is a necessary prerequisite. Sourander and Sjögren (1970) in a group of 60 patients suffering from Alzheimer's disease, found the syndrome to be nearly always present. They considered that the greater density of lesions found in the temporal lobes and the hippocampus, responsible for this syndrome, was specific of Alzheimer's disease and did not occur in 'simple' senile dementia. Unfortunately such a careful clinical examination was not performed in a group of patients suffering from senile dementia for the purpose of comparison.

The best argument for considering these two conditions as separate entities is the fact that both appear to breed true in the relatives of those affected (Sjögren et al., 1952; Larsson et al., 1963). Nevertheless other studies have cast some doubts concerning their total independence. Sjögren (1955) described a form of senile dementia with onset after the age of 65, with the typical focal features encountered in Alzheimer's disease but lacking extrapyramidal signs and with a tendency to exhibit restlessness rather than lack of spontaneity. Later Sourander and Sjögren (1970) considered this to be a form of Alzheimer's disease of late onset. A similar clinical picture, with focal features indicating parietal lobe dysfunction, has been described by McDonald (1969) in nearly half of a series of elderly demented women. Lauter and Meyer (1968) in a carefully examined group found dysphasia, dyspraxia and agnosia to be nearly always present, making the clinical distinction between Alzheimer's disease and senile dementia blurred. The same authors reported some families in which both senile and pre-senile forms coexisted.

In conclusion, there is little doubt that Alzheimer's disease can appear in patients over the age of 65. Doubts remain as to whether a 'simple' form of senile dementia exists as a separate entity or whether it is only a form of Alzheimer's disease of late onset with a clinical picture slightly different from the pre-senile variety. Only follow-up studies of a group of elderly demented patients could answer this question.

The relationship between senile dementia and dementia of vascular origin

The concept, long upheld, that 'arterio-sclerotic dementia' is a common cause of mental deterioration has come under attack recently. Hachinski *et al*. (1974), reviewing the problem, considered that dementia appears as a result of multiple small or large cerebral infarcts, commonly due to thromboembolic phenomena arising from the heart and the large vessels and is only rarely due to pathological lesions of the small intracerebral vessels. Dementia of vascular origin tends to appear earlier than senile dementia, is more common in men and is frequently associated with hypertension. Clinically it is characterized by abrupt episodes leading to residual weakness, slowness, dysarthria, dysphagia, small-stepped gait, brisk reflexes and extensor plantar responses. These are early signs which often precede the deterioration in memory. Exaggeration of emotional responses is a common feature. The term 'multi-infarct dementia' describes this condition more satisfactorily.

Although infarcted brain tissue appears in conjunction with the typical lesions of senile dementia (e.g. plaques and neuro-fibrillary tangles), a positive clinico-pathological correlation is present. Corsellis (1962) found that if a certain type of lesion was clinically suspected it was found at post mortem in 75% of cases in moderate or severe degree. Tomlinson *et al*. (1968) found that large infarcts (volume of softening greater than 50 ml) were only present in those patients with a clinical picture of 'multi-infarct dementia' and a high density of senile plaques (more than 14 per field) occurred almost exclusively in those patients with a clinical picture of senile dementia. Furthermore the choline acetyl transferase activity found to be selectively reduced in the brains of patients suffering from senile dementia appears to be normal in 'multi-infarct' dementia (White *et al.*, 1977).

'Multi-infarct dementia' is likely to account for a relatively small proportion of the dementias of the presenium and senium, probably less than a quarter, although the presence of vascular pathology may be a contributory factor in a large number of cases. This is of particular clinical significance as often the vascular pathology is the only one amenable to treatment (e.g. hypotensive drugs, endarterectomy, etc.).

The relationship between Parkinson's disease and dementia

Parkinson's disease of whatever aetiology is now considered to be a 'dopamine deficiency state' (Hornykiewicz, 1973). Cell loss in the substantia nigra and subsequent diminished concentration of dopamine in the striatum are the basis of some of the clinical symptoms. The advent of L-dopa has provided a new therapeutic dimension while at the same time its ability to produce or aggravate psychiatric symptoms has reawakened interest in the abnormal mental states that often accompany Parkinson's disease.

Mindham (1974) found depressive affect in 40% of an untreated group of patients. The degree of depression was related to the severity of the illness. Other abnormalities such as personality changes, delusional states, irritability, suspiciousness and obsessional disorders appeared to be less common. The administration of L-dopa has increased the severity and frequency of affective symptoms, even in the presence of physical improvement. Those patients with a previous history of depression were particularly at risk (Mindham, 1974; Mindham *et al.*, 1976).

Of particular interest here are the cognitive defects in Parkinson's disease and the wider overlap between extrapyramidal features and dementing illness.

Cognitive deficits in Parkinson's disease

Parkinson (1817) in his original description of the shaking palsy did not consider intellectual impairment to be part of the syndrome. Patrick *et al.* (1922), subscribed to the same view, but others (Gowers, 1886; Lewy, 1923; Mjönes, 1949) considered dementia to be a common feature of the disease. Recent studies have amply confirmed this view. Pollock and

Hornabrook (1966), in a population survey in Wellington, New Zealand, found evidence of dementia in 20% of those exhibiting the condition. Similarly Celesia and Barr (1970) and Mindham (1970) found it in about a third of patients suffering from Parkinson's disease admitted to a psychiatric hospital. The presence of intellectual impairment appears to be related to age, to the symptom of akinesia (Mettler and Crandell, 1959; Schwab, 1960; Garron et al., 1972) and is perhaps commoner in cases of 'arterio-sclerotic Parkinsonism'.

The intellectual deterioration found in Parkinson's disease involves a wide range of abilities. Striking discrepancies between scores in verbal intelligence and performance tests have been reported (Loranger et al., 1972) which cannot be explained solely in terms of motor deficits or affective changes. Reitan et al. (1971) using tests especially designed for the detection of brain damage (The Halstead Battery and the Trail Making Test) found attention and alertness, memory and abstract reasoning to be impaired. The performance was particularly poor in tests that required a coordination between several sensory modalities.

Extrapyramidal features in other dementing illness

The presence of extrapyramidal features in Alzheimer's disease has been repeatedly reported (Rothschild and Kasanin, 1936; Sjögren et al., 1952). More recently Pearce and Miller (1973) found parkinsonian signs in 60% of their 50 patients with radiological evidence of 'presenile cerebral atrophy'. Poverty of facial expression, positive glabella tap, akinesia of gait and limb movement were commonly found; tremor was often absent and only slight when present.

Extrapyramidal features are also present in Jakob-Creutzfeld disease (Jansen and Monrad-Krohn 1938), in the 'Parkinson-Dementia complex of Guam' (Hirano et al., 1961), and in progressive supranuclear palsy (Steele et al., 1964).

As a rule dementia results from a diffuse pathological process involving many different areas of the brain; the localization and degree of the lesions provided each individual syndrome with a characteristic constellation of symptoms. Clinically, extrapyramidal signs constitute a link between a variety of dementing illnesses. At one extreme of this spectrum we find progressive supranuclear palsy with lesions in the thalamic and subthalamic nuclei and relatively spared cortical mantle. The clinical picture is characterized by prominent parkinsonian features—apathy, inertia and a typical delay in carrying out intellectual functions—that is to say, disorders of timing and activation resulting most probably from lesions in the reticular activating system. Verbal and perceptual motor skills are well preserved. Albert *et al*. (1974) have appropriately named this syndrome 'subcortical dementia'. At the other end of the spectrum we find the predominantly 'cortical dementia' of Alzheimer's disease where focal cortical signs are more marked than extrapyramidal features.

The contribution of organic pathology to the functional psychosis of old age

Several follow-up studies have dealt with this problem (Kay *et al*., 1955, 1961; Kay, 1962; Post, 1962, 1965). In affective illness the risk of developing senile dementia is the same as for the general population and at post mortem Corsellis (1962) found no difference between this group and the normal elderly with regard to the presence and abundance of senile plaques and neuro-fibrillary tangles. The frequency of cerebro-vascular accidents in this group surpasses chance expectation. Strokes tend to precede the onset of depression acting as a precipitating factor, and in that sense they are comparable with other 'losses' (e.g. bereavement) known to be associated with the onset of depression in elderly patients (Post, 1962). However, once the depression has appeared the risk for subsequent cerebrovascular accidents does not seem to be greater than chance expectation, suggesting that a more specific aetiological relationship between the two is unlikely.

With regard to late onset schizophrenia the situation is less clear. In one follow-up study (Post, 1966) 22% of the patients appeared to have associated cognitive impairment. However, this high proportion may be an overestimate and may reflect the diagnostic difficulties encountered in this group of patients in whom sensory deficits were common, making assessment particularly arduous. Even so an association appears probable. Roth (1971) has postulated a causal relationship between late onset schizophrenia and organic brain pathology, similar to that between temporal lobe epilepsy and schizophrenia of early adult life, at least in a proportion of cases. The risk of cerebrovascular accidents in this group of patients does not appear to be increased.

Differential diagnosis—pseudodementia

It is not difficult to make a clinical diagnosis of dementia in the majority of cases. By the time patients are referred for assessment the dementing process has usually been present for several years, and severe cognitive impairment with affective and personality changes are nearly always present. The difficulties in diagnosis arise when the symptoms are atypical or in the very early stages of the illness; in such cases a few other psychiatric conditions closely resemble dementia. The term 'pseudo-dementia' is used here in a purely descriptive sense to encompass such conditions.

Depressive pseudodementia

The diagnostic difficulties arise when one is confronted with elderly depressed patients who appear retarded and perplexed, disorientated and with diminished awareness (Post, 1965). It appears that depression mimicking dementia may occur not infrequently. Kendell (1974), looking at stability of diagnosis in admissions to hospital in England and Wales, found that in 8·2% of the patients originally diagnosed as suffering from dementia the diagnosis was later changed to one of depression. Change in the opposite direction, from depression to dementia, was more rare (2·6%). Marsden and Harrison (1972), investigating a group of 106 patients originally diagnosed as suffering from dementia, found depression to be responsible for the symptoms in eight patients and mania in one. A higher proportion of misdiagnosed patients was found by Nott and Fleminger (1975) in a 10-year follow-up of a group of 35 patients originally thought to be suffering from pre-senile dementia. Twenty of these patients did not deteriorate as expected and in retrospect the authors felt that 'marked personality difficulties and neurotic symptoms or affective disorder' were the cause of the original picture.

From the clinical point of view attention has been focused on some of the similarities between the two conditions. About 12% of elderly patients with affective psychosis of acute onset have clouding of consciousness (Roth, 1955) and as many as 41% of elderly depressives show some clinical memory impairment when examined on admission (Post, 1965). The use of psychological tests confirms the clinical impression of memory impairment in some of these patients (Kendrick et al., 1965; Bolton et al., 1967).

Although as we have seen moderate degrees of intellectual impairment are common in elderly depressives, they appear to be different from those found in dementia. In depression the abnormalities are confined to rote learning and patients are able to handle considerable amounts of information provided that it is well structured. In dementia, on the contrary, the deficits are more widespread, affecting learning as well as logical memory, delayed recall and retrieval, and the patients are able to handle only very small amounts of material (Whitehead, 1973).

Fortunately the presence of mild degrees of memory impairment appears to be of little consequence in terms of prognosis. Post (1975) followed up 41 such patients and found that eight years later their outcome was not significantly different from that of a group without suspected cerebral pathology.

The best diagnostic guide in elderly depressives is the clinical history. A diagnosis of dementia should only be considered when there is a clear history of cognitive impairment preceding the onset of the affective symptoms. A tendency to perseveration, confabulatory answers and signs indicative of focal cortical damage (e.g. dysphasia, dyspraxia, etc.) are strongly in favour of dementia.

Patients with depression of late onset differ from those whose symptoms start in early adult life in that in the elderly group, neurotic premorbid personality is less common and the incidence of depression in relatives is lower. Hemsi et al. (1968), Cawley et al (1973) and Post (1975) have suggested that an alteration in cerebral functioning, perhaps related to ageing, may be a precipitating factor for depression in this group, and that when present may be the cause of depressive pseudodementia. Lowering of cerebral arousal or excitability could be such an abnormality. Diminished cerebral arousal is reflected by abnormalities in psychological tests and physiological measurements such as sedation and sleep thresholds. Clinical improvement is accompanied by a significant degree of normalization in psychological tests and physiological measurements. Although some aspects of this work have recently been criticized (Lader and Noble, 1975) on the grounds that sedation and sleep thresholds may not be adequate measurements of arousal and only reflect the state of the peripheral vascular system, the central hypothesis is of considerable interest and deserves further investigation.

The Ganser syndrome

Ganser first described, in 1897, a transient syndrome characterized by fluctuating levels of consciousness, hallucinations and peculiar verbal responses ('vorbeireden' or approximate answers). The symptom of approximate answers has attracted a great deal of attention and was best described by Anderson and Mallison (1941) as an answer that 'is never far from wrong and bears a definite and obvious relation to the question, indicating clearly that the question has been understood'. The syndrome which ends abruptly, leaving behind a period of amnesia, was thought to be precipitated by physical or emotional trauma. In the original three cases Ganser noticed the presence of 'hysterical stigma', i.e. widespread analgesia or hyperalgesia, not conforming to known anatomical distribution, and he considered the syndrome to be an 'hysterical twilight state'.

He was, from the beginning, opposed to the idea that malingering played a role in the causation of the syndrome.

The full syndrome, as originally described, appears to be rare. The symptom of the approximate answers, on the other hand, is more frequently seen. This dichotomy made Scott (1965) distinguish between the Ganser syndrome and the Ganser symptoms, the latter being often associated with functional or organic psychosis. This association has also been commented on by Whitlock (1967). Anderson *et al.* (1959) have documented its occurrence in dementia. The abrupt ending of the syndrome with total recovery, and its brief duration, should make differentiation from dementia possible.

Hysterical pseudodementia

This term is often made synonymous with Ganser's syndrome but it is better reserved for cases of malingering in people below average intelligence when trying to escape difficult situations by feigning mental illness. Anderson *et al.* (1959) and Curran and Partridge (1963) have emphasized the absence of clouding of consciousness which makes possible its separation from the Ganser syndrome.

Simulation

The simulation of dementia is probably very rare and when it appears is likely to occur in people of low intelligence while under stress (hysterical pseudodementia). Normal people when asked to feign mental illness tend to produce a picture of depression with or without paranoid features. Amnesia and feeblemindedness are seldom simulated (Anderson *et al.*, 1959). The symptoms produced by normal people bear only a resemblance to those seen in clinical practice, and some symptoms such as perseveration are rarely produced at all.

Anderson *et al.* (1959) described how experimental subjects simulating mental illness found increasing difficulty in sustaining the symptoms with the passing of time, tending to become more and more 'normal', in contrast with the psychiatric symptoms and performance in tests of cognitive function of patients suffering from organic dementia, both of which deteriorated in the course of the examination.

References

Albert, M. L., Feldman, R. G. and Willis, A. L. (1974). The 'subcortical dementia' of progressive supranuclear palsy. *J. Neurol. Neurosurg. Psychiat.* **37**, 121–130.

Anderson, E. W. and Mallison, W. P. (1941). Psychogenic episodes in the course of major psychoses. *J. Ment. Sci.* **87**, 383–389.

Anderson, E. W., Trethowan, W. H. and Kenna, J. C. (1959). An experimental investigation of simulation and pseudodementia. *Acta Psychiat. Neurol. Scand., Suppl.* 132.

Bollerup, T. R. (1975). Prevalence of mental illness among 70-year-olds domiciled in nine Copenhagen suburbs. *Acta Psychiat. Scand.* **51**, 327–339.

Bolt, J. M. W. (1970). Huntington's chorea in the West of Scotland. *Br. J. Psychiat.* **116**, 259–270.

Bolton, N., Savage, R. D. and Roth, M. (1967). The modified word learning test and the aged psychiatric patient. *Br. J. Psychiat.* **113**, 1139–1140.

Brothwood, J. (1971). The organisation and development of services for the aged with special reference to the mentally ill. *In* 'Recent Advances in Psychogeriatrics' (Eds D. W. K. Kay and A. Walk), pp. 99–112. Headley Bros, Ashford, Kent.

Cawley, R. H., Post, F. and Whitehead, A. (1973). Barbiturate tolerance and psychological functioning in elderly depressed patients. *Psychol. Med.* **3**, 39–52.

Celesia, G. G., and Barr, N. (1970). Psychosis and other psychiatric manifestations of levodopa therapy. *Archs Neurol.* **23**, 193–200.

Corsellis, J. A. N. (1962). 'Mental Illness and the Ageing Brain'. Maudsley Monograph No. 9. Oxford University Press, Oxford.

Curran, D. and Partridge, M. (1963). 'Psychological Medicine'. Livingstone, Edinburgh.

Dayan, A. D. (1970). Quantitative histological studies on the aged human brain. *Acta Neuropath. (Berlin)* **16**, 85–94.

Dayan, A. D. (1971). Comparative neuropathology of ageing: Studies on the brains of 47 species of vertebrates. *Brain* **94**, 31–42.

Ganser, S. J. (1898). On a peculiar twilight state. *Arch. f. Psychiat., Berlin* **30**, 633–640.

Garron, D. C., Klawans, H. L. and Narin, F. (1972). Intellectual functioning of persons with idiopathic Parkinsonism. *J. Nerv. Ment. Dis.* **154**, 445–452.

Gowers, W. R. (1886). 'A Manual of the Diseases of the Nervous System'. Churchill, London.

Hachinski, V. C., Lassen, N. A. and Marshall, J. (1974). Multi-infarct dementia. A cause of mental deterioration in the elderly. *Lancet* **ii**, 207–209.

Hanley, T. (1974). 'Neuronal fall-out' in the ageing brain. A critical review of the quantitative data. *Age and Ageing* **3**, 133–151.

Hemsi, L. K., Whitehead, A. and Post, F. (1968). Cognitive functioning and cerebral arousal in elderly depressives and dements. *J. Psychosom. Res.* **12**, 145–156.

Hirano, A., Kurland, L. T., Krooth, R. S. and Lessell, S. (1961). Parkinsonism-dementia complex, an endemic disease on the Island of Guam. I: Clinical features. *Brain* **84**, 642–662.

Hornykiewicz, O. (1973). Dopamine in the basal ganglia. *Br. Med. Bull.* **29**, 172–178.

Jansen, J. and Monrad-Krohn, G. H. (1938). On Creutzfeldt-Jakob's disease. *Z. Ges. Neurol. Psychiat.* **163**, 670.

Kay, D. W. K. (1962). Outcome and cause of death in mental disorders of old age. *Acta Psychiat. Scand.* **38**, 249–276.

Kay, D. W. K. and Roth, M. (1961). Environmental and hereditary factors in the schizophrenias of old age. *J. Ment. Sci.* **107**, 649–686.

Kay, D. W. K., Roth, M. and Hopkins, B. (1955). Affective disorders arising in the senium. *J. Ment. Sci.* **101**, 302–316.

Kay, D. W. K., Beamish, P. and Roth, M. (1964). Old age mental disorders in Newcastle-upon-Tyne: a study of prevalence. *Br. J. Psychiat.* **110**, 146–158.

Kendell, R. E. (1974). The stability of psychiatric diagnoses. *Br. J. Psychiat.* **124**, 352–356.

Kendrick, D. C., Parboosingh, R. C. and Post, F. (1965). A synonym learning test for use with elderly psychiatric subjects: a validation study. *Br. J. Soc. Clin. Psychol.* **4**, 63–71.

Lader, M. and Noble, P. (1975). Affective disorders. *In* 'Research in Psychophysiology' (Eds P. H. Venables and M. J. Christie), pp. 258–281. Wiley, Chichester.

Larsson, T., Sjögren, T. and Jacobson, G. (1963). Senile dementia: a clinical, sociomedical and genetic study. *Acta Psychiat. Scand., Suppl.* 167.

Lauter, H. and Meyer, J. E. (1968). Clinical and nosological concepts of senile dementia. *In* 'Senile Dementia' (Eds C. H. Muller and L. Ciompi), pp. 13–26. Hans Huber, Bern. Stuttgart.

Lewy, F. H. (1923). 'Die Lehre vom Tonus und der Bewegung'. Berlin.

Loranger, A. W., Goodell, H., McDowell, F. H., Lee, J. E. and Sweett, R. D. (1972). Intellectual impairment in Parkinson's syndrome. *Brain* **95**, 405–412.

Marsden, C. D. and Harrison, M. J. G. (1972). Outcome of investigation of patients with presenile dementia. *Br. Med. J.* **2**, 249–252.

Mettler, F. A. and Crandell, A. (1959). Relation between Parkinsonism and psychiatric disorder. *J. Nerv. Ment. Dis.* **129**, 551–563.

Miller, E. (1974). Dementia as an accelerated ageing of the nervous system: some psychological and methodological considerations. *Age and Ageing* **3**, 197–202.

Mindham, R. H. S. (1970). Psychiatric symptoms in Parkinsonism. *J. Neurol. Neurosurg. Psychiat.* **33**, 188–191.

Mindham, R. H. S. (1974). Psychiatric aspects of Parkinson's disease. *Br. J. Hosp. Med.* **11**, 411–414.

Mindham, R. H. S., Marsden, C. D. and Parkes, J. D. (1976). Psychiatric symptoms during L-dopa therapy for Parkinson's disease and their relationship to physical disability. *Psychol. Med.* **6**, 23–33.

Mjönes, H. (1949). Paralysis agitans: a clinical and genetic study. *Acta Psychiat. Scand., Suppl.* 54.

McDonald, C. (1969). Clinical heterogeneity in senile dementia. *Br. J. Psychiat.* **15**, 267–271.

Newton, R. D. (1948). The identity of Alzheimer's disease and senile dementia and their relationship to senility. *J. Ment. Sci.* **94**, 225–249.

Nott, P. N. and Fleminger, J. J. (1975). Presenile dementia: the difficulties of early diagnosis. *Acta Psychiat. Scand.* **51**, 210–217.

Parkinson, J. (1817). 'An Essay on the Shaking Palsy'. Sherwood, Neely and Jones, London.

Patrick, H. T. and Levy, D. M. (1922). Parkinson's disease: a clinical study of one hundred and forty-six cases. *Archs Neurol. Psychiat.* **7**, 711–720.

Pearce, J. and Miller, E. (1973). 'Clinical Aspects of Dementia'. Ballière Tindall, London.

Pilleri, G. (1966). The Klüver-Bucy syndrome in man. A clinico-anatomical contribution to the function of the medial temporal lobe structures. *Psychiat. Neurol., Basel* **152**, 65–103.

Pollock, M. and Hornabrook, R. W. (1966). The prevalence, natural history and dementia of Parkinson's disease. *Brain* **89**, 429–448.

Post, F. (1962). 'The Significance of Affective Symptoms in Old Age'. Maudsley Monograph No. 10. Oxford University Press, Oxford.

Post, F. (1965). 'The Clinical Psychiatry of Late Life'. Pergamon Press, Oxford.

Post, F. (1966). 'Persistent Persecutory States in the Elderly'. Pergamon Press, Oxford.

Post, F. (1975). Dementia, depression and pseudodementia. *In* 'Psychiatric Aspects of Neurological Disease' (Eds F. Benson and D. Blumer), pp. 99–120. Grune and Stratton, New York.

Reitan, R. M. and Bollit, J. (1971). Intellectual and cognitive functions in Parkinson's disease. *J. Consult. Clin. Psychol.* **37**, 364–369.

Riklan, M., Weiner, H. and Diller, L. (1959). Somato-psychologic studies in Parkinson's disease. *J. Nerv. Ment. Dis.* **129**, 263–272.

Roth, M. (1955). The natural history of mental disorders in the senium. *J. Ment. Sci.* **101**, 281–301.

Roth, M. (1971). Classification and aetiology in mental disorder of old age: some recent developments. *In* 'Recent Developments in Psychogeriatrics' (Eds D. W. K. Kay and A. Walk), pp. 1–18. Headley Bros, Ashford, Kent.

Rothschild, D. and Kasanin, J. (1936). Clinicopathologic studies of Alzheimer's disease: relationship to senile conditions. *Archs Neurol. Psychiat.* **36**, 293–321.

Schwab, R. S. (1960). Progression and prognosis in Parkinson's disease. *J. Nerv. Ment. Dis.* **130**, 556–566.

Scott, P. (1965). The Ganser syndrome, a peculiar hysterical state (trans. C. E. Schorer). *Br. J. Criminol.* **5**, 127–131.

Sjögren, H. (1955). Neuropsychiatric studies in presenile and senile diseases, based on a material of one thousand cases. *Acta Psychiat. Scand., Suppl.* 106, pp. 9–36.

Sjögren, T., Sjögren, H. and Lindgren, A. G. H. (1952). Morbus Alzheimer and Morbus Pick. *Acta Psych. Neurol. Scand., Suppl.* 82.

Sourander, P. and Sjögren, H. (1970). The concept of Alzheimer's disease and its clinical implications. *In* 'Alzheimer's Disease' (Eds G. E. W. Wolstenholme and M. O'Connor), pp. 11–32. J. A. Churchill, London.

Steele, J. C., Richardson, J. C. and Olszewski, J. (1964). Progressive supranuclear palsy: an heterogeneous degeneration involving the brain stem, basal ganglia and cerebellum with vertical gaze and pseudobulbar palsy, nuchal dystonia and dementia. *Archs Neurol. (Chicago)* **10**, 333–359.

Tomlinson, B. E., Blessed, G. and Roth, M. (1968). Observations on the brains of non-demented old people. *J. Neurol. Sci.* **7**, 331–356.

White, P., Goodhardt, M. J., Keet, P., Hiley, C. R., Carrasco, L. H., Williams, J. E. J. and Bowen, D. M. (1977). Neocortical cholinergic neurons in elderly people. *Lancet* **1**, 668–670.

Whitehead, A. (1973). Verbal learning and memory in elderly depressives. *Br. J. Psychiat.* **123**, 203–208.

Whitlock, F. A. (1967). The Ganser syndrome. *Br. J. Psychiat.* **113**, 19–29.

15 Social and transcultural psychiatry

Geoffrey G. Lloyd

Social psychiatry

There is no generally accepted definition of the term 'social psychiatry', which is not surprising since problems of definition abound in many areas of psychiatry. The absence of such a consensus, however, makes it all the more necessary for a writer to specify what he understands the term to mean. Hare (1969) has outlined the history of the term social psychiatry from its first appearance in the American literature in 1933 and has described the two main ways in which it has been used, with reference to the writings of Maxwell Jones on the one hand and Aubrey Lewis on the other. For Jones, social psychiatry was essentially a method of treatment, being an extension of the principles of group psychotherapy to larger numbers in the form of therapeutic communities. Lewis considered social psychiatry to have important implications for research and to be concerned with the investigation of social causes and social consequences of mental illness and with the various social methods which may be used to treat such illness. It is apparent from the more recent writings of Arthur (1971) and Wing (1971) that they are largely in agreement with Lewis and it is this viewpoint which will be adopted in this chapter.

Social psychiatry is not considered to be a single discipline but a method of approach concerned with all the social aspects of psychiatry. This chapter examines the principles of social psychiatry as they apply to adult mental illness. More detailed consideration of individual syndromes will be found in the appropriate chapters.

Social causes of psychiatric illness

It is generally assumed that most psychiatric disorders occur as a result of a complex interaction of biological, psychological and social factors. A considerable amount of research has been undertaken in recent years to discover which social factors are of aetiological importance or which may modify the course of such disorders. Implicit in the aims of research of this nature is the possibility of being able to prevent some mental illness or to reduce the resulting disabilities.

Much of this research has relied on epidemiological methods. *Epidemiology* may be broadly defined as the study of the relationship between a disease and the environment, and is particularly concerned with the distribution of diseases in defined population groups. In the calculation of rates of disease certain terms are used in a precise way so it is necessary to have an understanding of these.

The *prevalence* of a disease is the number of cases present in a unit of population at a given time (point prevalence) or during a given period (period prevalence).

The *expectancy* is the likelihood that an individual will develop the disease during a given period. It is a hypothetical figure derived from census data.

The *incidence* is the number of new cases appearing in a unit of population in a given period of time, usually one year. This rate, because it concentrates on new cases, is more likely to provide information about causal factors than are rates of prevalence or expectancy.

From the above definitions it is obvious that two closely related problems in epidemiology are, firstly, to establish criteria as to what constitutes a case, and secondly to identify the sick individual. These problems are especially pertinent in psychiatry where there is considerable disagreement, even between experts, over the diagnosis of certain categories such as the personality disorders and, to a lesser extent, the neuroses. In social psychiatry there are also problems related to the measurement of the various social factors which are being investigated. These difficulties contribute in large part to the inconsistent and contradictory findings reported in the literature.

Various sources of data have been used to identify patients, one of the most common being *hospital statistics* relating to admissions and out-patient attendances from a specified population. Such figures, however, are greatly influenced by local factors such as the number of available beds and the quality of services. In many areas, they are likely to represent only the most seriously ill. *Case registers* have been established in several centres in recent years, notably in Baltimore in the United States, and in Nottingham, Salford, Aberdeen and Camberwell in the United

Kingdom. By noting the contact of patients with various psychiatric agencies the progress of an individual patient can be followed over a period of time. The registers are cumulative and avoid duplication, and they are useful in the planning and evaluation of local psychiatric services (Wing and Hailey, 1972). However, they do not represent a complete picture of the rate of psychiatric illness in the community. On the basis of *general practice surveys* Shepherd *et al.* (1966) have estimated that during one year 14% of the population consult their doctor because of a psychiatric disorder, only one in five of this 14% being referred to a psychiatrist. This figure is likely to be an underestimate of the true prevalence since about a third of the psychiatric disorders in general practice are not detected by the doctor (Goldberg and Blackwell, 1970). In theory *population surveys* would be expected to provide the most accurate assessment of the prevalence of psychiatric illness in the community. Two North American studies, in the urban area of Midtown Manhattan (Srole *et al.*, 1962) and in the rural area of Stirling County (Leighton, 1959), revealed a very high prevalence of symptoms, over 80% in each case. Most afflicted individuals were considered to have only mild to moderate impairment but these studies obviously employed a wide definition of abnormality. They both used structured interviews administered by research assistants, the completed schedules then being assessed by psychiatrists. However, as Goldberg (1972) has emphasized, in the absence of objective criteria, interview by an experienced psychiatrist remains the ultimate method of case identification. This poses great practical problems because of the manpower and finance involved but Hagnell (1966) has successfully carried out such a study in Sweden in which he interviewed almost the entire population of a small rural area himself. Essen-Moller (1956) had interviewed the population from the same area 10 years previously so comparisons could be made. Hagnell found a history of mental disorder up to the present age of the subjects, the so-called life-time prevalence, of 1·7% for psychoses, 13·1% for neuroses and 1·2% for mental defiency. The rate of developing a mental illness using his criteria during the 10-year period of the study was 11·3% for men and 20·4% for women. Considerably lower figures were obtained if only admissions to psychiatric hospitals or attendances at clinics were considered. A more efficient method of case identification, which can be used on a large scale, is a two-stage procedure in which the population under survey is first screened by means of a suitably constructed questionnaire. Those subjects whose responses have marked them as possible cases can then be interviewed by trained psychiatrists using a standardized method. In practice, this approach encounters difficulties in obtaining a sample which is representative of the total population. Finlay-Jones and Burvill (1977) have discussed some sources of bias in the light of their

Australian survey using the General Health Questionnaire (Goldberg, 1972) as the means of case identification.

The social factors implicated as having causal significance in psychiatric illness include migration, economic poverty, patterns of family interaction, stressful life-events and social class. One of the earliest systematic studies, which has now become a classic, was that of Durkheim (1897) into the causes of suicide. He considered that suicide was related to the degree with which an individual was integrated into a social group, and that any factor which segregated the individual from the society in which he lived predisposed him to suicide. Durkheim's study relied heavily on statistical methods, as have many others attempting to identify social causes of illness. Unfortunately, there has been a tendency to equate statistical correlations with causal factors. Several social variables which have been associated with psychiatric illness have later been shown to be consequences of the illness rather than causes. Alternatively they have been shown to be a result of an intervening factor such as a life-long personality characteristic which may also precipitate the illness. The interpretation of social correlates of psychiatric illness should be made carefully since only rarely is this unambiguous. The discovery of such an association should lead to further research to unravel the nature of the link and the mechanism by which it has come to exist.

Migration is an event which exemplifies the dilemma over the interpretation of statistical associations. Despite a large volume of research, mainly finding that psychiatric illness, particularly schizophrenia, is more common in those who migrate between countries, firm conclusions still cannot be drawn. The association of psychiatric illness and migration may be due to migration causing illness, the stress hypothesis, or to the presence of certain premorbid personality traits which predispose both to illness and to migration, the selection hypothesis. Ødegaard (1932), in his pioneering study of Norwegian immigrants to Minnesota, concluded that the higher rate of hospital admission for psychiatric illness among the immigrant group was due to the selective migration of people predisposed to illness. Immigrants to New York State, both from overseas and from other American States, were found by Malzberg and Lee (1956) to have higher first admission rates than the native-born, it being their opinion that a combination of stress and selection factors was responsible for the differentials. Within a group of Hungarian immigrants to Great Britain after the 1956 uprising, Mezey (1960) showed that the rate of schizophrenia was significantly lower in those who gave a political reason for migrating than in those who migrated for non-political reasons. In a study based on the Camberwell Case Register, Clare (1974), while finding a higher referral rate among the Irish compared to the indigenous population for all psychiatric illness, noted that the referral rate for schizophrenia was approximately the same as that of the indigenous group. This was a surprising finding in view of the high reported rate of schizophrenia in Ireland (Walsh and Walsh, 1970) and prompted Clare to suggest a selective migration of individuals less predisposed to schizophrenia.

What emerges strongly from the literature on migration and psychiatric illness is that generalizations cannot be made on the basis of individual studies. The links vary according to the ethnicity of the group studied, the nature of the illness, the type of migration and the reasons for migrating. The time has passed when migration could be regarded as a unitary concept (Murphy, 1977).

The following sub-sections will consider some of the factors which have recently received most attention from research workers and about which some conclusions can be drawn.

Life-events

It now seems clear that potentially disturbing life events are experienced more commonly by certain psychiatric patients preceding the onset of their illness than by a normal population control group. Well defined crises and life changes were found to occur with greater frequency in the three-week period immediately prior to the onset of an acute episode of schizophrenia (Brown and Birley, 1968; Birley and Brown, 1970). In other three-week periods more distant from the onset there was no significant difference in the frequency of life events between the patient and control groups. Brown and Birley were careful to avoid some of the potential errors of this type of study by asking only standard questions about previously defined events. They also classified the events into 'independent' and 'possibly independent', thus excluding those events which might have been influenced or brought on by the illness.

Similar findings have since emerged with respect to depression (Paykel *et al.*, 1969; Brown *et al.*, 1973a), the events being characterized especially by threatened or actual loss, for example of a job through redundancy or of a close relative through bereavement. The depressed patients were subject to an increased rate of undesirable experiences for a much longer period prior to the onset of their symptoms than were the schizophrenics; markedly threatening events were found to be commoner for at least a year before onset in Brown's study. In a comparison of depressives and first admission schizophrenics (Jacobs *et al.*, 1974), the depressives reported more exit and other undesirable events in the six months before onset.

Having established a link between life events and onset of illness the nature of this link needs to be considered. Brown *et al.* (1973b) have produced evidence to suggest that in schizophrenia life events have a triggering effect, bringing forward in time an episode of illness which would have occurred quite soon even if the event had not taken place. On the other hand they have suggested that for at least a third of their depressed patients, life events have a formative effect and that without their influence depression would not have occurred for a long time, if at all.

Social class and social network

Studies of the social class distribution of schizophrenic patients have consistently shown that they are over-represented among the lower classes. Since the classic work of Faris and Dunham (1939) in Chicago showing high rates of schizophrenia in the culturally and economically impoverished central areas of the city, there has been a controversy over the reasons for this social class distribution. Schizophrenia has been attributed by some authors primarily to the poor socio-economic conditions experienced by members of the lower classes (Kohn, 1973), while others have explained the lower class distribution as being a result of the downward social drift consequent upon the effects of the illness (Goldberg and Morrison, 1963). Alternative theories have included those which suggest that failure to achieve an expected social class may produce stresses which cause illness (Turner and Wagenfeld, 1967) and that doctors employ different diagnostic and therapeutic practices towards the lower class sick (Hollingshead and Redlich, 1958). The controversy is by no means settled but recent work strongly supports the social drift hypothesis as far as schizophrenia is concerned (Hare et al., 1972).

Depression has been subject to less attention than schizophrenia but the evidence from recent studies indicates that the parental background of these patients does not differ from that of the normal population (Birtchnell, 1971; Hare et al., 1972). Birtchnell's study also found that the current social class of depressed patients presented a mixed picture, the patients being under-represented in social classes I and III, over-represented in class IV and V and slightly in excess in class II.

The above findings, and those of most other studies, relate to patients in contact with the psychiatric services. A community survey of women by Brown et al. (1975) has shown that, when current social class is considered, depression is more common in the working class. Compared to middle class women, the working class group suffered more life events which had severe, long-term, threatening implications and were more vulnerable to these events. The association between depression and life events was strengthened by the presence of certain factors which, however, had no association with depression in the absence of life events.

These factors were loss of mother before the age of 11, three or more children under 14 living at home, lack of an intimate, confiding relationship with husband or boyfriend, and lack of full-time or part-time employment. The first three of these factors were found to be more common in the working class and helped to account for the greater vulnerability of this group. This study represents a major contribution to social psychiatry, in particular to our recognition of the importance of the social network in protecting people from depression. It is supported by the work of Henderson *et al*. (1978) who have found deficiencies in the social network of non-psychotic out-patients and who are currently engaged in a prospective study to evaluate the provision of social relationships in such a group. If their findings are positive they may well be used, together with those of Brown, to form a small foundation of that long-cherished goal, preventive psychiatry.

Family factors

The importance attached by many writers to the quality of parent–child relationships during early childhood in influencing mental health has led to several investigations on the relationship between loss of a parent in childhood and later psychiatric illness, particularly depression. Granville-Grossman's review of this subject up to 1966 (Granville-Grossman, 1968) concluded that no consistent association between early bereavement and subsequent affective disorder had been demonstrated. Since that review Hill and Price (1967) have shown a higher rate of paternal death in depressed in-patients compared to other psychiatric in-patients, the difference being most marked for female patients. Birtchnell (1970), in contrast, found no difference in early parental death between depressives and other psychiatric patients, although he did show an increased rate for all psychiatric patients compared to normal population controls and also for severely depressed patients compared to those with moderate depression. These findings provide stronger evidence for childhood bereavement being a factor in the later development of depressive illness. Parental loss, from all causes, has been shown by Greer (1966) to be commoner during childhood in a group of psychiatric out-patients who attempted suicide compared to a control group of patients without a history of suicide attempt. A study by Bunch *et al*. (1971) of completed suicides did not reveal a higher rate of early parental death when compared with general population controls but there was a trend in the expected direction among those who had previously attempted suicide. Besides predisposing to depression, loss of family members may also exert a phenomenological influence in depressed patients. Such an association was found by Brown *et al.* (1977) in their community survey of depression in women. While finding a link between loss of mother before 11 and depression in adult life they discovered that, in the depressed group, psychotic symptoms were associated with past loss by death. In contrast, neurotic symptoms were associated with other types of past loss.

The family factors implicated in the causation of schizophrenia are more elaborate and speculative. The theories and contributions of Bateson, Lidz, Laing and others have been discussed at length in Chapter 11 and have also been reviewed by Hirsch and Leff (1975).

It was the conclusion of these authors that, with the exception of the work of Wynne and Singer, studies attempting to demonstrate an aetiological effect of deviant parental communication have been negative, contradictory or methodologically unsound. Wynne and Singer are of the opinion that, when compared with other groups, the speech of parents of schizophrenics is characterized by features which made it difficult to understand. These features include vagueness, irrelevancies, disruptions and lack of closure. Exposure to such speech over a period of several years is believed to predispose the offspring to schizophrenia. When a group of parents of British schizophrenics was examined, Hirsch and Leff were unable to replicate these findings and provide support for the hypothesis of Wynne and Singer. The reasons for this failure were not entirely clear but there was a suggestion that the characteristics of the two schizophrenic groups differed on such factors as diagnostic criteria and duration of illness.

The various theories that abnormalities of parental communication cause schizophrenia in offspring remain unproven. However, there is growing agreement that the type of family environment to which a patient returns after leaving hospital is important in influencing the future course of the illness (Brown *et al.*, 1972). The relapse rate has been shown to be higher in those schizophrenic patients who return to homes characterized by high emotional expression. In these circumstances the risks of relapse can be lessened by reducing the amount of face-to-face contact between patient and relatives. Vaughn and Leff (1976) have replicated these findings and have also shown that patients with neurotic depression are even more vulnerable than schizophrenics to high levels of expressed emotion.

Communicability of psychiatric illness

There are several conditions in clinical psychiatry in which it is claimed that psychopathology is transmitted from one ill person to others in the immediate social orbit, this transmission being compared by some to the spread of infectious diseases. A well known example is that of *folie à deux*, first described by Lasegue and Falret (1877). In this condition an initially well person acquires the false beliefs of a sick individual who is usually suffering from a paranoid psychosis. *Folie à deux* is said to occur only when the two have an intimate emotional relationship and when, for reasons of intelligence or personality, the psychotic individual exerts a powerful influence over the other. When the two individuals are separated the abnormal beliefs of the person who was not originally psychotic are usually relinquished. Sometimes a psychotic person can convince more than one other of the apparent veracity of his delusions and cases of *folie à trois* and *folie à quatre* have been reported.

Epidemic hysteria is another example of the transmission of psychopathology within a community from one member to another. Jaspers (1962), who said that these psychic epidemics 'gave a drastic illustration of the spread of psychic attitudes through unconscious infection', has commented on their rarity in modern times compared to the Middle Ages. Nevertheless, Sirois (1974) has collected reports of 78 distinct outbreaks from the world literature between 1872 and 1972. They were characterized by hysterical conversion symptoms which are precipitated by an event of emotional significance. The symptoms are initially confined to one individual or to a small group but thereafter spread to other members of the community. Females predominate in most of the reported outbreaks which have often been in schools, convents and hospitals. The exact nature of many of the reportedly hysterical symptoms has been questioned. An organic rather than a psychological cause has been proposed for some of the epidemics and the difference of opinion can rouse high feeling, as evidenced by the correspondence which followed the suggestion of McEvedy and Beard (1970) that the Royal Free Hospital epidemic of 1955 had a psychological aetiology. Benaim *et al.* (1973) have convincingly described a hysterical epidemic of falling in a class of London schoolgirls, claiming that the outbreak was triggered by news of the death after childbirth of a former class member. It was led by two intelligent, powerful and respected girls, spreading later to other pupils, but being virtually confined to an 'in group'.

Similarly the explosive increase of heroin abuse within an identifiable social network in an English town has been traced by de Alarcon (1969) to two main initiators. By establishing the date of first injection and identity of the initiator, de Alarcon was able to show that heroin abuse was introduced into the community by local boys who had acquired the habit elsewhere. Thereafter the abuse spread through long-standing or current links of school, neighbourhood or leisure activities.

Patterns of illness are constantly changing and while epidemics of hysteria are now relatively rare, one of the most striking recent trends in psychiatry has been a great increase in the incidence of attempted suicide, or parasuicide, as some writers call it. The work of Stengel and Cook (1958), among others, strongly suggests that this behaviour can serve as a means of communication between the patient and others in his environment. Usually this communication is an appeal for help. Kreitman and his colleagues have suggested that within contemporary society there exist sub-cultures in which the communicational aspects of attempted suicide are well defined and in which this type of behaviour is relatively acceptable. They have provided evidence compatible with this theory by showing that patients who attempt suicide are linked socially with greater frequency than would be expected by chance (Kreitman et al., 1970). Having demonstrated the existence of socially linked groups they speculated that the recent rise in attempted suicide might be at least partially due to case-to-case spread.

Illness behaviour

Apart from their significance in precipitating and influencing the course of psychiatric symptoms, social factors may also be important in determining whether individuals with such symptoms consult their doctor and become patients. In other words, social factors influence the adoption of the *sick role*. Parsons (1951) has formulated some of the consequences of the sick role as they affect the individual. The patient is exempt from many of the usual social responsibilities; he is not expected to be able to cure his illness by willpower; he should want to get well; he should seek medical help and co-operate with treatment. The way in which an individual perceives, evaluates and acts in response to his symptoms has been termed *illness behaviour* by Mechanic (1962). He has shown that the tendency to seek medical advice for symptoms is influenced by such factors as religious background, social class and degree of dependence on others. High levels of interpersonal stress were also associated with an increased tendency to medical consultation in his study.

It is more difficult to disentangle symptoms from illness behaviour in psychiatric disorders than it is in physical disorders but similar factors may be relevant. For example, in the study on depression by Brown et al. (1975) there was evidence that some of the factors which were associated with a high rate of depression, namely a poor marital relationship and three or more children under the age of 14, were paradoxically associated with a reduced chance of the woman seeking treatment from her doctor. These two conditions were more common among the working class group and would account for some of the social class differences in illness behaviour.

Social effects of psychiatric illness

Psychiatric illness has considerable social consequences not only for the individual patient, but also for the patient's family and the community at large. This is so especially for the chronic psychotic disorders and for the dementias.

The social adjustment of the individual is affected by the illness even after the more florid symptoms have been successfully treated. Features such as apathy, loss of energy, poor drive and impaired concentration are often found in schizophrenics who have recovered from an acute episode, and these features obviously have profound consequences on the individual's ability to work and to cope with the daily routine. These handicaps may lead to the patient having to take less demanding work, with a reduction in income, or eventually to unemployment. As a result the patient's confidence and morale are damaged and the family suffers financially. The downward social drift experienced by many schizophrenics has already been mentioned.

Some of these handicaps, as well as socially embarrassing behaviour, have been shown to be related partly to the poverty of the hospital environment in which patients are treated (Wing and Brown, 1970). As will be discussed in the next section, it has become the policy in recent years to avoid some of these undesirable effects by admitting patients to hospital for relatively short periods before discharging them back into the community. This policy sometimes involves discharging patients who still have florid symptoms such as delusions or hallucinations. For those patients who are discharged home to their families much of the responsibility for seeing that rehabilitation is continued falls to the immediate relatives. In some cases these patients can become a burden to their families and Wing *et al.* (1964) have described the strained relationships which occur within the families of discharged patients. In their group considerable distress was caused to relatives by certain forms of behaviour on the part of the patient, particularly threatened or actual violence, nocturnal overactivity, abnormal sexual behaviour and deterioration in personal habits. Frequently such behaviour led to a family crisis and re-admission of the patient. They considered the community services to be deficient in the prevention of such crises, contact with the services often being made only after a crisis had occurred. Stevens (1972) has also described the dependence of a group of severely handicapped patients on their relatives. Most of the patients studied by her were schizophrenics and many were living with elderly parents, either because they had never married or because their marriages had broken down. The patients had marked impairments in ability to communicate, in sociability and in use of their leisure time. Relatives expressed dissatisfaction with these impairments and most appeared to have suffered from some mental ill-health themselves as a result of looking after the patient. On the credit side, relatives often valued the company provided by the patient; several elderly parents would have been very isolated socially if the patient had not been living at home.

Creer and Wing (1974) have vividly amplified these findings in a series of interviews with members of the National Schizophrenia Fellowship, a charitable organization promoting the interests of patients and relatives, and also with a group of relatives of schizophrenic patients residing in an inner London suburb. Worries were chiefly related to the patients' poor social performance, unpredictable behaviour and uncertain long-term future. The relatives also felt depressed when their own efforts did not seem to help the patient and guilty when they believed others blamed them for failing in their responsibilities. Nearly half said that the effect on their own health and well-being of living with the patient had been severe. However, in spite of services which were regarded as inadequate, most relatives were tolerant and accepting in their attitudes, and complaints were few.

Neurotic illness has been studied less intensively than chronic psychosis but Cooper (1972) has shown in a general practice population that chronic neurosis is associated with social dysfunction. The ability to conduct social affairs and satisfaction with social roles were among the functions impaired and over all there was a relationship between the degree of social dysfunction and clinical severity of the neurosis. Cooper's study does not permit conclusions to be drawn about whether social dysfunction is secondary to neurosis or an aetiological factor.

Neurosis also appears to have ill-effects on the mental health of the other family members. Hagnell and Kreitman (1974) have reported a higher than expected rate of illness in both partners in a marriage and have suggested that this is due to the effects of neurosis on the originally healthy partner rather than to assortative mating. Wives appeared to be more susceptible than husbands to the effects of illness in the spouse. Children are also adversely affected by mental illness, of all sorts, in the parents (Rutter, 1966).

Whether relatives have to tolerate a greater burden in a community-orientated service than in one where admission to hospital is more commonly practised depends largely on the quality of support they receive. Grad and Sainsbury (1968), in a comparison of two contrasting services, found that the family burden was greater in the community service, the difference being due to the effect on their families of a group of mainly psychoneurotic patients under the age of 65 who had never been a severe burden. It was shown that the community service was not providing as much social support to the families of this group as the hospital-based service.

Social treatment of psychiatric illness

In the absence of definitive knowledge regarding the aetiology of psychiatric illness it is not yet possible to plan social changes to effect primary prevention. Claims have been made for the efficacy of various forms of social treatment for established illness, although not all of these have been adequately evaluated. Social treatment may be considered to embrace those measures which are taken to alter the patient's social environment thereby leading to a decrease in the severity of symptoms or handicaps.

Therapeutic communities

Since the Second World War there has been a vogue for organizing the potential benefits of the hospital environment along the lines of a therapeutic community, a term first used by Main (1946). The undesirable effects of institutionalization have been described by many writers, most graphically perhaps by Goffman (1961). One of the fundamental assumptions of the therapeutic community concept is that many of these undesirable effects can be prevented by altering the social structure of the traditional ward so that patients are encouraged to take a more responsible part in their own treatment. Hospital wards which are claimed to be therapeutic communities differ markedly from one another in their organization, and there is no agreement as to what constitutes such a community. Clark (1965) has pointed out that two different uses of the term have developed. The first, the therapeutic community approach, is related to the more liberal atmosphere pervading psychiatric hospitals in the last two decades, to the unlocking of doors and to the active rehabilitation and discharge of patients. Much of this has been made possible by the introduction of more effective psychotropic drugs. The second use of the term, the therapeutic community proper, is concerned with the type of unit developed and described by Maxwell Jones (1952, 1962). This is usually a unit of less than 100 persons where the aim is to remedy those difficulties in interpersonal relationships which are believed to be at the root of the patients' problems. Within such a community rigid hierarchies of authority are avoided and good patient–staff communication is fostered. Regular group meetings are held in which assumed therapeutic potentials of each patient are encouraged for the benefit of the rest of the group. In the therapeutic community for psychopaths at the Henderson Hospital (Whiteley, 1970) the group imposes its own rules and discipline. Individual patients are confronted with the effects of their mislearned patterns of social behaviour by the group and are encouraged to try out and adopt more acceptable behaviour. Craft (1965) has claimed success in the management of psychopaths of subnormal intelligence in a therapeutic community run on more authoritarian lines.

Proponents of therapeutic communities described by Jones are numerous and zealous but evaluation studies to justify their claims are lacking. It is difficult to accept that a particular ward milieu can be specifically therapeutic for all its patients who may have a wide variety of symptoms and handicaps. Those aspects of a ward environment which are therapeutic for some patients may be anti-therapeutic for others and it is important to identify these. Research in this area has been helped by the development of a Ward Atmosphere Scale (Moos and Houts, 1968) which assesses a variety of different dimensions of a ward's social and therapeutic environments as perceived by both patients and staff. In a study of large wards in American Veterans Administration hospitals (Moos and Schwartz, 1972) it was shown that wards with a high drop-out rate were perceived by staff as being low in support and involvement but high in anger and aggression. On the other hand, those wards with a high discharge rate were perceived by patients as being high in practical orientation and staff control and by staff as low in spontaneity. While the criteria chosen by these authors are not necessarily indicative of a good treatment outcome, the use of such a scale should promote the identification of the environmental factors which may be therapeutic for specific groups of patients.

Although the claims for therapeutic communities may have been over-stated, there is little doubt that changes in social environment can reduce a patient's disabilities. Wing and Brown (1970) showed that for chronic schizophrenics environmental poverty was associated with a clinical poverty syndrome characterized by social withdrawal, flatness of affect and poverty of speech. Enriching the social environment was followed by an improvement in these negative symptoms, the most important environmental change being a reduction in the amount of time the patients spent doing nothing. In the United States similar claims have been made by Gruenberg (1969) for comprehensive community psychiatric services in the prevention of the *social-breakdown syndrome*. This term has been applied to the secondary manifestations of psychotic disorders such as withdrawal, self-neglect, dangerous behaviour and failure to work.

If the environment is too stimulating, however, chronic schizophrenics tend to have a recurrence of positive symptoms such as delusions, hallucinations and thought disorder. Such patients do best in a social environment which is neither under-stimulating nor over-stimulating, one in which they are actively engaged in some task but which is routine, predictable and emotionally neutral. Consideration has also to be given to the social environment that the patient returns to after discharge from hospital. Homes in which there is a high level of expressed emotion are likely to induce recurrence of illness (Brown *et al.*, 1972; Vaughn and Leff, 1976) and patients from such families are often best advised to avoid excessive contact with their relatives. This may mean leaving home and living in lodgings or in a hostel. If living at home is unavoidable the patients can reduce contact with relatives by attending a day centre or, ideally, by obtaining a job.

Rehabilitation

The chronic handicaps associated with many psychiatric illnesses are usually only amenable to change when the patient has progressed through a planned programme of rehabilitation. Wing (1975) has defined three types of handicap accompanying schizophrenia: intrinsic handicaps are those which are assumed to be an integral part of the disease process (e.g. slowness); extrinsic handicaps include low intelligence, poverty and poor occupational skills; secondary handicaps form an intermediate group and include attributes such as low self-confidence and poor motivation which are thought to result from the patient's attitudes to his intrinsic handicaps. Rehabilitation aims at reducing such handicaps, or at least preventing their deterioration, so that the patient can be helped back towards employment. To be most effective a course of rehabilitation must include a careful assessment of each patient's handicaps, an assessment of the aims for the patient and the formulation of a series of attainable objectives. Such a programme can be started during the patient's hospital admission by establishing a regular pattern of attendance in the occupational therapy department. Thereafter the patient may progress to an Industrial Rehabilitation Unit (IRU) or to a hospital rehabilitation unit, the principles of which have been described by Bennett (1972). From there, many patients are able to move on to employment in the open market while others find work in sheltered workshops.

District psychiatric services

During the last twenty years there has been a great reduction in the number of psychiatric patients resident in hospitals in many Western countries. This has been achieved by discharging suitable long-stay patients and by increasing the out-patient and day-patient rehabilitation facilities. The traditional mental hospital has been criticized on account of its size, its old dilapidated buildings and the long distance which often separates it from the catchment area it serves. Such hospitals are now not considered to provide the ideal setting for the majority of the mentally ill who require in-patient treatment, and it is British government policy to establish smaller units in district general hospitals.

In England and Wales the change in the pattern of psychiatric care was given great impetus by the Mental Health Act, 1959, which was soon followed by similar legislation for Scotland and Northern Ireland. The Act was passed in recognition of the need for reform in the management of psychiatric illness because of advances in medical and social treatment. By abolishing the category of specially designated hospitals for the treatment of 'persons of unsound mind' it allowed patients to be admitted to units in general hospitals, with admission on a voluntary basis whenever possible. The Act also encouraged the establishment of a comprehensive network of out-patient facilities.

How many beds should remain to provide a comprehensive district service? This question has been the subject of debate for many years. A British study by Tooth and Brooke (1961) predicted that of all the long-stay patients in hospitals in 1954 none would remain by 1970. They also forecast that the needs of the mentally ill could be provided for with a bed ratio of 180 per 100,000 population. This figure was to include all psychiatric conditions except mental retardation. The predicted linear rate of decline of the in-patient population did not materialize and hundreds of old long-stay patients remain in hospital. However, for future needs many would consider the figure for the required number of beds to be too high. The current policy of the Department of Health and Social Security (Brothwood, 1973) is that, for a population of 100,000 there should be 50 hospital beds for the adult mentally ill and 25 day hospital places. For the aged with severe dementia there should be 30–40 beds and 10–20 places for day patients. It is also recommended that the local authority should provide 20–30 hostel places and 60 day centre places for those with social handicaps but who do not need continuous medical and nursing care. In addition the Department advises that units should be established on a regional or sub-regional basis for special groups such as children, adolescents, alcoholics, drug dependent patients and those in need of some degree of security.

The emphasis in this policy is on a shift in care from the hospital to the community. *Community care* has become a fashionable phrase but it is by no means certain that the community is prepared to assume more responsibility for its mentally ill members. Nor is it certain that for all discharged patients the community is any more therapeutic than the mental hospital environment. Much will depend on the quantity and quality of facilities available and there will probably be wide regional variations. A recent study (Mann and Cree, 1975) showed that long-stay patients continue to accumulate in hospitals. It was considered that of this new long-stay group, about a third would need continuing hospital care;

20% appeared likely to need supervised residential accommodation, such as a hostel; 15% were thought to need little or no supervision; and the remainder had a variety of specific needs, for example accommodation for the demented, blind or deaf. At present the appropriate supporting facilities in the community are inadequate or insufficient, as has been officially acknowledged (DHSS, 1975). More facilities will have to be provided if the larger mental hospitals are to be phased out, but until then admission and discharge policies will have to take into account the inadequacy of community services.

The position in the United States is somewhat similar. Because of a failure to establish a network of community services the policy of phasing out large state hospitals has become discredited in many states; in California the plan to close all state hospitals by 1982 has been abandoned after much public, professional and political opposition (Becker and Schulberg, 1976). There is likely to be an improvement in community services in future as a result of legislation passed in 1975 (Public Law 94–63) which requires that community mental health centres provide a range of 12 essential services. Federal funds are to be made available to finance these centres. Among the 12 services stipulated as essential, three which will have considerable influence on the phasing out of hospitals are (1) the provision of aftercare; (2) a programme of transitional half-way houses; and (3) screening of patients being considered for referral to the state hospital to determine whether alternative methods of treatment would be appropriate (Ochberg, 1976).

Are there sufficient psychiatrists?

Despite a fall in the number of hospital beds there has been an increase in re-admissions and out-patient attendances in the United Kingdom. A community-orientated service is likely to make more demands on the psychiatrists' time because of the greater therapeutic efforts needed to maintain patients in the community. In addition, as district general hospital units are established, more patients with neurotic or personality problems are likely to seek consultation. Liaison between psychiatrists and other medical specialists will further increase consultation for the psychiatrist. Doubts have been raised whether there will be sufficient psychiatrists to staff such a service (Russell, 1973) both because of the increased clinical demands and because of a relative decline in the number of trainees entering psychiatry.

At present little is known about the particular skills possessed by the psychiatrist. What is it that the psychiatrist, by virtue of his lengthy and expensive medical training, can do which the psychologist, nurse or social worker cannot do? In the face of a manpower shortage, there is a need for evaluative research to define the areas of particular competence so that the most efficient use can be made of the psychiatrist's time. It may well be that the role of the psychiatrist will have to change, becoming more consultative and advising primary care teams of general practitioners, nurses and social workers. The value of attaching a social worker to a general practice in terms of reducing the social disability and the symptoms of chronic neurosis has already been demonstrated on a small scale (Cooper *et al.*, 1975), as has the efficacy of specially trained nurses in the treatment of neurotic and sexual disorders using the techniques of behavioural psychotherapy (Marks *et al.*, 1975). The prevalence of psychiatric illness is such that most patients will never be referred to a specialist psychiatrist, so further evaluation of experimental primary care teams is clearly needed.

Transcultural psychiatry

If the examination of social factors can be expected to provide information about the aetiology and course of psychiatric illness, then the study of illness in different cultures should add further to our knowledge. This is one of the concerns of transcultural psychiatry, a branch of psychiatry which has grown vigorously in the last two or three decades and which recently has been the subject of two review monographs (Kiev, 1972; Yap, 1974). The difficulties involved in epidemiological surveys, referred to earlier in this chapter, apply with even greater force when comparisons are being made between different cultural groups. Treatment facilities and the concept of illness may differ widely between cultures, as may the criteria used to distinguish individual psychiatric syndromes from one another. Even between the United States and the United Kingdom, countries with a common language and which share many cultural values, there are significant discrepancies in diagnostic practice (Cooper *et al.*, 1972). There is also evidence that inhabitants from some developing countries discriminate less between different emotional states than do those from developed countries (Leff, 1973).

Reported transcultural variations in prevalence and incidence of psychiatric disorders therefore have to be viewed cautiously. Even if the figures are valid, their interpretation is difficult because it is not clear what particular components of culture are associated with any given pattern of symptoms. Culture is difficult to define and is often used as an umbrella term (Jablensky and Sartorious, 1975). Genetic and other biological factors, such as the effects of malnutrition and infections, have also to be taken into account when variations in rates of psychiatric illness are discovered. However, in spite of these reservations, sufficient data have been gathered to provide suggestions as to the role of cultural factors in the aetiology and course of psychiatric illness. Familiarity with these factors should no longer be regarded as the preserve of globe-trotting academics. Many areas of Great Britain now have large immigrant communities so that clinical problems modified by the effects of an alien culture already form part of the daily routine of the local psychiatric services (Cox, 1977).

It was previously widely believed that psychiatric illness was rare or non-existent in so-called primitive cultures and was introduced into a society as a result of contact with Western civilization. This rather naïve view is now known to be untrue. Psychiatric disorders occur ubiquitously, albeit with varying frequencies, and no culture has been described which is free of such disorders. Even when comparing groups from the inhabitants of Nova Scotia and the Yoruba people of Nigeria, Leighton *et al.* (1963) were more impressed by the similarities than by the differences. Psychotic disorders could be categorized into the recognized syndromes, although they were rare in both communities. Psychophysiological symptoms and psychoneurotic complaints were slightly more common among the Yoruba while drug addiction was absent in this group.

If a clear operational definition is used, schizophrenia can be recognized reliably in widely differing cultures (World Health Organization, 1973). With a few exceptions the reported prevalence of schizophrenia appears to be similar in different cultures (Jablensky and Sartorious, 1975) but there may be differences in the manifestations and content of the psychosis. Among illiterate Africans, schizophrenia in its early stages is often characterized by confusion, excitement, unsystematized delusions and transient auditory hallucinations, while in the better educated the picture is similar to that described in Europeans (German, 1972). Catatonic symptoms have been reported as being more common among Indian schizophrenics but it is uncertain whether this observation is related to a culture which encourages passivity and withdrawal or to the greater chronicity of the illness by the time patients reach hospital (Neki, 1973). The course of the illness may also differ from one culture to another. Results from the International Pilot Study of Schizophrenia showed that patients from centres in developing countries had a better outcome over a two-year period than those in centres in the developed countries (Sartorius *et al.*, 1977).

Previous reports about the rarity of depression in developing countries were probably incorrect. The condition was under-diagnosed because of the application of European criteria. Asuni (1962) has suggested that depression is common in Western Nigeria but that feelings of guilt, unworthiness and self-depreciation are infrequent and consequently suicide is rare. The clinical picture is more likely to be dominated by paranoid delusions, hypochondriasis and somatic complaints. Likewise, in a study of Indian patients, Teja *et al.* (1971) have noted the greater frequency of somatic symptoms, hypochondriasis, anxiety and agitation compared to British depressives.

The various neurotic disorders can also be recognized in widely differing cultures although somatic symptoms are probably more common in developing countries (Neki, 1973). Hysterical neuroses, with either conversion or dissociation symptoms are particularly common (German, 1972; Neki, 1973). Dissociative states resemble in many ways the trances and possession states which are deliberately sought in some cultures during religious and other ceremonies. These states, however, are of much shorter duration than the dissociative episodes and are recognized as normal by other members of the culture.

Transcultural studies in psychiatry suggest that there are constant patterns of symptoms in the major diagnostic categories, but there is no doubt that the content of the illness and behaviour pattern may vary, thus making it likely that the effect of culture on psychiatric disorder is more pathoplastic than pathogenic. Certain 'exotic' or *culture-bound* disorders have been reported in the literature. Although the pattern of symptoms is often unique to the particular culture, these disorders can be regarded as variants of the major psychoses and neuroses. The pathoplastic effect of cultural variable is seen at its greatest in these disorders, some of which are described below.

Koro occurs typically in Malaya and southern China. The patient becomes convinced that his penis is retracting into his abdomen and, in accordance with local belief, fears death will result if this happens. Somatic and psychic features of anxiety follow the conviction and the patient resorts to various practices to prevent retraction of the penis, such as placing a clamp on the organ or tying string around it. A few cases have been reported in women who fear retraction of the breasts or external genitalia. The syndrome is generally regarded as a form of an acute anxiety state occurring in those with unresolved sexual conflicts. Cultural factors almost certainly determine the nature of the fears and the consequent behaviour.

Amok was originally described in south-east Asia but is not exclusive to that region. It is virtually confined to men and is characterized by a prodromal period of depressive withdrawal followed by an outburst of rage in which the individual violently attacks people, animals or inanimate objects. Homicide is common and the episode often terminates with the person killing himself or being killed. Otherwise it ends in exhaustion and amnesia. Murphy (1973) has traced the declining incidence and changing psychopathology of amok. In its original form it was a recognized and endorsed instrument of social control being consciously directed at the superior members of society if traditional fair dealing was abandoned. With increasing trade with Europeans such drastic methods of social control became unnecessary and amok was rejected as acceptable behaviour. Only from this period, about the middle of the nineteenth century, did amok become a pathological syndrome, taking on the features of hysterical dissociation and sometimes occurring in the course of a chronic mental disorder.

Latah is considered to be a hysterical disorder which occurs mainly in the Far East and North Africa. The patients are usually middle-aged or elderly females who, after a sudden psychological trauma, develop a state similar to hypnotic suggestibility. There is often altered consciousness, echolalia, echopraxia and automatic obedience. Although these symptoms can last for several months schizophrenic features do not develop. Like amok, latah appears to be declining in incidence (Murphy, 1973).

Piblokto is a dissociative state occurring among Eskimo women. It is characterized by a period of depressive brooding, followed by sudden running into the snow and jumping into water. Self-destructive or homicidal behaviour may occur and amnesia is usually claimed for the whole episode when behaviour returns to normal.

Windigo psychosis occurs among the Cree and other North American Indian tribes in central and north-east Canada. The mythology of these people includes belief in a cannibalistic monster with a heart of ice, the windigo. The psychosis usually becomes manifest during times of food shortage and starvation. In the setting of a depressed mood the afflicted member of the tribe believes himself to have been transformed into the windigo and attacks of cannibalism on other members of the tribe may follow. Kiev (1972) considers this to be a classical depressive disorder, the depressive behaviour being influenced by the tribal mythology.

In concluding this chapter on social and transcultural psychiatry it seems appropriate to consider the provision of psychiatric care in developing countries. Earlier in the chapter reference was made to the problems of providing community services in the United Kingdom at a time of increasing demands on the available manpower. In particular it was suggested that more psychiatric treatment might have to be carried out by primary care teams of general practitioner, social worker and nurse. However, such recommendations hardly apply to countries with extreme shortages of all sorts of trained personnel. If psychiatric care is to be provided at all in these countries, which may have only one psychiatrist for every million people, then a new kind of health worker will have to be trained. These will probably be people with limited previous education and their training may last only a few months. Giel and Harding (1976), who have discussed the problems faced by developing countries

526   G. Lloyd

in the provision of psychiatric care, have suggested that the specialist's job will be to support and stimulate these community-based workers. In addition they have recommended that priority be given to the recognition and management of certain illnesses on the basis of their prevalence, seriousness, concern to the community and susceptibility to management. They selected epilepsy and the acute functional psychoses as being the psychiatric syndromes most worthy of priority, although they acknowledged that other conditions might require priority in certain countries, depending on factors prevailing locally.

Whatever the clinical priorities it is obvious that psychiatric services in developing countries cannot be modelled identically on those in Western countries, not only because of a deficiency in orthodox medical resources, but also, as Leff (1975) has reminded us, because many psychiatric disorders, especially those of neurotic type, may be effectively treated with folk remedies traditionally used in those cultures.

References

de Alarcon, R. (1969). The spread of heroin abuse in a community. *Bull. Narcot.* **21**, 17–22.
Arthur, R. J. (1971). 'An Introduction to Social Psychiatry'. Penguin, Harmondsworth.
Asuni, T. (1962). Suicide in Western Nigeria. *Br. Med. J.* **2**, 1091–1097.
Becker, A. and Schulberg, H. C. (1976). Phasing out state hospitals: a psychiatric dilemma. *New Eng. J. Med.* **294**, 255–261.
Benaim, S., Horder, J. and Anderson, J. (1973). Hysterical epidemic in a classroom. *Psychol. Med.* **3**, 363–373.
Bennett, D. (1972). Principles underlying a new rehabilitative workshop. *In* 'Evaluating a Community Psychiatric Service' (Eds J. K. Wing and A. M. Hailey). Oxford University Press, Oxford.
Birley, J. L. T. and Brown, G. W. (1970). Crises and life changes preceding the onset or relapse of acute schizophrenia: Clinical aspects. *Br. J. Psychiat.* **116**, 327–333.
Birtchnell, J. (1970). Early parent death and mental illness. *Br. J. Psychiat.* **116**, 281–288.
Birtchnell, J. (1971). Social class, parental social class and social mobility in psychiatric patients and general population controls. *Psychol. Med.* **1**, 209–221.
Brothwood, J. (1973). The development of national policy. *In* 'Policy for Action' (Eds R. Cawley and G. McLachlan). Oxford University Press, Oxford.
Brown, G. W. and Birley, J. L. T. (1968). Crises and life changes and the onset of schizophrenia. *J. Hlth Soc. Behav.* **9**, 203–214.
Brown, G. W., Birley, J. L. T. and Wing, J. K. (1972). Influence of family life on the course of schizophrenic disorders: a replication. *Br. J. Psychiat.* **121**, 241–258.
Brown, G. W., Sklair, F., Harris, T. O. and Birley, J. L. T. (1973a). Life-events and psychiatric disorders. Part 1: some methodological issues. *Psychol. Med.* **3**, 74–87.

Brown, G. W., Harris, T. O. and Peto, J. (1973b). Life-events and psychiatric disorders. Part 2: nature of causal link. *Psychol. Med.* **3**, 159–176.

Brown, G. W., Bhrolchain, M. N. and Harris, T. (1975). Social class and psychiatric disturbance among women in an urban population. *Sociology* **9**, 225–254.

Brown, G. W., Harris, T. and Copeland, J. R. (1977). Depression and loss. *Br. J. Psychiat.* **130**, 1–18.

Bunch, J., Barraclough, B., Nelson, B. and Sainsbury, P. (1971). Early parental bereavement and suicide. *Soc. Psychiat.* **6**, 200–202.

Clare, A. W. (1974). Mental illness in the Irish emigrant. *J. Ir. Med. Ass.* **67**, 20–24.

Clark, D. H. (1965). The therapeutic community—concept, practice and future. *Br. J. Psychiat.* **111**, 947–954.

Cooper, B. (1972). Clinical and social aspects of chronic neurosis. *Proc. Roy. Soc. Med.* **65**, 509–512.

Cooper, J. E., Kendell, R. E., Sharpe, L., Copeland, J. R. M. and Simon, R. (1972). 'Psychiatric Diagnosis in New York and London'. Oxford University Press, Oxford.

Cooper, B., Harwin, B. G., Depla, C. and Shepherd, M. (1975). Mental health in the community: an evaluative study. *Psychol. Med.* **5**, 372–380.

Cox, J. L. (1977). Aspects of transcultural psychiatry. *Br. J. Psychiat.* **130**, 211–221.

Craft, M. (1965). 'Ten Studies into Psychopathic Personality'. Wright, Bristol.

Creer, C. and Wing, J. K. (1974). 'Schizophrenia at Home'. National Schizophrenia Fellowship, Surbiton.

Department of Health and Social Security (1975). 'Better Services for the Mentally Ill'. HMSO, London.

Durkheim, E. (1897). 'Suicide' (Trans. 1952). Routledge and Kegan Paul, London.

Essen-Moller, E. (1956). Individual traits and morbidity in a Swedish rural population. *Acta Psychiat. Neurol., Suppl.* 100.

Faris, R. E. L. and Dunham, H. W. (1939). 'Mental Disorders in Urban Areas'. Hafner, New York.

Finlay-Jones, R. A. and Burvill, P. W. (1977). The prevalence of minor psychiatric morbidity in the community. *Psychol. Med.* **7**, 475–489.

German, G. A. (1972). Aspects of clinical psychiatry in Sub-Saharan Africa. *Br. J. Psychiat.* **121**, 461–479.

Giel, R. and Harding, T. W. (1976). Psychiatric priorities in developing countries. *Br. J. Psychiat.* **128**, 513–522.

Goffman, E. (1961). 'Asylums'. Anchor Books, New York.

Goldberg, D. P. (1972). 'The Detection of Psychiatric Illness by Questionnaire'. Oxford University Press, Oxford.

Goldberg, D. P. and Blackwell, B. (1970). Psychiatric illness in general practice. *Br. Med. J.* **2**, 439–443.

Goldberg, E. M. and Morrison, S. L. (1963). Schizophrenia and social class. *Br. J. Psychiat.* **109**, 785–802.

Grad, J. and Sainsbury, P. (1968). The effects that patients have on their families in a community care and a control psychiatric service: a two year follow-up. *Br. J. Psychiat.* **114**, 265–278.

Granville-Grossman, K. L. (1968). The early environment in affective disorders. *In* 'Recent Developments in Affective Disorders' (Eds A. Coppen and A. Walk). *Br. J. Psychiat.* Special Publication No. 2. Headley Bros, Ashford, Kent.

Greer, S. (1966). Parental loss and attempted suicide: a further report. *Br. J. Psychiat.* **112**, 465–470.

Gruenberg, E. M. (1969). From practice to theory: community mental-health services and the nature of psychoses. *Lancet* **1**, 721–724.

Hagnell, O. (1966). 'A Prospective Study on the Incidence of Mental Disorder'. Scandinavian University Books, Stockholm.

Hagnell, O. and Kreitman, N. (1974). Mental illness in married pairs in a total population. *Br. J. Psychiat.* **125**, 293–302.

Hare, E. H. (1969). The relation between social psychiatry and psychotherapy. *In* 'Psychiatry in a Changing Society' (Eds S. H. Foulkes and G. S. Prince). Tavistock, London.

Hare, E. H., Price, J. S. and Slater, E. (1972). Parental social class in psychiatric patients. *Br. J. Psychiat.* **121**, 515–524.

Henderson, S., Duncan-Jones, P., McAuley, H. and Ritchie, K. (1978). The patient's primary group. *Br. J. Pschiat.* **132**, 74–86.

Hill, O. W. and Price, J. S. (1967). Childhood bereavement and adult depression. *Br. J. Psychiat.* **113**, 743–751.

Hirsch, S. R. and Leff, J. P. (1975). 'Abnormalities in Parents of Schizophrenics'. Oxford University Press, Oxford.

Hollingshead, A. B. and Redlich, F. C. (1958). 'Social Class and Mental Illness: A Community Study'. Wiley, New York.

Jablensky, A. and Sartorius, N. (1975). Editorial: culture and schizophrenia. *Psychol. Med.* **5**, 113–124.

Jacobs, S. C., Prusoff, B. A. and Paykel, E. S. (1974). Recent life events in schizophrenia and depression. *Psychol. Med.* **4**, 444–453.

Jaspers, K. (1962). 'General Psychopathology'. Trans. J. Hoenig and M. W. Hamilton. Manchester University Press, Manchester.

Jones, M. (1952). 'Social Psychiatry'. Tavistock, London.

Jones, M. (1962). 'Social Psychiatry in the Community, in Hospitals and in Prisons'. Thomas, Springfield, Illinois.

Kiev, A. (1972). 'Transcultural Psychiatry'. Penguin, Harmondsworth.

Kohn, M. L. (1973). Social class and schizophrenia: a critical review and reformulation. *Schizophrenia Bull.* **7**, 60–79.

Kreitman, N., Smith, P. and Tan, E. S. (1970). Attempted suicide as language: an empirical study. *Br. J. Psychiat.* **116**, 465–473.

Lasegue, C. and Falret, J. (1877). La folie à deux ou folie communiquée. *Ann. Méd-psychol.* **18**, 321–335.

Leff, J. P. (1973). Culture and the differentiation of emotional states. *Br. J. Psychiat.* **123**, 299–306.

Leff, J. P. (1975). Editorial: Exotic treatments and Western psychiatry *Psychol. Med.* **5**, 125–128.

Leighton, A. H. (1959). 'My Name is Legion: The Stirling County Study of Psychiatric Disorder and Sociocultural Environment'. Basic Books, New York.

Leighton, A., Lambo, T. A., Hughes, C. C., Leighton, D. C., Murphy, J. M. and Macklin, D. G. (1963). 'Psychiatric Disorder Among the Yoruba'. Cornell University Press, Ithaca.

McEvedy, C. P. and Beard, A. W. (1970). Royal Free epidemic of 1955: a reconsideration. *Br. Med. J.* **1**, 7–11.

Main, T. F. (1946). The hospital as a therapeutic institution. *Bull. Menninger Clin.* **10**, 66–70.

Malzberg, B. and Lee, E. S. (1956). 'Migration and Mental Disease'. Social Science Research Council, New York.

Mann, S. and Cree, W. (1975). The 'new long-stay' in mental hospital. *Br. J. Hosp. Med.* **14**, 56–63.

Marks, I. M., Hallam, R. S., Philpott, R. and Connolly, J. C. (1975). Nurse therapists in behavioural psychotherapy. *Br. Med. J.* **3**, 144–148.

Mechanic, D. (1962). The concept of illness behaviour. *J. Chron. Dis.* **15**, 189–194.

Mezey, A. G. (1960). Personal background, emigration and mental disorder in Hungarian refugees. *J. Ment. Sci.* **106**, 618–627.

Moos, R. and Houts, P. (1968). The assessment of the social atmosphere of psychiatric wards. *J. Abnorm. Psychol.* **73**, 595–604.

Moos, R. and Schwartz, J. (1972). Treatment environment and treatment outcome. *J. Nerv. Ment. Dis.* **154**, 264–275.

Murphy, H. B. M. (1973). History and the evolution of syndromes: the striking case of Latah and Amok. *In* 'Psychopathology: Contributions from the Social, Behavioural and Biological Sciences' (Eds M. Hammer, K. Salzinger and S. Sutton). Wiley, New York.

Murphy, H. B. M. (1977). Migration, culture and mental health. *Psychol. Med.* **7**, 677–684.

Neki, J. S. (1973). Psychiatry in south-east Asia. *Br. J. Psychiat.* **123**, 257–269.

Ochberg, F. M. (1976). Community mental health centre legislation: flight of the phoenix. *Am. J. Psychiat.* **133**, 56–61.

Ødegaard, O. (1932). Emigration and insanity. *Acta Psychiat. Neurol., Suppl.* 4.

Parsons, T. (1951). 'The Social System'. Free Press, Chicago.

Paykel, E. S., Myers, J. K., Dienelt, M. N., Klerman, G. L., Lidenthal, J. J. and Pepper, M. P. (1969). Life events and depression: a controlled study. *Arch. Gen. Psychiat.* **21**, 753–760.

Russell, G. F. M. (1973). Will there be enough psychiatrists to run the psychiatric service based on the district general hospital? *In* 'Policy for Action' (Eds R. Cawley and G. McLachlan). Oxford University Press, Oxford.

Rutter, M. (1966). 'Children of Sick Parents'. Oxford University Press, Oxford.

Sartorius, N., Jablensky, A. and Shapiro, R. (1977). Two-year follow-up of the patients included in the WHO International Pilot Study of Schizophrenia. *Psychol. Med.* **7**, 529–541.

Shepherd, M., Cooper, B., Brown, A. C. and Kalton, G. W. (1966). 'Psychiatric Illness in General Practice'. Oxford University Press, Oxford.

Sirois, F. (1974). Epidemic hysteria. *Acta Psychiat. Scand., Suppl.* 252.

Srole, L., Langner, T. S., Michael, S. T., Opler, M. K. and Rennie, T. A. C. (1962). 'Mental Health in the Metropolis: The Midtown Manhattan Study', Vol. 1. McGraw-Hill, New York.

Stengel, E. and Cook, N. (1958). 'Attempted Suicide'. Oxford University Press, Oxford.

Stevens, B. (1972). Dependence of schizophrenic patients on elderly relatives. *Psychol. Med.* **2**, 17–32.

Teja, J. S., Narang, R. L. and Aggarwal, A. K. (1971). Depression across cultures. *Br. J. Psychiat.* **119**, 253–260.

Tooth, G. C. and Brooke, E. M. (1961). Trends in the mental hospital population and their effect on future planning. *Lancet* **1**, 710–713.

Turner, R. J. and Wagenfeld, M. O. (1967). Occupational mobility and schizophrenia: an assessment of the social causation and social selection hypotheses. *Am. Soc. Rev.* **32**, 104–113.

Vaughn, C. and Leff, J. P. (1976). The influence of family and social factors on the course of psychiatric illness: a comparison of schizophrenic and depressed neurotic patients. *Br. J. Psychiat.* **129**, 125–137.

Walsh, D. and Walsh, B. (1970). Mental illness in the Republic of Ireland: first admissions. *J. Ir. Med. Ass.* **63**, 365–370.

Whitely, J. S. (1970). The psychopath and his treatment. *Br. J. Hosp. Med.* **3**, 263–270.

Wing, J. K. (1971). Social psychiatry. *Br. J. Hosp. Med.* **5**, 53–56.

Wing, J. K. (1975). Impairments in schizophrenia: a rational basis for social treatment. *In* 'Life History Research in Psychopathology' (Eds R. D. Wirt, G. Winokur and M. Roff). University of Minnesota Press, Minneapolis.

Wing, J. K. and Brown, G. W. (1970). 'Institutionalism and Schizophrenia'. Cambridge University Press, Cambridge.

Wing, J. K. and Hailey, A. M. (1972). 'Evaluating a Community Psychiatric Service'. Oxford University Press, Oxford.

Wing, J. K., Monck, E., Brown, G. W. and Carstairs, G. M. (1964). Morbidity in the community of schizophrenic patients discharged from London mental hospitals in 1959. *Br. J. Psychiat.* **110**, 10–21.

World Health Organization (1973). 'Report of the International Pilot Study of Schizophrenia', Vol. 1. WHO, Geneva.

Yap, P. M. (1974). 'Comparative Psychiatry'. Toronto University Press, Toronto.

16 Forensic psychiatry

Peter Hill

Forensic psychiatry is concerned with the mentally disordered offender. An individual becomes an offender as a consequence of certain aspects of his behaviour which transgress the law. He is then likely to be further labelled in terms of his offence behaviour as an arsonist, murderer, paedophile, etc. Offence behaviour is, however, the final common pathway for the expression of a plethora of motives possessed by a variety of personalities acting in differing situations which offer opportunity or provocation to offend. Legally defined offences are not, and do not imply, psychiatric diagnoses.

Various studies have shown that, at least in the UK, very roughly one-third of prison inmates would be diagnosed as having a psychiatric disorder (see Gunn, 1977). A North American study by Guze (1976) found about half of a prison population to suffer from a psychiatric disorder other than 'sociopathy'. Gunn (1977) reports his application of a principal components analysis to his sample as a whole and the finding that two dimensions resulted: psychiatric disturbance, and recidivism. Property offences loaded heavily on the recidivist factor, not on the psychiatric, whereas violent, sexual, and drug offences loaded heavily on the psychiatric factor.

Viewed from the opposite side it would seem that personality disorder (including 'psychopathy', alcoholism and drug addiction) and mental subnormality are those clinical conditions whose prevalence among prison inmates is excessive. Whether this is similarly true for all offenders is unconfirmed but it is plain from the reports of Rollin (1969) from a psychiatric hospital, and Tidmarsh and Wood (1972) from a reception centre, that certain men are cursed with both psychiatric handicap (commonly schizophrenia in Rollin's series) and a recidivist career, repeatedly offending in a trivial manner and circulating between a variety of institutions: hospital, prison or reception centre. Probably it is the existence of such persons that raises the possibility in the psychiatrist's mind of a special association between psychiatric disorder in general and criminal behaviour in general but, taking psychiatric patients as a whole, there would seem to be no evidence that they are more likely to behave criminally than the general population.

Juvenile delinquency

Delinquency means law-breaking behaviour, no more. As such it is very common. Various studies (e.g. Christie *et al.*, 1965; Belson, 1968) confirm that a majority of young persons admit to offending but, of course, only a minority are caught. Even so, the minority is a sizeable one. In London, two surveys have shown that 20–25% of male adolescents are convicted at some time (West and Farrington, 1973; Power *et al.*, 1972). The question arises as to how the minority is selected; clearly factors such as mode of dress, social manner, particular school attended or previous contact with the police will affect an individual's liability to be arrested. However, over and above this one is probably justified in assuming that those law-breakers who are arrested tend to be those who break the law most frequently since in West and Farrington's (1973) study a significant correlation was found between the number of confidentially admitted undetected delinquent acts and court appearance.

In the United Kingdom, criminal responsibility does not apply below the age of 10, but half of all indictable (i.e. severe) crimes are committed by individuals under 21. In large cities, one boy in five will be convicted by the age of 21 most commonly between 14 and 18, and just under a half of all first offenders re-offend (though most criminal careers die out before the individual is far into his twenties). It is clear, then, that juvenile delinquency merits particular consideration both in the extent of adolescent criminality and the severity of offences. Adult crime is predominantly non-indictable.

It has become a cliché to state that the aetiology of delinquency (subsequently used to imply juvenile delinquency) is multifactorial. This is not only the result of the heterogeneity of delinquent behaviour and delinquents themselves, but reflects a quantitative aspect of delinquent behaviour. Certain levels of aggression or selfish appropriation are acceptable, others are not. Legality becomes illegality at a point on a continuum of antisocial behaviour which extends from mild to severe. In addition there are the circumstances of the crime.

The classic study of Hartshorne and May (1928), in which children thought they could steal or cheat undetected, demonstrated that no single trait of honesty or dishonesty existed for all situations and that dishonest behaviour was more closely linked with the situation and the opportunities within it than with any characteristic of the individual. Most subjects were dishonest in some situations though which particular situations varied from person to person. The point deserves reiteration: in considering criminal behaviour one is concerned with individuals acting in particular circumstances. Objective studies suggest factors likely to predispose individuals to act criminally; the meaning of the particular act to the individual and the precipitants in the situation are less amenable to scientific enquiry but require assessment in the individual case.

Considering the psychiatrist's role in all this, it will be clear that his involvement will be dependent upon his ability to understand abnormal psychology rather than upon his knowledge of formal mental illness; the contribution of the latter to juvenile delinquency is minute. When considering the individual case, the circumstances of the crime are vital; when considering the aetiology of delinquency as a whole, one is generally talking about personal predisposition. For simplicity, three headings are used; social, individual and family factors.

1 Social factors

The explanation of delinquency may be couched in any of the languages of the various disciplines involved in its study. Sociology has recently been concerned with studying the processes considered to operate in the creation of deviance or delinquency, e.g. labelling, alienation and identification. It is beyond the scope of this book to do justice to such views though this is not to dismiss them. Much criminology on the other hand has tended to be concerned with the explanation of the variation in the prevalence of delinquency and the significance of social factors derived from objective measurement. This led, in the 1960s, to debate as to the importance of so-called delinquency areas. It had been well known for years that delinquency rates are higher in some areas of cities than others and the question arose as to which characteristics of the areas were relevant. Mays' (1954) account of life in Liverpool's dockland suggested that the social environment there sanctioned or encouraged various delinquent acts in that shop-lifting, rowdiness, lorry-skipping, etc. were so common as to be considered normal and appropriate activities for adolescents seeking excitement or to enhance their status. This interpretation implicates the sub-culture and the attitudes or rewards therein as the significant factor rather than, say, the physical characteristics or poverty of the area. This would be in accordance with the theories of Cloward and Ohlin (1961) and Cohen (1955) whereby the social identifications offered within the North American delinquent gang satisfy individuals' needs while sanctioning antisocial behaviour.

Re-examination of the characteristics of high delinquency areas has questioned the significance of the once-hallowed correlates of low social class, poverty and overcrowding. For example, Little and Ntsekhe (1959) found a considerably smaller excess of delinquents among lower social classes than previously assumed, and Palmai et al. (1967) reported a fairly even distribution of young offenders throughout all social classes. Rutter and Madge (1976, p. 180) have argued that the real association between poverty and crime is not directly causal but that poverty 'predisposes to a variety of family difficulties and troubles more directly associated with delinquency'. Similarly there is an evident interaction between over-crowding and large family size which leads to a blurring of significance.

Differences in delinquency rates exist not only between city boroughs but between electoral wards within boroughs (Power et al, 1972) and between streets (Jephcott and Carter, 1954). Whilst the latter study shows that this was largely due to particular families one has also to explain why delinquent areas remain stable over time (Wallis and Maliphant, 1967). Selective immigration or physical dilapidation do not seem to be sufficient explanation (Rutter and Madge, 1976). A partial answer is suggested by the studies of Power (e.g. 1967) wherein it has been demon-strated that there are marked differences in delinquency rates between schools even when schools draw their pupils from the same geographical area, and that these differences remain stable over a 10-year period. Selective intake of delinquent children provides part but by no means all the explanation and it seems likely that the ethos of some particular schools is conducive to delinquency amongst their pupils, perhaps in terms of standards demanded, models of behaviour provided by staff, discipline, or staff–family–pupil relationships.

2   Individual factors

There is a problem which arises in considering the environmental or social contribution to delinquency. If the criminal behaviour of individ-uals is seen as responsive to factors in the sub-culture, social class, physical environment, school and so on, are such individuals necessarily also psychologically disturbed? The risk is that, even in posing the ques-tion, subsequent research assumptions may be couched in inappropriate terms. Stanley Cohen (1971) has been rightly scornful of the tendency to label deviance as secondary to psychological abnormality and sees the attempts to predict future delinquency on individual characteristics alone, isolated from its social context, as futile. It is clearly necessary, however, to assess the importance of the contribution of individual predisposition to the interaction between the individual and his social environment.

Mays (1954) described most of his Liverpool offenders as being essentially normal personalities and it has been a widespread assumption that the more 'socialized' the delinquency, the more normal the individual. This is well expressed by Scott (1965):

> there are, on the one hand fringe or formes frustes delinquents, comprising those who are reacting to the local subcultural influences, as well as those showing minor degrees of predisposition (licked rather than bitten, as one might say), while on the other hand there are the hard core delinquents who unlike the first category, will not respond to simple measures.

Similarly, Rutter *et al.* (1970) argued that the essential difference between socialized and unsocialized delinquents is one of deviance of personality rather than that of neighbourhood or the fact that crime was committed in company.

However, Stott (1966) and Conger and Miller (1966) found little difference in rates of emotional disturbance according to whether the delinquents in question were from high or low delinquency areas or were 'deprived' or 'not deprived'. Given that areas with high delinquency rates tend to be those with high rates of child psychiatric referral (Gath *et al.*, 1977) it seems reasonable to conclude that delinquency is one aspect of 'personal maladjustment' in Stott's phrase and that area differences relate to 'personal maladjustment' of which crime is one manifestation.

Relevant to this is the phenomenon of recidivism. Nearly half of all adolescents appearing in court re-offend but less than one in 10 will go on to *repeatedly* offend. Stott and Wilson (1977) demonstrated a quantitative relationship between the degree of non-delinquent maladjustment and the number of convictions. Knight and West (1975) showed that those who continue criminal activities into adult life differ from those who do not in that they come from more disturbed and deprived backgrounds with more criminality in their families of origin. Roughly speaking, there appears to be a continuum of severity whereby the likelihood of associated social, familial, emotional and behavioural abnormality increases as one progresses from 'unofficial' delinquency detected only on self-report through delinquency (single offence) to recidivism. This is a likely partial explanation for the well-established finding that the best predictor of future delinquency is the extent of past delinquency.

Using longitudinal approach a variety of studies, in particular Conger and Miller (1966) in retrospective, and West and Farrington (1973) in prospective surveys, have shown that future delinquents were likely to be identifiable by their teachers during primary schooling. Such pre-delinquent misbehaviour was typified by disobedience, aggression, quarrelsomeness and truancy. Nevertheless, Rutter and Madge (1976) have stressed that there are discontinuities as well as continuities; most children who display behavioural abnormalities in early childhood do not become delinquent and at least half of all delinquents do not show behavioural deviance when younger.

Twin studies have repeatedly demonstrated little if any difference in the concordance rate for juvenile delinquency within MZ as opposed to DZ pairs (Shields, 1977). This is in contrast to the higher concordance rate for MZ rather than same sex DZ pairs when criminality in adults is considered (Christiansen, 1970). In Hutchings and Mednick's (1974) Danish study, 1145 men aged 30–44 adopted outside their family of origin during early childhood were compared with a control group of the same size matched for sex, age, social status and locality of residence. The criminal records for each group and for the biological and adoptive fathers were examined (see Table I). Clearly the data suggest that for a sizeable

Table I   *Criminality of male adoptees (Hutchings and Mednick, 1974)*

	Per cent criminal (rounded figures)
Neither biological nor adoptive father criminal	10
Adoptive father (only) criminal	11
Biological father (only) criminal	21
Both fathers criminal	36

minority of criminals a genetic effect operates though the use of sibling controls would have yielded clearer evidence. An environmental effect is also evident though it would appear that it operates on a genetically vulnerable group and that the interactive effect is greater than mere summation. It is not clear from the study reports how many of the adoptees' crimes were committed below the age of 21 but in that it was indictable offences (roughly speaking) that were recorded it seems likely that a significant proportion would have been committed by juveniles. If this is so it is difficult to reconcile with the previously noted absence of genetic effect detected in the twin studies. Possibly the defining limit of juvenile delinquency as a single offence obscures any possible genetic effect operating predominantly on recidivists who would be likely to continue their criminal careers into adult life.

The eight-fold male predominance in delinquency rates and the XYY phenomenon point to ways in which chromosomal constitution *may* be significant. However, most boys and most XYYs are not convicted delinquents. The familiar over-representation of mesomorphs in a population of delinquents (Glueck and Glueck, 1956) further suggest the operation of constitutional factors.

As a group, delinquents have a below-normal mean IQ. This seems to be almost entirely due to the low scores of recidivists (Douglas *et al.*, 1968), one-time offenders differing little from non-offenders. Furthermore, IQ represents the result of an interaction between inherited endowment and environment and, obviously, a depriving environment tends to be depriving in many respects.

Organic brain disease may be held to be a predisposition in that it may sensitize the individual to an adverse psychosocial environment or promote learning or temperamental difficulties (q.v. Chapter 5). The association between epilepsy and crime is discussed elsewhere in this chapter.

3   Family factors

Familial criminality

Many studies have demonstrated that delinquency tends to run in families. For example both Ferguson (1952) and West and Farrington (1973) have shown that delinquents were just over twice as likely as non-delinquents to have criminal fathers. Where both parents have criminal records the delinquency rate among their sons rises to about 60% (West and Farrington, 1973) which, although impressive, still means that delinquency in the sons in such a family is by no means inevitable. In Ferguson's study delinquency was more strongly linked with delinquency in brothers than with paternal criminality.

It is extremely difficult to disentangle the mechanisms involved. West and Farrington (1973) found that most of the criminal parents were no longer criminally active during the period of child-rearing so that modelling of behaviour by parents seems unlikely. Neither, in the same study, was there much suggestion that erstwhile criminal parents were anything but censorious toward delinquency in their offspring.

There remain three other possible mechanisms (at least):
(a) parental criminality is associated with poor parenting behaviour;
(b) criminal parents transmit permissive attitudes toward e.g. property ownership or aggressive interpersonal behaviour by more subtle means;
(c) a genetic link.

Poor parenting behaviour is considered below. It is worth noting in passing that when West and Farrington took poor parental supervision into account only a slight association remained between paternal criminality and filial delinquency. The transmission of attitudes by covert encouragement of overtly proscribed antisocial behaviour has been clinically described by Johnson (1949) in terms of 'superego lacunae' though the extent of such mechanisms remains uncertain.

Family size

Various surveys have confirmed the association between large family size (say five or more children) and delinquency. Whether this represents a causal relationship is more problematic. Large family size correlates highly with low income, paternal unemployment, poor material care of children, etc. and may be merely an index of social disadvantage which in turn correlates with parental conflict and poor parental supervision (West and Farrington, 1973). Large families tend to be associated with poor educational attainment and low IQ in the children (Douglas *et al.*, 1968) and it can be argued that, whereas by no means all large families produce disadvantaged or delinquent children, where family resources are stretched by social disadvantage the presence of a large family group means that discipline becomes less discriminatory, supervision less intense, and parent–child interactions less frequent.

Poor parenting behaviour

It is well established that poor parental supervision, over-indulgent or inconsistent discipline, or over-harsh punishment characterize the families of delinquents (McCord and McCord, 1959; Glueck and Glueck, 1950). Clearly such factors will interfere with satisfactory social training in that appropriately discriminating rewards and punishments will not be applied in such a way that the child may clearly appreciate social expectations of his behaviour.

Family discord

The relationship between quarrelling parents and inconsistent parental discipline is obvious, but is not the whole explanation of the relationship repeatedly demonstrated between family discord and delinquency (see e.g. McCord and McCord, 1959; Glueck and Glueck, 1950; West and Farrington, 1973). Parental rejection, hostility or unremitting criticism unmitigated by praise or warmth expressed towards the child is strongly associated with aggression and delinquency. The general finding is that discord exists at several levels within the family; thus marital and parent–child conflict frequently co-exist. A hostile attitude towards the child influences the relative proportions of punishment and praise meted out by the parent and the child fails to experience sufficient approval for his positive activities. A poor parent–child relationship minimizes the chances of satisfactory identification with the parents and their principles and leads to a negative self image fostering, in its turn, role-confirming 'bad' behaviour by the child. This is fertile breeding ground for deviant behaviour of all kinds: low self-esteem, high levels of aggression, poor educational prowess, failure to identify with social mores, and psychiatric disturbance.

Classification

Because delinquency is defined by the dictates of the law for a particular time, place, and social group it is not surprising that delinquents, defined as they are by the transgression of contemporaneous laws, do not form a homogeneous group. Generalizations tend to become accordingly banal or speculative. Some classificatory schemes tend to categorize people or personalities rather than delinquents, for example, the I scale of the Grants (Sullivan *et al.*, 1957). This determines a number of levels and sublevels of maturity in interpersonal relationships. Most delinquents fall into the lower middle range, higher levels representing sophisticated perceptions of other people. The Jesness Inventory (Jesness, 1962, 1963) enables an individual to be located on the scheme and suggests broad treatment approaches likely to prove appropriate according to the experience of the California Youth Authority Project (e.g. Warren, 1969).

The best known, and simplest, scheme is that of Hewitt and Jenkins (1946) viz:

(a) socialized (association with gangs, conforming to delinquent sub-culture).
(b) unsocialized (cruel, destructive, anti-authoritarian).
(c) overinhibited (seclusive, neurotic).

Various studies in the UK have found this less useful than its apparent face validity and in particular Field (1967) found that it does not predict family background as originally claimed.

Scott's (e.g. 1965) types have an obvious clinical appeal but the scheme is untried epidemiologically:

(a) well trained to antisocial standards ('subcultural');
(b) badly trained (the result of ineffectual or inconsistent discipline);
(c) reparative (delinquency compensating for feelings of inadequacy or conflicts between basic drives and repressive training);
(d) maladaptive (a stereotyped, repetitive response to conflict situations according to the experimental neurosis paradigm).

An exception to the general rule of not classifying from offence behaviour (as this is the final expression of a variety of motives) is Rich's (1956) validated typology of theft:

   (a) marauding (unplanned theft by a group);
   (b) proving (demonstration of skill or manhood to peers);
   (c) comforting (impulsive, solitary, often from parents and associated with feelings of rejection);
   (d) secondary (planned and deliberate);
   (e) miscellaneous (theft on instruction from parent etc.).

Management

The psychiatrist stands in an ambiguous position with respect to the delinquent. When he is asked to prepare a report for the court the position is simple enough: what is required is comprehensible formulation and the implications this holds for sentencing. Knowledge of the powers of the court in question is essential and communication with any social worker or probation officer likely to be involved is mandatory. The increasing use of supervision orders and intermediate treatment orders by juvenile courts suggests that the psychiatrist will be called upon increasingly to advise on the content of such measures after the juvenile leaves court.

The situation becomes more complex when the psychiatrist has been asked (usually covertly) to abolish the illegal behaviour. Most commonly this arises in drug and sexual offences but it is also likely to occur in connection with recidivism. Some modesty in the claim that might be made for psychiatric intervention is advisable. Indeed, if the question is put bluntly as to what psychiatric or psychiatrically inspired measures can abolish offence behaviour, good answers are sparse. Obviously no single measure is sufficient or universally applicable.

Using re-offence rates as a parameter of therapeutic success, it is important to note that individual counselling for juvenile offenders once or twice weekly for nine months within a medium security unit (the PICO project) was successful with suitable candidates: those who were bright, verbal, anxious and motivated to change. Treated unsuitable candidates did worse if anything than untreated controls and re-offended significantly more often on 30-month follow-up (Adams, 1961). This illustrates the importance of selecting appropriate cases for appropriate treatment. When this is not done it is well known that practically all measures, penal, social and psychiatric, produce practically the same dismal results.

Further exploration of the differential application of treatment regimes (probation, day attendance for 'guided group interaction', vocational guidance, group homes, etc.) to *selected* delinquents by *selected* staff was the theme of the California Youth Authority Community Treatment Project. The allocation of a delinquent to a particular treatment programme was determined by the I level of the Jesness Inventory. Such reports as have been published (e.g. Warren, 1969) show a lower reconviction rate for experimental subjects than for controls but the major interest is the attempt within the project to apply differential staffing. This is a sophisticated extension of the discovery by the Grants (1959) that mature offenders were successfully rehabilitated by 'mature' but not by 'immature' staff. One might also cite the manner in which it was the black rather than the white youths in the Highfields Project who benefited from the guided group interaction (Weeks, 1958) and the finding of Craft *et al.* (1964) at Balderton that, within a hospital, a paternalistic regime proved superior to a therapeutic community approach when immature, unintelligent delinquents were randomly allocated to each.

Psychopathy

Accurate definition of psychopathy is so elusive it is legitimate to question whether the term should survive. Psychiatrists continue to use the term, frequently pejoratively, and it is enshrined in the English Mental Health Act—though not in the Scottish or Northern Irish Acts. It is clear that several criticisms can be made:

(a) there is no general agreement as to its meaning;
(b) its definition (MHA) is circular in that mental abnormality is inferred from antisocial conduct, yet is used to explain antisocial conduct;
(c) as a diagnostic label it has (partly as a function of its low reliability) low information content when applied to the individual;
(d) the largely judgemental element contained in the descriptions of psychopathic deviance.

Gunn and Robertson (1976) described the impossibility of extracting a single factor of psychopathy from the social and pathological data on prisoners sent to Grendon Underwood Prison with the diagnosis of psychopathy. It thus becomes questionable whether psychopaths have anything in common beyond the diagnostic label and a certain unpopularity with psychiatrists.

The historical development of the concept is succinctly reviewed by Lewis (1974). The roots of the current label in the older ideas of moral defect and moral insanity are evident if a contemporary definition is considered, for example that of 'antisocial personality disorder' (which includes psychopathic disorder in MHA terms) in the ICD Glossary (1968):

a deviation of personality . . . not a result of a psychosis or any other illness . . . confined to those individuals who offend against society, who show a lack of sympathetic feeling and whose behaviour is not readily modifiable by experience, including punishment. They are affectively cold and callous. They may tend to abnormally aggressive and seriously irresponsible conduct.

One can immediately cavil: the inability to profit by experience applies to antisocial and certain interpersonal behaviours only. Many psychopaths seem remarkably adept at learning coping skills in institutional environments. Nor should it be assumed that psychopaths cannot foresee the consequences of their actions; frequently they predict only too well the consequences of future antisocial acts from which they nevertheless find themselves unable to refrain when particular situations arise.

Scott (1960) comments that all major definitions of psychopathy contain four common elements:

(1) An excluding clause: no primary psychosis or subnormality.
(2) An emphasis on duration: persistent from an early age.
(3) A description of the behaviour: abnormally aggressive or inadequate, seriously irresponsible, asocial, antisocial.
(4) Society is impelled to do something about it (i.e. treatment).

Some of the contradictions and ambiguity which pervade the use of the term are illustrated within the (Butler) Report of the Committee on Mentally Abnormal Offenders (Home Office and DHSS, 1975). Their proposed amendment to section 60 of the 1959 Mental Health Act states that an offender 'suffering from psychopathic disorder with dangerous antisocial tendencies' shall not be committed to hospital unless the court is satisfied that there is a relevant mental or organic illness or relevant psychological defect and that therapeutic benefit will result from hospital admission.

Aetiology

The hypothesis that genetic factors are significant is supported by Schulsinger's (1972) study in which 57 Danish psychopaths who had been adopted were precisely matched with 57 control adoptees. The incidence of mental disorder in adoptive and biological relatives of each group was then determined blindly. More psychopathy was found among biological relatives of index cases than among adoptive relatives (see Table II).

It is often stated that posterior temporal slow waves on the EEG are especially common among psychopaths (see Hill and Watterson, 1942). This is generally equated with a maturation delay.

Bowlby's original (and subsequently revised) proposition that maternal deprivation in the first three years of life could result in psychopathic disorder has been generally refined to a considered view that interference with attachments and bond formation in infancy is likely to result in defective socialization and difficulties with interpersonal behaviour subsequently (see Rutter, 1972). It should be emphasized that this is far from the invariable fate of children institutionalized since birth.

Within families one can observe the adverse consequences of discord and rejection on the behaviour and socialization of children but the invulnerability of many children is as striking as the fact that such factors are common in the retrospective histories of adult psychopaths.

Three attitudes characterize dynamic explanations:

(1) The emphasis on the tendency to find release in 'acting out' behaviour rather than forming intrapsychic defences against turmoil induced by frustration.
(2) The immaturity of interpersonal, emotional and moral development summarized tersely by epithets such as selfish, childish.
(3) Stressing of the need of the psychopath for external controls in view of defective superego development.

Table II *Incidence (in rounded figures) of mental disorders in the relatives of 57 psychopathic adoptees (Schulsinger, 1972)*

Mental disorders in relatives	Psychopaths		Controls (also adopted)	
	Biological relatives (%)	Adoptive relatives (%)	Biological relatives (%)	Adoptive relatives (%)
Any	19	14	13	12
Psychopathy (strict)	4	1	1	1
Psychopathy (loose definition)[a]	14	8	7	5
Psychopathy (strict) in fathers	9	2	2	0

[a] Includes doubtful psychopathy, criminality, alcoholism, hysterical personality disorder as well as strictly defined psychopathy (non-psychotic, inappropriate, impulse-ridden, acting-out behaviour in adult life).

Management

Out-patient counselling

Current complaints and problems are listed and disentangled. Crises are mapped so that patterns may be derived to enable anticipatory action to be taken. Great care is taken to avoid being made responsible as 'the doctor'. The object is to enable some insight to be gained by the patient and his relatives. Gunn (1971) has advocated the pursuit of similar activities within special centres staffed by a variety of disciplines to avoid confusions between involved agencies and provide long-term, consistent care and support.

Therapeutic community in-patient

Hospitals such as the Henderson achieve a success rate of about 40% (as judged by ex-patients being self supporting and out of trouble—Whiteley, 1970). Some selection towards normal or superior intelligence usually obtains. This is the model for Grendon Underwood Prison. Against this one may set the finding by Gibbens et al. (1959) that 24% of psychopaths identified in prison had stayed virtually out of trouble on eight-year follow-up.

Authoritarian in-patient

The Balderton experiment (Craft et al., 1964) demonstrated that a paternalistic regime benefited a group of psychopaths with subnormal intelligence significantly more than a therapeutic community approach when subjects were alternatively allocated to either regime. Craft's unit at Conway, run on paternalistic lines achieves a 40% success rate (Craft, 1968).

Prognosis

Several studies have demonstrated that the presence or absence of 'psychopathy' does little to alter the prognosis in terms of re-conviction when prisoners with similar criminal records are considered (e.g. Gibbens et al., 1959). In general the tendency to overt aggressive or antisocial behaviour diminishes with time but the psychopath may continue to wreak havoc within his marriage and family. Alcoholism and an early death are quite likely (Robins, 1966). Curiously enough the presence of an abnormal EEG was associated with an improved prognosis in Gibbens et al.'s study.

The 47 XYY karyotype

The Carstairs study (Jacobs et al. 1965, 1968) revealed that nine of the 315 inmates of this Scottish special security hospital had an XYY sex-chromosome constitution. Confirmation of a rate of about 3% within British special hospitals was provided by Casey *et al.* (1971). Various surveys of the chromosome status of neonates have shown rates of around one to two per 1000 live born males (see e.g. Ratcliffe *et al.*, 1970). The attrition rate through death is unknown as there are no satisfactory total population studies of adult males. It has been a repeated finding that the prevalence of XYY men in maximum security hospitals in Great Britain and the USA is significantly raised above that level predicted for the general population from neonate studies. Whilst noting that several British special hospitals admit both mentally subnormal and normally intelligent mentally ill patients, it is generally held that the prevalence in subnormality hospitals and in ordinary prisons is lower than in special hospitals though higher than in the general population. Hunter (1977) demonstrated a rate of 0·7% among 1811 mentally handicapped males in subnormality hospitals in Northern England.

The height of 47 XYY individuals is a distinctive characteristic. Half (but only half) of Pitcher's (1970) sample were over 183 cm (6 feet) tall, the mean being 181 cm with a standard deviation of 6·7 cm. The shortest was 161 cm (5 feet 3½ in.).

It has been suggested that abnormalities of sexual development are more prevalent among XYY men (see Pitcher's (1971) review) but this is not a universal characteristic. The possibility that some reportedly Y chromosomes are fragmented X chromosomes cannot be overlooked.

The population study of Witkin *et al.* (1976) provides important information. From a total population sample of nearly 29,000 men all those within the top 15·9% of the height distribution (using a cut-off point of 184 cm) were traced and 91% provided material for chromosomal analysis. It is important to note that many XYYs will have been missed by using this cut-off. However, the sample yielded 12 XYY, 16 XXY and 4111 XY males. Intelligence, educational achievement, criminal record and EEG were among the variables considered; 42% of the XYYs, 19% of XXYs and 9% of XYs had criminal records (of, roughly speaking, indictable offences). The excess of XYY over XY is statistically significant, the other differences are not. The offences committed by XYYs were *not* particularly acts of aggression, neither were their crimes especially serious. This is in accordance with the Carstairs findings but not with other assertions that aggressive behaviour is characteristic (see Pitcher, 1971).

For both the XYY and XXY groups the intellectual level was significantly lower than XY controls though some XYY individuals scored within the normal range. This variable of intelligence was felt to be highly important, though when held constant along with parental social status and height (which had correlated negatively with criminality among XY controls), an elevation of XYY over XY crime rate persisted.

Comparison of EEGs showed XYYs to have a significantly lower average frequency of alpha rhythm than matched XY controls. This may be interpreted as a development lag, and as such, commensurate with the low intelligence finding.

It is probably fair to say that, the more systematic the study, the weaker the proposition that an XYY 'syndrome' within which a *necessary* association between 47 XYY constitution, tall stature, and violent behaviour holds. Rather, one is left with a presumptive hypothesis that the 47 XYY genotype tends to be associated with tall stature, an increase in the likelihood of criminal conviction, and (vide Witkin) lower intelligence. Most XYY individuals go unconvicted.

Violence

Destructive aggressive acts wherein the determined pursuit of an objective is accompanied by force are seen by courts and the general public as products of abnormally powerful motivation or abnormally weak self-control and the psychiatrist frequently is invited to comment and explain. Violence is hardly a unitary phenomenon and the similarities between pathological jealousy, football hooliganism, and child abuse are not obvious. Suitable reviews are provided by Gunn (1973) and Harrington (1972) which demonstrate a multiplicity of hypotheses and a plurality of mechanisms which may combine to explain or produce a violent act.

The model suggested by Megargee (1966) whereby violence is most likely at each end of a continuum from over-control of impulses with rigid inhibitions to under-control and habitually aggressive behaviour, is often cited, but has received only qualified support from experimental study (e.g. Blackburn, 1970). Nevertheless the exercise whereby controls and impulses are separately analysed would appear potentially useful as a model for appraisal of the individual case.

Crimes of violence

The peak age for crimes of violence against the person is between 17 and 21—somewhat older than the peak age for all convictions, as theft and similar offences against property are by far the most common crimes at all ages and are especially rife amongst youths of 14 to 17.

Murder

Unlawful killing with a particular *mens rea* (i.e. 'malice aforethought') carries, on conviction, a mandatory sentence of life imprisonment. Various mitigating circumstances such as provocation or diminished responsibility indicate that certain unlawful homicides are to be considered as the lesser crime of manslaughter with sentence at the judge's discretion.

Nearly all murderers who come to trial are male and, in the majority of instances, their motives are emotional and the victims are relatives or close associates. Only a minority are motivated by straightforward criminal gain (e.g. robbery or sexual adventure). Typically, murderers are young adults from lower socio-economic backgrounds. In England, victims are twice as likely to be female (wives are most vulnerable) and the common settings are quarrels, rages, paranoia or suicidal despair, less commonly morbid jealousy or child abuse. Nearly one in two murderers are found to be suffering from mental abnormality, especially personality disorder, subnormality and schizophrenia, at trial (Driver *et al.*, 1974).

The above generalizations are valid for the UK (Gibson and Klein, 1961, 1969) and would not be true for the substantial minority (as much as one-third according to West, 1965) who commit suicide after murder. West found that this group was less socially deviant, contained a larger minority of women, was even more domestic and resembled in demographic terms a population of suicides. Conversely, the experience in North America and the West of Scotland has shown that in those areas suicide only rarely follows murder (Gillies, 1976).

In the United States it would appear that the setting is less likely to be domestic. Wolfgang (1958) has argued for a 'subculture of violence' and has shown that perhaps a quarter of homicides are victim-precipitated by, for example, a would-be murderer having the tables turned on him. Victims, in his study, had similar general characteristics to their killers and were *not* weak, passive people. Gillies (1976) has drawn attention to the manner in which Glasgow murderers resemble their urban American counterparts, especially in their tendency to be mentally normal though frequently drunk. It has been demonstrated that there is an association between drinking and murder in up to a half of all instances (see e.g. Virkkunen, 1974).

In a rich descriptive essay, Brittain (1970) has portrayed the sexually sadistic murderer as male, uncommunicative, shy, somewhat ascetic, and with a precarious self-esteem yet powerful fantasy. He is likely to be sexually feeble and may show deviant orientation: homosexuality, paedophilia or transvestism. Commonly there is a burning interest in Naziism, black magic, or monsters and this is usually expressed in an extensive collection of books on such subjects, many of which shade into sadistic pornography. Typically he is emotionally blunted in his response to his own cruelty and tends to make an exception for himself. Numerically, sadistic murderers are rare and would seem qualitatively distinct from most murderers who in general act within chronic domestic stress or explosively and carelessly in an already violent setting.

Rape

The legal definition of 'unlawful [extra-marital] sexual intercourse with a woman without her consent' does not mention the use of force. Thus, if one studies a cohort of men convicted of rape, it is inevitable that a sizeable minority will be heterosexual paedophiliacs who have had intercourse with a girl too young to have been able to exercise judgement and give consent. If the paedophiles are excluded one is left with a group of individuals who have used force in their quest for carnal knowledge. Many of these are selfish, predatory, sexually well-adjusted young men who snatch not only sex but property too and who rape as 'part of a general cycle of aggression' (Gibbens et al., 1977). The remainder are a remarkably heterogeneous group including would-be rape-murderers and sexual novitiates who misread their partner's signals.

Various attempts have been made at classifying forcible rape, usually using motive as the differentiating factor. Perhaps the most concise is ultimately derived from Gebhard et al.'s (1965) massive survey.
  (1) Aggressive aim (sexual behaviour is in the service of anger and humiliates the victim).
  (2) Sexual aim (aggression in the service of achieving sex).
  (3) Sadistic men who need an element of cruelty to achieve sexual satisfaction.

The prognosis for rape is well illustrated by Gibbens et al. (1977) 12-year follow-up (see Table III). Their 'aggressive' group refers to individuals with a general propensity toward aggressive behaviour, the 'remainder' group is a heterogeneous miscellany.

Table III

	Paedophiliac	Aggressive	Remainder
% reconvicted for standard list offences (including sex offences)	63	85	28
% reconvicted of sexual offences	20	20	3

Arson

Nineteenth century views of arson as a disease entity (pyromania) have been replaced by the concept of fire-setting as a behavioural symptom.

Lewis and Yarnell (1951) published the authoritative work which suggested the basis for the following categories:

(1) Accidental–subnormality, confusional states, intoxication.
(2) Acting on delusions or hallucinations.
(3) Revenge–on employer, wife or society.
(4) Erotic–fire fetishism with simultaneous masturbation.
(5) Heroic–wanting adulation for *extinguishing* fire, etc.
(6) Excitement–attempt to dispel tension or misery.
(7) Cry for help–'wiping slate clean', attention-attracting, forcing imprisonment.
(8) Criminal intent to defraud insurance company or conceal evidence.

Characteristics of arsonists studied generally appear to parallel the institution wherein they are discovered (special hospitals, etc.) though it is widely suggested (e.g. Hurley and Monahan, 1969) that most are young men, half of whom are subnormal and half, not necessarily the *other* half, alcoholic. Most have been active fire-setters since puberty or before and have convictions for other offences against property. Imprisoned arsonists have a high incidence of social and sexual maladjustment though it would be naïve to reduce arson to a unifying level of sexual metaphor. Certainly many arsonists do masturbate while watching the flames but it would seem most likely that, in many instances, sexual behaviour is a response to excitement rather than vice versa. Similarly, erections and ejaculations occur in house-breakers, combat troops and men in other situations in which fear and excitement with high levels of psychophysiological arousal occur.

Traditionally, arsonists recidivate though the low reconviction rate shown by Soothill and Pope (1973) in a 20-year cohort follow-up challenges this.

Non-accidental injury to children

Child abuse is not any single entity but a term used to describe a variety of acts by parents ranging from frank explosive assault—the battered child in Kempe's original phrase—to overpunitive discipline or irresponsible neglect. Scott (1973) has itemized the various ways in which children may meet death at the hands of a parent—intentional ridding of an unwanted encumbrance, mercy killing, the specific consequence of parental delusion, displacement of parental anger onto the child, and finally, the classic child-provoked battering. It would seem reasonable to extend such multiplicity of motive and mechanism toward explanation of the non-fatal child abuse where injury results. Taken thus, it becomes apparent that non-accidental injury to children represents a description of the consequence of certain parental behaviours, variously determined, rather than being a 'clinical' entity with uniform characteristics, antecedents and prognosis.

Some generalizations can nevertheless be made. Various estimates of incidence have been made from which one might suggest a rate of roughly 0.5% of children under three per year. Kempe (1971) estimates 40,000 cases per annum in the USA, a *Lancet* editorial (1973) suggests 3000 cases p.a. in the UK. In one series (Oliver, 1975) the death rate among battered children was 10% over a two-year period. According to Skinner and Castle (1969) the risk of an injured child being battered again is of the order of 60% and where the first sib is battered the chance of subsequent sibs being likewise assaulted is 13 to one. Put another way, Smith *et al.* (1973) found that 19% of the abused child's siblings had also been battered. This questions simple scape-goating theory whereby only one child in any family would be at risk for abuse.

Detection of child abuse will naturally increase with the suspicion of the examining doctor. Cameron (1970) provides a review of typical injuries. One may cite as items that must arouse suspicion:

(a) multiple bruises, burns or lacerations of various ages especially bite marks, fingertip bruises and laceration of the inner aspect of the upper lip;

(b) multiple fractures, sub-periosteal haematomata, and epiphyseal separations on X-ray;

(c) subdural haematomata, retinal injury, or rupture of abdominal viscera;

(d) delay reporting injury or seeking help by parents (by more than six hours, say);

(e) discrepant or vague history of injury.

Factors combining to produce child abuse may be summarized under three headings.

1   *Relevant to the child.* Battered children are likely to be the product of a pre-marital pregnancy or illegitimacy (Smith *et al.*, 1974). Traditionally they are said to be either only children or the youngest of a family—an unwelcomed start or addition to a family. If one considers that it is predominantly infants who are at risk the statement becomes somewhat tautological as children of such an age usually are occupants of such ordinal positions. Certain individual differences, easy waking at night or a piercing cry, seem on anecdotal grounds to increase the vulnerability of the child. Ounsted *et al.* (1974) are among the workers who have pointed out how early separation of the newborn baby from mother by, say, admission to a special care unit because of neonatal problems, may prejudice satisfactory bonding between mother and child and sow the seeds of later rejection and violence.

2   *Relevant to the parents*. The various assertions as to the characteristics of abusing parents have not always been tested against controls. An exception is the study by Smith *et al.* (1973) which found among the parents of battered children:

   (a) an excess of low social class;
   (b) a marked tendency for the mother to be unmarried and the biological father to be absent;
   (c) a younger maternal age at birth of first child;
   (d) a high prevalence of unsatisfactory marriages;
   (e) 'gross personality defect' in one-third of the fathers;
   (f) subnormal intelligence in nearly half of the mothers;
   (g) a criminal record possessed by nearly one-third cf the fathers;
   (h) severe mental illness in only a small minority of parents who typically had inflicted bizarre injuries.

It is well known that battering parents have often themselves been victims of parental violence. Oliver and Taylor (1971) describe a family within which five generations of children had been abused.

3   *Relevant to the family's social situation*. The single most relevant factor would appear to be social isolation (see e.g. Davoren, 1968). Other popularly cited associations such as paternal unemployment or financial problems seem to be insignificant when appropriate controls are selected (Smith *et al.*, 1974).

Management of the problem, once detected, must necessarily involve both emergency action and judiciously considered help to child and family in the longer term. A Place of Safety Order may be needed if the parents will not readily agree to hospitalization and this should be followed by a case conference to establish the key worker and a surveillance network which can be used as a therapeutic vehicle. Where a local authority possesses an 'at risk' register the child's name must be admitted to it and consideration borne as to whether other siblings should be included thereupon. If appropriate, a Care Order should be sought by the Social Services. The child, if allowed home, will probably need placement in a day nursery to alleviate the caretaking burden and allow supervision.

Further work is arduous where rehabilitation of the child within the family is attempted. The NSPCC group (Baher *et al.*, 1976) claimed considerable success from intensive supportive psychotherapeutic work with the parents as do workers such as Ounsted *et al.* (1974) using an in-patient setting for counselling selected abusing families. The relative superiority of various intervention strategies is not established. Time and again one returns, in treatment, to correcting the distorted expectations of parents, well documented by Helfer and Kempe (1968), that the child should satisfy the needs of the parent in a situation of reversed dependency, exaggerated by the echoes of a punitive childhood experience by the parent who is trapped in a disharmonious unsatisfying marriage or isolated from community and family of origin.

Those children who experience non-accidental injury do not fare well even if they survive. Intracranial and retinal damage, probably from shaking, leads to mental subnormality in perhaps one-quarter of assaulted children (see review by Scott, 1977). The emotional damage can only be guessed at, though the transmission of patterns of child abuse across generations has already been noted.

Exhibitionism

The typical exhibitionist is a young man who exposes his genitals to a woman as an end in itself. Such activity renders him liable to conviction under the Vagrancy Act 1824 when he is usually said to be guilty of indecent exposure. Other persons may be guilty of indecent exposure without being exhibitionists as such; they may have exhibited their genitals as a prelude, inviting or threatening, to further sexual activity such as intercourse. Rooth (1971) provides the authoritative review. He considers that the individual exhibitionist is typically a passive person with little capacity for the appropriate expression of anger and with generally poor social skills. Emotional immaturity combines with gauche unassertiveness to create a boyish impression with an inner, frail egocentricity, vulnerable to setbacks and discouragement. Such a man may be married but in general would be expected to have a poor capacity for heterosexual relationships and activities.

In common with many disorders of sexual orientation and behaviour it is said that exhibitionists have experienced a close but ambivalent relationship with their mother and a poor relationship with a distant, despised father. Family attitudes to sex are restrictive. The usual dynamic formulations stress castration fears exaggerated by the close relationship with the mother. Thus the victim's response to the exposure provides him with reassurance as to his own masculinity and potency. By extension, the act may also be seen as an invitation for the victim to expose herself and prove she is not castrated. It is difficult to square the classical formulations with the observation that in many societies genital exposure is a grave insult (as indeed is expressed by the Vagrancy Act 1824: 'wilfully, openly, lewdly and obscenely exposing his person with intent to insult any female') or with the clinical impression that many exhibitionists store the memory of their victim's response in their personal psychic attics as material for future fantasy for masturbation or to power an erection suitable for marital intercourse.

The actual offence behaviour is a risky business. The favourite haunts of exposures tend to be reasonably public places that afford some cover—parks, streets at night, parked cars. Many exhibitionists expose repeatedly as if to obtain a 'perfect' response. Rooth (1971) observes that the urge to expose often mounts at times of stress and that apprehension under such circumstances may produce a feeling of considerable relief for the exposer. It is unclear whether such relief is a consequence of the assuaging of unconscious guilt or the relief from a stressful, intolerable social situation. Typical victims are young women or children, never acquaintances, and the cherished responses those of fear or disgust. The successful act of exposure is apparently a moment of power and assertion in a life of timid inferiority.

'Cure' for many is apparently provided by the first court appearance as only 10–20% go on to a second conviction. Subsequent convictions are progressively associated with worsening prognosis and would seem to indicate psychiatric referral though it would seem that psychiatry can offer little for seriously recidivist exhibitors. Benefit apparently follows from both group therapy and aversive techniques though in the absence of controls it is impossible to comment constructively. Nevertheless it is interesting to note that Jones and Frei (1977) have described apparent short-term success with a treatment package including the prohibition of masturbation to deviant imagery, the encouragement of sexual inter-course with wives and a series of sessions in which the subject undresses in front of an interrogative group and video recorder while describing one of his exposing episodes. Subsequently he views the video tape and is invited to comment on his feelings.

Epilepsy and crime

The medical defence of automatism (see below) is often said to apply specially to offences committed during or possibly just after an epileptic fit. Gunn (1977) elicited a prevalence rate of epilepsy among prisoners in the prisons of England and Wales of 7·2 per 1000 in 1967, considerably higher than general population rates. Gunn and Fenton (1971) then went on to examine the records of imprisoned epileptics to see if any of the offences resulting in imprisonment could have been committed during a period of impaired consciousness. Only one possible case in the general prison population and three within a special hospital could be found. Clearly automatism cannot explain the apparent association between epilepsy and crime. Further examination of cases (Gunn, 1974) displayed evidence for each of four possible mechanisms acting to produce the association when this is not just fortuitous:

(a) organic brain disorder responsible for *both* epilepsy and offence behaviour;
(b) organic brain disorder causing epilepsy with consequent social rejection and sense of inferiority leading to offence behaviour;
(c) adverse social factors leading to both epilepsy and antisocial behaviour (e.g. battered child);
(d) a tendency to reckless and antisocial behaviour which leads to offences *and* accidents which may injure brain and cause post-traumatic epilepsy.

The assertion that a substantial proportion of murderers have abnormal EEGs (see e.g. Winkler and Kove, 1962; Hill and Pond, 1952) loses force when suitable controls are used. Driver *et al.* (1974) were unable to demonstrate an excess over controls of EEG abnormalities in 150 murderers including 23 whose crimes were 'motiveless'. In both murderers and controls the rate of EEG abnormalities was about 10% even though nearly half of those charged with murder were psychiatrically abnormal.

Shop-lifting

Shop-lifting is one of the few offences where women predominate over men. Most only offend once but 10% are reconvicted, usually for further shop-lifting. It seems that women shop-lifters in the UK may be divided into two groups (Gibbens *et al.*, 1971). The majority, perhaps two-thirds, are British and usually middle-aged. Characteristically they suffer from a multiplicity of minor physical symptoms—insomnia, headache and the like. At the time of the offence they feel that their life ahead seems barren and not infrequently they suffer from persistent depressive mood. On follow-up (Gibbens *et al.*, 1971) they were more frequently admitted to a mental hospital than controls and were usually diagnosed as depressed. The implication is that, in a middle-aged woman, shop-lifting may be a sign of a developing depression. One is reminded of Alexander's acting out concept whereby the commission of a minor offence provides a rationale and expiation for guilt originating from internal psychic processes.

A minority of one-third are foreign born though not always tourists. Usually young and of blameless upbringing, they appear to view themselves as committing a technical offence akin to exceeding the speed limit and often seem to have seen themselves as relatively poor and isolated in alien surroundings.

Male shop-lifters are markedly different. Half steal books—an activity virtually unknown in women—and as a group they are much more likely to be recidivist. Among juveniles, stealing from shops tends to be a 'marauding' activity though occasionally with a 'proving' element. In such circumstances it tends to be a transient phenomenon.

Assessment of amnesia

It is not uncommon for a person on remand to deny any memory for his (alleged) offence. Obviously malingering is likely but other possibilities must necessarily be considered:

(1) Intoxication by alcohol or drugs.
(2) Hypoglycaemia, including that induced by alcohol.
(3) Epilepsy—a very rare association with peri-ictal events (q.v.).
(4) Transient global amnesia: acute transient confusional state with subsequent amnesia including retrograde amnesia of up to a few hours previously. Usually in men over 50 who are obviously atherosclerotic and may have previously indulged in abnormal exercise or unusual neck movements (e.g. at air displays).
(5) Head injury, usually obvious. Activity that is already initiated, as in a brawl, is continued but novel behaviours would not be initiated during concussion. Beware the subsequent subdural haematoma.
(6) Psychogenic. Many murderers cannot recall the dramatic events of their killing even if they plead guilty. Extreme emotional pre-occupation at the time of the offence is demonstrable, i.e. not in embezzlement cases. The mechanism may be dissociation, defective registration or subsequent repression.

It will be necessary to obtain a full account of the maximum recall possible and to repeat this on subsequent days. The report must then be examined for inconsistencies or any favourable bias in recall and checked against the depositions, particularly looking for any suggestion of an abnormal level of consciousness. Any evidence of premeditation would weigh against a genuine amnesia. Naturally a low threshold for investigations such as an EEG, skull X-ray, fasting blood sugar, etc., must be maintained.

Court reports

No space is available for advice as to the compilation and organization of a report; the articles by Scott (1953), Gibbens (1974) and Briscoe (1975) are required reading. The principles of stating sources, arguing from cited facts or documented observations, and eschewing jargon deserve re-iteration. Some knowledge of the powers of the court and of possible psychiatric 'defences' is required and is outlined below.

Criminal responsibility

In general, a person is guilty of a criminal act only if both his guilty act (*actus reus*) and his guilty intent (*mens rea*) can be established. Some crimes of 'strict liability', such as possessing adulterated tobacco, are exceptions to this rule and proven commission of the act alone is sufficient for the person to be guilty. A further exception is provided by the instances of children who have not yet reached their tenth birthday and consequently are held to be *doli incapax*, incapable of criminal intent and therefore entirely exempt from criminal responsibility though not, of course, from care proceedings under the Children's and Young Persons Act 1969. Between their tenth and fourteenth birthdays children are exempt from criminal responsibilities unless it can be proved that they caused an *actus reus* with *mens rea* and that they did so with *mischievous discretion*, i.e. that they were capable of discerning good from evil at the time of the offence—evil in this case meaning moral rather than legal wrongness. Beyond the fourteenth birthday a person (although an infant in the eyes of the law until the age of 18) is presumed fully responsible for his actions. The necessity for *mens rea* to be established for most severe offences allows the possibility of entering a psychiatric 'defence' in any of five ways:

(1) Unfit to plead.
(2) Incapacity to form an intent (automatism).
(3) McNaghton mad—not guilty by reason of insanity.
(4) Diminished responsibility $\Big\}$ for murder only.
(5) Infanticide

Unfit to plead on arraignment
(Criminal Procedure (Insanity) Act 1964)

This may be raised by either party or the judge at any point in trial proceedings before the defence case opens and concerns the defendant's sanity *at the time of the trial*. It is not to be lightly entered into as a trial of fitness to plead is held in front of a separate jury and, if upheld, results in admission of the defendant to a (special) hospital as though under Sections 60 and 65 where he is regarded as 'under disability' without limitation of time until considered fit for trial by consent of the Home Secretary. A person who is fit to plead must be able to: understand the charge against him and the significance of his plea; challenge a juror; examine a witness; instruct counsel; follow the progress of the trial. Where the issue is raised by the defendant the onus of proving that he is unfit to plead rests with him but is established on the balance of probabilities. If the issue is raised by the prosecution or by the judge the case must be proved beyond reasonable doubt. It should be noted in passing that under Section 73 of the 1959 Mental Health Act it is possible for the Home Secretary, acting on the advice of two doctors, to detain a person remanded in custody for trial and ascertained to be mentally ill or severely subnormal in hospital *before* his trial commences.

Automatism

It will be evident that consciousness must be so clouded as to be all but obliterated before the capacity to form an intent is lost and the act regarded as involuntary. Immense intoxication just short of stupor might be allowed but the more usual relevant conditions are hypoglycaemia, concussion and epilepsy. True epileptic automatisms are exceptional as the settings for offence behaviour (q.v.) but the question may arise over post-ictal confusion. It is a difficult defence to use successfully and renders the defendant liable (though not automatically so) to indefinite hospitalization under Sections 60 and 65.

Not guilty by reason of insanity

Following the shooting of Sir Robert Peel's secretary by Daniel McNaghton (who spelled his name in various ways) acting on a delusional belief that the Tories were plotting against his life, the Law Lords in 1843 set forth the following rules for the special verdict which until 1964 was 'guilty but insane' but since the Criminal Procedure (Insanity) Act 1964 is 'not guilty by reason of insanity':
  (1) Everyone is 'presumed to be sane and to possess a sufficient degree of reason to be responsible for his crimes, until the contrary be proved to (the Jury's) satisfaction'.
  (2) At the time of the act, the accused must have been 'labouring under such a defect of reason, from disease of the mind, as not to know the nature and quality of the act he was doing or, if he did know it, that he did not know he was doing what was wrong'.
  (3) Where a man commits a crime under an insane delusion his responsibility shall be assessed as though 'the facts with respect to which the delusion exists were real'.

Whether a particular psychological condition amounts to a 'disease of the mind' as enshrined above is a legal question. Since the 1957 Homicide Act and also the abolition of capital punishment the use of this as a defence in murder cases—formerly its principal arena—has become rare. Naturally it may be invoked as a defence against other charges but is usually reserved for instances where a 'not guilty' verdict would be valuable for insurance or emigration purposes as the 'conviction' is not recorded. Where the verdict (which, when the matter is raised by the defence, is on the balance of probabilities) is found, the court must order that the accused be admitted to a hospital to be specified by the Home Secretary—almost always a special hospital.

Diminished responsibility (Homicide Act 1957)

Conviction for murder carries an automatic life sentence. Against a charge of murder, a successful defence on the grounds of diminished responsibility results in a verdict of *guilty of manslaughter* with the resulting sentence at the discretion of the judge. The jury decides on the basis of medical evidence whether the accused was suffering from

> such abnormality of mind (whether arising from a condition of arrested or retarded development of mind or any inherent causes or induced by disease or injury) as substantially impaired his mental responsibility for his acts and omissions in doing or being a party to the killing.

It is a defence that can only be entered against the charge of murder and is frequently used. 'Abnormality of mind' means that the reasonable man would term it abnormal. It can include the situation where the (overwhelming) difficulty the accused found in controlling his impulse to commit a physical act was substantially greater than an ordinary man, not suffering from mental abnormality, would experience in similar circumstances. Substantial need not mean total but means more than trivial. The usual sentence is hospitalization under Section 60 and 65 but the judge may specify any of a range of sentences from probation to life.

Infanticide (Infanticide Act 1938)

A woman who kills her child within a year of its birth may have a charge of murder reduced to that of infanticide and dealt with as if guilty of manslaughter, thus avoiding an automatic life sentence, if it can be shown that the 'balance of her mind was disturbed . . . by . . . the effects of giving birth or by . . . lactation consequent upon the birth'.

Responsibility for non-criminal acts

It is convenient to mention here the assessment of the capacity of mentally disordered individuals to manage their own affairs.

Testamentary capacity

A person making a will must have a 'sound disposing mind'. This may be established by the following questions:
(1) Does he know the nature and extent of his property?
(2) Does he know which persons have a claim on it?
(3) Can he form a judgement on the relative strengths of these claims?
(4) Has he expressed himself legibly, clearly and without ambiguity?
It follows that a person may be quite deluded but still capable of drawing up a sound will. Assessment is for the will in question—mild dementia would invalidate a complex will but not a simple one.

The Court of Protection

Composed of various 'Masters' (in Lunacy), this body manages the property and affairs of those who, because of their mental disorder, cannot do so themselves. An application from a relative or similar is heard and medical evidence is assessed. If appropriate, a Receiver—usually a relative or close friend—is appointed who will have control over the person's property. This arrangement cannot be revoked by the patient in the same way as can a Power of Attorney authorization, which in any case relies for its validity on the patient understanding what he is doing when he signs the authorization.

Lord Chancellor's visitors

Four officers appointed by the Lord Chancellor visit persons who are under the jurisdiction of the Court of Protection and report as to whether their affairs are being managed appropriately. Three are medical and have statutory access to medical records.

The powers of the court

A mentally disordered offender may be dealt with by the court by invoking the normal penal sentences: fines, imprisonment etc. If the court wishes to take the mental disorder specifically into account, several courses of action are available. If the offender agrees to receive treatment, or if compulsory admission under part IV of the 1959 Mental Health Act has been arranged, the court may absolutely or conditionally discharge the offender.

Alternatively, the offender may be required to receive treatment as a condition of probation. Under the Powers of Criminal Courts Act 1973 (or, as is still widely referred to, under the Criminal Justice Act 1948) a doctor approved under Section 28 of the 1959 Mental Health Act may provide medical evidence that the offender's mental disorder requires medical treatment and that such treatment is available. The offender must be willing to comply with the requirements of the order. Should he default he may be brought back to the court by the supervising probation officer. The court may discontinue the treatment requirement if the doctor responsible advises so. Under the Criminal Justice Act 1972 the maximum duration of such an order is three years.

Offenders below the age of 17 may be committed to the care of a Local Authority. The Children and Young Persons Act 1969 provides that a supervision order may include a condition of submission to treatment for not more than 12 months and not beyond the offender's eighteenth birthday.

Section 60 of the 1959 Mental Health Act enables a higher (Crown) or lower (Magistrates) Court to make an order consigning a person to hospital for treatment of mental disorder or (less commonly) to the guardianship of a Local Authority or other person. The court must be satisfied by two doctors, one of which must be approved under Section 28 of the Act as having special experience in the diagnosis or treatment of mental disorder, that:

(1) The convicted person is suffering from mental disorder.
(2) That a particular hospital (or Local Authority) will admit him within 28 days.
(3) That hospital treatment (or reception into guardianship) is appropriate.

Such an order cannot be made until the court is satisfied that the defendant is guilty, i.e. not until after conviction as far as Crown Courts are concerned. Thus, if the defendant is unfit to plead he can only be held 'under disability' and a hospital order cannot be invoked. Further circumstances debarring the use of a Section 60 order are where the penalty for the offence is fixed by law (such as 'life' for murder) or, as far as Magistrates' Courts are concerned, where the offence is not punishable by imprisonment.

Once admitted to hospital an offender cannot be transferred to prison though under Section 72 of the 1959 Mental Health Act a person in prison or Borstal may be transferred to a psychiatric hospital for treatment and, if necessary, returned to prison when treatment is completed. There is nothing in theory to prevent a hospital receiving an offender on a Section 60 order (alone) one day and discharging him the next. Under Section 63 of the Act the nearest relative cannot discharge the patient though may appeal to a Review Tribunal annually on the patient's behalf. The patient may appeal himself to the Tribunal within six months of the order being made.

Section 61 of the Act allows similar orders to be made on children.

A higher court may add a restriction order to a hospital order under Section 65 of the Act provided that one of the two doctors gives oral evidence to the court. Such an order means that the powers of discharge, transfer and the granting of leave may only be exercised with the consent of the Home Secretary. Furthermore, the patient and his relatives have no direct access to the Mental Health Review Tribunal though the Home Secretary does and may be requested to do so every two years after the first 12 months; he must comply. A restriction order may be for a specified period of time or without limit of time—the judge decides. The latter does not mean the person can never leave hospital but rather that he can only do so with the consent of the Home Secretary who can recall him to any psychiatric hospital at any time without going through the court. Appeal against Section 60 and 65 may be made (once only) through the courts under normal legal appeals procedure.

References

Adams, S. (1961). The PICO Project. *In* 'The Sociology of Punishment and Conviction' (Eds N. Johnston *et al.*), Chapter 32. Wiley, New York.

Baher, E., Hyman, C., Jones, C., Jones, R., Kerr, A. and Michael, R. (1976). 'At Risk'. Routledge and Kegan Paul, London.

Belson, W. A. (1968). The extent of stealing by London boys. *Advancement Sc.* **25**, 171–184.

Blackburn, R. (1970). 'Personality Types Among Abnormal Homicides'. Special Hospitals Research Report No. 1. Broadmoor Hospital, Special Hospitals Research Unit.

Briscoe, O. V. (1975). Assessment of intent—an approach to the preparation of court reports. *Br. J. Psychiat.* **127**, 461–465.

Brittain, R. P. (1970). The sadistic murderer. *Med. Sci. Law* **10**, 198–207.

Cameron, J. M. (1970). The battered baby. *Br. J. Hosp. Med.* **4**, 769–778.

Casey, M. D., Blank, C. E., Mobley, T., Kohn, P., Street, D. R. K., McDougall, J. M., Gooder, J. and Platts, J. (1971). 'Patients With Chromosome Abnormality in Two Special Hospitals'. Special Hospitals Research Report No. 2. Broadmoor Hospital, Special Hospitals Research Unit.

Christiansen, K. O. (1970). Crime in a Danish twin population. *Acta Genet. Med. Gemellol.* **19**, 323–326.

Christie, N., Andeneas, J. and Skirbeck, S. (1965). A study of self-reported crime. *In* 'Scandinavian Studies in Criminology' (Ed. K. O. Christiansen), Vol. I, pp. 86–116. Tavistock, London.

Cloward, R. A. and Ohlin, L. E. (1961). 'Delinquency and Opportunity'. Routledge and Kegan Paul, London.

562   P. Hill

Cohen, A. K. (1955). 'Delinquent Boys: The Culture of the Gang'. Routledge and Kegan Paul, London.
Cohen, S. (Ed.) (1971). 'Images of Deviance'. Penguin, Harmondsworth.
Conger, J. J. and Miller, W. C. (1966). 'Personality, Social Class and Delinquency'. Wiley, New York.
Craft, M. (1968). Psychopathic disorder: a second trial of treatment. Br. J. Psychiat. 114, 813–820.
Craft, M., Stephenson, G. and Granger, C. (1964). A controlled trial of authoritarian and self-governing regimes with adolescent psychopaths. Am. J. Orthopsychiat. 34, 543–554.
Davoren, E. (1968). The role of the social worker. In 'The Battered Child' (Eds R. Helfer, and C. Kempe). Chicago University Press, Chicago.
Driver, M. V., West, L. R. and Faulk, M. (1974). Clinical and EEG studies of prisoners charged with murder. Br. J. Psychiat. 125, 583–587.
Douglas, J. W. B., Ross, J. M. and Simpson, H. R. (1968). 'All Our Future'. Peter Davies, London.
Ferguson, T. (1952). 'The Young Delinquent in His Social Setting'. Oxford University Press, Oxford.
Field, E. (1967). A Validation Study of Hewitt and Jenkins' Hypothesis. Home Office Research Unit Report No. 10. HMSO, London.
Gath, D., Cooper, B., Gattoni, F. and Rockett, D. (1977). 'Child Guidance and Delinquency in a London Borough'. Oxford University Press, Oxford.
Gebhard, P., Gagnon, J., Pomeroy, W. and Christenson, C. (1965). 'Sex Offenders'. Harper and Row, New York.
Gibbens, T. C. N. (1974). Preparing psychiatric court reports. Br. J. Hosp. Med. 12, 278–284.
Gibbens, T. C. N., Pond, D. A. and Stafford-Clark, D. (1959). A follow-up study of criminal psychopaths. J. Ment. Sci. 105, 108–115.
Gibbens, T. C. N., Palmer, C. and Prince, J. (1971). Mental health aspects of shop-lifting. Br. Med. J. iii, 612–615.
Gibbens, T. C. N., Way, C. and Soothill, K. L. (1977). Behavioural types of rape. Br. J. Psychiat. 130, 32–42.
Gibson, E. and Klein, S. (1961). 'Murder'. HMSO, London.
Gibson, E. and Klein, S. (1969). 'Murder 1957 to 1968'. HMSO, London.
Gillies, H. (1976). Homicide in the West of Scotland. Br. J. Psychiat. 128, 105–127.
Glueck, S. and Glueck, E. T. (1950). 'Unraveling Juvenile Delinquency'. The Commonwealth Fund, New York.
Glueck, S. and Glueck, E. T. (1956). 'Physique and Delinquency'. Harper Bros, New York.
Grant, J. D. and Grant, M. Q. (1959). A group dynamic approach to the treatment of nonconformists in the Navy. Ann. Am. Acad. Pol. Soc. Sci. 322, 127–135.
Gunn, J. (1971). Forensic psychiatry and psychopathic patients. Br. J. Hosp. Med. 6, 260–264.
Gunn, J. (1973). 'Violence'. David and Charles, Newton Abbot.
Gunn, J. (1974). Social factors and epileptics in prison. Br. J. Psychiat. 124, 509–517.
Gunn, J. (1977). Criminal behaviour and mental disorder. Br. J. Psychiat. 130, 317–329.
Gunn, J. and Fenton, G. (1971). Epilepsy, automatism and crime. Lancet i, 1173–1176.

Gunn, J. and Robertson, G. (1976). Psychopathic personality: a conceptual problem. *Psychol. Med.* **6**, 631–634.
Guze, S. B. (1976). 'Criminality and Psychiatric Disorders'. Oxford University Press, New York.
Harrington, J. A. (1972). Violence: a clinical viewpoint. *Br. Med. J.* **i**, 228–231.
Hartshorne, H. and May, M. A. (1928). 'Studies in Deceit'. Macmillan, New York.
Helfer, R. E. and Kempe, C. H. (1968). 'The Battered Child'. Chicago University Press, Chicago.
Hewitt, L. E. and Jenkins, R. L. (1946). 'Fundamental Patterns of Maladjustment—The Dynamics of their Origin'. Michigan Child Guidance Institute, State of Illinois.
Hill, J. D. N. and Pond, D. A. (1952). Reflections on one hundred capital cases submitted to electro-encephalography. *J. Ment. Sci.* **98**, 23–43.
Hill, J. D. N. and Watterson, D. (1942). Electro-encephalographic studies of psychopathic personalities. *J. Neurol. Neuropsychiat.* **5**, 47–65.
Home Office and DHSS (1975). Report of the Committee on Mentally Abnormal Offenders. HMSO, London. (Cmnd. 6244).
Hunter, H. (1977). XYY males. *Br. J. Psychiat.* **131**, 468–477.
Hurley, W. P. and Monahan, T. M. (1969) Arson: the criminal and the crime. *Br. J. Criminol.* **9**, 4–21.
Hutchings, B. and Mednick, S. A. (1974). Biological and adoptive fathers of male criminal adoptees. *In* 'Major Issues in Juvenile Delinquency'. World Health Organization, Copenhagen.
(ICD) General Register Office (1968). 'A Glossary of Mental Disorders. Based on the International Statistical Classification of Diseases, Injuries and Causes of Death'. HMSO, London.
Jacobs, P. A., Brunton, M., Melville, M. M., Brittain, R. P. and McClemont, W. F. (1965). Aggressive behaviour, mental subnormality and the XYY male. *Nature (Lond.)* **208**, 1351–1352.
Jacobs, P. A., Price, W. H., Court Brown, W. M., Brittain, R. P. and Whatmore, P. B. (1968). Chromosome studies on men in a maximum security hospital. *Ann. Hum. Genet.* **31**, 339–358.
Jephcott, A. P. and Carter, M. P. (1954). 'The Social Background of Delinquency'. University of Nottingham, Nottingham.
Jesness, C. F. (1962). The Jesness Inventory: Development and Validation. California Youth Authority Research Report No. 29, Sacramento.
Jesness, C. F. (1963). Redevelopment and Revalidation of the Jesness Inventory. California Youth Authority Research Report No. 35, Sacramento.
Johnson, A. M. (1949). Sanctions for superego lacunae of adolescents. *In* 'Searchlights on Delinquency' (Ed. K. Eissler). International Universities Press, New York.
Jones, I. H. and Frei, D. (1977). Provoked anxiety as a treatment of exhibitionism. *Br. J. Psychiat.* **131**, 295–300.
Kempe, C. H. (1971). Pediatric implications of the battered baby syndrome. *Arch. Dis. Child.* **46**, 28–37.
Knight, B. J. and West, D. J. (1975). Temporary and continuing delinquency. *Br. J. Criminol.* **15**, 43–50.
Lancet (1973). Editorial: violent parents. *Lancet* **ii**, 1017–1018.
Lewis, A. J. (1974). Psychopathic personality: a most elusive category. *Psychol. Med.* **4**, 133–140.

Lewis, N. D. C. and Yarnell, H. (1951). 'Pathological Firesetting'. Nervous and Mental Diseases Monograph, No. 83. Coolidge Foundations, New York.

Little, W. R. and Ntsekhe, V. R. (1959). Social class background of young offenders from London. *Br. J. Delinq.* **10**, 130–135.

McCord, W. and McCord, J. (1959). 'Origins of Crime'. Columbia University Press, New York.

Mays, J. B. (1954). 'Growing Up in the City'. Liverpool University Press, Liverpool.

Megargee, E. I. (1966). Under-controlled and over-controlled personality types in extreme antisocial aggression. *Psychol. Monogr.* **80**, No. 3.

Oliver, J. E. (1975). Statistics of child abuse (correspondence). *Br. Med. J.* **iii**, 99.

Oliver, J. E. and Taylor, A. (1971). Five generations of ill-treated children in one family pedigree. *Br. J. Psychiat.* **119**, 473–480.

Ounsted, C., Oppenheimer, R. and Lindsay, J. (1974). Aspects of bonding failure: the psychopathology and psychotherapeutic treatment of families of battered children. *Dev. Med. Child Neurol.* **16**, 447–456.

Palmai, G., Storey, P. B. and Briscoe, O. (1967). Social class and the young offender. *Br. J. Psychiat.* **113**, 1073–1082.

Pitcher, D. (1970). A study of subjects with an XYY sex-chromosome constitution and their families. M. Phil. Dissertation, London University.

Pitcher, D. (1971). The XYY syndrome. *Br. J. Hosp. Med.* **5**, 379–393.

Power, M. J., Benn, R. T. and Morris, J. N. (1972). Neighbourhood, school and juveniles before the courts. *Br. J. Criminol.* **12**, 111–132.

Power, M. J., Ash, P. M., Schoenberg, E. and Sirey, E. C. (1974). Delinquency and the family. *Br. J. Soc. Work.* **4**, 13–38.

Power, M. J., Alderson, M. R., Phillipson, C. M., Schoenberg, E. and Morris, J. N. (1967). Delinquent schools? *New Society* **10**, 542–543.

Ratcliffe, S. G., Stewart, A. L., Melville, M. M., Jacobs, P. A. and Keay, A. J. (1970). Chromosome studies on 3500 newborn male infants. *Lancet* **i**. 121–122.

Rich, J. (1956). Types of stealing. *Lancet* **i**, 496–498.

Robins, L. (1966). 'Deviant Children Grown Up'. Williams and Wilkins, Baltimore.

Rollin, H. R. (1969). 'The Mentally Abnormal Offender and the Law'. Pergamon, Oxford.

Rooth, F. G. (1971). Indecent exposure and exhibitionism. *Br. J. Hosp. Med.* **6**, 521–533.

Rutter, M. (1972). 'Maternal Deprivation Reassessed'. Penguin, Harmondsworth.

Rutter, M. and Madge, N. (1976). 'Cycles of Disadvantage'. Heinemann Educational, London.

Rutter, M., Tizard, J. and Whitmore, K. (1970). 'Education, Health and Behaviour'. Longman, London.

Schulsinger, F. (1972). Psychopathy: heredity and environment. *Int. J. Ment. Hlth* **1**, 190–206.

Scott, P. D. (1953). Psychiatric reports for Magistrates' Courts. *Br. J. Delinq.* **4**, 82–98.

Scott, P. D. (1960). The treatment of psychopaths. *Br. Med. J.* **i**, 1641–1646.

Scott, P. D. (1965). Delinquency. *In* 'Modern Perspectives in Child Psychiatry' (Ed. J. G. Howells). Oliver and Boyd, London.

Scott, P. D. (1973). Parents who kill their children. *Med. Sci. Law* **13**, 120–126.

Scott, P. D. (1977). Non-accidental injury in children. *Br. J. Psychiat.* **131**, 366–380.

Shields, J. (1977). Polygenic influences. *In* 'Child Psychiatry: Modern Approaches' (Eds M. Rutter and L. Hersov). Blackwell, Oxford.

Skinner, A. E. and Castle, R. L. (1969). '78 Battered Children: A Retrospective Study'. NSPCC, London.

Smith, S. M., Hanson, R. and Noble, S. (1973). Parents of battered babies: a controlled study. *Br. Med. J.* **iv**, 388–391.

Smith, S. M., Hanson, R. and Noble, S. (1974). Social aspects of the battered baby syndrome. *Br. J. Psychiat.* **125**, 568–582.

Soothill, K. L. and Pope, P. J. (1973). Arson: a twenty year cohort study. *Med. Sci. Law* **13**, 127–138.

Stott, D. H. (1966). 'Studies of Troublesome Children'. Tavistock, London.

Stott, D. H. and Wilson, D. M. (1977). The adult criminal as juvenile. *Br. J. Criminol.* **17**, 47–57.

Sullivan, C., Grant, M. Q. and Grant, J. D. (1957). The development of interpersonal maturity: applications to delinquency. *Psychiat.* **20**, 373–385.

Tidmarsh, D. and Wood, S. (1972). Psychiatric aspects of destitution. *In* 'Evaluating a Community Psychiatric Service' (Eds J. Wing and A. Hailey). Oxford University Press, Oxford.

Virkkunen, M. (1974). Alcohol as a factor precipitating aggression and conflict behaviour leading to homicide. *Br. J. Addiction* **69**, 149–154.

Wallis, C. P. and Maliphant, R. (1967). Delinquent areas in the county of London: ecological factors. *Br. J. Criminol.* **7**, 250–284.

Warren, M. Q. (1969). The case for differential treatment of delinquents. *Ann. Am. Acad. Pol. Soc. Sci.* **381**, 47–59.

Weeks, H. A. (1958). 'Youthful Offenders at Highfields'. University of Michigan Press, Ann Arbor, Michigan.

West, D. J. (1965). 'Murder Followed by Suicide'. Heinemann, London.

West, D. J. and Farrington, D. P. (1973). 'Who Becomes Delinquent?'. Heinemann Educational, London.

Whiteley, J. S. (1970). The psychopath and his treatment. *Br. J. Hosp. Med.* **3**, 263–270.

Winkler, G. E. and Kove, S. S. (1962). The implications of electroencephalographic abnormalities in homicide cases. *J. Neuropsychiat.* **3**, 322–330.

Witkin, H. A., Mednick, S. A., Schulsinger, F. *et al.* (1976). Criminality in XYY and XXY men. *Science* **193**, 547–555.

Wolfgang, M. E. (1958). 'Patterns in Criminal Homicide'. University of Philadelphia Press, Pennsylvania.

17 Psychiatry in general practice

Anthony Clare and Gaius Davies

Psychiatry is concerned with forms of illness as varied and widespread as those of physical medicine. Although there have been many therapeutic developments during the past thirty years, there are still, for example, almost as many hospital beds in Western Europe and North America occupied by psychiatric patients as by patients suffering from all other disorders. It is clear, too, that a large part of the population suffers from psychiatric disturbances which do not require in-patient treatment. Mental disorders are as diverse as the individuals who suffer from them and it is only by intentionally ignoring most of what is individual about these illnesses that a few common types can be recognized, comparable to the 'diseases' of somatic medicine.

The ways in which a human being can become mentally ill are determined by the structural and functional patterns inherent in the human organism. Diversity arises through their becoming manifest under the influence of each individual's social environment and in combination with his other inherited tendencies. Diversity, therefore, can be due to a combination of hereditary causes and to the effect of each individual's environment throughout his life upon his development and behaviour. There is always an interplay between inheritance and environment.

Likewise there is always an interplay between psychological and somatic factors in the genesis of illness. There is, therefore, no dividing line between somatic medicine and psychiatry. The human being is not composed of two discrete and independent parts, a rarified mind existing within a solid body, but is an organism all of whose subsidiary functions contribute to the highest function, his mind, which brings him not only consciousness but also an integrated behaviour in relation to his surroundings. Disturbances, transient or long-lasting, of these part-functions, such as in the sensory apparatus or in the circulatory system, will exert some effect on his state of mind. Alterations in the central nervous system represent the most obvious example of this but the endocrine organs, the autonomic nervous system and the metabolic processes are often of marked significance in the various maladjustments summed up as mental disorder.

It is also clear, however, that emotion may plan an important part in the chain of events that cause or aggravate physical diseases and the interplay between psychological and physical events may influence the outcome of many a surgical or other illness. Much of the resurgent interest in 'psychosomatic' medicine reflects the belated recognition of these clinical facts. It is plain, therefore, that psychiatric issues must be the concern of all physicians and not merely the preserve of psychiatrists. Thus the practice of psychiatry is inseparable from the general practice of medicine. Patients increasingly present with overt psychological problems to general practitioners, while a proportion of apparently physical problems prove to have a psychosocial cause in whole or in part. In addition, most people with physical illness or injuries or handicaps are either anxious or depressed to varying extents. There is no more profound base for the identification of this psychiatry than is found in primary care and every general practitioner and family physician inevitably faces these problems.

The body of this chapter is effectively divided into two sections. The first reviews the relationship between psychiatry and family medicine or general practice and concerns itself with those studies which have significantly contributed to a better understanding of the extent and the nature of psychiatric morbidity in this field and the relationship between psychiatric and physical health and social factors. The second section draws attention to those psychiatric disorders which have particular relevance to the general practitioner, but concentrates on recent developments in the organization, delivery and content of psychiatric treatment in the general practice setting.

Psychiatric morbidity in general practice

In the past, reported prevalence rates of psychiatric disorders have varied enormously. However, there is growing evidence to suggest that once methods of recording and classification of psychiatric disorders can be standardized, closer agreement on psychiatric incidence and prevalence can be obtained, even among psychiatrists from different countries.

However, cross-national studies of the psychiatric diagnosis habits of family physicians are lacking. In addition the diversity of national health care systems means that the extent to which psychiatric disorders are encountered and recognized by family physicians varies considerably. A Czechoslovakian survey, for example, found that fewer than 20% of psychiatric cases had been seen initially by district physicians (Polachek, 1972) whereas in the United Kingdom the general practitioner is the first medical contact for almost all patients who come to psychiatric clinics. From British studies of patients registered under the National Health Service, it appears that 60–70% consult their doctor in any one year and that the proportion of patients who have not consulted for two years or longer is only about 10%. These figures strongly reinforce the view that such a practitioner is well placed to monitor psychiatric disorders in the general population and to identify those serious enough to warrant treatment. Such assumptions cannot be made in health systems where services are based chiefly on private practice, since many patients will be unable or unwilling for financial reasons to seek medical aid. However, even where medical advice and treatment are freely available, selective features will continue to operate. Some relate directly to the illness. A phobic patient, for example, may be unable to make the journey to visit the doctor, a paranoid patient be unwilling to do so. Socially deteriorated schizophrenics and alcoholic patients have, as a rule, poor motivation to solicit medical advice and little perception of physicians as helping agents. For such individuals, the family physician is less likely to be the doctor of first contact than for the anxious, depressed and hypochon-driacal patients who occupy so much of his daily routine.

In the United Kingdom, the view that between one-quarter and one-third of all illnesses treated by general practitioners fall into the various categories of mental disorder has been supported by studies of industrial sickness records (Fraser, 1947). On the basis of such reports, it was computed that in the 1950s about 80 million days work were lost each year in Britain, a country of some 50 millions, through mental illness. It has been pointed out (Shepherd, 1974) that comparable findings have been reported from other studies which have taken a global look at the community care of the mentally ill. Data are presented (Table I) which are abstracted from a report of the Royal College of General Practitioners (1972) and which refer to the registered patients of an average general practitioner.

Global statistics of this kind, while affording a useful perspective, may conceal important differences between diagnostic groups. It is convenient to consider psychiatric morbidity under the two broad headings of 'major' and 'minor' disorder, while bearing in mind the shortcomings of such a dichotomy. In the former category, which includes the major organic and functional psychoses, severe mental retardation, chronic alcoholism and

Table I *Psychiatric disorders and social pathology in a hypothetical average practice population of 2500. Modified from Royal College of General Practitioners (1972). Present state and future needs of general practice*

Acute major disorders	Cases per annum
Severe depression	12
Suicide attempts	3
Completed suicide	one every three years
Chronic mental illness	55
Severe mental handicap	10
Neurotic disorders	300
Social pathology	
Chronic alcoholism (known cases)	5
Chronic alcoholism (unknown cases)	25
Juvenile delinquency	5–7
Problem families	5–10
Broken homes (one parent families with children under 15)	60

narcotic addiction, the patient manifests conspicuous abnormality and social impairment. In the latter group, comprising the neuroses, most character disorders and the milder forms of mental retardation, the patient usually remains a visible social unit. It is clear that whereas the type of morbidity cannot be equated simply with the type of medical care, the division does correspond roughly to what falls to the psychiatric specialist and general medical services respectively. The most important aspects of psychiatric research in family medicine are those dealing with the 'minor' disorders since, at the present time, the great majority of these conditions remain outside specialist care. The findings of a number of investigations carried out in Britain over the past twenty-five years are summarized in Table II.

Table II *Psychiatric referral rates from general practice and community surveys in England and Wales. From Kaeser and Cooper (1971)*

Authors	Year	Size of population	Survey period (years)	Referral rate per 10,000 at risk	Proportion of psychiatric cases referred
Bodkins et al.	1953	14,000	1	72·9	—
Hopkins	1958	1,400	3	160·6	—
Martin et al.	1957	17,250	1	29·0	5·3
Fry	1959	5,500	1	61·8	5·0
Rawnsley and Loudon	1961	18,500	9	17·7	—
Taylor and Chave	1964	40,000	3	31·5	5·4
Shepherd et al.	1966	15,000	1	71·4	5·1

Over the past fifteen years, a series of studies have been mounted by the General Practice Research Unit at the Institute of Psychiatry to study the nature and extent of psychiatric morbidity in general practice. Much of this work has been focused understandably on 'conspicuous' morbidity, defined as 'illnesses or disabilities severe enough to lead to medical consultation and conforming to recognized clinical patterns for identification by the practitioner'. In general, however, the whole range of the so-called 'minor' mental disorders is comprehensively covered by the general practitioner survey which, furthermore, has the additional advantage of helping the investigator tackle one of the more intractable problems in the sphere of mental disorder, namely the detection of a 'psychiatric' case. For operational purposes, this becomes an individual whose symptoms, behaviour, distress or discomfort leads to a medical consultation at which a psychiatric diagnosis is made by a qualified physician. Shepherd (1974) has summarized the more important findings of this programme of research.

Of some 15,000 patients at risk during a 12-month period, rather more than 2000, approximately 14% consulted their doctor at least once for a condition diagnosed as entirely or largely psychiatric in nature. The bulk of these patients would be classifiable in the International Classification of Diseases as suffering from neurotic or personality disorders which therefore take their place among the commoner conditions in practice;

No more than about 1 in 20 of the patients identified in the survey had been referred to any of the mental health facilities despite what the family practitioners freely acknowledged to be the unsatisfactory nature of the treatment which they were able to provide;

The demographic, social and diagnostic contours of this population are quite different from those provided by hospital statistics. Corresponding discrepancies are found in respect to outcome and therapeutic responses. Thus the data show that a large proportion of psychiatric morbidity encountered in family practice is made up of chronic disorders and in a 7-year follow-up study more than half the cohort exhibited a very poor outcome in terms of recurrence or chronicity;

Emotional disorders were found to be associated with a high demand for medical care. Those patients identified as suffering from psychiatric illness attended more frequently and exhibited higher rates of general morbidity and more categories of illness per head than the remainder of patients consulting their doctors.

Since the publication of these findings, similar findings have been furnished by workers as far apart as Australia (Stoller and Krupinski, 1969) and Austria (Strotzka, 1969).

Neuroses form a much larger proportion of psychiatric morbidity in family practice than in hospital psychiatric practice. Neuroses constituted 63% and character disorders 4% of the psychiatric disorders seen by Shepherd and his colleagues (1966) in their study of 46 London general practices. Corresponding figures for all out-patients at the Maudsley Hospital, London, a psychiatric hospital, were 40% and 37% and for in-patients 29% and 26% respectively. Only a small proportion of neurosis is dealt with by psychiatrists and an even smaller proportion by in-patient services. By contrast the psychoses formed 4% of the total psychiatric morbidity in the survey by Shepherd and his colleagues compared with 25% of the Maudsley Hospital out-patient cases and 72% of first admissions to mental hospitals in England and Wales in 1957 (Marks, 1973).

There is evidence, however, that not all those patients who suffer from psychiatric illness and who attend their general practitioners are actually detected. Of 200 patients attending a London general practitioner, 93 were clinically psychiatrically ill, yet one-third of these were unkown to the practitioner until their responses to a questionnaire were examined (Goldberg and Blackwell, 1970). Most of the psychiatric problems were classified as 'minor affective illnesses'. At six-months follow-up, two-thirds of these problems had remitted. The bulk of the morbidity in this practice was thus short-lived. Cooper (1972), in a study of eight general practices in London, found that anxiety and depression accounted for 80% of chronic neuroses. Whereas anxiety neurosis occurred to a comparable extent in either sex, two-thirds of those with depressive neurosis were women. Specific neurotic problems, such as phobias, obsessions and hypochondriasis, were found in only 2·8% of cases. Non-specific anxiety states and depressive neuroses are less easy to differentiate in a general practice sample than in a sample of psychiatric out-patients or in-patients.

Not enough is known about the normal course and outcome of the neuroses and related non-psychotic disorders. One extensive review of the subject (Greer and Cawley, 1966) concluded that 'it is not possible to make legitimate generalisations about the prognosis of neurotic disorders from the published data'. Longitudinal studies of psychiatric illness in general practice populations suggest that the previous duration of illness is the most important prognostic factor for the neuroses and that a rough dichotomy can be established between chronic disorders of poor prognosis on the one hand and short-term situational reactions on the other.

Psychiatric and physical morbidity

Patients with psychiatric disorder not only consult more frequently and maintain higher levels of demand for medical care than the average, they also present more physical symptoms and are more often referred to medical and surgical departments. Indeed, over the short-term many psychiatric illnesses appear to be misdiagnosed because of their somatic presentation. It may of course be argued that the degree of physical morbidity of the neurotic patient is equivalent to that of non-psychiatric patients but that the latter tend to complain more and consult more frequently. Conversely, patients who habitually consult their doctors may well be labelled 'neurotic' whatever the true nature of their complaints.

To illuminate the positive correlation between physical and psychiatric morbidity, Eastwood (1970) embarked upon an extensive study as part of a health screening survey in general practice. Those invited to participate comprised one-half randomly selected of all patients aged 40–65 years registered with a large group-practice. Of a possible 2000 patients, just over two-thirds took part. Each patient underwent a battery of tests, including morphological measurements, blood pressure readings, ventilatory function tests, electrocardiogram and a number of blood and urine tests. In addition, a questionnaire including 20 items selected from the Cornell Medical Index was completed by each patient. Two weeks later, the patient was physically examined by the family physician who by this time had received a report of the test results. At their first attendance, patients whose questionnaire scores suggested a possible psychological disturbance were given a standardized psychiatric interview: as a result, 124 (8·2%) were classified as confirmed psychiatric cases. A control group, matched with these 124 patients by age, sex, marital status and social class, was drawn from among those patients whose questionnaire responses gave no indication of mental disturbance; any 'false negatives' were excluded at the interview stage.

When these two matched groups were compared in respect of the screening survey findings, the index group proved to have a significant excess of major physical disease. Physical disorders appeared to 'cluster' together in some individuals and this occurred to a significantly greater extent in the psychiatric group. Thus 17% of the psychiatric group had had two major plus several minor physical conditions compared with only 2·4% of the controls. These findings agree with those of Hinkle and his colleagues (Hinkle and Wolff, 1957; Hinkle et al., 1958) who found in a variety of ethnic and socio-economic groups that members of these adult populations exhibited differences in their general susceptibility to illness of all types so that some persons experienced a greater number of illnesses per unit time than others. On average, 25% of the members of these populations had experienced 50% of the episodes of illness over a 20-year period whereas a further 25% had suffered less than 10% of the episodes.

As Eastwood and Trevelyan (1972) observe, the idea that individuals have a generalized psychophysical propensity to disease appears to be a valuable alternative model to that which seeks only specific single cause and effect relationships. The notion of multiple aetiology in disease and multiple responses by man to agents threatening his health reflects a greater acceptance of the realities of the ecology of ill-health. It is also a notion which general practitioners, regularly confronted by patients in whom psychological and physical disturbances appear inextricably intermingled, can readily comprehend.

Social factors and psychiatric morbidity

The social component of psychiatric disorders in family practice is as important as their clinical features and it is necessary to employ a socio-medical framework to classify and describe them (Sylph *et al.*, 1969; Fitzgerald, 1970; Cooper, 1972). In one study of the social functioning and psychiatric status of 20 general practice patients defined as 'chronic neurotics' and compared with those of a matched control group, a signifi-cant correlation was found between social difficulties and neurotic illness (Sylph *et al.*, 1969). The neurotic patients tended to have limited or conflict-ridden relationships with neighbours, relatives and workmates, an excess of problems with spouses and children and a significantly less satisfactory adjustment to their life situation, as measured by ratings of satisfaction and dissatisfaction with several of its important aspects such as housing, occupation and social role. As Bloom (1975) among others has pointed out, there is an extensive sociological literature testifying to a positive association between certain global variables, such as social class, and mental illness, a literature which has been ably summarized by Dohrenwend and Dohrenwend (1969, 1974). More recently, Brown and his colleagues have suggested that the experience of depression may be associated with major stressful life occurrences (Brown et al., 1975). Cooper and Sylph (1973) have shown that new cases of neurotic illness in general practice are distinguished from controls by a marked excess of life events immediately preceding onset. The findings of these British studies broadly agree with those on the social role-performance of depressed women reported by an American research group (Weissman and Paykel, 1974).

While an association between social status and prevalence of psy-chiatric disturbance has often been reported, little has been established about aetiology or its significance for social class differences (Harris, 1976). In one survey of a random sample of women living in South London, a large class difference in the prevalence of depression was found not to be primarily associated with greater frequency of life events and difficulties but more to protective factors affecting individual vulner-ability (see Chapter 12) (Brown et al., 1975). Why certain factors tend to be protective remains unclear and requires further research.

Aspects of specific psychiatric disorders in general practice

The psychoses include the organic psychoses, schizophrenia and related paranoid states and manic-depression. Such disorders are encountered infrequently but usually occasion concern as a result of the associated social disturbances and florid clinical picture and represent about 4% of the overall psychiatric morbidity in general practice. Those mental disorders that occur in the elderly are comprised of the organic dementias and the functional disorders, of which the most common is depression.

There is now substantial evidence that large numbers of elderly people in the community do suffer from mental illness of a degree which in many instances matches the clinical severity of those admitted to hospitals or institutions. Psychogeriatric disorders (see Chapter 14) are often unrecognized by the patient's family physicians and are not referred to mental health and welfare services (Harwin, 1973). As the number of those aged 65 and over is predicted to increase considerably, the need to establish a means of identifying those elderly patients whose psychiatric disorders are often unrecognized or untreated becomes a matter of some importance. It has been suggested that ancillary medical personnel such as home nurses could be used specifically to identify psychiatric disorder among the elderly. In one practice survey in which a group of home nurses were asked to assess the mental state of elderly patients with physical illness living at home, a substantial majority of patients, subsequently confirmed by specialized psychiatric examination, were successfully identified by the nurses (Harwin, 1973). Few severe cases were missed. Such results encourage the prospects of paramedical staff being employed in this fashion. However, it is probably necessary that they should receive more specialized training if their efficiency in identification is to be increased. In the study mentioned, the nurses initiated very little in the way of medico-social action except in instances of acute social distress or clinical crises, partly because they appeared to accept psychiatric symptoms as being an understandable reaction to social or physical adversity or else an inevitable accompaniment of old age for which there is little hope of therapeutic intervention.

Under the heading of schizophrenia are included those illnesses which are characterized from the outset by a fundamental disturbance of the personality involving its most basic functions and which give the normal person his feeling of uniqueness, self-direction and individuality. A detailed consideration of the schizophrenia syndrome is presented in Chapter 11 but aspects particularly apposite to general practice will be discussed here.

Specialized treatment in a psychiatric hospital or clinic is usually necessary at some stage in the disorder and must be decided chiefly by the social risks and the severity. The major phenothiazines—chlorpromazine, promazine and trifluoperazine—and the butyrophenones, of which haloperidol is the main example, are often beneficial during the acute stage of a schizophrenic illness. However, their too early and enthusiastic use may obscure rather than clarify the clinical picture and there is much to be said for the family physician, suspicious of a schizophrenic illness, withholding medication pending a consultant opinion or the development of unequivocal schizophrenic symptoms in the setting of clear consciousness and physical health.

Chlorpromazine is still the drug of choice, but for those patients who show marked volitional disturbances and intense delusional activity trifluoperazine and related phenothiazine derivatives may be more effective. The value of maintaining patients on phenothiazines after they have made a symptomatic recovery has for some time been questioned although more evidence in favour of such an approach has been provided by a number of studies (Pasamanick et al., 1964; Leff and Wing, 1971). The use of long-acting phenothiazines in the maintenance treatment of schizophrenic patients, who for one reason or another do not take oral medication and relapse, is now a well established feature of this condition. Such drugs have enabled many patients to return to and be maintained in the community. The duration of such maintenance therapy is of importance to the family physician who often is taxed by the task of supervising treatment. The placebo-controlled, double-blind trial conducted by Hirsch and his colleagues (1973) suggested that some patients might require treatment indefinitely, yet a third of the comparable population in this trial remained out of hospital while receiving placebo alone.

The transfer of care from the hospital service to the patient's relatives and the community services, intrinsic to maintenance-treatment programmes, poses problems for the patient's family and physician. A number of studies (Stevens, 1972; Creer and Wing, 1974) have shown that the burden shouldered by relatives can be heavy, not least because many patients, while losing the symptoms exhibited in hospital, can show other symptoms when at home, especially a passivity and absence of initiative which render their lives rigid and uniform. Long-acting phenothiazines in common with the short-acting variety, can produce unpleasant side-effects, particularly extrapyramidal reactions, and often require concomitant corrective administration of anti-Parkinsonian drugs. For these reasons, it is important that patients maintained on long-acting drugs should be carefully monitored. This may be done by the general practitioner himself or by special clinics run by district or community nurses under the supervision of hospital-based psychiatrists or general practitioners (Shepherd and Watt, 1974).

Manic-depressive psychosis is characterized by profound disturbances of affect (i.e. feelings and emotions). The illness usually appears unprovoked but may occasionally follow some stress. The psychosis has a strong tendency to recur, attacks may be repetitious, alternating and cyclical with depression and elation (see Chapter 12). Severe affective psychosis whether of a manic or depressive nature almost certainly will require the diagnostic and treatment resources of specialized psychiatric services. However, after specialist out- or in-patient treatment the general practitioner is often involved in prophylactic maintenance treatment utilizing antidepressant drugs or lithium, and this necessitates that he is carefully informed concerning the side-effects and toxic effects which may be anticipated. Given the need to monitor the serum levels of lithium in patients maintained on the drug, it is mandatory that such patients be under the supervision of a psychiatric clinic.

It is often thought convenient to differentiate so-called 'endogenous' cases of affective disorder from psychogenic or reactive cases. However, it is more likely that depressive illnesses are best regarded as continua extending between the classical psychotic archetype, manic-depressive psychosis, and the neurotic archetype, neurotic depression. On such a basis there is not a great deal of purpose, apart from administrative convenience, in trying to diagnose affective disorder from psychogenic depression, anxiety neurosis or involutional melancholia; these can quite properly be seen as subdivisions of affective disorder in which the age of onset, reactivity, severity or chronicity is being stressed. The family physician, for the most part, sees patients who do not present with the classical picture of psychotic or neurotic depression but with a mixture of depressive and anxiety symptoms which vary in severity.

Affective disorders carry a high risk of suicide and suicidal behaviour. Official statistics and epidemiological studies indicate those individuals in the general population who are most at risk and hence provide possible clues to causes and prevention (see Chapter 12). The role of the family physician is clearly important in view of the relationship between overdoses and the prescription of certain types of drugs. One study of 100 suicides (Barraclough *et al.*, 1974) found that 40% had visited their general practitioner in the week before they died. Over 70% had done so in the previous three months. The doctor apparently recognized in most cases that the patient was psychologically disturbed because he prescribed tranquillizers or barbiturates to approximately 80% of them. However, the patient's depression was not usually recognized for relatively few were given antidepressant drugs and then mostly in deficient doses. Forty-five per cent died from barbiturate poisoning and 15 of the 17 patients categorized in this study as 'impulsive' killed themselves with barbiturates recently prescribed by their general practitioners. It has been emphasized that a substantial proportion of suicides could be prevented if family doctors were as well trained in their recognition and management of depression and of other psychiatric conditions associated with high rates of suicide as they are in the diagnosis and treatment of basic medical conditions (Sainsbury, 1973).

The non-psychotic psychiatric disorders constitute the bulk of psychiatric morbidity which presents in general practice. These disorders are composed largely of minor affective illness in which there is often an inextricable intermingling of depression, anxiety and somatic symptoms. There is often no clear distinction between neuroses and personality disorder as seen in the general practice setting and the family doctor will often see anxiety states, various phobic, obsessional and hysterical illnesses as well as a variety of abnormal illness behaviour which ranges from hypochondriasis to frank malingering (see Chapter 7).

Studies of the natural history of neurotic disorders presenting in family practice are relatively few. One study of acute 'mild affective disorder' reported a very good prognosis (Goldberg and Blackwell, 1970), two-thirds of the patients having remitted by six-month follow-up. However, the prognosis in more chronic cases is less satisfactory and there is evidence that psychiatric patients in general practice whose symptoms have not remitted by the end of one year tend to have illnesses which continue for many years (Kedward, 1968). Fry (1960) reported that 27% of the males and 43% of the females in his practice diagnosed as suffering from neurotic disorders required further treatment for their symptoms over a three-year follow-up period. A seven-year follow-up (Cooper et al., 1969) confirmed the more favourable outcome for men. The patterns of consultation and diagnosis over the years suggested a varying prognosis with a minority of short-term cases of good outcome and a majority of chronic or recurrent cases. These authors speculated that the former group was composed largely of 'situational reactions' and the latter of constitutionally vulnerable individuals.

The general practitioner along with other sources of primary care has an increasing role to play in the treatment of alcohol dependence (Cartwright et al., 1975). The average family practitioner in the United Kingdom can be expected to know of five chronic alcoholics in his practice (see Table I), but Wilkins (1974), a Manchester based general practitioner, using a questionnaire designed to reveal patients at risk to alcoholism, showed that the average practitioner misses four times as many alcoholics as he detects, and demonstrated the alcohol prevalence rate in the practice population aged between 15 and 65 to be 18·2 per 1000. General practitioners can play a major part in assessment and long-term support of alcoholics (Acres, 1977), and Pollak (1974) has shown how alcoholic clinics can work effectively from a general practice base.

The role of the general practitioner in the treatment of drug dependence is more complex as the presenting problem is often one of multiple drug taking. In the past in the United Kingdom a small number of unscrupulous or misguided general practitioners helped to create an illicit market of opiates and amphetamines, and consequently since 1968 maintenance prescribing of opiates and cocaine to addicts has been restricted to Home Office licensed doctors who are usually psychiatrists specializing in drug dependence. Although the general practitioner is able to offer the addict the opportunities of a long-term therapeutic relationship, he is also one of the major sources of misused drugs, in particular barbiturates (Edwards, 1977).

As has been pointed out in Chapters 5 and 6 the role of the family practitioner with regard to the psychiatric disturbances of childhood and mental handicap heavily emphasizes his status as the link between the individual patient, his family and the health, education and social services. Given his position, he is well placed to record the diagnosis, monitor progress and ensure the provision of adequate special medical and social services care. The severely mentally handicapped inevitably require institutional care but the family physician's role in advising and supporting families caring for mildly subnormal children and adults can be crucially important, particularly his role as coordinator of the various specialist services and skills, medical, educational and social, available to such families.

Strategies of treatment

Broadly speaking there are three principal modes of treatment open to the general practitioner: (a) the psychological (including behavioural), (b) those procedures aimed at modifying directly the patient's social environment and (c) the pharmacological. Each is destined to occupy an indispensable role in future programmes of primary health care. However, it is worth recalling the judgement of a World Health Organization report on this topic:

> Transcending in importance these three broad methods of treatment, there are certain general needs, such as a tolerant attitude, dependability, continuity, an interest that allows a doctor to take even minor disorders seriously, and attention to the needs of close relatives of the patient.
>
> (World Health Organization, 1961)

The time consuming nature of many psychiatric problems makes it difficult for the general practitioner to take an active role in treatment. The average practitioner in Britain for example is consulted two to four times per year for each patient on his list; a doctor with 2500 patients under his care might provide between 5000 and 10,000 consultations for all medical problems annually. It is therefore not surprising to find that the average consultation time in general practice is not much more than five minutes and rarely over ten (Shepherd *et al.*, 1966). The attitudes of family physicians to psychiatric patients vary from intense personal interest to active dislike. In the London general practice survey, the practitioners' attitudes were found generally to reflect a tolerant indifference although there were a number of exceptions:

> One was altogether averse to psychiatry, and blamed psychiatrists for encouraging neurotic patients to avoid their responsibilities; the second states that the neurotic patients on his list were so few and so easily identifiable as to render any systematic study unnecessary; the third commented simply that all neurotic patients were ungrateful and that there was nothing that could be done for them.   (Shepherd *et al.*, 1966)

All observers agreed that there are great variations of attitude to psychiatric and sociomedical problems among general practitioners. Younger doctors, those more recently qualified and those expressing a special interest recognize more psychiatric cases (Rawnsley and Loudon, 1962). On the whole, practitioners feel confident in their ability to recognize serious psychiatric disturbances but less able to relate them to causal or precipitating factors (Shepherd *et al.*, 1966). Although many regard the treatment of neuroses as their business, they tend to feel inadequately trained. It is worth noting that in one study a majority of doctors reported that they found psychiatric work more irksome than other aspects of practice and were apprehensive of any increase in the number of chronic patients under their care (Rawnsley and Loudon, 1962).

Psychological methods of treatment include psychotherapy and behavioural techniques. Implementation of formal methods of psychotherapy within the general practice situation has proven difficult and has led to a number of attempted adaptations. Perhaps the strongest single influence in Western Europe has been that advocated most forcefully by Balint and developed by a number of his colleagues (Balint, 1957; Balint and Norell, 1973). In his book, 'The Doctor, his Patient and the Illness', a new approach to the patient seen in general practice was described. Taking any patient that a general practitioner might wish to discuss, Balint's technique was to show the relevance of psychological understanding to practical management. The book, like subsequent publications, was the practical outcome of regular meetings between a group of interested practitioners with Balint acting as the leader of the 'research seminars'. The aim was to study the public counter-transference of the doctors—those feelings and attitudes towards their patients which they were willing to discuss freely, rather than their private counter-transferences. Balint hoped this might achieve definite but limited changes in the doctor's personality. He sought to show that the drug most often prescribed was the doctor himself and that careful attention should be paid to how this was done.

Originally, Balint advocated the use of a long interview of some 40 minutes. The general practitioner was encouraged to listen and observe so that the meaning of a symptom pattern might be accurately assessed. A more useful therapeutic relationship was thus expected to develop, but a major handicap for most practitioners was the lack of adequate time. In the United Kingdom, the time available in group practices with appointment systems is barely six minutes per patient per consultation. The most recent development from the Balint seminars (Balint and Norell, 1973) faces this fact realistically and offers the 'flash technique' as a possible answer. By the flash is meant an experience—within the brief interview—of an intuitive understanding by the patient and doctor (either separately or together) of the meaning for the patient of his symptoms. This may occur within a framework of a more traditional diagnostic formulation, but lead to insight, and sometimes to an interpretation which helps both patient and doctor. Focal psychotherapy has also been part of the Balint approach. The doctor, by a process of 'selective attention and neglect' may guide his patient to look at those areas where help is required.

Since Balint's death in 1971 his influence has inspired a movement which grows internationally and begins to make inroads into the whole of medicine (Hopkins, 1976). It is more difficult to assess the influence of his work specifically in the general practice situation in the United Kingdom. It has certainly enlightened and informed the teaching of general practice, and is part of that phenomenon of the last twenty years whereby general practitioners have identified and defined their professional role as general specialists. At present less than 1% of British general practitioners are trained in the Balint method compared with 15% of Dutch practitioners and, although not of proven therapeutic effectiveness, Balint training has been demonstrated to increase sensitivity (Steel, 1976). At its best it allows the practitioner to maintain a balanced and insightful approach to the whole person whether he presents with psychiatric or somatic symptoms, or both; at its worst it leads to sloppy psychologizing and seeks to identify causal mechanisms of even physical disease as disturbance in the person's psychodynamic system.

As a response to the peculiar circumstances of the general practice interview Balint's flash technique has its equivalents in the single long interview and the so-called 'twenty minute hour' practised in the United States. A closely related line of development has been the application to family practice of the theories of transactional analysis (Browne and Freeling, 1967). The tendency for the family physician to become a specialized psychotherapist is not always easy to avoid, and in a number of countries, such as the Federal Republic of Germany, family physicians are able to take a diploma in psychotherapy. However, it tends to be a small, often somewhat atypical group of practitioners who use psychodynamic techniques and many have an atypical patient clientele. There is little evidence as yet that such methods are permeating the main body of clinical practice, and indeed Sir Denis Hill, in an important essay, has cautioned the general practitioner: 'least of all, I think should he aspire to be a psychotherapist although he needs to share with all those in the caring professions a common psychological understanding' (Hill, 1969). Commenting on the present position of psychotherapy *vis-à-vis* family medicine, a World Health Organization Working Group on psychiatry and primary health care observed:

> The drift of a small number of general practitioners into psychotherapy, as into other specialities, is unavoidable, and relatively unimportant. The crucial point is that the great majority of general practitioners, with no special interest in psychotherapy, should be competent to understand and tolerate their patients' behaviour, even when markedly deviant; and that they should be prepared to give sympathy, advice and reassurance in all cases. The extent to which individual practitioners fulfill these requirements varies enormously, and must be considered a product of personality, training and conditions of service. The most important need appears to be increased attention to behavioural studies in both undergraduate and postgraduate education.   (World Health Organization, 1973)

The common mixed affective disorders can impose considerable emotional demands on the family physician and the essential requisites for effective management can prove elusive. At one extreme, the family physician may be expected to share the patient's intense distress and deal with intractable life situations. At the other he may have to endure displays of hostility and irritability or deal with what appears to be a succession of trivial or incomprehensible complaints. Each type of confrontation has the potential to engender attitudes of helplessness, despair or exasperation. However, the majority of non-psychotic psychiatric disorders can be effectively treated by discusssion, reassurance and attention to environmental factors. In this regard, it is relevant that a recent study of the effects of maintenance antidepressant drug treatment and psychotherapy on symptoms of depression (Paykel *et al.*, 1975) showed that psychotherapy produced no significant advantages over simple support and supervision in terms of symptomatic improvement although it did improve ratings of social adjustment. Formal psychotherapy in general practice, however, is precluded by lack of time and training. Psychodynamic interpretations may be invalid, detrimental or too painful for the patient to tolerate and are best given by those who have received some formal training in this field. Nevertheless, selection of a few cases by practitioners for special interviews, particularly in the context of general discussions with other interested colleagues, can be instructive and rewarding for the family physician concerned. The term 'psychotherapy', however, is ill-defined and is currently applied not merely to formal methods of psychodynamically based intervention but to the provision of support and reassurance through listening, advising and explaining. The personality and attitudes of the practitioner are powerful influences in treatment and an optimistic manner about the outcome of the patient's illness helps generate relief.

The development of specialized behavioural techniques has been the major advance in the management of the more severe and lasting forms of anxiety, phobias and obsessional states (Marks, 1974). These techniques include desensitization, modelling and flooding and are described at length in Chapter 22. Such procedures are most effective in the relatively circumscribed and severe neurotic disorders seen in psychiatric out-patient departments and mental hospital wards but Rachman and Philips (1954) have argued that they have a certain place in general practice. The chronic anxiety state, commonly seen in general practice, is less amenable to such psychological techniques. Social anxieties have been modified using training in social skills (McFall and Lillesand, 1971), but as Marks (1974) points out, most work in this area has been uncontrolled and the rather complex therapeutic techniques required are still evolving. Whether such techniques should be reserved for psychiatrists and clinical psychologists or should be extended to family physicians, social workers, community nurses and health visitors, remains to be determined.

The strong association between the clinical symptoms of neurotic disorders in general practice and various problems of social adjustment referred to earlier underlines the need for attention to be directed at the social aspects of these disorders in treatment. A number of studies of collaboration between general practitioners and social workers have consistently advocated the need for closer liaison between the general medical, psychiatrists and social services (Collins, 1965; Goldberg and Neill, 1973; Forman and Fairbairn, 1968). Collins, for instance, analysed 319 situations dealt with over the course of a year in a four doctor Cardiff practice with 9000 patients. She found that of all consultations, 42% needed a specialist social worker, 33% a generic social worker and 20% only practical help. Although the Seebohm Report recommended in 1968 that collaboration between social worker and general practice was to be encouraged, it also removed the specialist social worker which appears to be so essential in the psychiatric area. Cooper (1971) has proposed four functions of the social worker in general practice: (1) assessor of social work difficulties; (2) as links and coordinators with other agencies; (3) as casework therapist; and perhaps (4) sponsoring co-operation with medical care.

General practitioners have only slowly taken up a social work contribution in the primary health care team, and to date there has been little in the way of evaluation. However, one evaluative study (Cooper *et al.*, 1975) has assessed the possible therapeutic value of attaching a social worker to a metropolitan group practice in London in the management of chronic neurotic illness. The psychiatric and social status of a group of patients before treatment and after one year was compared with a control group treated more conventionally over the same period. The results indicate that the experimental service conferred significant benefit on the patient population.

> Patients in both the experimental and control groups of this study received medication from their own doctors as usual and could be referred to specialist agencies in the normal way. In the event, only 5·4% of the experimental patients were referred to the psychiatric services during the year compared with 18·5% of the control patients. Similarly, only 30% of the experimental patients were in touch with any outside social agency as against 40% of the controls. Comparison of general practitioner treatment for the two groups was confined to their prescribing of psychotropic drugs and indicates that the experimental group had received less medication of this kind than the control group. The overall changes in psychiatric state and social adjustment during the follow up period show that while the initial clinical and social scores of the two groups were closely similar, those of the experimental group fell significantly more during the follow up year.

There have been very few controlled attempts to evaluate medico-social intervention in the community and none to have demonstrated benefit, however small, to so notoriously resistant a group of patients as those suffering from chronic neurotic disorders (Segal, 1972; Fischer, 1973; Goldberg, 1973). For these reasons alone, the results of the investigation by Cooper and his colleagues carry some general implications which extend well beyond the findings themselves, limited as they are by the extent of the follow-up (Cooper *et al.*, 1975). As the authors themselves point out, the most significant conclusion may well be 'the demonstration that evaluative research in the mental health field can be carried out in an extramural setting'. Such studies also touch on the question of the psychiatrist's contribution to the primary health care team. With the growth of health centres and large group practices, it is to be expected that there will be a growing participation in primary health care by both psychiatrists and psychiatric nurses.

For psychosocial disorders to be managed effectively, not merely the social worker but the health visitor and district nurses must play an active role alongside the general practitioner (Brook and Cooper, 1975). There appear to be strong arguments in favour of such a development in which the primary health care team would come to be regarded more and more as the keystone of community psychiatry (World Health Organization,

1973). However, the discovery of a significant amount of social difficulties among neurotic patients in general practice does not inevitably imply that social work intervention should be mobilized in every case. Some social problems appear intractable, others beyond the resources of society to deal with. At the present time, too little is known about how those problems which could be alleviated might be identified. 'Attractive as the concept of multidisciplinary work at the primary health care level might be', observes a recent *Lancet* editorial, 'it still requires more painstaking inquiry and evaluation if it is to develop into something more substantial than a pious exhortation at the national level' (*Lancet*, 1975).

Psychotropic drugs currently account for just under one in five of all prescriptions dispensed by chemists under the National Health Service in Britain. These prescriptions, issued by general practitioners, represent about 3000 million tablets or capsules, about 60 million every week. Overall from 1961 to 1971 there was a 48·8% increase in prescriptions for these drugs. Analysis shows that 41% of psychotropic drugs dispensed in 1971 were hypnotics, 38% tranquillizers, 15% antidepressants and 6% appetite suppressants or stimulants (Parish, 1973; Parish *et al.*, 1976). Over one in three of all psychotropic drugs prescriptions dispensed by National Health Service pharmacists in England and Wales in 1971 were for chlordiazepoxide ('Librium'), diazepam ('Valium') or nitrazepam ('Mogadon').

The phenomenal increase in the prescribing of hypnotics and the minor tranquillizers is not easy to explain. Parish (1971) collected some relevant data from a retrospective analysis of the medical records of 48 general practitioners. The benzodiazepines were found to be the drugs of choice for 'anxiety neurosis', 'neurotic depression' and 'tension headaches' and to figure prominently in the treatment of 'affective psychosis', 'nervous dyspepsia' and 'insomnia'. Such a wide spectrum of morbidity suggests that these drugs are being prescribed less for the treatment of specific conditions than as the favoured form of medication for the alleviation of anxiety in general. It also needs to be noted that the benzodiazepines can induce dependence, a hazard of some importance if they are misused.

A more disturbing feature of Parish's study is that although a wide range of powerful psychotropic drugs is available many practitioners did not use them in the most effective way. Choice of drugs was often haphazard and both dose and length of treatment inadequate. In two-thirds of the cases, psychotropic drugs were given for less than a month. There was no contact between doctor and patient in almost a quarter of the cases. The doctors' notes showed no reference to quantity prescribed and 43% contained no entry of the strength of the preparation used.

If Watts' (1966) estimate that in 20 years he has seen 10% of his practice present with depressive illness is anything to go by it is not surprising that there is wide use in general practice of potent antidepressant medication, in particular tricyclic drugs and monoamine oxidase inhibitors. Both these classes of drugs have profound side-effects (see Chapter 9) and produce serious consequences when taken in overdose. The effective daily therapeutic antidepressant doses are often fairly high and a fortnight's supply given to a patient with suicidal ambivalence may not always be sound clinical judgement, and may indeed encourage some practitioners to prescribe smaller 'safer' amounts, but in essentially non-therapeutic doses. Clearly, adequate therapeutic doses given in non-lethal amounts necessitate regular short spaced appointments at the practice, but a study in Manchester of 73 patients with new episodes of depressive illness makes it clear that patients do not always receive the best treatment available (Johnson, 1973). This study showed that the much-prized doctor–patient relationship was not effectively used: there was a low consultation rate, over half the patients only seeing their practitioner on one occasion in the first six weeks. Medication was neither adequately prescribed, but in the absence of adequate support, nor was it regularly taken. Johnson is very critical of the poor use of drugs and stresses the need for a supportive role by the practitioner before chemotherapy can be effective.

It is worth noting that minor emotional illnesses are notoriously subject to suggestion or reassurance and responsive to change. They are thus sensitive to placebo and display a high rate of spontaneous remission. Patients in general practice with minor emotional states display a placebo response of around 50% in various drug studies compared to active drug response rates of about 75% (Wheatley, 1972). Blackwell points out that it is more than likely that the busy general practitioner who makes a habit of ending each interview with a prescription will be gratified and rewarded by the response that many patients report. 'Too often neither the patient nor the doctor pauses to examine the role played by inquiry, discussion and reassurance' (Blackwell, 1973).

Psychiatric referral from general practice

In the United Kingdom, the great majority of patients seen by psychiatric specialists are referred by their general practitioners. However, it is now widely accepted that the general practitioner sends to psychiatrists only a small proportion of the patients whom he himself regards as disturbed. Shepherd and his colleagues (1966) found that only 5·1% of patients regarded by their general practitioners as psychiatrically disturbed were referred and confirmation of referral figures ranging between 5 and 10% has come from a number of other studies in Great Britain (Rawnsley and

Loudon, 1962; Kessel, 1960) and from other European countries (Strotzka *et al.*, 1969; Bentsen, 1970; Øgar, 1972), a referral rate similar to that for specialist referral of physical illnesses.

Depending on the existing medical service structure, the bulk of such referrals may be made to psychiatrists based at hospitals or polyclinics, to private practice specialists, or to community mental health services. The evidence is still extremely limited about which cases family physicians refer in terms of diagnostic categories. Indeed, one group of researchers (Mowbray *et al.*, 1961) found that patients were referred less on the basis of a diagnostic appraisal than because of abnormalities of conduct, the existence of social problems and inappropriate responses to medical treatment. Both Watts (1958) and Shepherd and his colleagues (1966) found that more patients with psychosis than with neurosis were referred, 25% with psychosis compared with 4·8% with neurosis and 0·6% for psychosomatic problems. Most studies seem to agree that more younger patients are referred than older but there is conflicting evidence concerning sex differences and concerning the relative proportions of new and chronic cases referred. Older physicians refer more cases than younger ones (Shepherd *et al.*, 1966; Mowbray *et al.*, 1961) while younger physicians recognize more psychiatric problems for what they are (Rawnsley and Loudon, 1962; Mowbray *et al.*, 1961). Shepherd and his colleagues found that 'high reporting' practices referred 4·8% of cases compared with a rate of 5·7% for 'low reporting' practices ('high reporting' practices recognize more psychiatric morbidity in their practices).

How useful is psychiatric referral? A valid comparison of the results of care by the psychiatrist and the GP is extremely difficult to mount. In one single-handed study based on a semi-rural group practice referring patients to a provincial mental hospital and its clinics in peripheral general hospitals (G. Davies, 1976 personal communication) 108 patients were randomly divided into two groups. Each group contained similar psychiatric patients with predominantly affective disorders, neurotic illnesses and personality disorders and a minority of psychotic patients. They were assessed before treatment and at six months and one year. At one year and six months there was no significant difference in the numbers who had improved. The main result—that some 70% of both groups showed a good outcome at one year—is strikingly similar to the results of follow-up studies of neurotic disorders based on general practice and hospital populations.

To date, attempts to relate physicians' diagnostic and referral habits to their personal characteristics have had mixed results. One small study of a group of Scottish physicians (Mowbray *et al.*, 1961) suggested that a physician's age, length of time in practice, size of practice and interest in psychiatry all influence his classification of problems as psychiatric but other studies have failed to confirm all but the last of these as relevant factors.

A number of general hospital studies have been undertaken on communication between family physicians and hospital (King Edward's Hospital Fund, 1963; De Alarcón and Hodson, 1964). Though little attention has been paid to the special problems of psychiatric referral, one study of referrals to an emergency clinic (Birley and Heine, 1966) found that few of the doctors' referral letters contained information about the family or social setting, fewer than half gave details of medication prescribed and most did not make it clear whether or not the family physicians wanted the hospital to take over clinical responsibility. The authors concluded that the referral letters were an ineffective means of communicating either the facts about the patient or the practitioner's expectations of the hospital service. It is worth emphasizing that such a failure of communication need not be ascribed simply to neglect or disinterest. In the study in question it frequently transpired that the family physician had taken considerable pains over the case and knew a great deal which he had not set down. The investigators speculated that inadequate letters represented a form of withdrawal by the practitioner, perhaps occasioned by his unsureness of his diagnosis and treatment and a consequent fear of being criticized by the hospital. On the other hand, the family physician may be seriously dissatisfied with his communication or lack of communication with the hospital-based psychiatrist. In a study of practitioners who used the services of the Maudsley Hospital, it was found that whilst the clinical service was satisfactory, practitioners complained that they were often unable to speak with the hospital doctor in clinical charge of the patient. When offered a choice of either a short discharge letter, a detailed summary or a long letter, the practitioners chose the fairly detailed, but not over-inclusive, long letter (Davies and Noble, 1966). In another survey of practitioners in a London borough (Harwin et al., 1970), enquiry was made at interview about their experience of the local psychiatric service. Complaints were frequent on two topics, unnecessary domiciliary visits by the psychiatrists as a means of arranging hospital admission and inadequate after-care supervision of discharged mental hospital patients.

In a wide-ranging review of referral to specialist psychiatric services, Kaeser and Cooper (1971) emphasize the difficulties inherent in any attempt to determine the factors at work. Most physicians believe that personal referral, from one colleague to another, is preferable. It may be that the generally poor standard of communication and co-operation between family physicians and psychiatrists in modern urban societies can be attributed largely to their lack of direct professional contact. On the other hand, it is accepted that many more severely disturbed patients require the full resources of an organized psychiatric service. Clearly the question of how personal communication with the family physician can be established and maintained by hospital-based psychiatrists is a vital one for the future of the mental health services.

Crisis intervention and the general practitioner

Examples of crises where the general practitioner may be called to help are: bereavement reactions, or family and community disasters; battering of children or wives; attempted suicides; reactions to retirement. The relevance of crisis theory to the possible ways of helping patients in the United Kingdom has been recently reviewed (Brandon, 1970; Morrice, 1976).

The clearest example is that of grief reactions: Lindemann and Caplan of Harvard have described how the process of mourning can give rise to acute distress or longstanding disability when the grief work is not facilitated and completed. Caplan (1964) describes four phases of crisis: in the first, there is a rise in tension as a threatening situation is perceived and coping mechanisms are called into action. The second phase is accompanied by increased anxiety and the patient's behaviour may become disorganized and his attempts at problem-solving less effective. The third phase shows attempts to mobilize resources (both internal and external) to solve the problems, or re-define them, or produce temporary solutions—which may be maladaptive and incomplete. Phase four may follow, with breakdown in social behaviour, or episodes of acute neurotic or psychotic symptoms.

In the second phase the patient is more suggestible and dependent: the need for support and direction is greater and may prove more fruitful at this stage. The patient turns to a number of different agencies for help, and multiple brief interventions are of value. This has been shown in the management of premature babies, and evidence of a similar kind shows the value of the same approach in helping parents who have a problem either in actually battering their children or in fears of doing so. The family practitioner by his own intervention and in facilitating that of other agencies, can have a key role in resolving some of the crisis situations (Morrice, 1976).

Other periods of crisis in development such as puberty, engagement, marriage, pregnancy and the menopause are the daily concern of the general practitioner. Many crises arise in association with the common changes which occur in the lives of their patients: a thorough knowledge of how best to handle developmental crises may, in the view of Caplan and others, have great relevance to the prevention of psychiatric breakdown. Clearly the general practitioner may be able to identify the vulnerable patient and mobilize supportive networks. The success claimed by the Samaritans for clients described as despairing may be understood as showing the value of help in crisis given by workers with relatively little training. The general practitioner has frequently means of integrating the help of priest or minister, health visitor or social worker—all to provide brief, frequent supportive contacts. They are seen, on this view, to be preferable to the use of drugs or admission. Crisis care and better co-operation between family practitioner and hospital requires a willingness to work as a member of a team. Traditionally in the United Kingdom this had not been a feature of the general practitioner's approach. Since 1977, a hospital-based three-year vocational training scheme for general practice includes six months of psychiatric training. Some 1000–1500 doctors are expected to participate and they may well in due course make a considerable difference to the psychiatric aspects of primary health care.

The future: research and practice

It has been authoritatively concluded (World Health Organization, 1973) that the most significant trend in primary medical care today is the appearance in several countries of the multidisciplinary health team. In Eastern Europe, primary medical care has long been based on the district enabling a high degree of co-operation to develop between clinicians, public-health workers and nurses. In many Western European countries as well as in Australia, Canada and the United States, single-handed practices are giving way to the formation of group practices, largely in response to changing urban conditions. The growth of primary medical care teams augurs well for the mental health services. The resulting opportunities for closer co-operation between physicians, health visitors and home nurses, social workers and psychologists should prove wholly beneficial for the care of the mentally ill in the community. There are some disadvantages, not the least being the gradual dilution in the strength of the doctor–patient relationship which occurs with the transformation of single-handed into group practices. For this reason it has been suggested that a group of five or six doctors with adequate nursing and ancillary support offers a suitable compromise and is able to provide comprehensive care, including specialist cover, while avoiding the worst dangers of impersonal, fragmented care (Department of Health and Social Security, 1971). There is more general agreement about the composition of the team which should comprise, in addition to family physicians, health visitors, home nurses, practice nurses, receptionists, secretaries and some part-time attached workers such as midwives (Brook and Cooper, 1975). Many authorities now accept that a social worker should be an integral member of the team.

With the development of group practice and health centres has come the opportunity for specialists to undertake clinical sessions outside the hospital setting. There are obvious advantages for the psychiatric patient in meeting the psychiatrist in familiar surroundings, introduced by his own doctor and without the stresses of a hospital visit. These may well be decisive factors in bringing specialist care to the child, the elderly person, the morbidly anxious or suspicious person. Closer liaison with psychiatrists offers the family physician the opportunity of increasing his clinical knowledge and confidence in this field.

A prominent feature of nurse attachment schemes in Britain has been the increased involvement of health visitors and public health nurses in psychosocial problems. A survey of over 2000 home visits by 72 health visitors found that 'mental health' and 'social care' together accounted for nearly half the topics discussed; among elderly patients and those referred by family physicians, the proportion was even higher (Clark, 1973). It is possible that in future health visitors will devote more time to high-risk groups such as old people living alone and families suffering from bereavement.

In no European country to date has there been any large-scale attachment of social workers to family practices. One of the side-effects of the current trends towards community care of the mentally ill will be to highlight the serious shortage of trained social workers in most parts of Europe. Even in countries relatively well supplied with social workers, progress in the attachment of social workers to family practices has been slow and only small local schemes have been reported.

Family physicians have a solid tradition of working with and through local community groups and agencies on behalf of their patients. Much help for the mentally sick and their families can be mobilized through churches, voluntary bodies and social organizations. Community action groups, now becoming an accepted feature of modern urban life, represent another potential source of help for the senile, the mentally ill and the chronically handicapped.

The family physician, in the course of his daily work, functions as an effective screening agent, but in no systematic way. Many patients do not attend for long periods and, even if they do, it is not likely that their disease would often be detected at the pre-symptomatic stage. Whether he should carry out more systematic and effective screening is much debated at the present time (World Health Organization, 1973). Screening for mental illnesses poses special problems. The model of the disease process that can be detected at the pre-symptomatic stage is not entirely appropriate but there are notable exceptions, as Wilkins (1974) has shown in the detection of the excessive drinker. Any approach to screening would have to concentrate on the detection of existing symptoms (most commonly depression, anxiety, tension, fatigue) not previously recognized. Even if such screening procedures were widely adopted, there is little agreement at the present time about the correct or optimum management of these detected cases. Many experienced practitioners believe in the principle of 'healthy neglect' provided no serious functional impairment exists.

In such circumstances, screening of psychiatric disturbance in family practice is still regarded as an experimental procedure. The testing of standardized questionnaires, designed for use in this field, represents a useful development. Considerable work has gone into the development of a standard psychiatric interview for use in community and general practice surveys (Goldberg et al., 1970) and one questionnaire, the General Health Questionnaire, constructed and validated for use as an initial psychiatric screening instrument, appears to be of greater validity than previously available instruments of this type (Goldberg, 1972). In addition, it has also proved possible to construct a validated version of a social interview schedule (Clare and Cairns, 1978) which has proved valuable in identifying the social correlates of psychiatric disorder in the community (Cooper, 1972).

The use of such screening tools in a variety of studies confirms that mental illness in the community constitutes a major public health problem which is ripe for further epidemiological enquiry. Meanwhile, for the social administrator, the findings continue to underline the conclusion reached a decade ago:

> Administrative and medical logic alike . . . suggest that the cardinal requirement for improvement of the mental health services . . . is not a large expansion and proliferation of psychiatric agencies but rather a strengthening of the family doctor in his therapeutic role.   (Shepherd et al., 1966)

These profound changes in the general practive setting, and in particular the changing quality of the doctor–patient relationship, have not gone unnoticed by medical sociologists (Cartwright, 1969; Stimson and Webb, 1975). The doctor–patient interaction as identified in primary care services has always been a target for sociological analysis and comment, particularly when the interaction is telescoped into a short consultation. Sociologists rightly ask what kind of medical care or doctoring can take place in a five-minute interview. Here the concept of illness behaviour becomes important (Dingwall, 1976), and Stimson and Webb (1975) have shown in their study of doctor–patient interaction how illness behaviour and the language used to describe symptoms and convey medical need is very different in the surgery waiting room, or afterwards back at home, as compared with in the surgery itself. The social interaction of the interview is often seen as a battle for control between doctor and patient, a technical negotiation over access to resources of medical facility, but also to personal concern and sensitivity. These workers found that the emotional element in problems tended to be 'played down' by both doctor and patient so there is almost an emotional flatness in the consultation. Fears were rarely brought into the open and there was a strong element of complicity in the consultation, a form of mutual good manners and doctor–patient etiquette. This kind of empirical research serves to remind us that there is a long way to go before general practitioners achieve their full potential in dealing with emotional and psychiatric problems. Elsewhere, Stimson (1977) has argued that although general practice has taken upon itself responsibilities over emotional and more broadly social therapy, as has been detailed in this chapter, practitioners have partly failed in the clinical setting because they are not prepared to grasp the nettle of the social and political implications of health needs and their own responses.

Notwithstanding the caveats of the sociologists, it does appear that to strengthen the family practitioner and the primary care of psychiatric problems, implies a recognition on the part of the participants in the multidisciplinary team of the extent of the knowledge, skills and attitudes essential for general practice. A Working Party of the Royal College of General Practitioners (1972) has gone so far as to enunciate the broad goals of training for the future general practitioner. He should be able:

(1) To make diagnoses about his patient which are expressed simultaneously in physical, psychological and social terms.

(2) To demonstrate how his recognition of the patient as an unique individual modifies the ways in which he elicits data and makes hypotheses about the nature of the illness and its management.

(3) To demonstrate that he can make decisions about every problem which his patients present to him.

(4) To demonstrate his understanding and use of the time scale which is peculiar to general practice.

(5) To demonstrate his understanding of the way in which interpersonal relationships within the family can cause illness or alter its presentation, course and management.

(6) To demonstrate his understanding of the relationship between health and illness on the one hand and the social characteristics of patients on the other.

(7) To demonstrate his knowledge and use of the wide range of interventions available to him.

(8) To demonstrate the knowledge and appropriate skills of practice management.

(9) To demonstrate that he recognizes his continuing educational needs.

(10) To demonstrate that he understands the basic methods of medical research as applied to general practice.

(11) To demonstrate that he is willing and able critically to audit his own work.

In boldly stating such a job definition, the Working Party has provided a most useful opportunity for all those involved in the planning, administration and implementation of primary health care services to subject the roles of the other paramedical professionals to similar scrutiny. Given the extent of the psychosocial problems which present to the primary health care team, it is becoming increasingly necessary for various participating parties to have a clear understanding of their respective areas of expertise.

References

Acres, D. I. (1977). The primary health team in alcoholism. In 'New Knowledge and New Responses' (Eds G. Edwards and M. Grant). Croom Helm, London.

Balint, E. and Norell, J. S. (1973). 'Six Minutes for the Patient'. Tavistock, London.

Balint, M. (1957). 'The Doctor, his Patient and the Illness'. Pitman Medical, London.

Barraclough, B., Bunch, J., Nelson, D., and Sainsbury, P. (1974). A hundred cases of suicide: clinical aspects. Br. J. Psychiat. 125, 355–373.

Bentsen, B. G. (1970). 'Illness and General Practice'. Universitetsforlaget, Oslo.

Birley, J. L. T. and Heine, B. (1966). The psychiatric emergency clinic: an enquiry into the process of referral and disposal. (Unpublished paper.)

Blackwell, B. (1973). Psychotropic drugs in use today: the role of diazepam in medical practice. J. Am. Med. Ass. 225, 13, 1637–1641.

Bloom, B. L. (1975). 'Changing Patterns of Psychiatric Care'. Human Sciences Press, New York.

Brandon, S. (1970). Crisis theory and the possibilities of therapeutic intervention. Br. J. Psychiat. 117, 627–633.

Brook, P. and Cooper, B. (1975). Community mental health care: primary team and specialist services. J. Roy. Coll. Gen. Pract. 25, 93–110.

Brown, G. W., Brolchain, N. W. and Harris, T. O. (1975). Social class and psychiatric disturbance of women in an urban population. Sociology 9, 225–254.

Browne, K. and Freeling, P. (1967). 'The Doctor-Patient Relationship'. Livingstone, Edinburgh and London.

Caplan, G. (1964). 'Principles of Preventive Psychiatry'. Tavistock, London.

Cartwright, A. (1969). 'Doctors and their Patients'. Routledge and Kegan Paul, London.

Cartwright, A. K. J., Shaw, S. J. and Spratley, T. A. (1975). Designing a comprehensive community response to problems of alcohol abuse. Report by the Maudsley Alcohol Pilot Project to DHSS, London.

Clare, A. W. and Cairns, V. E. (1978). Design, development and use of a standardized interview to assess social maladjustment and dysfunction in community studies. Psychol. Med. 8, 4, 589–604.

Clark, J. (1973). 'A Family Visitor. A descriptive analysis of health visiting in Berkshire'. Royal College of Nursing, London.

Collins, J. (1965). 'Social Casework in a General Medical Practice'. Pitman, London.

Cooper, B. (1971). Social work in general practice: the Derby scheme. *Lancet* I, 539–542.

Cooper, B. (1972). Clinical and social aspects of chronic neurosis. *Proc. Roy. Soc. Med.* **65**, 509–512.

Cooper, B. (1972). Social correlates of psychiatric illness in the community. *In* 'Approaches to Action' (Ed. G. McLachlin), pp. 65–70. Oxford University Press for Nuffield Provincial Hospital Trust, Oxford.

Cooper, B. and Sylph, J. (1973). Life events and the onset of neurotic illness: an investigation in general practice. *Psychol. Med.* **3**, 421–435.

Cooper, B., Fry, J. and Galton, G. (1969). A longitudinal study of psychiatric morbidity in general practice population. *Br. J. Prev. Soc. Med.* **23**, 210–217.

Cooper, B., Harwin, B. G., Depla, C. and Shepherd, M. (1975). Mental health care in the community: an evaluative study. *Psychol. Med.* **5**, 4, 372–380.

Creer, C. and Wing, J. K. (1974). 'Schizophrenia at Home'. Institute of Psychiatry, London.

De Alarcón, R. and Hodson, J. M. (1964). Value of the general practitioner's letter. A further study in medical communication. *Br. Med. J.* **2**, 436–438.

Davies, G. and Noble, P. (1966). Unpublished Data.

Dingwall, R. (1976). 'Aspects of Illness'. Martin Robertson, London.

Department of Health and Social Security (1971). The Organization of Group Practice. HMSO Welsh Office, London.

Dohrenwend, B. P. and Dohrenwend, B. S. (1969). 'Social Status and Psychological Disorder: A Causal Enquiry'. Wiley, New York.

Dohrenwend, B. P. and Dohrenwend, B. S. (1974). Social and cultural influences on psychopathology. *Ann. Rev. Psychol.* 417–452.

Eastwood, M. R. (1970). Psychiatric morbidity and physical state in a general practice population. *In* 'Psychiatric Epidemiology' (Eds E. H. Hare and J. K. Wing). Oxford University Press for the Nuffield Provincial Hospital Trust, Oxford.

Eastwood, M. R. and Trevelyan, M. H. (1972). Relationship between physical and psychiatric disorder. *Psychol. Med.* **2**, 363–372.

Edwards, G. (1977). Clinical review of dependence. *General Practitioner* 15 April, 13–28.

Fischer, J. (1973). Is casework effective? A review. *Social Work* **1**, 5–20.

Fitzgerald, R. (1970). The social worker and general practice. *Update* **2**, 219–224.

Forman, J. A. S. and Fairbairn, E. M. (1968). 'Social Casework in General Practice'. Oxford University Press, Oxford.

Fraser, J. (1947). The incidence of neurosis among factory workers. MRC Industrial Health Research Board, Report No. 90. HMSO, London.

Fry, J. (1960). What happens to our neurotic patients? *Practitioner* **185**, 85.

Goldberg, D. P. (1972). 'The Detection of Psychiatric Illness by Questionnaire'. Maudsley Monograph No. 21. Oxford University Press, Oxford.

Goldberg, D. P., Cooper, B., Eastwood, M. R., Kedward, H. B. and Shepherd, M. (1970). A standardised psychiatric interview for use in community surveys. *Br. J. Prev. Soc. Med.* **24**, 18–23.

Goldberg, D. P. and Blackwell, B. (1970). Psychiatric illness in general practice. A detailed study using a new method of case identification. *Br. Med. J.* **2**, 439–443.

Goldberg, E. M. (1973). Service for the family. *In* 'Roots of Evaluation' (Eds J. K.

Wing and H. Hafner), pp. 281–296. Oxford University Press for the Nuffield Provincial Hospital Trust, Oxford.

Goldberg, E. M. and Neill, J. E. (1973). 'Social Work in General Practice'. Allen and Unwin, London.

Greer, S. and Cawley, R. H. (1966). 'Some Observations on the Natural History of Neurotic Illness'. Archdall Medical Monograph No. 3. Australasia Medical Publishing Company, Sydney.

Harris, T. (1976). Social factors in neurosis, with special reference to depression. In 'Research in Neurosis' (Ed. J. M. van Praag), pp. 22–39. Bohn, Scheltema and Holkema, Utrecht.

Harwin, B. G. (1973). Psychiatric morbidity among the physically impaired elderly in the community. In 'Roots of Evaluation' (Eds J. K. Wing and H. Hafner), pp. 269–278. Oxford University Press, Oxford.

Harwin, B. G., Cooper, B., Eastwood, M. R. and Goldberg, D. P. (1970). Prospects for social work in general practice. Lancet 2, 559–561.

Hill, D. (1969). 'Psychiatry in Medicine: retrospect and prospect'. Nuffield Provincial Hospitals Trust, London.

Hinkle, L. E., Jr., and Wolff, H. G. (1957). Health and social environment: Experimental investigations. In 'Explorations in Social Psychiatry' (Eds A. H. Leighton, J. A. Clausen, and R. N. Wilson). Basic Books, New York.

Hinkle, L. E., Jr., Christenson, W. N., Kane, F. D., Ostfield, A., Thetford, W. N. and Wolff, H. G. (1958). An investigation of the relation between life experience, personality characteristics, and general susceptibility to illness. Psychosom. Med. 20, 278–295.

Hirsch, S. R., Gaind, R., Rohde, P. D., Stevens, B. C. and Wing, J. K. (1973). Out-patient maintenance of chronic schizophrenic patients with long-acting fluphenazine: double-blind placebo trial. Br. Med. J. 1, 633–637.

Hopkins, P. (1976). Holistic medicine and the influence of Michael Balint. In 'Integrated Medicine: The Human Approach' (Ed. H. Maxwell). Wright, Bristol.

Johnson, D. A. W. (1973). Treatment of depression in general practice. Br. Med. J. 2, 18–20.

Kaeser, A.·C. and Cooper, B. (1971). The psychiatric patient, the general practitioner, and the out-patient clinic: an operational study and a review. Psychol. Med. 1, 312–325.

Kedward, H. B. (1968). The outcome of neurotic illness in the community. Soc. Psychiat. 4, 1–4.

Kessel, W. I. N. (1960). Psychiatric morbidity in a London general practice. Br. J. Prev. Soc. Med. 14, 16–22.

King Edward's Hospital Fund for London (1963). Report on Communications and Relationships between General Practitioners and Hospital Medical Staff.

Lancet (1975). Editorial: psychiatrists, social workers and family doctors. Lancet ii, 805–806.

Leff, J. P. and Wing, J. K. (1971). Trial of maintenance therapy in schizophrenia. Br. Med. J. 3, 599–604.

Marks, I. M. (1973). Research in neurosis: a selective review. 1. Causes and courses. Psychol. Med. 3, 4, 436–454.

Marks, I. M. (1974). Research in neurosis: a selective review. 2. Treatment. Psychol. Med. 4, 1, 89–109.

McFall, R. M. and Lillesand, D. B. (1971). Behaviour rehearsal with modelling and coaching in assertion training. J. Abnorm. Psychol. 77, 313–323.

Morrice, J. K. W. (1976). 'Crisis Intervention: Studies in Community Care'. Pergamon, London.

Mowbray, R. M., Blair, W., Jubb, L. G. and Clarke, A. (1961). The general practitioner's attitude to psychiatry. *Scot. Med. J.* **6**, 314–321.

Øgar, B. (1972). Psykiatri i almenpraksis. En pilotunderspkelse. *T. norske Laegeforen,* **12**, 905.

Parish, P. A. (1971). The prescribing of psychotropic drugs in general practice. *J. Roy. Coll. Gen. Pract.* **21**, *Suppl.* 4.

Parish, P. A. (1973). What influences have led to increased prescribing of psychotropic drugs? *In* 'The Medical Use of Psychotropic Drugs'. *J. Roy. Coll. Gen. Pract.* **23**, *Suppl.* 2.

Parish, P. A., Stimson, G. V., Mapes, R. E. A. and Cleary, J. (1976). Prescribing in general practice. *J. Roy. Coll. Gen. Pract.* **26**, *Suppl.* 1.

Pasamanick, B., Scarpitti, F. R., Lefton, M., Dinitz, S., Wernert, J. J. and McPheeters, H. (1964). Home versus hospital care for schizophrenics. *J. Am. Med. Ass.* **187**, 177–181.

Paykel, E. S., Dimascio, A., Haskell, D. and Prusoff, B. A. (1975). Effects of maintenance amitriptyline and psychotherapy on symptoms of depression. *Psychol. Med.* **5**, 1, 67–77.

Polachek, A. (1972). On problems of professional training and qualification of the primary contact physician. Department of Health Organization and Economics, Bratislava.

Pollak, B. (1974). Clinics for alcoholics. *Hospital Update*, March.

Rachman, S. and Philips, C. (1975). 'Psychology and Medicine'. Temple Smith, London.

Rawnsley, K. and Loudon, J. B. (1962). Factors influencing the referral of patients to psychiatrists by general practitioners. *Br. J. Prev. Soc. Med.* **16**, 174.

Royal College of General Practitioners (1972). The future general practitioner. BMA, London.

Sainsbury, P. (1973). Suicide: opinions and facts. *Proc. Roy. Soc. Med.* **66**, 579.

Seebohm Report (1968). Committee Report on Local Authority and Allied Personal Social Services. Cmnd 3707, HMSO, London.

Segal, S. P. (1972). Research on the outcome of social work therapeutic interventions: a review of the literature. *J. Hlth Soc. Behav.* **13**, 3–17.

Shepherd, M. (1974). General practice, mental illness and the British National Health Service. *Am. J. Pub. Hlth* **64**, 3, 230–232.

Shepherd, M. and Watt, D. C. (1974). Impact of long-term neuroleptics on the community: advantages and disadvantages. *Neuropsychopharmacology*, Excerpta Medica International Congress Series No. 359.

Shepherd, M., Cooper, B., Brown, A. C. and Kalton, G. W. (1966). 'Psychiatric Illness in General Practice'. Oxford University Press, Oxford.

Steel, R. (1976). General practice, the team approach and social services. *In* 'Comprehensive Psychiatric Care' (Ed. A. A. Baker). Blackwell, Oxford.

Stevens, B. (1972). Dependence of schizophrenic patients on elderly relatives. *Psychol. Med.* **2**, 17–32.

Stimson, G. V. (1977). Social care and the role of the general practitioner. *Soc. Sci. Med.* **11**, 485–490.

Stimson, G. V. and Webb, B. (1975). 'Going to see the Doctor: the Consultation Process in General Practice'. Routledge and Kegan Paul, London.

Stoller, A. and Krupinski, J. (1969). Psychiatric disturbances. *In* 'Report on a National Morbidity Survey'. NHMRC, Canberra.

Strotzka, H. et al. (1969). 'Kleinburg: eine sozialpsychiatrische Feldstudia'. Austrian State Publishers, Vienna and Munich.

Sylph, J., Kedward, H. B. and Eastwood, M. R. (1969). Chronic neurotic patients in general practice. A pilot study. *J. Roy. Coll. Gen. Pract.* **17**, 162–170.

Watts, C. A. H. (1958). General Registrar Office/Royal College of General Practitioners Morbidity Survey. Morbidity Statistics from General Practice, Vol. 111. Studies on medical and population subjects 14.

Watts, C. A. H. (1966). 'Depressive Disorders in the Community'. Wright, Bristol.

Weissman, M. M. and Paykel, E. S. (1974). 'The Depressed Woman: A Study of Social Relationships'. University of Chicago Press, Chicago.

Wheatley, D. (1972). Evaluation of psychotropic drugs in general practice. *Proc. Roy. Soc. Med.* **65**, 317–320.

Wilkins, R. H. (1974). 'The Hidden Alcoholic in General Practice'. Elek Science, London.

World Health Organization (1961). The undergraduate teaching of psychiatry and mental health promotion. Technical report series 208. WHO, Geneva.

World Health Organization (1973). 'Psychiatry and Primary Medical Care'. Copenhagen.

18 Psychiatry in a general hospital

Joseph Connolly

The earlier sequestration of the psychologically disordered under the care of an alienist in large mental hospitals situated away from population centres has been partly reversed in Europe and North America by the establishment of psychiatric facilities within communities. These include the provision of new psychiatric units for in-, out- and day-patients in general hospitals (Kaufman, 1965; Little, 1974).

Those who champion such units cite as advantages the opportunities for stigma-reduction (encouraging earlier referral), recovery close to home and relatives, employment possibilities after rehabilitation not available 'out in the sticks'. Furthermore these units allow cross-consultation and investigation of both physical illness and psychological disorder which occur in the same people more frequently than chance allows (Eastwood and Trevelyan, 1972; Eastwood, 1975). There are several possible reasons for this interesting concurrence. Life 'stressors' could conceivably contribute to cause both physical illness and psychological disorder. Either of them might cause the other, and the handling (by medication or hospitalization) of either might cause the other (Lloyd, 1977).

Liaison psychiatry has been growing in acknowledgement of this concurrence at rates variably influenced by such local factors as the attitudes and availability of personnel involved. In-patient referrals to psychiatrists in general hospitals have varied between 0·5 and 10% of admission (Crisp, 1968; Anstey, 1972a); 2·5% of the patients attending the casualty department of one London teaching hospital were referred for psychiatric evaluation (Anstey, 1972b).

Critics believe that the management of disturbed patients in general hospitals presents recurrent difficulties that can only bring psychiatry into disrepute. Some colleagues in medicine, surgery and nursing dread lest the patients from the hospital's psychiatric ward intrude on other units, disrupt their working and interfere with the care of seriously ill patients, that screaming and violence will fracture the night, that tubes and drips will be pulled out and untold damage done. The fantasy goes beyond the facts but is fed by small incidents. Confused patients do wander; psychotic patients do behave in incomprehensible ways along corridors; noise can be a problem.

By and large neurotic patients cause little difficulty for the physically ill in neighbouring wards, and psychotic patients are not too hard to contain while their treatment goes forward. However, patients with severe personality disorder, especially if at all intelligent, can find defects in the system of a ward that is run on at all liberal lines. There is no law of nature that units in general hospitals can deal with all comers; they can deal with most (Little, 1974). Transfer to a traditional psychiatric hospital, or even to a regional secure unit of violent patients with either severe personality disorders or psychoses, has not been entirely superseded.

Critics fear too, that psychiatrists working in general hospitals will squander time on the less grave psychiatric problems, usually dealt with by general practitioners (Shepherd *et al.*, 1966), which come to medical notice in hospital and are referred to the now less-than-alien alienist who rises in response, delighted at the recognition that he is almost a proper doctor. Paradoxically, the medical skills of psychiatrists working in such hospitals may atrophy because of the ease of referral to better medical and surgical opinions than their own on the premises.

Like an airport, a general hospital cannot choose who comes to it. The airport will cater for the mobile (mostly), the hospital will cater for the physically ill (mostly), including those who are to die during their admission. Other groups of special interest to the psychiatrist include those who are not ill but believe themselves so, or those who want others to believe them ill. The psychiatrist in either airport or general hospital will meet many problems he is familiar with elsewhere. Neuroses, functional psychoses, personality disorders, may emerge in juxtaposition to physical illness as they may to air travel. Many of the problems encountered will, however, spring from the human experience of illness and from the peculiarities of the setting itself.

Attendance at hospital, hospitalization itself, most medical and many nursing manoeuvres are accompanied by potentially overwhelming emotions like fear, anger, depression, arising from threat posed to life and future (Chesser, 1975). Most patients and staff manage these situations without being overwhelmed. The 'good' patient becomes aware that something is wrong, signals it credibly with culturally acceptable emotion, accepts the offer of investigation and treatment, bears any pain involved with some stoicism, is appropriately grateful if the outcome is good and not too reproachful or litigious if it is bad. The 'good' doctor or nurse shows interest in the patient, is evidently competent, assured and communicates some awareness of the impact of the disease and therapeutic ministrations on the person. Any marked deviation from these stereotypes may lead either patient or doctor to consider psychiatric referral of the other. Referrals by doctors have so far predominated, though, in Britain, implementation of the Merrison Committee's recommendations on the sick doctor may redress the balance a little (Merrison, 1975).

Some of the factors which lead to psychiatric consultation in a hospital can be identified. The objectives of the patient and staff ussally overlap with regard to, for example, the amelioration if not the cure of illness. Patients with Munchausen syndrome manifestly do not share the objectives of staff (Blackwell, 1968), and subject themselves to multiple hospitalizations and often operations with diverse and skilfully simulated illnesses. One young woman I encountered had had both a tracheostomy and a craniotomy. Blackwell (1968) notes the association in these patients of criminal activities, colourful lying and wanderlust, sexual immaturity and knowledge of illness from occupation or personal experience. Detecting such patients, itself no easy matter, is easier than understanding their motives entirely, or detaching them from their chosen career.

Nursing staff, social workers, physiotherapists and occupational therapists increasingly provide the impetus for psychiatric referral. When an unusually large cluster of referrals arrived during one week from one surgical ward its explanation became clear in the irritation of the nursing staff with what they construed as the preoccupation of the surgeons with wound-healing and their disregard of the psychological and social factors in the lives of patients. These the nurses, during their long hours with patients, had recognized. None of the patients referred had serious psychiatric disorder. The psychiatrist had been involved as the ward 'emotions man'.

Experienced hospital staff ordinarily have a very wide tolerance for deviation from the stereotype of 'good' patient, and for the range of emotions thought appropriate to accompany physical disease—though less with the thwarting of therapeutic objectives. The psychiatrist tends to be consulted, with varying reluctance, if certain limits are overstepped. He will be brought to see the too sad, the too glad, the too bad and the too mad. He will be asked to manage the deviance and, increasingly, to help in its understanding. Short of removal of a patient to a psychiatric ward, for which there will often be pressure and sometimes justification, he may aim to diminish the deviance or increase staff tolerance to it (Lipowski, 1976).

Conceptualization of the problems will be coloured by beliefs about aetiology. The psychoanalytically orientated may see the hospital as a temple dedicated to, and permeated by, castration anxiety with, to say the least, very unusual people attracted to work in it as staff. Communications to the staff along such lines require a certain delicacy if they are to be understood at all. Figure 1 outlines a time-based model about which there is likely to be more agreement between professionals and with patients.

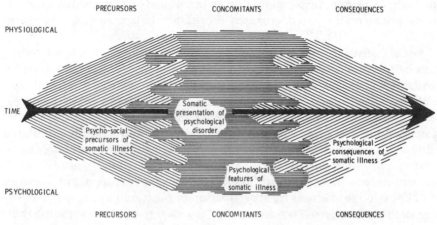

Fig. 1 Illness-related areas of psychiatric interest.

Precursors of illness (like bereavement), its concomitants (like the delirium of pneumonia or the hyperventilatory tetany of anxiety) and its consequences (like post-gastrectomy syndrome) can be studied for convenience by physiological or psychological methods. It might be trivial and impractical to measure the amount of tear fluid shed after a bereavement whose psychological impact on the person is of greater interest but, naturally, phenomena are occurring in the same person in both fields of study at the same time.

The major, though indistinctly divided, domains into which a psychiatrist will be drawn in a general hospital are also outlined in Fig. 1. This chapter is concerned with extracerebral illness and no attempt is made to be exhaustive. Neurological disorders are dealt with elsewhere in the volume.

The psychosocial precursors of physical illness

In several illnesses—some would say all—the discovered physical factors in causation appear, even if necessary, insufficient and enquiry into possible psychosocial contributors continues. Three strands of research can be perceived—those concerned with the influence on disease (mediated by perhaps neural and/or humoral mechanisms) from societal forces, from personality and from so-called life events. These lines of research will be exemplified in several physical illnesses. The liaison psychiatrist's evaluation will be incomplete unless considerable attention is given to these areas in the lives of all his patients.

Peptic ulcer

What is known about the causation of duodenal ulcer can be summarized easily. In especially younger patients, blood group O, the non-secretion of ABH substances into saliva, the ability to taste dilute concentrations of PTC are all over-represented suggesting, with the strong family incidence of the condition, a vulnerability of genetic origin. Patients' stomachs are large and many secrete large amounts of acid and pepsin—whether ulcers are active or healed. Serum pepsinogen levels are high. Smoking and alcohol intake, perhaps because they increase secretion, alter mucus production or mucosal vascularity, are accepted as adverse influences.

There are secular changes this century in the condition with a fall in incidence and a reversal of the sex ratio—males now predominating about four to one. Both observations are difficult to dismiss as artefacts of ascertainment practices.

Patients with gastric fistulae, studied now over two centuries, show changes in secretion, vascularity and motility with emotion. Whether this is any more than an analogue of the facial blush or whether it could lead to structural disease is by no means clear. Gastro-duodenal ulceration in monkeys after electrical stimulation of brain (French *et al.*, 1957) in electrically shocked 'executive' monkeys (Brady, 1958) or in 'yoked' rats (Weiss, 1968) may or may not be extrapolable to man—but the temptation for creative and dissatisfied physicians to speculate is clear.

Varieties of an ulcer-prone 'driven' personality and the presence in patients of a specific conflict over dependence linked with oral gratification have been alleged. Genetically determined gastric hypersecretion was hypothesized to lead to augmented infantile demand for nourishment, with rage and further hypersecretion if unsatisfied. A table of possible mismatches in infants' demands and maternal capacity (and/or inclination) to respond has even been constructed (Engel, 1975). Conflict over dependence in mismatched, unsatisfied infants is then seen as contributing to personality development producing either the passive and resentful or, by overcompensation, the excessively self-reliant. Both, the story goes, will hypersecrete and ulcerate if this conflict is heightened by life situations.

United States army recruits undergoing their initial 16-week training were identified, blind, on a battery of psychological tests, as either showing this alleged conflict or not. Their serum pepsinogen levels (as a parameter of pepsin production) were measured (Weiner *et al.*, 1959). Four duodenal ulcers were found on radiography at intake and new ulcers appeared in five other soldiers. All nine were 'conflicted' on testing and were serum pepsinogen hypersecretors. Weiner has himself assembled the criticism against his work and it is now clear that peptic ulceration is not a homogeneous category. Ulcers vary in site, chronicity and have all possible associations with hyper- and hypo-secretion, whether basal or maximally stimulated (Ackerman and Weiner, 1976).

As so often in this field, the paper edifice erected on shallow foundations is too big to be durable. Curiously the hardest data are old. If the same factors that extend ulceration also initiate it, the increase in peptic ulcer perforation in both Glasgow and London during the 1940 blitz (Illingworth *et al.*, 1944) seems to indicate that an externally imposed, threatening environmental event was associated with a structural change in some patients that was both life-threatening and could escape medical notice only with great difficulty. Unfortunately the rise in perforations seen at the same time in non-belligerent Stockholm makes interpretation less than simple (Lewis, 1954).

Hypertension

The genetic influence on essential hypertension is accepted but the transient, weeks-long elevation of both systolic and diastolic blood pressure in front-line troops together with the evanescent blood pressure elevation in normals, angered or under physical or psychological pressure in laboratories, continues to promote the idea that environmental conditions may contribute to sustained 'essential' hypertension. Suggestions are that the patient may experience (or even by inarticulable processes actually select) feeling states in response to environmental happenings over the years and that if these states are accompanied by increased peripheral resistance and/or cardiac output, physiologically induced hypertension will lead to secondary renal vascular change, in time, with essential hypertension as a result.

Personality measures on patients attending hypertensive clinics show them scoring higher on neuroticism (N) and extraversion (E) on the EPI. The high N score is probably a consequence of their being patients for it is only the high E score that emerged in one population survey of the non-patient hypertensives, who also have fewer health complaints than normotensives (Tibblin *et al.*, 1972). A more recent study showed no significant differences in measurable psychiatric disorder between non-hypertensives and patients with moderate hypertension, whether aware or not yet aware of that diagnosis (Mann, 1977).

Migrants have more hypertensives among them than the base population from which they were drawn. 'Failure to aculturate' with its emotional sequelae is speculated on as cause but other explanations (as for ischaemic heart disease below) are possible. Population surveys throughout the world show that hypertension rises more steeply with age in societies where the old have, in their lives, encountered greater social and political instability (Henry and Cassel, 1969).

Recurrent illness

In recurrent, traditionally 'psychosomatic' illnesses like peptic ulcer, rheumatoid arthritis, ulcerative colitis, eczema, psoriasis and urticaria, there is no shortage of clinical reports of an anecdotal nature suggesting their susceptibility to environmental or emotional influence (Rees, 1976). The difficulty that limits credence is that the onset of an episode in these conditions is difficult to pinpoint. The psychosocial environment may itself be the consequence of an insidious onset rather than the cause of illness or even the consequence of a previous episode.

The psychological precipitation and amelioration of asthma is well documented. Everyone knows the story of the rose pollen asthmatic whose asthma could be precipitated by an artificial rose. The placebo response in some asthmatics has been ingeniously explored (Luparello *et al.*, 1968) and, in a controlled trial, asthmatic children hypersensitive to house dust did as well in their own homes, if the rest of the household were sent on a paid holiday, as did matched patients who were hospitalized (Purcell *et al.*, 1969).

Prevalence of asthma among some groups seems unduly high. White Protestant children in Maryland USA and University students in Britain both have twice the national prevalence. Societal influence, personality differences and ascertainment practices compete in explanation. The modification of asthma either by psychotherapy or by such behavioural approaches as deconditioning is under extensive investigation.

Ischaemic heart disease

Both the physical (Epstein, 1967; Keys *et al.*, 1972) and psychosocial precursors (Jenkins, 1971, 1976; Theorell, 1970; Connolly, 1974) of ischaemic heart disease (IHD) have had an extensive coverage but the quantitation of the relative contributions to causation is still a long way off.

Sociological studies

The different IHD rates between rural and urban communities, during urbanization (Tyroler and Cassell, 1964) among the occupationally or geographically mobile (Syme et al., 1964) or the 'emancipated from tradition' (Wardwell et al., 1964) has evoked much speculation.

Studies correlating socio-economic status with myocardial infarction have found all types of relationship including curvilinear ones of opposite concavity. Secular changes may be occurring too for, in Sweden, employers had the national incidence of first myocardial infarctions between 1935 and 1949 but significantly more between 1950 and 1954 (Biörck et al., 1958).

In a study of status incongruity in the US seven parameters of a person's standing in society were measured—education, occupation, income, dwelling, neighbourhood, religion and membership of voluntary organization. Manifestations of ischaemic heart disease correlated with no one parameter but increased with increasing incongruities between them (Shekelle et al., 1969).

Japanese Americans experienced the high US rates for IHD and not the low rates prevalent in Japan (Gordon, 1967). Boston Irishmen manifested ischaemic heart disease significantly more often than their brothers who stayed in Ireland, though whether acculturation factors, personality characteristics of the migrant or diet are responsible remains unclear (Clancy et al., 1963).

Personality

In the late 1940s personality profiles for patients who had such conditions as angina, myocardial infarction, peptic ulcer or hypertension had a considerable vogue. Initial, necessarily retrospective, delineations of such profiles gave way to prospective studies using standardized instruments. Thus the MMPI and Catell 16PF have been used on cohorts before any manifestations of IHD. Those who were to become anginal scored—before it—higher on the Hs (hypochondriasis), K (test-taking attitudes) and Hy (Hysteria) scales of the MMPI and lower on the Catell C scale (affected by emotion vs emotionally stable) than those who were to experience a myocardial infarction with the non-IHD population scoring between them. Non-survivors of the infarction would be differentiated from survivors—for example they scored higher on the Catell 'happy go lucky vs glum' scale (Lebovitz et al., 1967; Shekelle et al., 1969).

The correlation between the now well-known time-pressured Type A behaviour (Friedman and Rosenman, 1959) and subsequent IHD could not be explained in prospective studies by any other recognized physical risk factor correlation (Rosenman *et al.*, 1970).

The sons of Type A behaviour men are significantly more often themselves Type A behaving than are the sons of Type B behaviour men (Bortner *et al.*, 1970), but whether Type A behaviour, in all its degrees of development, predicts only ischaemic heart disease remains to be seen (Mertens and Seegers, 1972).

Happenings and illness

It is artificial to separate happenings like death, birth, marriage, job loss, and moving house from the personality and cultural setting of those who experience them. Provided it is realized that life events interact with other psychosocial and probably physical precursors of disease, the reasons for a rigorous approach to their measurement will become clear.

Mortality of bereavement

Widowers over the age of 55 die in the first six months after bereavement at 40% above the expected rate for age-matched married men. For the following eight and a half years their mortality rates are as expected. The admittedly imprecise death certificate diagnosis showed that 'Arteriosclerotic and Degenerative Heart Disease' was attributed as cause of death by physicians 67% in excess of expectation for those widowers (Parkes *et al.*, 1969).

The death of a close relative appeared in another study to carry its own mortality—some seven times that of close relatives (matched for age, sex and marital status) of patients who had not died in the same semi-rural Welsh general practice (Rees and Lutkins, 1967). This apparent mortality of bereavement is of unmatched objectivity in this area of research. A precisely datable illness-outcome (death) follows a precisely datable happening—the initial death. Other happenings may be important for illness but as a life event death is hard to beat.

Following the description of the clustering of illness after 'unsatisfactory years' (Hinkle and Wolff, 1957) with half of all illness clustering in an unfortunate third of persons, some attempt at quantitation of life changes before illness was made by Seattle researchers (Holmes and Rahe, 1967). On a normative population they enquired how much adjustment between zero and infinity would be needed for 43 happenings like death and illness in the family, job changes, rows and purchases,

provided that marriage scored 500. Averages were obtained, divided for
convenience by 10 (with marriage now at 50) and called Life Change Units
(LCU). Patients with various illnesses were questioned about their
experience of the 43 adjustments. A fairly common pattern emerged in
the reported build-up from baseline levels of LCU in the one or two years
before such conditions as diabetes mellitus, tuberculosis, hernia operations, pregnancy and myocardial infarction with a return to baseline over
the year to follow. Non-surviving patients of myocardial infarction, on
the accounts of their close relatives, had higher LCU scores than did
survivors in the 6–18 months before infarction (Theorell and Rahe, 1971).
This Swedish finding was confirmed in one later Finnish study (Rahe et
al., 1974) but not in Theorell's later investigation (1975).

Prospective studies on US Naval personnel have yielded only modest
correlations (0·1–0·2) between reported LCU and subsequent treatment-
seeking. Criticism of the LCU methodology has included the failure to
define events rigorously enough to allow the normative and patient
populations to report and score comparably, e.g. 'major illness in family
member'. The 'effort after meaning' in a patient recovering from an illness
may prove a source of over-reporting of happenings unless controlled.

Myocardial infarction has attracted considerable research attention
because its onset is precisely known and if happenings can be precisely
dated they can be related to that onset.

An excess of events undoubtedly antedating an illness (whose onset is
also indisputable) which are beyond the control of a patient would convince most sceptics of a contributing role for life's happenings in physical
illness. When events are specified with some precision (and they are
counted only if they happen to the patient, first degree relatives and
household members), provided enough information is gathered to allow
decision as to whether they were independent of the control of patients,
their measurement is taken out of the hands of patients and put into those
of the researchers (Brown and Birley, 1968; Brown and Harris, 1978;
Brown et al., 1973 a, b).

With this approach, which may well lose data because of its rigour, 121
men between the ages of 35 and 65 were interviewed in a coronary care
unit, within three days of infarction, about the occurrence of the pre-
designated events. Ninety-one men proved to have sustained a myocardial infarction and they were matched for age and occupation level with
91 men who were similarly interviewed at work after random selection
from a 7000-strong payroll. Both groups matched, by chance, on marital
status and household size as groups. Significantly more men reported at
least one of these rather sizable and memorable events ($p < 0·01$) than did
comparison subjects (Connolly, 1976) only in the three weeks before
infarction, whether this occurred unexpectedly or in an anginal setting.

Further, most events appeared beyond the control of both patients and comparison subjects (Fig. 2).

Researchers, too, however, have their biases about the role of such events in illness and definitive prospective studies have yet to be effected and will prove difficult—especially if event-reporting has to be as frequent as this study suggests.

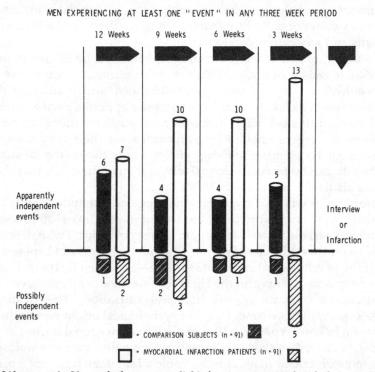

Fig. 2 Life events in 91 men before myocardial infarction contrasted with their comparison subjects' experience.

Theorell (1970) has delicately bypassed this difficulty with his measurement of 'perceived work load' in men over 45 and initially free of IHD. In the one or two years following, those who perceived either too much or too little work load (which makes no pretence at estimating actual work load) experienced a myocardial infarction significantly more often than those without such problems.

The somatic presentation of psychological disorder

Practitioners in all branches of medicine recognize the 'calling card syndrome' where professional attention is procured with gastro-intestinal, respiratory or cardio-vascular symptoms, for example, when really the patient has a problem in living. Awareness of this will vary widely both among patients and their doctors. Organic symptoms may be preferred as currency for the patient/doctor transaction by either or both. Patients of lower socio-economic standing are more likely, initially, to present non-psychological complaints to their doctors. Exclusion of organic disease, reassurance, possibly 'placebation' with not too harmful a medication may satisfy either or both. Problems in living are then dealt with (as most problems are) without medical assistance.

Dissatisfaction with this as outcome of the transaction invites attention to accessible causes of anxiety (with its palpitations, sweating, tremor, hyperventilation, urinary frequency, diarrhoea and giddiness) or of depression (with its lassitude, disinterest, poor appetite, decreased libido and sleep disturbance). High proportions of patients attending general practitioners' surgeries have no organic cause for their symptoms, and even in reputable gastro-enterology clinics where the search for such an abnormality can be pursued extensively, none is found in a majority of the patients (Dally and Gomez, 1977).

Some patients will be affronted by the suggestion that their complaints have their cause not in structural disease but in psychological processes. This may be particularly so where pain is the complaint. The patient is an almost incontrovertible authority on whether he is or is not experiencing pain. If the psychological experience—pain—is caused by trauma, infection or neoplasia, its siting on the Fig. 1 schema is evidently removed from that occupied by pain of psychological causation. The distinction occupies much medical time. Pain of psychological origin was found not to conform to known patterns (like the colics) or neuronal territories (like sciatica), to last longer than organically caused pains, rarely to wake from sleep, to be described in as unremarkable a language (and not a bizarre one) and to respond better to psychotropics than to analgesics (Merski and Spear, 1967).

A common clinical situation is that of pain in part determined by structural disorder, as in low back pain (Wolkind, 1976), but the severity reported and the disability caused are greater than that normally associated with the structural abnormality. Of 50 men with low back, 23 whose pain was unimproved after six hospital treatment sessions differed from the 27 who had improved, on initial Middlesex Hospital Questionnaire replies. The replies of the 23 men were closer to neurotic population replies (with loss of libido and appetite) making the best prediction of non-improvement (Forrest and Wolkind, 1974).

Pain clinics run, for example, by an anaesthetist, physician and psychiatrist jointly are now widely found. Medication, psychotherapy and increasingly therapy, based on operant conditioning principles designed to change the ways chronic pain responds to or operates on the domestic environment, are finding usage and being evaluated (Stern-bach, 1977).

The advantages of disability (as below in hysteria) including sometimes compensation, may satisfy the doctor as explanation but the proposition being put, however gently and circuitously, to the patient is that, though there is pain, life is in some way pain-evoking or pain-worsening. Some patients will find this acceptable and may find the model helps them to live with pain, or welcome attempts to elevate mood or decrease anxiety in order to make pain less obtrusive. Others will find the idea incredible, question its scientific standing and ask how its validity could be tested.

Chronic hyperventilation is claimed to be present in 6–10% of medical out-patients. Lum (1976) reviewed the syndrome and reported on 640 of his own cases. Symptoms are experienced in all bodily systems and attributed to neural dysfunction due to the respiratory alkalosis. Whether anxiety causes or is caused by the hyperventilation, an approach which viewed it as a habit disorder requiring the retraining of breathing rendered 70% of patients asymptomatic.

Hysteria

Kendell (1974) described the several usages of the term hysteria. As a diagnosis it is followed by more face-reddening revisions than most (Slater, 1965; Reed, 1975). Yet clinicians continue to need it as a diagnosis, perhaps to halt expensive, painful and hazardous investigations when the likelihood of discovering pathological processes is becoming remote while the decreasingly credible complaints continue and their advantages to the patient become clearer.

The fascination of the physician with the symbolism of, say, an hysterical paralysis may not be matched by his patient's receptivity to the idea. Kendell recommends weighting the balance of advantages of the 'healthy role' over those of the 'sick role' (Parsons, 1952; Mechanic, 1962) as the therapeutic aim. This management presupposes that the diagnosis of hysteria can be made more securely now than it was by skilled earlier clinicians. The coaxing of the 'acting sick' into 'acting healthy' can be as great a challenge for the physician as any in medicine.

Hypochondriasis

Preoccupation with bodily function and sensation (and repeated complaints about them) may be a durable personality characteristic, the symptoms of a serious psychiatric disorder (like psychotic depression), or even a psychiatric condition in its own right which is highly resistant to treatment of any kind (Kenyon, 1964, 1976). Hypochondriacal attitudes are probably learnt early in family life and can be expected to change with height of anxiety or depth of depression, each leading to enteroceptive vigilance and yet another medical consultation. Psychiatric referral rarely brings joy to either patient or psychiatrist, unless there is a clear-cut psychiatric disorder like severe depression or marked anxiety which are eminently treatable.

Like obesity, anorexia nervosa (p. 134) exemplifies the difficulties of a dualist concept of psyche and soma. It may be viewed as the somatic presentation of a psychological disorder with body image distortion and weight phobia (Crisp, 1970). It may have its own psychosocial precursors in parental attitudes, premorbid personality and obesity. Alternatively the frequent antedating menstrual disorder can be taken as evidence of a hypothalamus-cortex (somatic) disorder responsible for the psychological consequences. It would be hard to prove that either neuronal or psychological events preceded the other.

Suicide and overdosing

Suicide is described in more detail on pp. 426–430. The current epidemic of overdosing with therapeutic substances has not yet peaked, but the liaison psychiatrist seems powerless to halt it. About 15% of acute medical admissions to hospitals in London are for overdoses and one in seven prescriptions for psychotropic drugs or hypnotics is used for overdosing (R. Farmer, 1978, personal communication). The attitudes of the hospital staff in the face of this therapeutic impotence and the increasing workload it represents have been explored (Bancroft et al., 1977) and succinctly described as 'counter-transference hate'.

Psychological concomitants of physical illness

There is a distinction, though a difficult one to draw, between on the one hand the reaction of the patient with anxiety over an impending serious operation, or with depression at the knowledge of near-future death, and on the other hand the mental states imposed, as it were, by some illnesses. Examples of the latter might be the delirium of pneumonia, the dysmnesic state of hypoglycaemia, the exogenous psychoses of endocrinopathy, the depression which precedes other signs of pancreatic cancer, the sub-acute confusional state described as herald to bronchial cancer, or the anxiety-like features of incipient thyrotoxicosis. If the former are called 'person-reactions' and the latter 'brain-reactions', the terms are recognized as less than satisfactory. The contribution from a person's experience to, for example, the content of delirious and psychotic delusions is as evident as is the brain's contribution to the person's reaction to life-threatening illness.

What the patient *knows* and *feels* are, because of their interdependence, not quite the latitude and longitude of the mental state. Together, if accessible, they help to explain what he *does*. In the person-reactions, over- or under-modulation of emotions is intimately linked with patients' appraisals of their illnesses that range between maximization and minimization. The modulation will usually follow patterns fashioned during adversities of earlier life. Inappropriate modulation and appraisal may lead to dangerous activities during illness. Thus over-modulation among the minimizers (to which the putative extra-conscious defence mechanisms of denial, repression and overcompensation may contribute) can lead to neglect of a breast lump or blood in the urine and the rejection of essential treatment. The under-modulating maximizers *know* that the admittedly low mortality of an operation will include them and may refuse it in terror.

Anxiety states and 'neurotic, reactive' depression on this model are seen as modulation-failure. About a quarter of seriously ill medical patients who completed the Beck inventory (Paykel and Moffic, 1975) were clinically depressed, judged appropriately so for illness-severity though less depressed than matched psychiatric patients, who incidentally contemplated suicide more. Defective modulation of the externally directed anger or suspicion that sometimes accompanies illness may involve the liaison psychiatrist when, for example, medical or surgical ward staff have been antagonized, ill-advised discharge is threatened by the patient or petulant non-cooperation endangers a home dialysis programme.

Dying

Hospitals are increasingly places to die. A growing literature (Hinton, 1976) attests the attempts to make the process of dying less awesome. With the decline of religion more patients are looking not for a priest to ease their passage to eternity but for a physician to prepare them for extinction.

Both Hinton (1976) and Cassem and Stewart (1977) have reviewed the relevant research. The association of depression, anxiety and confusional states with dying has been quantified and the person-reactions to dying appear to be determined by such factors as progress of the fatal disease, the effects of treatment, the patient's awareness of oncoming death which may be suspected, shielded or shared, interactions with significant people, the setting and personality characteristics. The last only weakly predicted (Hinton, 1975) the emotional state accompanying the dying and how it was handled.

The crucial question is, how best will this person spend the dying time? The answers are likely to be highly individual and not necessarily in the psychiatric sphere. Some will want human contact, others solitude, some will prefer activity while it is possible, others will want to talk—but about anything except death. Many may come to be glad to break the conspiracy of silence and ventilate the disappointment, fear and anger that surrounds the realization of death—perhaps in time with spouse or children. Some will want renonciliation, others recrimination.

The usefulness of delineating a sequence of attitudes such as death-denying, death-defying, bargaining, depression and death-accepting (Kübler Ross, 1970) or the concept of the patient's erratic 'trajectory' from social death with isolation to psychic, biologic and physiological deaths (Pattison, 1975) remains to be seen.

Is it an abdication by the responsible doctor and a pre-mortem affront to the patient to involve a psychiatrist in care of the dying? Are they simply involved as professionals who will listen? Does the suggestion that they should operate only in an educative role for the responsible nursing and medical staff exemplify the 'those who can, do: those who cannot, teach' principle? There are more interesting questions than clear answers in this area.

Psychotropics have no indications which are different from normal and the outcome of psychotherapy with patient (Feigenberg, 1975) or family is as difficult to evaluate here as in situations more remote from death.

Brain reactions

With few exceptions the clinical features of brain-reactions do not help identify their causes and very little is known about pathogenetic mechanisms (Heller and Kornfeld, 1975). The depressions of hypocalcaemia, hypothyroidism or nicotinimide deficiency are indistinguishable, as is the delirium of heart failure from that of atropine-toxicity. The confusional state of dialysis disequilibrium has no special features to separate it from that of hypoxia. An exogenous psychosis in a patient with systemic lupus erythematosus who was taking amphetamines would create an aetiological puzzle for the clinician that would have to await amphetamine withdrawal for its solution. The phenomena would not help him.

The mood psychoses of hypothalamus-pituitary-adrenal cortex origin or during steroid medication in the medical ward may mimic exactly the functional psychoses in the psychiatric unit. The presence of a cognitive deficit on mental state examination (oneirophrenia and depressive pseudodementia notwithstanding) will alert one to an organic cause though rarely point to its nature. Exogenous psychoses in clear consciousness without such deficit are, however, well recognized.

Four organically determined and overlapping syndromes of confusion, dysmnesia, delirium and psychosis are met repeatedly in hospital practice. Some of their recognized extracerebral causes are shown in Table I.

Table I *Well recognized causes of confusional, dysmnesis, delirious or psychotic states originating extracerebrally*

Trauma
  Hypothermia.   Heat injury.
  Fat embolism.   Open heart surgery.   Cataract surgery.

Poisons
  (iatrogenic and otherwise)
  CNS depressants like alcohol and barbiturates and their withdrawal.
  Carbonmonoxide
  CNS stimulants like amphetamines and the hallucinogens.
  Corticosteroids, INH, cycloserine, opiates, anticholinergics, L-dopa.

Infections
  Pneumonia.   Abcess.   Systemic infections like typhoid and typhus.

Degenerations
  Athero and arterio-sclerosis of coronary, renal and peripheral vessels.

Major Organ Failure
  Heart.   Lung.   Liver.   Kidney.

Metabolic disorders
  Deficiency or excess of:
  Oxygen, water, glucose, sodium, calcium or the hormones of anterior pituitary, thyroid, parathyroid, or adrenal cortex.
  Deficiency of:
  Thiamine, riboflavine, nicotinamide, pyridoxine, cyanocobalamine.

  Diabetes mellitus.   Acute intermittent porphyria.

Neoplasms
  Especially of bronchus and pancreas and with carcinomatous hypercalcaemia.

Autoimmune disease
  Systemic Lupus Erythematosus.

Certain high technology settings in modern medicine have frequently featured such brain-reactions. The open heart recovery room always produced more confusional states and delirium than did the coronary care unit (Kornfeld *et al.*, 1965). Hypoxia, especially during time on bypass, anaesthesia and analgesia are likely contributors. In both settings, attention to patient's perception, cognition and emotion has decreased the disturbed psychological states. Provision of windows, daylight, clock and calendar, care with lighting and a familiar nursing staff aware of its role in gently anchoring patients in reality, supportive psychotherapy and tranquillizing medication, have all had their impact.

The multiple factors contributing in renal dialysis units to the depressive and anxiety states, confusion, delirium and sometimes frank, often paranoid, psychoses have been indicated (Neary, 1976). They include rapid change in nitrogenous metabolites, sodium depletion, water intoxication, pH change, hypertension, heart failure, intercurrent infections, anaemia, medications and dietary deficiencies. If analgesic abuse has itself been responsible for the renal failure, previous psychiatric vulnerability and abuse of other drugs may colour the clinical features (Murray, 1973).

Rapid biochemical change during treatment is responsible for the dialysis disequilibrium syndrome—a transient confusional and delirious state seen with both haemo- and peritoneal-dialysis. The results of rapid metabolic change have also been reported in thyrotoxicosis, where not only may a highly agitated delirious presentation (thyroid storm) be seen but, in its treatment with carbimazole, a paranoid psychosis has been described. This remitted when medication was discontinued and then resumed at a lower dosage (Greer and Parsons, 1970).

The lack of specificity of cause in the illness-imposed brain-reactions has some exceptions. An otherwise non-specific delirious or psychotic state accompanying obscure abdominal pain, nausea and vomiting and limb weakness may lead to enquiry for recent exposure to barbiturates, sulphonamides or alcohol, the search for porphobilinogen and delta-amino-laeuvulinic acid in the urine and the triumphant, if rare, diagnosis, of acute intermittent porphyria.

The anxiety-like state of incipient thyrotoxicosis repeatedly exercises both psychiatrists and physicians. Compared with naturally occurring anxiety states, it is seen in patients with a later age of onset, no perceptible emotional precipitant, few hysterical features, lower neuroticism score on the EPI, warm extremities, increased cold tolerance and weight loss in spite of good appetite (Gurney *et al.*, 1966).

Patients who are phobic of blood, tissue injury, injections and illness are exceptional among phobics in that they faint with bradycardia when confronted with phobic stimulation (Connolly *et al.*, 1976). The condition may interfere with necessary treatment and can be successfully treated using a behavioural approach (Marks *et al.*, 1976; Lloyd and Deakin, 1975).

Carroll (1976) has reviewed psychoendocrine relationships of the hypothalamus-pituitary-adrenal axis. Patients with primary depression closer to the endogenous profile secrete more cortisol than normals especially around midnight when normal secretion is at its lowest. Serious depression is seen more in Cushing's disease than in his (peripherally caused) syndrome, but is also recognized in Addison's disease. No parsimonious explanation (in the shape of high ACTH or corticotrophin releasing factor levels) yet accounts for all of the findings, which include mania-like states as well as depressions in all these naturally occurring conditions as well as with steroid medication.

Depression has been described following the use of several hypotensive agents possibly due to a depletion (by reserpine for example) of or interference with (alpha methyl dopa, guanethidine, bethanidine) the putative neurotransmitter activity of biogenic amines. Treatment follows orthodox lines after drug discontinuation. Interactions of these and other drugs with antidepressants may prove at best a nuisance (tricyclic plus guanethidine) and at worst extremely hazardous (MAOI plus pethidine).

Management of person-reactions and of illness-imposed states will be directed where feasible towards their causes. Often it will, as elsewhere in psychiatry, be aimed necessarily only at symptom-relief. Major tranquillizers, antidepressant treatment, anxiolytics, all have their customary place alongside some form of supportive and, more rarely, interpretive psychotherapy. Explanation and support for the family of the patient and other professionals involved in care will be an integral part of such management.

Disorders of pregnancy and puerperium

Pregnancy itself, at least when well established, has the reputation of decreased incidence of psychological disorder, though this is currently under more systematic investigation (Kumar and Robson, 1978). More disorder appears in the three months after delivery than in any other three months in the two years before or the two years after it (Kendell *et al.*, 1976). 'Postpartum Blues', possibly related to decreased tryptophan turnover, affects about two-thirds of women, is transient and usually clears without intervention. About 10% of women go on to manifest clinical depression with 'neurotic' and 'reactive' features. This is responsive to antidepressants but, untreated, lasts in almost half for more than a year (Pitt, 1968).

Puerperal psychosis is seen in one in 500 to 1000 deliveries. Primiparae over the age of 30 carry a higher risk. Now that trauma, haemorrhage and infection are less common in childbirth, frankly organic syndromes are encountered less frequently and the obstetric complications are as infrequent in those who manifest psychoses as in those who do not. The syndrome is in phenomenology, family history and outcome hard to distinguish from non-puerperium-linked psychoses. About one in six subsequent puerperia will be similarly complicated. Over two-thirds are emotion-dominant psychoses and a third has the worse prognosis of a schizophrenia—albeit one of acute onset and precipitation. Management includes special provision (often in mother-and-baby units) for the child while the mother is psychotic and for her gradual restoration to mothering as she improves, carefully supervised in hospital and later in the commmunity.

Psychological consequences of physical illness

Depressions following infections like influenza, infective hepatitis and brucellosis have long been known. Post-infective depression may follow an influenzal illness of any severity and while the depression is most often not grave, it tends to last several weeks. Some exceptions have been known to go on to stupor and to respond only to ECT.

Infectious mononucleosis was followed in 13 out of 20 women by a measurable clinical depression in the year following diagnosis (Cadie *et al.*, 1976). The depression had antedated the diagnosis in four, perhaps contributing, in the less severe illnesses, to the initial consultation and giving an erroneous impression of how often it is a sequel. Similar findings were not evident among men.

Elderly patients with paranoid psychoses are significantly more often deaf especially with severe middle ear disease than are age- and sex-matched patients with affective psychoses. Deafness may owe its pathogenicity to the isolation it imposes which is not as apparent in patients who have visual defects (Cooper *et al.*, 1976).

The immediate adverse psychological consequences of amputation may not be conspicuous in younger patients following trauma. In older patients, with co-existing peripheral and cerebrovascular disease, confusional and delirious states are often encountered in the post-operative period. Some degree of depression is noted by nurses in almost every patient. Predictive or poor long-term adjustment to amputation, as the patient learns to live with a prosthesis and leave hospital to take up family, occupational, social and sexual life again, are inadequacies in these spheres pre-operatively, but prolonged illness or multiple operations before amputation, life- or limb-threatening illness following it, rigidity and/or compulsive self-reliance, a heroic post-operative period, and stump or phantom pain within three weeks of operation also all predict poor outcome. A realistic yet determined approach to convalescence, in spite of some sadness, appears healthiest (Parkes, 1973).

Late consequences include prolonged pain in phantom and/or stump for which no local cause can be found. Such pain appears more likely if there has been prolonged pre-operative pain from, for example, osteomyelitis or ischaemia and is particularly resistant to treatment including neuronal section even as far up as the thalamus. Treatment by such physical manoeuvres as vibration or distraction have been only modestly successful (Morganstern, 1970). The emergence of pain in stump or phantom long after amputation strongly suggests depression and sometimes responds well to antidepressants. Such pain, while most often seen in those who have made a poor adjustment to limb loss (and believed by some patients to be responsible for that poor adjustment), is sometimes seen in highly successful amputees. It can be very resistant to any therapeutic intervention.

An excess of depressive disorder is seen in hysterectomized patients—for example, two and a half times more frequently than after cholecystectomy in women (Barker, 1968). Previous psychiatric disorder and alcoholism were indicators of poor outcome. It has been suggested that patients who come for hysterectomy and are found to have no distinct uterine pathology have measurable psychiatric disorder—perhaps contributing to their presentation for surgery (Ross and Tyrer, 1976).

The consequences of termination of pregnancy remain contested. Some believe there are no psychiatric grounds for the procedure and that the greater the apparent psychiatric indications the more likely are psychiatric complications, with post-abortive psychoses apparently carrying a worse prognosis than puerperal ones (Sim, 1968). Estimates of patients' regret and guilt following termination range between 25 and 51% in earlier decades (Ekblad, 1961; Seigfried, 1951). Attitudes to the procedure seem to determine whether psychiatric sequelae are found and these may have been changing in recent years.

One prospective study (Lask, 1973) looked at the six months following termination with the finding that about two-thirds of patients showed a favourable outcome. Psychiatric sequelae in the other third correlated with desertion by the partner, age 21–30, multiparity, a previous psychiatric history, being farm-born and having distinct ambivalence about the operation.

Three hundred and sixty women were followed after first trimester termination of pregnancy performed in accordance with the British 1967 Abortion Act. 'Interpreted liberally' this allows the procedure if continued pregnancy is judged likely to risk injury to mother's mental health. Sixty per cent of the women were available for follow-up a mean of 18 months after termination and were reported to be improved in psychosocial and sexual adjustment with adverse sequelae rare. Whether the untraced 40% would differ was, of course, unknown (Greer *et al.*, 1976).

Following myocardial infarction the patient's perception of his disability, measured by self-report and, indirectly, by how soon he returns to work, is often inconsonant with his cardiologist's appraisal. Severely breathless or anginal older patients may return to work early and see themselves as relatively fit especially if of higher socio-economic standing and with good previous work records. Unskilled and semi-skilled men with poor work records before infarction, are more likely to be off work for prolonged periods and report marked disability in the absence of objective evidence of it (Cay *et al.*, 1973).

Ninety per cent of patients who came to gastric surgery because of complications like haemorrhage, stenosis, perforation and penetration do well following it. Of those who had surgery for intractable pain only 60% do well and the remaining patients tolerate dumping and discomfort badly (Small and Cay, 1973). The notion of 'earning' gastric surgery by years of pain did not help in predicting who will do well with operations but marked personality disorder, salicylate dependency, alcoholism and high neuroticism predict a poor response as do the patients' reports before operation of poor maternal warmth towards them in childhood and their current perceived 'emotional deprivation' (Thoroughman *et al.*, 1964; Pascal *et al.*, 1966; McColl, 1964).

The consequences of illness are not limited to the patient. The family are usually involved, and in many illnesses this will carry management implications easy to overlook. Children with a parent who has a severe chronic disability have behaviour disorders above expectation (Rutter, 1962). Marriages of patients on chronic haemodialysis are markedly abnormal, patient-centred with high tension, poor communication and unvoiced hostility (Maurin and Schenkel, 1975).

The important point is that many illness-consequences are predictable from the illness-precursors. Hence the indistinct edging of the domains pictured in Fig. 1.

Summary

Some of the facets of psychiatry in a general hospital setting have been described. The advantages and disadvantages of psychiatric units in such hospitals are outlined together with some of the factors that lead to psychiatric consultation in the physically ill. The principal domains into which the psychiatrist working in this setting will find himself drawn are indicated—with those whose psychiatric experience has been gained elsewhere specially in mind.

References

Ackerman, S. H. and Weiner, H. (1976). *In* 'Modern Trends in Psychosomatic Medicine' (Ed. O. W. Hill), Vol. 3. Butterworths, London.

Anstee, B. H. (1972a). Psychiatry in the casualty department. *Br. J. Psychiat.* **120**, 625–629.

Anstee, B. H. (1972b). The problem of psychosomatic referrals in a general hospital. *Br. J. Psychiat.* **120**, 631–634.

Bancroft, J., Skrimshire, A., Casson, J., Harvard-Watts, O. and Reynolds, F. (1977). People who deliberately poison or injure themselves. *Psychol. Med.* **7**, 289–303.

Biörck, G., Blomquist, G. and Stevens, J. (1958). Studies on myocardial infarction in Malmö, 1935–1954. *Acta Med. Scand.* **161**, 21–32.

Blackwell, B. (1968). The Munchausen syndrome. *Br. J. Hosp. Med.* **1**, 98–105.

Bortner, R. W., Rosenman, R. H. and Friedman, M. (1970). Familial similarity in pattern A behaviour: father and sons. *J. Chron. Dis.* **23**, 39–43.

Brady, J. V. (1958). Ulcers in 'executive monkeys'. *Sci. Am.* **199**, 95–100.

Brown, G. W. and Birley, J. C. T. (1968). Crises and life changes and the onset of schizophrenia. *J. Hlth Soc. Behav.* **9**, 203–214.

Brown, G. W. and Harris, T. (1978). 'Social Origins of Depression'. Tavistock, London.

Brown, G. W., Sklair, F., Harris, T. O. and Birley, J. L. T. (1973a). Life events and psychiatric disorders, Part 1. *Psychol. Med.* **3**, 74–87.

Brown, G. W., Harris, T. O. and Peto, J. (1973b). Life events and psychiatric disorders, Part 2. *Psychol. Med.* **3**, 159–176.

Cadie, M., Nye, F. J. and Storey, P. (1976). Anxiety and depression after infectious mononucleosis. *Br. J. Psychiat.* **128**, 559–561.

Carroll, B. J. (1976). Psychoendocrine relationships in affective disorders. *In* 'Modern Trends in Psychosomatic Medicine' (Ed. O. W. Hill), Vol. 3. Butterworths, London.

Cassem, N. H. and Stewart, R. S. (1977). Management and care of the dying patient. *In* 'Psychosomatic Medicine' (Eds Z. J. Lipowski, D. R. Lipsitt and P. C. Whybrow). Oxford University Press, New York.

Cay, E. L., Vetter, N., Philip, A., and Dugard, P. (1973). Return to work after a heart attack. *J. Psychosom. Res.* **17**, 231–243.

Chesser, E. S. (1975). Psychosocial reactions to investigation and treatment of organic disease. *Medicine* **10**, 447–452.

Clancy, R. E., Truslson, M. F. and Hegsted, D. M. (1963). Comparison of Irish-born Bostonians with their brothers living in Ireland. Conf. Cardiovascular Disease Epidemiology, Chicago.

Connolly, J. (1974). Stress and coronary artery disease. *Br. J. Hosp. Med.* **11**, 297–302.

Connolly, J. (1976). Life events before myocardial infarction. *J. Hum. Stress* **2**, No. 4, 3–17.

Connolly, J., Hallam, R. S. and Marks, I. M. (1976). Selective association of fainting with blood-injury-illness fear. *Behav. Ther.* **7**, 8–13.

Cooper, A. F., Garside, R. F. and Kay, D. W. K. (1976). A comparison of deaf and non-deaf patients with paranoid and affective psychoses. *Br. J. Psychiat.* **129**, 532–538.

Crisp, A. H. (1968). The role of the psychiatrist in a general hospital. *Postgrad. Med. J.* **44**, 267–276.

Crisp, A. H. (1970). Psychological aspects of some disorders of weight. In 'Modern Trends in Psychosomatic Medicine' (Ed. O. W. Hill), Vol. 2. Butterworths, London.

Dally, P. J. and Gomez, J. (1977). Psychologically mediated abdominal pain in surgical and medical out patient clinics. Br. Med. J. 1, 1451–1453.

Eastwood, M. R. (1975). 'The Relation Between Physical and Mental Illness'. University of Toronto Press, Toronto.

Eastwood, M. R. and Trevelyan, M. H. (1972). Relationship between physical and psychiatric disorder. Psychol. Med. 2, 363–372.

Ekblad, M. (1955). Induced abortion on psychiatric grounds. Acta. Psychiat. Neurol. Scand., Suppl. 99.

Engel, G. L. (1975). In 'American Handbook of Psychiatry' (Ed. S. Arieti), Vol. 4, p. 669. Basic Books, New York.

Epstein, F. H. (1967). Predicting coronary heart disease. J.A.M.A. 201, 795–800.

Feigenberg, L. (1975). Care and understanding of the dying: a patient-centred approach. Omega 6, 81–89.

Forrest, A. J. and Wolkind, S. N. (1974). Masked depression in association with low back pain. Rheum. Rehab. 13, 148–153.

French, J. D., Porter, R. W., Cavanagh, E. B. and Longmire, R. L. (1957). Experimental gastroduodenal lesions induced by stimulation of the brain. Psychosom. Med. 19, 209–220.

Friedman, M. and Rosenman, R. H. (1959). Association of a specific overt behavioral pattern with blood and cardiovascular findings, J.A.M.A. 169, 1286–1296.

Glaser, B. G. and Spanes, A. L. (1968). 'Time for Dying'. Aldine, Chicago.

Gordon, T. (1967). Further mortality experience among Japanese Americans. Pub. Hlth Rpt 82, 973–984.

Greer, H. S., Lal, S., Lewis, S. C., Belsey, E. M. and Beard, R. W. (1976). Psychiatric sequelae of therapeutic abortion. Br. J. Psychiat. 128, 74–79.

Greer, S. and Parsons, V. (1968). Schizophrenia-like psychosis in thyroid crisis. Br. J. Psychiat. 114, 1357–1362.

Gurney, C., Roth, M. and Harper, M. (1966). Quoted in Mayer Gross, W., Slater, E. and Roth, M. 'Clinical Psychiatry' (1969), p. 96. Baillière, Tindall and Cassell, London.

Heller, S. S. and Kornfeld, D. S. (1975). In 'American Handbook of Psychiatry' (Ed. S. Arieti). Basic Books, New York.

Henry, J. P. and Cassel, J. C. (1969). Psychological factors in essential hypertension. Am. J. Epidemiol. 90, 171–200.

Hinkle, L. E. and Wolff, H. G. (1957). The nature of man's adaptation to his total environment and the relation of this to illness. Arch. Int. Med. 99, 442–460.

Hinton, J. (1976). Approaching death. In 'Modern Trends in Psychosomatic Medicine' (Ed. O. W. Hill), Vol. 3. Butterworths, London.

Hinton, J. M. (1975). The influence of previous personality on reactions to having terminal cancer. Omega 6, 95–102.

Holmes, T. H. and Rahe, R. H. (1967). The social readjustment rating scale. J. Psychosom. Res. 11, 213–218.

Illingworth, C. F. W., Scott, L. D. W. and Jamieson, R. A. (1944). Acute perforated ulcer: frequency and incidence in the West of Scotland. Br. Med. J. 2, 617–623, 655–658.

Jenkins, C. D. (1971). Psychological and social precursors of coronary disease. N.E.J.M. 284, 244–255, 307–317.

Jenkins, C. D. (1976). Recent evidence supporting psychological and social risk factors for coronary disease. *N.E.J.M.* **294**, 987–994, 1033–1038.

Kaufman, M. R. (Ed.) (1965). 'The Psychiatric Unit in the General Hospital'. International Universities Press, New York.

Kendell, R. E. (1974). A new look at hysteria. *Medicine* (1st ser.) 1780–1783.

Kendell, R. E., Wainwright, S., Hailey, A and Shannon, B. (1976). The influence of childbirth on psychiatric morbidity. *Psychol. Med.* **6**, 297–302.

Kenyon, F. E. (1964). Hypochondriasis—a clinical study. *Br. J. Psychiat.* **110**, 478–488.

Kenyon, F. E. (1976). Hypochondriacal states. *Br. J. Psychiat.* **129**, 1–14.

Keys, A., Aravanis, C. and Blackburn, H. (1972). Probability of middle aged men developing coronary heart disease in five years. *Circulation* **45**, 815–828.

Khan, A. U., Bonk, C. and Gordon, Y. (1974). Non-allergic asthma and the conditioning process. *Ann. Allergy* **32**, 245–254.

Kidson, M. A. (1973). Personality and hypertension. *J. Psychosom. Res.* **17**, 35–41.

Kornfeld, D. S. L., Zimberg, S. and Malm, J. R. (1965). Psychiatric complications of open heart surgery. *N.E.J.M.* **273**, 287–292.

Kübler-Ross, E. (1970). 'On Death and Dying'. Tavistock, London.

Kumar, R. and Robson, K. (1978). Neurotic disorders in pregnancy and the puerperium. *In* 'Mental Illness in Pregnancy and the Puerperium' (Ed. M. Sandler). Oxford University Press, Oxford.

Lask, B. (1975). Short term psychiatric sequelae to therapeutic termination of pregnancy. *Br. J. Psychiat.* **12**, 173–177.

Lebovitz, B. Z., Shekelle, R. B., Ostfeld, A. M. and Paul, O. (1967). Prospective and retrospective psychological studies of coronary heart disease. *Psychosom. Med.* **29**, 265–272.

Lewis, A. (1954). Aspects of psychosomatic medicine. *Recenti Progressi in Medicina* **16**, 434–453.

Lipowski, Z. J. (1968). Review of consultation psychiatry and psychosomatic medicine. *Psychosom. Med.* **29**, 153–171, **29**, 201–224, **30**, 395–422.

Lipowski, Z. J. (1976). *In* 'Modern Trends in Pychosomatic Medicine' (Ed. O. W. Hill), Vol. 3, p. 16. Butterworths, London.

Lipowski, Z. J. (1977). Psychosomatic medicine in the seventies: an overview. *Am. J. Psychiat.* **134**, 233–244.

Little, J. C. (1974). 'Psychiatry in a General Hospital'. Butterworths, London.

Lloyd, G. G. (1977). Psychological reactions to physical illness. *Br. J. Hosp. Med.* **18**, 352–358.

Lloyd, G. G. and Deakin, G. (1975). Phobias complicating treatment of uterine carcinoma. *Br. Med. J.* **4**, 440.

Lum, L. C. (1976). The syndrome of habitual chronic hyperventilation. *In* 'Modern Trends in Psychosomatic Medicine' (Ed. O. W. Hill), Vol. 3. Butterworths, London.

Luparello, T., Lyons, H. A., Bleecker, E. R. and McFadden, E. R. (1968). Influences of suggestion on airway reactivity in asthmatic subjects. *Psychosom. Med.* **30**, 819–825.

Maltsberger, J. T. and Buie, D. H. (1974). Counter transference hate in the treatment of suicidal patients. *Arch. Gen. Psychiat.* **30**, 625–633.

Mann, A. (1977). The psychological effect of a screening programme and clinical trial for hypertension upon participants. *Psychol. Med.* **7**, 431–438.

Marks, I. M., Hallam, R. S., Connolly, J. and Philpot, R. (1976). 'Nurses in Behavioural Psychotherapy'. Royal College of Nurses, London.

Maurin, J. and Schenkel, J. (1975). A study of the family unit's response to haemodialysis. *J. Psychosom. Res.* **20**, 163–168.

McColl, D. (1964). Peptic ulceration and work. *Trans. Ass. Indust. Med. Offrs.* **14**, 20–23.

Mechanic, D. (1962). The concept of illness behaviour. *J. Chron. Dis.* **15**, 189–197.

Merrison, A. W. (1975). Report of the Committee of Inquiry into the Regulation of the Medical Profession. HMSO, London.

Merski, H. and Spear, F. G. (1967). 'Pain: Psychological and Psychiatric Aspects'. Baillière, Tindall and Cassell, London.

Mertens, C. and Seegers, M. J. (1971). *In* 'Neural and Psychological Mechanisms in Cardiovascular Disease' (Ed. A. Zanchetti). Casa Editrice, Milano.

Morganstern, F. S. (1970). *In* 'Modern Trends in Psychosomatic Medicine' (Ed. O. W. Hill), Vol. 2. Butterworths, London.

Murray, R. (1973). The origins of analgesic nephropathy. *Br. J. Psychiat.* **123**, 99–106.

Neary, D. (1976). Neuropsychiatric sequelae of renal failure. *Br. J. Hosp. Med.* **15**, 122–130.

Parkes, C. M. (1973). Factors determining the persistence of phantom pain in the amputee. *J. Psychosom. Res.* **17**, 97–108.

Parkes, C. M., Benjamin, B. and Fitzgerald, R. G. (1969). Broken heart: a statistical study of increased mortality among widowers. *Br. Med. J.* **1**, 740–743.

Parsons, T. (1952). 'The Social System'. Free Press, New York.

Pascal, G. R., Thoroughman, J. C., Harvis, J. R. and Jenkins, W. O. (1966). Early history variables in predicting surgical success for intractable duodenal ulcer patients. *Psychosom. Med.* **28**, 207–215.

Pattison, E. M. (1975). Help in the dying process. *In* 'American Handbook of Psychiatry' (Ed. S. Arieti). Basic Books, New York.

Paykel, E. S. and Moffic, H. S. (1975). Depression in medical in-patients. *Br. J. Psychiat.* **126**, 346–353.

Pitt, B. (1968). 'Atypical' depression following childbirth. *Br. J. Psychiat.* **114**, 1325–1335.

Purcell, K., Biddy, K., Chai, H., Muser, J., Molk, L., Gordon, N. and Mears, J. (1969). The effect on asthmatic children of experimental separation from the family. *Psychosom. Med.* **31**, 144–164.

Rahe, R. H., Romo, M., Bennett, L. and Siltanen, P. (1974). Subjects' recent life changes and sudden death in Helsinki. *Arch. Int. Med.* **133**, 221–239.

Reed, J. L. (1975). Hysteria. *Br. J. Hosp. Med.* **5**, 237–247.

Rees, W. L. (1976). Stress, distress and disease. *Br. J. Psychiat.* **128**, 3–18.

Rees, W. D. and Lutkins, S. G. (1967). Mortality of bereavement. *Br. Med. J.* **4**, 13–16.

Rosenman, R. H., Friedman, M., Strauss, L., Jenkins, C. D., Zyzanski, S. J. and Wurm, M. (1970). *J. Chron. Dis.* **23**, 173–187.

Ross, J. and Tyrer, S. (1976). *In* 'Psychosexual Problems' (Eds H. Milne and S. Hardy). Crosby Lockwood Staples Press, St Albans.

Rutter, M. L. (1962). Illness in Patients and Children, pp. 207–224. M.D. Thesis, University of Birmingham.

Shekelle, R. B., Ostfeld, A. M. and Paul, O. (1969). Social status and the incidence of coronary heart disease. *J. Chron. Dis.* **22**, 381–394.

Shepherd, M., Cooper, B., Brown, N. C. and Kalton, G. W. (1966). 'Psychiatric Illness in General Practice'. Oxford University Press, Oxford.

Siegfried, S. (1951). Psychiatrische Untersuchungen über die Folgen der

Kunstlichen Schwangerschaftsunter-brechung. *Schweiz Arch. Neurol. Psychiat.* **67**, 365–369.

Sim, M. (1968). 'Guide to Psychiatry', p. 893. Livingstone, Edinburgh.

Slater, E. (1965). Diagnosis of 'hysteria'. *Br. Med. J.* **1**, 1395–1399.

Small, W. P. and Cay, E. L. (1973). Emotional aspects of peptic ulcer surgery. *In* 'Emotional Factors in Gastrointestinal Illness' (Ed. A. E. Lindner). American Elsevier Co., New York.

Sternbach, R. A. (1977). Psychophysiology of pain. *In* 'Psychosomatic Medicine' (Eds Z. J. Lipowski, D. R. Lipsitt, and P. C. Whybrow). Oxford University Press, New York.

Stroebel, C. F. (1969). *In* 'Circadian Rhythms in Non-Human Primates' (Ed. F. H. Rohles). Bibliotheca Primatologica 9, Karger, Basle.

Syme, S. L., Hyman, M. M. and Enterline, P. E. (1964). *J. Chron. Dis.* **17**, 277–289.

Theorell, T. (1970). 'Psychosocial Factors in Relation to the Onset of Myocardial Infarction'. Karolinska Institutet, Stockholm, Sweden.

Theorell, T. and Rahe, R. H. (1971). Psychosocial factors and myocardial infarction: I An inpatient study in Sweden. *J. Psychosom. Res.* **15**, 25–31.

Theorell, T., Lind, E. and Floderus, B. (1975). The relationship of disturbing life changes and emotions to the early development of myocardial infarction and some other serious illnesses. *Rév. Epidem. Santé Publ.* **24**, 41–59.

Thoroughman, J. C., Pascal, G. R., Jenkins, W. O., Crutcher, J. C. and Peoples, I. C. (1964). Psychological factors predictive of surgical success in patients with intractable duodenal ulcer. *Psychosom. Med.* **26**, 618–624.

Tibblin, G., Lindstrom, B. and Ander, S. (1972). *In* 'Physiology, Emotion and Psychosomatic Illness' (Ed. R. Porter). Elsevier Excepta Medica, North Holland.

Tyroler, H. A. and Cassel, J. (1964). Health consequences of culture change. *J. Chron. Dis.* **17**, 167–178.

Wardwell, W. I., Hyman, M. and Bahnson, C. B. (1964). Stress and coronary heart disease in three field studies. *J. Chron. Dis.* **17**, 73–84.

Watson, J. P., Bennett, D. H. and Isaacs, A. D. (1970). Psychiatric units in general hospitals. *Lancet* **1**, 511–514.

Weiner, H. (1972). Some comments on the transduction of experience by the brain. *Psychosom. Med.* **34**, 355–380.

Weiner, H., Thaler, M., Reiser, and Mirsky, I. A. (1959). Etiology of duodenal ulcer. *Psychosom. Med.* **19**, 1–10.

Weiss, J. M. (1968). Effects of coping responses on stress. *J. Comp. Physiol. Psychol.* **65**, 251–260.

Wolkind, S. N. (1976). Psychogenic low back pain. *Br. J. Hosp. Med.* **15**, 17–24.

19 The basis of drug treatment in psychiatry

Peter Tyrer

Kipling once said that words were the most powerful drug used by mankind and one might surmise that words about drugs would be the most powerful of all. Certainly over the past thirty years there has been no shortage of words, most of them polysyllabic, about the subject which is now dignified by the name of clinical psychopharmacology. I shall not attempt to ape the many excellent and comprehensive accounts of the subject (Shepherd, *et al.*, 1968; Joyce, 1968; Silverstone and Turner, 1974; Lader, 1976; Simpson, 1976) and in this chapter shall try to illustrate the scope of the subject and its relevance to clinical psychiatry. The aims of clinical psychopharmacology are fairly simple and can be expressed in words of one syllable:
(a) to find out which drugs are good for ills of the mind and which are not (efficacy);
(b) to make sure drugs are safe (safety—including drug and other interactions);
(c) to note the changes caused by drugs in man (pharmacodynamics);
(d) to find out what goes on when drugs pass in and out of the body (pharmacokinetics);
(e) to use drugs to find out how ills are caused (investigation).
These aims are basically the same as those of clinical pharmacology and therapeutics in medicine but it is only recently that clinical psychopharmacology has attained respectability in psychiatry. There are several reasons for this delayed maturity, but perhaps the most important is that the track record of the subject is hardly an impressive one. Not a single advance in drug treatment has been made by design; they have all come

by accident, or to use the synonym of the moment, serendipity. A clinician has used a drug for the treatment of psychiatric patients, usually on quite false theoretical grounds, and found clinical effects that he had never predicted. Such is the stuff of advance in many medical disciplines but when all advances are made in this way it is fair to doubt the scientific status of the subject. Nevertheless, it would be wrong to assume that there is no need for clinical psychopharmacologists. The late Dr Henry Miller once described the good psychiatrist as a superlative physician (Miller, 1967), a paragon with such acumen that he could detect all organic illness presenting in his patients even when it presented in a psychological guise. Few would argue with this as an ideal, but it could never become commonplace. Similarly, it may be ideal for every psychiatrist to be a trained psychopharmacologist, but this can never be achieved in practice. Even if further advances in drug treatment are made by accident, we need the clinical psychopharmacologist to dot the 'i's' and cross the 't's' following the discovery, to make sure that the advance is used to its full effect and that any untoward dangers are immediately recognized. It took many years to progress from the initial evidence that lithium carbonate controlled manic excitement (Cade, 1949) to the conclusion that the compound was not only effective in controlling hypomania but also preventing relapse in manic-depressive psychosis (Melia, 1970; Coppen *et al.*, 1971; Hullin *et al.*, 1972). It is doubtful whether this could have been achieved without careful attention to monitoring plasma levels and detailed evaluation of the drug's effects by workers well versed in clinical psychopharmacology.

The subject also has to cope with other critics, many of whom are within psychiatry and have powerful voices. One which is now heard more faintly claims that drugs are ineffective and merely place the patient in a chemical strait-jacket which prevents other treatments from being used effectively. It is hard to see how any impartial observer looking at treatment in psychiatry today could conclude that the sum effect of drug treatments in psychiatry has been an adverse one. Drugs are the most effective symptomatic treatment available and the main doubts revolve round their long-term effects and whether or not they produce good personal and social adjustment. Nevertheless there is good evidence that, once symptomatic improvement has occurred, the patient is more amenable to psychotherapy (Klerman *et al.*, 1974).

Another criticism of the use of drugs for the treatment of mental disorders runs something like this. 'We do not know how drugs work and we are ignorant of many of the changes that occur in mental disorders. As the brain is such a complex organ it is wrong to interfere with its function unless we are absolutely sure of a drug's mechanism of action.' If this anti-empirical standpoint was adhered to closely no psychotropic drugs would be prescribed at all. In practice all drugs are used before full knowledge of their mechanism of action is known and apart from conditions such as pernicious anaemia and scurvy for which treatment involves replacement of a naturally occurring bodily substance all drug treatments have an element of the unknown about them. Argument still revolves around the mechanism of action of aspirin, even though it has been in clinical use for nearly a century.

The most serious difficulty in judging the use of drug treatment in psychiatry is our ignorance of the aetiology of most mental disorders. It is logical to treat a patient whose symptoms are all due to poor cardiac function with digoxin, a drug which improves the efficiency of the heart, but to treat a patient with depression with an antidepressive drug can only be justified if depression is regarded as an illness in its own right. If convincing evidence can be produced that depression is merely a symptom of an underlying disturbance then the argument that symptomatic treatment just masks the real problem carries much more weight. In its simplest form, most psychiatric symptoms can be postulated to be hysterical (Bonhoeffer, 1911). The patient responds to intolerable conflict by 'splitting off' symptoms which are presented to the psychiatrist for treatment. Concentration of treatment on symptom removal merely colludes with the patient and is counter-productive. Any symptom which is removed is soon replaced by a different symptom as the underlying conflict remains unresolved. The Freudian concept of 'symptom substitution' is an excellent example of an explanation that is so plausible that it is accepted as true. Careful investigations into the phenomenon have failed entirely to validate the concept (Marks, 1971; Feather and Rhoads 1972) and any apparently new symptoms turn out to be the emergence of old ones (Crisp, 1966). It is better to take an agnostic view of symptom formation, 'the mechanisms by which symptoms develop are an attribute of the human make-up, and to show that they are at work is not to explain their appearance' (Sargant and Slater, 1954). Drug treatment alleviates, suppresses or removes symptoms, and provided that this is not equated with cure, it can be justified if it relieves suffering, restores normal function and does no harm. If clinical psychiatrists are to use drugs effectively, however, they must be given judiciously and with at least a passing knowledge of their pharmacological actions and therapeutic spectra. The abuse of psychotropic drugs by doctors and patients alike is now common knowledge and if we are not to be indicted as doctors who 'pour drugs of which they know little, to treat diseases of which they know less, into human beings of whom they know nothing' (Stevens, 1974) we need to be rational in our therapies. In the rest of this chapter I hope to show that the aims of clinical psychopharmacology can help to achieve this.

Efficacy

No subject is likely to arouse greater argument in psychiatry than the best way to establish the effectiveness of a treatment procedure. Most psychiatric conditions have variable natural histories and any improvement over time may depend on several factors, of which the treatment given by a doctor is only one. Nowadays doctors will not accept that treatment X is effective merely because doctor Y has administered it to one or more patients and found improvement. The statement that, for example, 80% of patients improve on a specific treatment gives no useful information and can be positively misleading if the same percentage of patients improve if they receive no treatment whatsoever. The standard way of allowing for extraneous factors is to compare specific treatments under a controlled evaluative procedure, the double-blind clinical trial. Although the merits and demerits of this approach are widely discussed throughout all therapeutics there are several aspects that are more specific to psychiatry. Some of the criticisms of the double-blind procedure are given below and in answering them one can judge the place of this approach in determining the value of a drug therapy.

(i) 'It fails to prove what everyone knows.' At the outset it must be made clear that a double-blind therapeutic trial is not carried out to prove the efficacy of a treatment. It does the opposite; it tests the null hypothesis that there is no difference between the effectiveness of two or more treatments. If the results show differences which are statistically significant the null hypothesis has to be discarded, but only for the treatments given under the conditions of the trial. Thus, treatment X may be shown to be superior to treatment Y in a study, but only when given for a set period in a certain dose. When fun is poked at the results of several controlled trials of a treatment because they contradict each other it is often found that the results differ because the conditions of treatment also differed. For example, in 12 controlled trials of the monoamine oxidase inhibitor, phenelzine, and placebo in the treatment of depressive and phobic disorders six showed phenelzine to be superior and six found no difference between phenelzine and placebo. Retrospective analysis of these trials showed that dose and duration were important variables in determining clinical response, the higher the dose and the longer the duration of the treatment the greater the efficacy of the active drug (Tyrer, 1976a).

(ii) 'The principles of medical ethics prevent (orthomolecular) psychiatrists from withholding from half their patients a treatment that they consider to be valuable. Controlled tests can be carried out only by skeptics.' This statement (Pauling, 1974) was made by the famous molecular biologist, Linus Pauling, whose advocacy of orthomolecular treatment in psychiatry is well known (Pauling, 1968). It shows that misconceptions about controlled trials are not confined to non-scientists. Controlled trials can be carried out by anyone who is prepared to put their beliefs to the test, however strong those beliefs happen to be. The ethical consideration frequently confuses belief and knowledge. It may be unethical to give a known inferior treatment to a patient but not one which is merely believed to be inferior. Those who feel strongly that a placebo control is unethical in a drug trial may not be aware how powerful are its therapeutic effects (Beecher, 1955), and it is chastening to remind ourselves that the 'history of medical treatment is the history of the placebo effect' (Shapiro, 1959). Unfortunately perhaps, it is only those who become involved in controlled trials who are reminded of the extent of this effect. When patients severely handicapped by chronic agoraphobia become almost symptom-free after eight weeks of placebo treatment and remain well two years later (Tyrer and Steinberg, 1975) one develops a new respect for the dummy pill.

With the acceptance of the principles of controlled evaluation it could now be regarded as unethical not to carry out a double-blind study of a new treatment soon after open clinical studies have indicated that it may be of value. True, any treatment, if genuinely effective, will be recognized as such in the fullness of time no matter how poorly designed were its original studies, but the speed of acceptance is greatly accelerated if properly designed trials are performed at the outset. When Professor Joseph Lister asked his houseman, Dr McFie, to place a strip of lint soaked in carbolic acid over the open fracture of a young boy in June 1863, he could not have predicted that it would take sixteen years before the principles of antiseptic surgery became accepted (at the Sixth International Medical Congress at Amsterdam). One can predict with some confidence that if a properly designed trial comparing antiseptic techniques with traditional methods was carried out soon after Lister's discovery then much of the succeeding controversy would never have taken place. Indeed, a leading article in 1867 asked for confirmation of Lister's findings 'by experiment and observation' (*Lancet*, 1867) at just the time when a controlled trial would have been appropriate. Not to carry out a controlled trial may produce unnecessary delay. As Sir Austin Bradford Hill has commented (1966) 'the process of (clinical) learning might be a little less long if it were supported by the experimental method and attitude of mind' and, provided that these attitudes enjoy a healthy symbiosis with clinical observation the results can only be of value to patients.

(iii) 'We are never going to learn how to treat depression properly from double-blind sampling in an MRC statistician's office' (Sargant, 1965). I was working as a psychiatric house physician when this observation was made, and at the time I thoroughly approved of it. After all, it has face validity; how can a statistician compete with a clinician on the latter's territory? The mistake is to assume that the two are in competition. In the healthy symbiosis referred to above the two work closely, the qualitative observations made by the clinician on individual patients being converted to quantitative data by the statistician (or clinician) in a way that allows comparison between groups. Provided that the data conversion is done properly none of the clinician's expertise is lost. The generalization from the individual to the throng worries many psychiatrists because of the complexity of human behaviour. The controlled trial is criticized because, to paraphrase Tennyson,

> So careful of the group it seems
> So careless of the single case.

Although there is a place in psychiatry for the careful study of individual patients it is mandatory to study groups of patients with similar disorders before any predictions about the efficacy of a treatment can be made. If homogeneity can be achieved in the selection of patients for study then a controlled trial is feasible. Homogeneity involves selection, which depends on sound classification of the disorders under study. Unfortunately psychiatry has only recently begun to get its diagnostic house in order, and much of the argument about efficacy revolves around selection procedures. For example, Dr Sargant's above comment was made in response to the findings of a multi-centre controlled trial carried out under the auspices of the Medical Research Council, which showed that in depressed in-patients ECT was significantly superior to imipramine and that both these treatments were superior to placebo and the mono-amine oxidase inhibitor, phenelzine (Medical Research Council, 1965). Phenelzine (and other MAOIs) had been claimed by Dr Sargant and others to be a valuable treatment of depression, anxiety neurosis, and phobic anxiety (West and Dally, 1959; Rees and Davies, 1961; Sargant and Dally, 1962; Sargant and Slater, 1964), and its poor showing in the MRC trial (it was less effective than placebo in women) led to Dr Sargant's indictment. What was at fault was not the controlled trial nor even the statisticians employed by the MRC, but the poor state of classification of depressive disorders. In retrospect, the MRC trial was correct in its findings for depressed in-patients, and Dr Sargant was also correct in regarding phenelzine as effective in different populations, the characteristics of which have been shown by others in controlled trials (Lipsedge et al., 1973; Robinson et al., 1973; Solyom et al., 1973; Tyrer et al., 1973; Ravaris et al., 1976).

(iv) 'It is not possible to gain a valid evaluation of a drug, and eliminate the clinical skill and judgement of the investigator, just as it is not possible to obtain a valid picture of the effectiveness of psychoanalysis without considering the clinical skill of the analyst' (Barsa, 1963). This is a common criticism of the controlled trial, and is particularly popular among those who claim that psychiatry is primarily an art rather than a science. It has no substance, for controlled evaluation can account for clinical skill, judgement and innumerable other factors that are not the main purpose of the investigation. It may be that a drug used in the hands of a certain physician may account for only 10% of the clinical improvement shown by a group of patients; personal charisma, spontaneous improvement, placebo effect and psychotherapy accounting for the remainder. This does not make a controlled trial invalid, it merely means that many more patients will need to be studied before significant differences in efficacy will be demonstrated between active drug and a placebo. Some are quite happy to compare drug therapy in this way but feel that the psychotherapies are sacrosanct. There is no logic in this, it is just that the achievement of double-blind procedure is much more difficult with these treatments. Controlled studies are now well established in behaviour therapy (Marks and Gelder, 1968; Feldman and McCulloch, 1971; Crowe, 1976), and it is equally feasible to compare the effectiveness of formal psychotherapy under controlled conditions. It is problems of selection rather than inadequacy of trial design that has prevented this being exploited fully (Candy *et al.*, 1972). Some recent studies in the United States have successfully compared drug therapy, psychotherapy and social therapies under carefully controlled conditions. The comparison has favoured drug therapy in the treatment of schizophrenia (Hogarty *et al.*, 1973; Chien, 1976) and depressive illness (Covi *et al.*, 1974; Klerman *et al.*, 1974), although in the long term social adjustment appears to be helped more by psychotherapy (Weissman *et al.*, 1974; Weissman, 1976). Intelligent combinations of these different treatments are usually the most effective (Klerman, 1976; May, 1976).

I have dwelt at length on the controlled trial because psychopharmacology deserves most of the credit for introducing it to psychiatry. Despite its many critics, it is now an established part of the evaluation of treatment. Acceptance of this should not blind us to its limitations. The controlled trial is excellent in testing hypotheses, but poor in generating them. Most major advances in this quarter are made by isolated observations which lead to a major reappraisal of accepted views. Many of these observations are made by gifted observers, and others by cranks who produce one good idea among a hundred nonsensical ones. The initial stages of an important discovery are radical and anti-Establishment. The controlled trial is very pro-Establishment; the careful examination of hypotheses by a group of trained investigators using accepted procedures. It is wasteful of time and personnel (Joyce, 1968) and the road to completion can be a hazardous one (Blackwell and Shepherd, 1967). It leads to the shuffling advance of knowledge instead of the giant stride. Nevertheless, it is a necessary antidote to a subject which has never been short on theory but has often failed to deliver the facts. The pace of the shuffler may seem interminably slow, but, like the sapper in a minefield, it is better to be absolutely certain of the territory ahead before moving forward. The controlled trial is also of major importance in aiding the widespread use of a new treatment. It transforms personal knowledge to the body of accepted knowledge, and does so much more quickly than the trial-and-error approaches of the past. Its advocates echo the words of Konrad Lorenz (1966),

> the scientist knows very well that he is approaching ultimate truth in an asymptotic curve and is barred from ever reaching it; but at the same time he is proudly aware of being indeed able to determine whether a statement is a nearer or less near approach to truth. This determination is not furnished by any personal opinion nor by the authority of an individual, but by further research proceeding by rules universally accepted by all men of all cultures and all political affiliations.

Safety

The dictum 'primum non nocere' applies to all treatment, and a completely effective drug is of no value if it carries dangers. Toxicology is a major part of pharmacology and before any drug can be released for general clinical use it needs approval from the Committee on Safety of Medicines in Britain (or the Foods and Drugs Administration in the United States). Many toxic compounds are detected in animal pharmacological studies but others slip through and their adverse effects are found in the pilot phase of clinical assessment, when routine studies of haematological, renal and hepatic function are made together with other investigations such as the ECG. Acute toxic effects are usually found quickly, but ones which only make their appearance after many months are much more elusive, and depend on the perceptive clinician rather than the pharmacologist for their detection. It took over ten years of widespread experience with the phenothiazines before the drug-induced complications of tardive dyskinesia and ocular pigmentation were recognized, and even longer before lithium-induced hypothyroidism was detected (Schou et al., 1968; Candy, 1972). Detection of such effects takes longer if they occur in unexpected organ systems or if the only adverse effects are teratogenic. The thalidomide tragedy has made all doctors more aware of the dangers of prescribing drugs in pregnancy, even if they have been marketed for many years. No drug can be said to be completely safe until it has been used extensively for several decades, and by then, if no dangers are known, it is most likely to be proved to have no more than a placebo effect. 'Choose old established remedies' may seem a reactionary axiom, but in the case of drugs it is certainly safest, and is needed to counteract the frenetic advertising of some pharmaceutical companies, which often seems to imply that the latest drug is best solely on the basis of recency.

Pharmacodynamics

The effects that drugs have in man form the major part of clinical pharmacology, and, strictly speaking, efficacy should be included under this heading as well. However, the knowledge that a drug may be effective for a named condition is of little value unless one has some ideas when improvement is likely to occur, what is the correct dosage, the route and frequency of administration of the drug, which unwanted effects may complicate progress, and for how long treatment needs to be continued. Drug effects need to be considered separately for three phases of treatment; the acute phase (which lasts until the expected therapeutic effects occur), maintenance phase, and the withdrawal phase (which begins when the drug is reduced or stopped and lasts till the time that all traces of the drug (and its metabolites) have been eliminated from the body). How knowledge of these effects is helpful (one might say essential) to the prescribing clinician can be illustrated by the use of three well-established drugs in common clinical situations; chlorpromazine in the treatment of schizophrenia, diazepam in the treatment of acute anxiety and phenelzine in the treatment of agoraphobia.

In the acute phase chlorpromazine may be given intravenously, intramuscularly or by mouth. Although the intramuscular and intravenous routes may be used in the emergency control of disturbed behaviour, unwanted effects occur more seriously and postural hypotension in particular may be a major problem. Antipsychotic activity takes several days to develop and is not accelerated by intramuscular or intravenous administration so there is no gain from using these routes in the alleviation of schizophrenic symptoms. Dosage may be increased from 200 mg to 2000 mg a day but there is little advantage in increasing beyond this level unless the patient is acutely ill and under 40 years old (Prien and Cole, 1968). There is also no indication for giving long acting injectable phenothiazines as an initial treatment. During the acute administration of chlorpromazine many unwanted effects may occur, including over-sedation, photosensitivity, postural hypotension, jaundice and extrapyramidal effects, most of which tend to lessen in severity as treatment proceeds. Extrapyramidal effects include dystonia, pseudo-Parkinsonism, akathisia and oculogyric crises, and, when detected, will need the simultaneous administration of an anti-Parkinsonian drug. There is great variation in the incidence of extrapyramidal effects and it is wrong to automatically prescribe an anti-Parkinsonian agent whenever chlorpromazine is given.

In maintenance treatment a lower dose of chlorpromazine will usually be needed, and at this level anti-Parkinsonian medication may not be necessary. Dosage schedules may be altered to once or twice daily, most drug being given at night in view of its sedative effects, and further adjustment may be needed so that antipsychotic activity is maintained but initiative and interest are allowed expression. Interactions with monoamine oxidase inhibitors (Goldberg, 1964), hypotensive drugs (Janowsky et al., 1972) and alcohol (Hollister, 1972) may augment unwanted effects and reduce the therapeutic ones. Although immediate withdrawal effects are uncommon with chlorpromazine, a drug which had no addictive potential, drug action continues for several weeks after stopping treatment. Tardive dyskinesia may develop at this time (Marsden et al., 1975) and in such instances chlorpromazine therapy may need to be restarted. Ocular pigmentation may also occur late in treatment (Prien et al., 1970).

Diazepam is currently the most prescribed drug in the world and its chief use is for the alleviation of anxiety. In acute dosage it exerts its anxiety-reducing effects after about one hour when given orally (Tyrer and Lader, 1974) and within seconds or minutes after intravenous administration (Kelly et al., 1973). It is a sedative in larger dosage and the amount required to relieve anxiety without producing excessive sedation will have to be chosen carefully after initial response. The drug also has independent muscle relaxing properties in therapeutic dosage (Matthews, 1966). A paradoxical release of aggression may sometimes occur during treatment (Feldman, 1962), and occasionally this may require stopping the drug. Performance in driving and in other tasks may be impaired, often without the subject's knowledge (Betts et al., 1972) and the patient will need to be warned of these effects. Other unwanted effects which occur in less than 1% of patients include confusion, hypotension and ataxia (Miller, 1973). In maintenance therapy there are sound reasons for preferring a flexible dosage regime to a fixed dosage one (Tyrer, 1975a) and most patients are responsible enough to monitor their therapy effectively. Care must be taken with other drugs which may potentiate sedation, particularly alcohol and hypnotic agents (Fujimori, 1965). Tolerance and dependence may occur in a small number of patients and stopping the drug may lead to marked withdrawal symptoms (Gordon, 1967; Clare, 1971; Fruensgaard, 1976). To avoid the dangers of tolerance and habituation it is best to prescribe the drug for a defined period with a specific aim in view.

In the acute phase of treatment with phenelzine in agoraphobia it is important to emphasize the drug and dietary restrictions that need to be observed with all of the monoamine oxidase inhibitor drugs. Of these the drug restrictions are perhaps more important, as there have been no fatalities due to the simultaneous administration of tyramine-containing foodstuffs and phenelzine, the main dangers being due to the interaction of indirectly acting sympathomimetic drugs and a monoamine oxidase inhibitor. Many of these compounds, such as phenylpropanolamine, may be purchased in chemists without a prescription. The patient will also need to be warned about autonomic side-effects, particularly dry mouth, postural hypotension and constipation, and that these effects will be noted early whereas therapeutic ones may be delayed for up to eight weeks (Tyrer, 1975b). In maintenance treatment special care must be taken that any other drugs prescribed do not interact with phenelzine. If the drug is stopped too early the patient is likely to relapse (Lipsedge *et al.*, 1973; Solyom *et al.*, 1973) and in most cases therapy should be continued to several months. If this continues for over a year, however, there may be difficulties in withdrawing the tablets. Occasionally, tolerance may develop with a tendency to increase the dose (Bridges, 1972) and frank withdrawal symptoms may occur on stopping the drug (Pitt, 1974). Once the drug is stopped the dietary and drug restrictions need to be continued for at least three weeks because of persistence of the drug in the body.

These are but a few of the many pharmacological effects of these three drugs, and I have confined myself to those which are of immediate clinical relevance. The informed reader will doubtless find nothing new in these bald statements and may wonder why it is worth repeating them. I have done this to illustrate that the prescribing of a drug in psychiatry is rarely a single event, and that certain skills and knowledge are necessary to use drugs effectively and safely. It is unfortunate that many psychiatrists regard the initial prescription of a drug as their responsibility but its maintenance and withdrawal as of less importance, to be left to the general practitioner. I have often wondered what general practitioners must think when they receive letters from psychiatrists which end 'please reduce and stop drug X at your discretion'. Why should some personal idiosyncratic discretion which is unlikely to be based on pharmacological or psychiatric principles be the basis of this important decision? Would the same cavalier advice be given about the continuation of an antibiotic or hypotensive drug? The usual reason for this curious abrogation of responsibility is the ignorance of correct procedures of maintaining and withdrawing psychotropic drugs, so that in practice the psychiatrist's opinion is of no more value than that of a general practitioner. Tricyclic antidepressants were in general use for over ten years before a careful study of maintenance therapy was made, showing that relapse in depressive illness was much less likely if imipramine or amitriptyline rather than placebo was prescribed for six months after recovery (Mindham *et al.*, 1973). With knowledge like this clinical discretion about continuation of treatment can be relevant and rational. The necessity for adequate knowledge of drug effects and dangers throughout a course of treatment seems to be forgotten by those who advocate the extension of the power of prescribing psychotropic drugs to social workers and other paramedical personnel (Office of Health Economics, 1975). Such groups are not equipped to prescribe responsibly and appropriately and will not be unless pharmacology and therapeutics become an essential part of their training curriculum.

Pharmacokinetics

The sub-specialty of pharmacokinetics within clinical pharmacology has come to the fore in recent years. Pharmacokinetics is concerned with the absorption, distribution, metabolism, and excretion of drugs and already there is a considerable literature on its importance in psychiatry (Lader, 1976) although, gratifyingly, not yet enough to justify the neologism, psychopharmacokinetics. As the pharmacological activity of a drug is dependent primarily oñ the concentration of drug available at the site of action it is an important part of clinical pharmacology. As may be gathered from the term 'pharmacokinetics', the subject is concerned with the mathematical analysis of drug distribution and concentration within the body and does not appeal to many clinicians because it is not directly concerned with drug effects. Nevertheless, it is important in pharmacology because it explains many of the pharmacodynamic effects of drugs which would otherwise only have an empirical basis. Knowledge of pharmacokinetics can also explain the great variation in response to drugs between individuals (Smith and Rawlins, 1973). The value of pharmacokinetics can be illustrated using the three examples of clinical drug use previously discussed.

Following a single dose of chlorpromazine there is a rapid rise in plasma level which reaches a peak after two hours. Much lower plasma levels are found after oral administration than after intramuscular injection, and pharmacokinetic data suggests that some of the orally administered chlorpromazine does not enter the systemic circulation (Curry *et al.*,

1970). *In vitro* experiments have shown that chlorpromazine is destroyed in the intestinal wall and a similar process may occur *in vivo* in man (Curry *et al.*, 1971). The practical implications of this are that oral and intramuscular doses of chlorpromazine are not equivalent. One frequently finds on prescription cards that a dose of chlorpromazine (or similar antipsychotic drug) may be given orally or intramuscularly depending on whether or not the patient is co-operative. It has to be realized that if the intramuscular route is chosen that more active drug will be absorbed. About 90% of chlorpromazine is bound in plasma (i.e. it is not available for action at receptor sites because it is tied to plasma proteins) and there are up to 10-fold inter-individual differences in the degree of this binding (Curry, 1970). This is one of the chief factors accounting for the wide variation in dosage regimens between patients. During the first two weeks of treatment with chlorpromazine there is a fairly good correlation between plasma concentration of the drug and clinical response (Curry *et al.*, 1972). After this time, however, plasma levels show little relationship to clinical improvement and higher doses are needed to maintain the same plasma level (Curry, 1976). As mentioned earlier, many patients on chlorpromazine do not need the simultaneous administration of anti-Parkinsonian drugs. There is some evidence that anti-Parkinsonian medication induces liver microsomal oxidase enzymes (Loga *et al.*, 1975). These enzymes are involved in the metabolism of chlorpromazine and so when they are induced metabolism is increased. Part of the action, therefore, of anti-Parkinsonian drugs in reducing extrapyramidal side-effects may be due to a lowering of plasma chlorpromazine levels by increasing the metabolism of the drug. In long-term therapy one of the metabolites of chlorpromazine, 7-hydroxychlorpromazine, which has half the potency of chlorpromazine (Barry *et al.*, 1974), becomes important. There is some evidence that plasma levels of this metabolite are more clearly related to clinical effects in such patients (Sakalis *et al.*, 1972; MacKay *et al.*, 1974). The persistence of such metabolites after stopping therapy may account for the continuation of clinical effects long after the drug has been stopped.

The initial administration of diazepam by any route leads to a rapid rise in plasma level, reaching a peak after about one hour (Dasberg *et al.*, 1974). There is great variation in the absorption and distribution of the drug in the body and there are seven-fold differences in the amount of drug in the body between individuals after a single dose (Van Der Kleijn, 1971). During maintenance therapy a steady state is achieved in which dose and plasma levels are more closely related (Rutherford *et al.*, 1978). The longer diazepam is prescribed the more important do some of its active metabolites become in their contribution to clinical effects. The major active metabolite is *N*-desmethyldiazepam, which is an effective

hypnotic and anti-anxiety drug in its own right (Robin *et al.*, 1974; Tansella *et al.*, 1975). This drug has a long half-life and so it accumulates after repeated administration. In patients taking diazepam over many months the plasma level of desmethyldiazepam is about twice that of diazepam (Rutherford *et al.*, 1977) and probably much more important in determining anti-anxiety effects. A regular dose of diazepam taken at night is
— therefore likely to give anti-anxiety effects throughout the next day. Pharmacokinetics also does us a service in illustrating that many of the benzodiazepine drugs currently marketed are metabolites of other benzodiazepine drugs and represent no real advance (Tyrer, 1974). There is little point in changing from diazepam to oxazepam in the treatment of anxiety as oxazepam is one of the major metabolites of diazepam and its prescription will confer little new apart from the placebo effect of a different coloured tablet (Schapira *et al.*, 1970).

One of the factors which may account for the delayed or absent clinical improvement with phenelzine in agoraphobic patients is acetylator status. It is thought that phenelzine is primarily metabolized by acetylation although the evidence is circumstantial (Marshall, 1976) as estimation of its metabolites is difficult. Approximately half the population are slow acetylators and the other half fast acetylators, determined by polygenic inheritance (Price-Evans *et al.*, 1960). Slow acetylators break down drugs that are normally metabolized by acetylation slowly and so adequate levels of the drug accumulate in the body leading to clinical response. Fast acetylators may metabolize the drug so rapidly that therapeutic levels are never achieved. There is clinical evidence that slow acetylators respond to phenelzine better than fast acetylators (Johnstone and Marsh, 1973; Johnstone, 1976), and have more side-effects (Price-Evans *et al.*, 1965) and determination of acetylator status has been suggested as a useful clinical test before a decision is made to prescribe a hydrazine monoamine oxidase inhibitor.

From these examples it can be seen how knowledge of the pharmacokinetics of a drug can help to make its use more rational and lead to better understanding of pharmacological effects. It has been of most value in the study of well established drugs but recently plasma levels have often been carried out in the initial evaluation of a drug in human subjects. Most of the findings of pharmacokinetics in psychiatry have not yet altered clinical practice, the one exception being the estimation of plasma levels of lithium. The value of regular monitoring of plasma lithium levels in maintenance treatment is now well established and before long it may become equally important with other drug therapies. A word of caution is necessary in interpreting pharmacokinetic data. Because measurement in psychiatry is not as exact as in some other medical disciplines it is often thought that an objective measurement, such as a plasma level, is a more valid measure. This is not true, for a plasma level, or distribution volume, or biological half-life of the drug is of no clinical use unless it is correlated with pharmacological effects. A complex series of pharmacokinetic data is of no value on its own, and if one attempts to interpret clinical findings from this data one can go sadly awry. For example, the pharmacological classification of barbiturates into short, medium and long-acting has not been substantiated clinically and most of these drugs are equally effective hypnotics with similar duration of action (Hinton, 1961). Biological responses to drugs are exceedingly complex and have to be recorded independently of pharmacokinetic data if useful clinical deductions are to be made (Dollery, 1973; Turner, 1974). Pharmacokinetic estimations may be particularly valuable when a patient shows an unexpected response to a drug; it is unlikely to be necessary as a routine in all patients.

Investigation

The use of drugs to investigate mechanisms of disease is of recent origin. In psychiatry the problems associated with this approach are tremendous because our knowledge of normal psychological function is so inadequate. Nevertheless, the use of drugs in clinical practice has indirectly led to some valuable hypotheses. For example, the monoamine hypothesis of affective disorders, which postulated that depression occurred when there is a relative deficiency of cerebral catecholamines and that mania resulted when there was a relative abundance of such amines (Schildkraut, 1965) developed out of clinical observations of depression with anti-hypertensive drugs and from the pharmacological activity of antidepressant drugs. It is unlikely to be true in its simplest form but has proved a very useful hypothesis for those investigating biological abnormalities in affective disorders. Similarly, the demonstration that many antipsychotic drugs were also dopamine-blocking drugs (Carlsson and Lindqvist, 1963), had led over the years to the dopamine hypotheses of schizophrenia, which postulate that there is an excess of dopaminergic activity in schizophrenic patients. Although investigations are still at a relatively early stage, it is proving fruitful and tentative support has been given from a number of sources (Randrup, 1970; Anden, 1972; Crow *et al.*, 1976). Investigation in psychiatry is not confined to disturbances of brain function. The relationship between the bodily symptoms of anxiety and its accompanying mental changes has been studied with beta-adrenoceptor blocking drugs. These drugs block some of the peripheral responses to sympathetic stimulation and the results of several studies suggest that in some pathologically anxious patients somatic symptoms due to sympathetic activation may be the prime mover in maintaining pathological mood (Tyrer, 1976b).

Conclusion

In deciding on the place of drugs in mental disorders the psychiatrist faces bewildering contradictions. At one level it is quite inappropriate to deal with problems of psychosocial integration and interpersonal relationships with drug therapy. Similarly it appears equally inappropriate to treat an episodic psychotic disorder in someone whose usual psychosocial integration shows no impairment, with psychological forms of treatment. Unfortunately decisions about treatment are often based more on personal prejudice and unsound theories than on knowledge of the relative efficacy of the different treatments available. It is wrong to regard this empirical knowledge as less useful than knowledge which has a sounder theoretical basis. It is still one of the major functions of medicine to alleviate suffering and if we possess the wherewithal to relieve suffering, provided it is not associated with new adverse effects, then no theoretical argument can prevent its use. By all means follow up theoretical views and develop them into testable hypotheses, but in the last resort the effectiveness of any treatment has to be compared with another one by the cold scrutiny of a clinical trial. If the drug repeatedly fails to better an existing treatment in any respect it has to be discarded or modified. If a treatment is to be used well, its prescriber needs to know as much as possible about its nature, its mechanism of action, and all its effects, both wanted and unwanted.

In this account I have concentrated on those aspects of psychopharmacology which illustrate the principles behind rational drug therapy. For many psychiatric disorders such therapy is the most effective in our present knowledge. Treatment is in a constant state of flux, and doubtless there will be great variation in psychiatric therapy even within the space of a few years. This does not matter, provided that such changes are made on the basis of adequate evidence, and not because a philosophical trend, a political creed, or public opinion decrees it so. The hospital physician does not go through agonies of self-doubt whenever he has to prescribe a drug for a particular disorder. He does not think of drug therapy in general terms, he considers a specific disorder and chooses an appropriate therapy, which may be a pharmacological one. The same attitude needs to be taken by psychiatrists, and although this is encouraged by the multi disciplinary training we receive, all too often it is lost when training is completed.

References

Anden, N. E. (1972). Dopamine turnover in the corpus striatum and the limbic system after treatment with neuroleptic and anti-acetylcholine drugs. *J. Pharm. Pharmacol.* **24**, 905–906.

Barry, H., Steenberg, M. L., Manian, A. A. and Buckley, J. P. (1974). Effects of chlorpromazine and three metabolites on behavioral responses in rats. *Psychopharmacologia* **34**, 351–360.

Barsa, J. (1963). The fallacy of the 'double-blind'. *Am. J. Psychiat.* **119**, 1174–1175.

Beecher, H. K. (1955). The powerful placebo. *J.A.M.A.* **159**, 1602–1606.

Betts, T. A., Clayton, A. B. and Mackay, G. M. (1972). Effects of four commonly-used tranquillizers on low-speed driving performance tests. *Br. Med. J.* **4**, 580–584.

Blackwell, B. and Shepherd, M. (1967). Early evaluation of psychotropic drugs in man: a trial that failed. *Lancet* **ii**, 819–822.

Bonhoeffer, K. (1911). Wie weit kommen psychogene Krankheitzustände und Krankheitprozesse vor, die nicht der Hysterie zuzurechnen sind? *Allg. Z. Psychiat.* **68**, 371–386. [English translation by H. Marshall *in* 'Themes and Variations in European Psychiatry' (Eds S. R. Hirsch and M. Shepherd, pp. 53–64.]

Bridges, P. K. (1972). Psychosurgery today: psychiatric aspects. *Proc. Roy. Soc. Med.* **65**, 1104–1108.

Cade, J. F. J. (1949). Lithium salts in the treatment of psychotic excitement. *Med. J. Aust.* **36**, 349–352.

Candy, J. (1972). Severe hypothyroidism—an early complication of lithium therapy. *Br. Med. J.* **3**, 277.

Candy, J., Balfour, S. H. G., Cawley, R. H., Hildebrand, H. P., Malan, D. H., Marks, I. M. and Wilson, J. (1972). A feasibility study for a controlled trial of formal psychotherapy. *Psychol. Med.* **2**, 345–362.

Carlsson, A. and Lindqvist, M. (1963). Effect of chlorpromazine or haloperidol on formation of 3-methoxytryptamine and normetanephrine in mouse brain. *Acta Pharmacol. Toxicol.* **20**, 140.

Chien, C. (1976). Drugs and rehabilitation in schizophrenia. *In* 'Drugs in Combination with Other Therapies' (Ed. M. Greenblatt), pp. 13–34. Grune and Stratton, New York.

Clare, A. W. (1971). Diazepam, alcohol and barbiturate abuse. *Br. Med. J.* **4**, 340.

Coppen, A., Noguera, R., Bailey, J., Burns, B. H., Swani, M. S., Hare, E. H., Gardner, R. and Maggs, R. (1971). Prophylactic lithium in affective disorders. *Lancet* **ii**, 275–279.

Covi, L., Lipman, R. S., Derogatis, L. R., Smith III, J. E. and Pattison, J. H. (1974). Drugs and group psychotherapy in neurotic depression. *Am. J. Psychiat.* **131**, 191–198.

Crisp, A. H. (1966). 'Transference', 'symptom emergence' and 'social repercussion' in behaviour therapy. *Br. J. Med. Psychol.* **39**, 179–196.

Crow, T. J., Deakin, J. F. W., Johnstone, E. C. and Longden, A. N. (1976). Dopamine and schizophrenia. *Lancet* **ii**, 563–566.

Crowe, M. J. (1976). Behavioural treatment in psychiatry. *In* 'Recent Advances in Clinical Psychiatry' (Ed. K. Granville-Grossman), Vol. 2., pp.169–199. Churchill Livingstone, Edinburgh.

Curry, S. H. (1970). Plasma protein binding of chlorpromazine. *J. Pharm. Pharmacol.* **22**, 193–197.

Curry, S. (1976). Plasma level studies in psychotropic drug evaluation. *Br. J. Clin. Pharmacol.* **3**, *Suppl.* 1, 20–28.

Curry, S. H., Marshall, J. H. L., Davis, J. M. and Janowsky, D. S. (1970). Factors affecting chlorpromazine plasma levels in psychiatric patients. *Arch. Gen. Psychiat.* **22**, 209–215.

Curry, S. H., D'Mello, A. and Mould, G. P. (1971). Destruction of chlorpromazine during absorption in the rat in vivo and in vitro. *Br. J. Pharmacol.* **42**, 403–411.

Curry, S. H., Lader, M. H., Mould, G. P. and Sakalis, G. (1972). Clinical pharmacology of chlorpromazine. *Br. J. Pharmacol.* **44**, 370–371P.

Dasberg, H. H., Kleijn, E. Van Der, Guelen, P. J. R. and Praag, H. M. van (1974). Plasma concentrations of diazepam and of its metabolite N-desmethyldiazepam in relation to anxiolytic effect. *Clin. Pharmacol. Ther.* **15**, 473–483.

Dollery, C. T. (1973). Pharmacokinetics—master or servant. *Eur. J. Clin. Pharmacol.* **6**, 1–2.

Evans, D. A. P., Manley, K. A. and McKusick, V. A. (1960). Genetic control of isoniazid metabolism in man. *Br. Med. J.* **2**, 485–491.

Evans, D. A. P., Davison, K. and Pratt, R. T. C. (1965). The influence of acetylator phenotype on the effects of treating depression with phenelzine. *Clin. Pharmacol. Ther.* **6**, 430–435.

Feather, B. W. and Rhoads, J. M. (1972). Psychodynamic behaviour therapy. *Arch. Gen. Psychiat.* **26**, 496–511.

Feldman, P. E. (1962). An analysis of the efficacy of diazepam. *J. Neuropsychiat.* **3**, *Suppl.* 1, 62–67.

Feldman, M. P. and McCulloch, M. J. (1971). 'Homosexual Behaviour—Therapy and Assessment'. Pergamon Press, Oxford.

Fruensgaard, K. (1976). Withdrawal psychosis: a study of thirty consecutive cases. *Acta Psychiat. Scand.* **53**, 105–118.

Fujimori, H. (1965). Potentiation of barbital hypnosis as an evaluation method for central nervous system depressants. *Psychopharmacologia* **7**, 374–378.

Goldberg, L. I. (1964). Monoamine oxidase inhibitors. *J.A.M.A.* **190**, 456–462.

Gordon, E. B. (1967). Addiction to diazepam (Valium). *Br. Med. J.* **1**, 112.

Hill, A. B. (1966). Reflections on the controlled trial. *Ann. Rheum. Dis.* **25**, 107–113.

Hinton, J. M. (1961). The action of amylobarbitone sodium, butobarbitone, and quinalbarbitone sodium upon insomnia and nocturnal restlessness compared in psychiatric patients. *Br. J. Pharmacol.* **16**, 82–89.

Hogarty, G. E., Goldberg, S. C. and The Collaborative Study Group, Baltimore (1973). Drugs and sociotherapy in the aftercare of schizophrenic patients: one year relapse rates. *Arch. Gen. Psychiat.* **28**, 54–64.

Hollister, L. E. (1972). Psychiatric and neurologic disorders. *In* 'Clinical Pharmacology' (Eds K. L. Melmon and H. F. Morelli). Macmillan, New York.

Hullin, R. P., McDonald, R. and Allsopp, M. N. (1972). Prophylactic lithium in recurrent affective disorders. *Lancet* i, 1044–1046.

Janowsky, D. S., El-Yousef, M. K., Davis, J. M., Fann, W. E. and Oates, J. A. (1972). Guanethidine antagonism by antipsychotic drugs. *J. Tennessee Med. Assoc.* **65**, 620–622.

Johnstone, E. C. (1976). The relationship between acetylator status and inhibition of monoamine oxidase, excretion of free drug and antidepressant response in depressed patients on phenelzine. *Psychopharmacologia* **46**, 289–294.

Johnstone, E. C. and Marsh, W. (1973). Acetylator status and response to phenelzine in depressed patients. *Lancet* i, 567–570.

Joyce, C. R. B. (1968). Psychological factors in the controlled evaluation of therapy. *In* 'Psychopharmacology—dimensions and perspectives' (Ed. C. R. B. Joyce), pp. 215–242. Tavistock, London.

Kelly, D., Pik, R. and Chen, C. (1973). A psychological and physiological evaluation of the effects of intravenous diazepam. *Br. J. Psychiat.* **122**, 419–426.

Kleijn, E. van der (1971). Pharmacokinetics of distribution and metabolism of ataractic drugs and an evaluation of the site of antianxiety activity. *Ann. N. Y. Acad. Sci.* **179**, 115–125.

Klerman, G. L. (1976). Combining drugs and psychotherapy in the treatment of depression. *In* 'Drugs in Combination with Other Therapies' (Ed. M. Greenblatt), pp. 67–81. Grune and Stratton, New York.

Klerman, G. L., Dimascio, A., Weissman, M. M., Prusoff, B. and Paykel, E. S. (1974). Treatment of depression by drugs and psychotherapy. *Am. J. Psychiat.* **131**, 186–191.

Lader, M. (1976). Clinical psychopharmacology. *In* 'Recent Advances in Clinical Psychiatry' (Ed. K. Granville-Grossman), Vol. 2, pp. 1–30. Churchill Livingstone, Edinburgh.

Lancet (1867). Leading article. *Lancet* **ii**, 234–235.

Lipsedge, M. S., Hajioss, J., Huggins, P., Napier, L., Pearce, J., Pike, D. J. and Rich, M. (1973). The management of severe agoraphobia: a comparison of iproniazid and systematic desensitization. *Psychopharmacologia* **32**, 67–80.

Loga, S., Curry, S. and Lader, M. (1975). Interactions of orphenadrine and phenobarbitone with chlorpromazine: plasma concentrations and effects in man. *Br. J. Clin. Pharmacol.* **2**, 197–208.

Lorenz, K. (1966). 'On Aggression', pp. 248–249. Trans. M. Latzke. Methuen, London.

Mackay, A. V. P., Healey, A. F. and Baker, J. (1974). The relationship of plasma chlorpromazine to its 7-hydroxy and sulphoxide metabolites in a large population of chronic schizophrenics. *Br. J. Clin. Pharmacol.* **1**, 425–430.

Marks, I. M. (1971). Phobic disorders four years after treatment: a prospective follow up. *Br. J. Psychiat,* **118**, 683–689.

Marks, I. M. and Gelder, M. G. (1968). Controlled trials in behaviour therapy. *In* 'The Role of Learning in Psychotherapy' (Ed. R. Porter), pp. 68–81. J. A. Churchill, London.

Marsden, C. D., Tarsy, D. and Baldessarini, R. J. (1975). Spontaneous and drug-induced disorders in psychotic patients. *In* 'Psychiatric Complications of Neurological Diseases' (Eds D. F. Benson and D. Blumer). Grune and Stratton, New York.

Marshall, E. F. (1976). The myth of phenelzine acetylation. *Br. Med. J.* **2**, 817.

Matthews, W. B. (1966). Ratio of minimum H reflex to maximum M response as a measure of spasticity. *J. Neurol. Neurosurg. Psychiat.* **29**, 201–204.

May, P. R. A. (1976). Rational treatment for an irrational disorder; what does the schizophrenic patient need. *Am. J. Psychiat.* **113**, 1008–1012.

Medical Research Council, Report of Clinical Psychiatry Committee (1965). Clinical trial of the treatment of depressive illness. *Br. Med. J.* **1**, 881–886.

Melia, P. I. (1970). Prophylactic lithium: a double-blind trial in recurrent affective disorders. *Br. J. Psychiat.* **116**, 621–624.

Miller, H. (1967). Depression. *Br. Med. J.* **1**, 257–262.

Miller, R. R. (1973). Drug surveillance neutralizing epidemiologic methods: a report from the Boston Collaborative Drug Surveillance Program. *Am. J. Hosp. Pharmac.* **30**, 584–592.

Mindham, R. H. S., Howland, C. and Shepherd, M. (1973). An evaluation of continuation therapy with tricyclic antidepressants in depressive illness. *Psychol. Med.* **3**, 5–17.

Office of Health Economics (1975). Medicines which affect the mind. No. 54. Office of Health Economics, London.

Pauling, L. (1968). Orthomolecular psychiatry. *Science* **160**, 265–271.

Pauling, L. (1974). On the orthomolecular environment of the mind: orthomolecular theory. *Am. J. Psychiat.* **131**, 1251–1257.

Pitt, B. M. N. (1974). Withdrawal symptoms after stopping phenelzine? *Br. Med. J.* **2**, 332–333.

Prien, R. F. and Cole, J. O. (1968). High dose chlorpromazine therapy in chronic schizophrenia. *Arch. Gen. Psychiat.* **18**, 482–495.

Prien, R. F., Delong, S. L., Cole, J. O. and Levine, J. (1970). Ocular changes occurring with prolonged high dose chlorpromazine therapy. *Arch. Gen. Psychiat.* **23**, 464–467.

Randrup, A. (1970). Role of brain dopamine in the antipsychotic effects of neuroleptics. Evidence for studies of amphetamine-neuroleptic interaction. *Modern Problems Pharmacopsychiat.* **5**, 60–65.

Ravaris, C. L., Nies, A., Robinson, D. S., Ives, J. O., Lamborn, K. R. and Korson, L. (1976). A multiple-dose, controlled study of phenelzine in depression-anxiety states. *Arch. Gen. Psychiat.* **33**, 347–350.

Rees, L. and Davies, B. (1961). A controlled trial of phenelzine (Nardil) in the treatment of severe depressive illness. *J. Ment. Sci.* **107**, 560–566.

Robin, A., Curry, S. H. and Whelpton, R. (1974). Clinical and biochemical comparison of chlorazepate and diazepam. *Psychol. Med.* **4**, 388–392.

Robinson, D. S., Nies, A., Ravaris, C. L. and Lamborn, K. R. (1973). The monoamine oxidase inhibitor, phenelzine, in the treatment of depressive-anxiety states. *Arch. Gen. Psychiat.* **29**, 407–413.

Rutherford, D., Okoko, A. and Tyrer, P. (1978). Plasma concentrations of diazepam and desmethyldiazepam during chronic diazepam therapy. *Br. J. Clin. Pharmacol.* **6**, 69–73.

Sakalis, G., Curry, S. H., Mould, G. P. and Lader, M. H. (1972). Physiologic and clinical effects of chlorpromazine and their relationship to plasma level. *Clin. Pharmacol. Ther.* **13**, 931–946.

Sargant, W. (1965). Antidepressant drugs. *Br. Med. J.* **1**, 1495.

Sargant, W. and Dally, P. J. (1962). Treatment of anxiety states by anti-depressant drugs. *Br. Med. J.* **1**, 6–9.

Sargant, W. and Slater, E. (1954). 'Physical Methods of Treatment in Psychiatry', (3rd edn). Churchill Livingstone, Edinburgh (4th edn, 1964).

Schapira, K., McClelland, H. A., Griffiths, N. R. and Newell, D. J. (1970). Study on the effects of tablet colour in the treatment of anxiety states. *Br. Med. J.* **2**, 446–449.

Schildkraut, J. J. (1965). The catecholamine hypothesis of affective disorders: a review of supporting evidence. *Am. J. Psychiat.* **122**, 509–522.

Schou, M., Amdisen, A., Eskjaer Jensen, S. and Olsen, T. (1968). Occurrence of goitre during lithium treatment. *Br. Med. J.* **3**, 710–713.

Shapiro, A. K. (1959). The placebo effect in the history of medical treatment: implications for psychiatry. *Am. J. Psychiat.* **116**, 298–304.

Shepherd, M., Lader, M. and Rodnight, R. (1968). 'Clinical Psychopharmacology.' English Universities Press, London.

Silverstone, T. and Turner, P. (1974). 'Drug Treatment in Psychiatry'. Routledge and Kegan Paul, London.

Simpson, L. L. (Ed.) (1976). 'Drug Treatment of Mental Disorders'. Raven Press, New York.

Smith, S. and Rawlins, M. (1973). 'Variability in Human Drug Response'. Butterworth, London.

Solyom, L., Heseltine, G. F., McClure, D. J., Solyom, C., Ledwidge, B. and Steinberg, G. (1973). Behaviour therapy versus drug therapy in the treatment of phobic neurosis. *Can. Psychiat. Ass. J.* **18**, 25–32.

Stevens, A. (1974). *The Guardian*, May 6th.

Tansella, M., Siciliani, O., Burti, L., Schiavon, M., and Zimmermann Tansella, C. H. (1975). N-desmethyldiazepam and amylobarbitone sodium as hypnotics in anxious patients. Plasma levels, clinical efficacy and residual effects. *Psychopharmacologia* **41**, 81–85.

Turner, P. (1974). Blood level or pharmacological response? *Br. J. Clin. Pharmacol.* **1**, 11.

Tyrer, P. (1974). The benzodiazepine bonanza. *Lancet* **ii**, 709–710.

Tyrer, P. (1975a). Use and abuse of tranquillisers. *In* 'Advanced Medicine, Topics in Therapeutics, 1' (Ed. A. M. Breckenridge), pp. 242–254. Pitman Medical, Kent

Tyrer, P. (1975b). Length and treatment with monoamine oxidase inhibitors in phobic anxiety states. *In* 'Neuropsychopharmacology, Proceedings of the IX Congress of the Collegium Internationale Neuropsychopharmacologicum', pp. 800–807. Excerpta Medica, Amsterdam.

Tyrer, P. (1976a). Towards a rational therapy with monoamine oxidase inhibitors. *Br. J. Psychiat.* **128**, 354–360.

Tyrer, P. (1976b). 'The Role of Bodily Feelings in Anxiety'. Maudsley Monograph, No. 23, Oxford University Press, Oxford.

Tyrer, P. J. and Lader, M. H. (1974). Physiological and psychological effects of ± propranolol, + propranolol and diazepam in induced anxiety. *Br. J. Clin. Pharmacol.* **1**, 379–385.

Tyrer, P. and Steinberg, D. (1975). Symptomatic treatment of agoraphobia and social phobias: a follow up study. *Br. J. Psychiat.* **127**, 163–168.

Tyrer, P., Candy, J. and Kelly, D. (1973). A study of the clinical effects of phenelzine and placebo in the treatment of phobic anxiety. *Psychopharmacologia* **32**, 237–254.

Weissman, M. M. (1976). Psychotherapy and behaviour therapy. *Lancet* **ii**, 45.

Weissman, M. M., Klerman, G. L., Paykel, E. S., Prusoff, B. and Hanson, B. (1974). Treatment effects on the social adjustment of depression. *Arch. Gen. Psychiat.* **30**, 771–778.

West, E. D. and Dally, P. J. (1959). Effect of iproniazid in depressive syndromes. *Br. Med. J.* **1**, 1491–1494.

20 Psychosurgery and electroconvulsive therapy

Anthony Clare

Psychosurgery

Definition

A World Health Organization publication (1976) defines psychosurgery as 'the selective surgical removal or destruction . . . of nerve pathways . . . with a view to influencing behaviour'. This definition has provoked a critical response from Bridges and Bartlett (1977) who point out that much modern psychosurgery is concerned with the treatment of intractable affective illnesses without any intended effect on behaviour at all and they suggest as an alternative definition 'the surgical treatment of certain psychiatric illnesses by means of localized lesions placed in specific cerebral sites'. However, this too seems an inadequate definition for it fails to account for those operations which are intended to modify behaviour and for those where there does not appear be any specific cerebral target. The recent report of the US National Commission for the Protection of Human Subjects of Biomedical and Behavioral Research (1977) acknowledged these difficulties and eventually adopted the following definition for use in its exhaustive survey of the available literature and its final assessment of the efficacy of operative procedures:

> Psychosurgery means brain surgery on (1) normal brain tissue of an individual who does not suffer from any physical disease, for the purpose of changing or controlling the behavior or emotions of such individual, or (2)

diseased brain tissue of an individual, if the primary object of the performance of such surgery is to control, change or affect any behavioral or emotional disturbance of such individual.

Within the terms of this definition, surgery with a dual purpose, for example the relief of epileptic seizures as well as relief of emotional disorders, would be classifiable as psychosurgery if the predominant reason for performing the operation was to affect the behavioral or emotional disturbance.

History

In 1875, the British neurologist, Sir David Ferrier, described how the removal of a large portion of the frontal lobes in monkeys appeared to have little or no effect on sensory or motor abilities but produced a remarkable change in 'the animals' character and disposition', the monkeys becoming more tame and docile (Ferrier, 1875). The first published account of a psychosurgical intervention in man was that of Burckhardt who in 1891 attempted to interrupt the connecting fibres between the frontal lobes and the rest of the brain in severely disturbed and actively hallucinating patients. However, his results were poor and he encountered fierce opposition from his medical colleagues.

While the study of the relationship between brain function and behaviour in man was initially restricted to observing changes in those individuals who had suffered cerebral damage, usually of a frontal lobe variety, active experimentation in animals flourished. In this century, the work by Lashley on cortical learning, Kluver's experiments on the temporal lobes and Jacobsen and Fulton's research showing how frustrational responses in chimpanzees could be modified by frontal lobe surgery led to a resurgence of interest on the part of neurosurgeons concerning the possible application in man. In 1936, on the advice of Egaz Moniz, Almeida Lima performed the first series of psychosurgical interventions and an enthusiastic account of this work in 20 patients was published. The Americans, Freeman and Watts, modified Moniz's surgical procedure and devised the so-called 'standard leucotomy' (Fig. 1) which was to be widely used until early in the 1950s. By that time, Freeman and Watts had operated on over 1000 patients. The estimated figure for all US operations by this time was of the order of 40,000 while in England and Wales Tooth and Newton (1961) summarized the results on 10,365 patients leucotomized between 1942 and 1954.

The standard leucotomy consisted of making a burr hole in the temporal regions, inserting a cutting instrument and sweeping it in an arc in the coronal plane, thereby dividing as much white matter as possible. The operation was crude and the indiscriminate division of frontolombic connections often led to intellectual impairment, loss of self control, euphoria and aggressive outbursts. The associated mortality (approximately 6%) and the many side-effects resulted in its eventual abandonment as a routine procedure.

Initial claims for leucotomy were enthusiastic but gradually psychiatrists became disillusioned and this together with the development of the phenothiazines and an increasing interest in and awareness of the importance of social rehabilitation of chronic patients led to a steady decline in the number of operations. By 1961 only 11 British hospitals reported performing more than 10 leucotomies apiece, their collective sum being 189 or 45% of the national total. However, two developments, one technical and one theoretical, stimulated a renewed interest in psychosurgery. The technical impulse derived from the introduction of improved surgical techniques and particularly of stereotactic procedures. The theoretical impulse derives from the growth of knowledge concerning brain circuits, derived mainly from animal studies. Particular attention has been drawn to the limbic circuits proposed by Papez (1937), and Yakovlev (1948). Based on anatomical and functional considerations, a distinction is frequently made between medial and lateral limbic circuits in the brain.

> The *medial limbic circuit* is said to include (among other structures) the medial frontal cortex, the cingulate gyrus, the anterior thalamic nucleus, and connecting fibre systems. The *lateral limbic circuit* is believed to include (among other structures) the orbital frontal cortex, the dorsomedial thalamic nucleus, the amygdala and connecting fibre systems.

Damage to the medial limbic system often produces states of motor and psychic hypoactivity whereas stimulation or irritative disorders often produce signs of motor and psychic hyperactivity, such as restlessness, irritability and anxiety. The lateral limbic circuit appears to be involved in a broad spectrum of disorders including depression, perceptual and hallucinatory disturbances and uncontrolled aggression. Broadly speaking, psychosurgical lesions of the medial frontal area, the anterior cingulate region or closely related fibre systems are said to be most effective in syndromes characterized by psychic hyperactivity such as is seen in patients suffering from tension, anxiety,. restlessness and obsessive-compulsive behaviour. Lesions involving the orbital frontal cortex and closely related fibre systems are reportedly most effective in syndromes characterized by various mainfestations of depression. Lesions of the amygdala are thought to be most beneficial in patients in whom hyperkinetic activity and/or unprovoked assaultive behaviour is the major behavioural problem.

However, Valenstein (1977) found considerable disagreement concerning the specificity of brain targets in psychosurgery in a limited survey of leading neurosurgeons and neuropsychiatrists in the US. Many respondents, who often had a great many years of experience observing psychosurgical patients, indicated that there was no evidence that brain targets should be varied as a function of psychiatric syndromes. Other, equally experinced clinicians believe that they can justify varying the brain targets. 'It seems clear', observes Valenstein, 'that with such strong and significant disagreement among those who practise psychosurgery, it cannot be convincingly argued that our understanding of the physiological basis of psychosurgery has advanced very far'. Such knowledge as has accumulated over the years is mainly empirical. There is some agreement about the brain targets that are most likely to produce the best results and a reasonable amount of agreement about the patients most likely to be helped. Here, too, however there are definite areas of disagreement.

Contemporary procedures

Psychosurgery has developed from crude procedures for destroying poorly defined areas of the frontal lobes to fairly precise techniques aimed at ablating relatively specific targets throughout the brain. The most significant development has been the gradual introduction of stereotactic instruments. Basically, such an instrument positions the head in a fixed plane and with the aid of three-dimensional maps it becomes possible to place electrodes or other devices through small skull holes into almost any area of the brain. In 1949, Spiegel and Wycis of Temple University first described the use of the stereotactic instrument to destroy a circumscribed region in the dorsomedial thalamus of psychotic patients. Gradually, the use of the instrument gained acceptance and today most operations use some variation of the basic principle of this approach. In current practice, the accuracy of such surgery is increased by information gained from brain-scanners, electrical recording and on-line X-rays.

Another major development concerns the method of destroying brain tissue. Initially, psychosurgical operations were performed with a knife or leucotome. Later, psychosurgeons used a suction technique for removing tissue. The use of stereotactic procedures has led to the development of a remarkable array of destructive techaniques. Gildenberg (1975) suggests that over 70% of neurosurgeons in the US and Canada using stereotactic techniques produce brain lesions with radio frequency waves. Other methods include the use of a cryoprobe (freezing), a leucotome, electro-cautery, radio-isotopes (including the implantation of radioactive yttrium seeds), proton beams, ultrasound, compression and thermocoagulation. Brain tissue has also been destroyed using injections of alcohol and an inert oil or wax.

The areas of the brain identified in Fig. 1 represent the main brain targets for psychosurgical operations currently being practiced around the world. Particular procedures are favoured by particular psychosurgeons. Lesions may be placed in the connections of the hippocampus and hypothalamus (Sano *et al.*, 1972), in the cingulum bundle (Lewin, 1973; Ballantine *et al.*, 1967) the amygdala (Narabayashi *et al.*, 1963; Kim and Umbach, 1973), the corpus callosum (Laitinen, 1972), the subcaudate area (Bridges and Bartlett, 1977) and the medial quadrants of the frontal lobes (Kelly *et al.*, 1973). As mentioned above, consensus is lacking concerning the specificity of many of these approaches. Thus for example, Lewin (1973) concludes that open cingulectomy (the removal of the cingulate gyrus on each side) is not beneficial in cases of depression whereas Foltz and White (1962) and Ballantine and his colleagues (1967), using a stereotactic approach, claim that it is. Wherein lies the difference

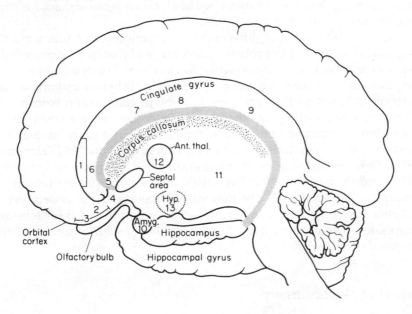

Fig. 1 Approximate brain targets of current psychosurgical procedures.
Frontal lobe procedures: (1) Bimedial leucotomy; (2) Yttrium lesions in subcortical white matter; (3) Orbital undercutting; (4) Basal tractotomy and substantia innominotomy; (5) Anterior capsulotomy (destruction of fibers of internal capsule); (6) mesoloviotomy (similar to rostral cingulotomy, but lesion invades genu knee of corpus cellosum). *Cingulotomies*: (7) anterior cingulotomy; (8) mid-cingulotomy; (9) posterior cingulotomy. *Amygdalectomy*: (10) amygdalectomy or amygdalotomy. *Thalatomies*: (11) Dorsomedial, centromedian, parafascicular nuclei (12) anterior thalatomy. *Hypothalotomy*: (13) posterior, ventromedial, and lateral hypothalamic targets.

between the open and the stereotactic approach? Lewin concludes that the stereotactic approach does not actually destroy the cingulum alone but also interrupts connecting fibres with the medial limbic system. (His remarks seem to indicate that the specificity of stereotactic techniques is not universally acknowledged.)

Knight and his colleagues in Britain have been enthusiastic advocates for the use of radioactive yttrium seeds, placing them on each side of the posterior orbital aspect of the frontal lobe, the so-called 'subcaudate tractotomy'. Good results have been claimed in severely and chronically depressed and obsessional patients (Knight, 1969; Bridges et al., 1973). Beneficial results have also been reported with stereotactic lesions placed in the anterior part of the cingulum and the medial quadrant of the frontal lobe in patients with anxiety, depression or obsessional symptoms (Kelly et al., 1973). Partial removal of both temporal lobes or removal of the posterior portion of the cingulate gyrus in cases of serious and persisting aggression has been reported to be effective (Turner, 1972) while Hitchcock and his colleagues use sterotaxic bilateral amygdalotomies for similar conditions (Hitchcock et al., 1972).

There are international differences in psychosurgical practices. For example, there is a greater relative percentage of frontal lobe procedures performed in the UK compared with the US whereas in the latter country cingulotomies are more frequently performed. When cingulotomies are performed in Britain they are usually done in conjunction with frontal lobe operations resulting in a combined procedure often termed 'limbic leucotomy'. Excluding limbic leucotomies, there is a much greater tendency to perform multiple target psychosurgery in the US (Valenstein, 1977). Data abstracted from all articles published on psychosurgery since 1971 confirm the conclusion that, with the exception of operations for intractable pain in the US, the majority of operations are undertaken in patients suffering from anxiety, obsessive-compulsive disorders and depression. There is a relatively higher number of schizophrenic patients operated on in the US.

Extent of psychosurgery

Valenstein (1977) points out that only a relatively small number of those neurosurgeons who practise psychosurgery actually publish their results. In addition, many of the published articles summarize the results of operations performed over a number of years. It is not possible, therefore, to obtain a valid estimate of the extent of psychosurgery from a literature survey alone. A questionnaire survey undertaken on behalf of the Task Force on Psychosurgery of the American Psychiatric Association found a decline in the number of psychosurgeons in the US and Canada performing psychosurgery over the three years studied, 1971–1973, a decline attributed to the deterrent effect of the public controversy over the subject in addition to the effect of several well-publicized law suits against neurosurgeons. On the basis of this survey's results and those of Gildenberg (1975) Valenstein (1977) suggests that the average number of psychosurgical procedures performed is very likely to have been between 400 and 500 per year during the years 1971–1973. The average number of such operations per year seems to have decreased after 1973 but there is a lack of reliable data available. Robin and Macdonald (1975) have estimated that approximately 200 procedures were performed in Britain in 1974. However, this is very much in the nature of an informed guess—there is no British agency with reliable and comprehensive statistics on the amount of psychosurgery performed.

Indications

There is general agreement that patients suffering from severe disturbances of mood and emotion are most likely to benefit from psychosurgery. The more intense and persistent the emotional responses, the more appropriate, it is argued, is the referral for psychosurgery (Bridges and Bartlett, 1977). Crippling phobias, ritualistic and compulsive behaviours, and profound, intractable and suicidal depression figure most prominently in the mental state reports of patients referred for psychosurgical treatment. Such disturbances are usually described as being of long duration and resistant to alternative treatments such as psychotherapy, electrical treatment and drugs. However, the criteria whereby psychiatrists refer patients for treatment (in those countries, such as the UK and the United States, where most if not all psychosurgical candidates are psychiatrically referred) and the criteria whereby neurosurgeons accept them are only rarely made explicit. The declaration commonly made to the effect that 'all therapeutic alternatives have been exhausted' lacks precision. One Canadian psychiatrist (Lehmann, 1973) has attempted to be more specific about the criteria and has suggested that, for example, a patient referred for psychosurgical treatment of anxiety and depression should have had at least one but preferably two courses of ECT, disabling symptoms for at least two years, adequate doses of both minor and major tranquillizers and psychotherapy by a trained therapist for a minimum period of six months. Kelly (1976), in his less specific description of selection criteria, tends to agree broadly with such recommendations.

While there is general agreement concerning the possible beneficial effects of psychosurgery in the management of intractable *depression*, chronic *anxiety* and crippling *obsessive-compulsive disorders*, there is much controversy over its role in the treatment of *schizophrenia*. Those who question its value insist that it has no beneficial effect on the thought disorders of these patients or on severe delusions and hallucinations. Others believe that it is helpful in patients with high levels of anxiety, depression and obsessional symptoms. Some of the disagreement is related to the lack of clarity of diagnostic labels currently used in psychiatric practice.

There is disagreement too over those categories of patients for whom psychosurgery is contraindicated. Kelly (1976) reflects a fairly orthodox view when he argues that patients who have 'very poor impulse control', psychopaths, alcoholics, drug addicts and patients with diffuse brain damage, should not be considered for operation. Others, while not dis-agreeing on the importance of the patient's motivation to get well, have insisted that criminals, psychopaths and sexual deviants do benefit. In Germany, ventromedial hypothalamic ablations have been performed on paedophilic homosexuals and individuals who have committed violent sexual crimes (Dieckmann and Hassler, 1975; Roeder *et al.*, 1972). Critics have argued that the amelioration of behaviour problems results from a partial 'functional castration' and a significant reduction in all sexual expression (Valenstein, 1973). The ethics of performing such operations, particularly on persons either in prison or during the time when they are facing imprisonment, are discussed below.

A small number of patients with severe obesity secondary to excessive eating have been treated by destroying the lateral hypothalamic area of the brain (Quaade, 1974; Quaade *et al.*, 1974). These operation, performed in Denmark, have been criticized because of the dangers of causing endocrine disorders, serious disturbances in sensory and motor function and decrements in general motivation (Marshall, 1974; Valenstein, 1975). The appropriateness of psychosurgery for aggressive and assaultive behaviour is also controversial. There are patients in whom aggressive-ness appears related to clear-cut brain damage who sometimes show an impressive response to surgery. The position with regard to violent patients who do not show any evidence of cerebral pathology is less clear. This has not, however, prevented psychosurgical operations, particularly amygdalectomies, from being carried out on violent patients who showed no evidence of brain damage.

There is understandable disquiet concerning the issue of psycho-surgery performed on children. The number of children involved may actually be relatively small. Valenstein (1977), on the basis of a survey of the world literature, concluded that there were references to 156 opera-tions on children under 15 performed throughout the world. Seventeen of these were performed in the US, seven of them after 1970. Two of these had epilepsy in addition to behaviour disorders. A comparable analysis revealed that there were 11 US operations on individuals aged between 15 and 20 mentioned in the literature published after 1970. Nevertheless, while the number of children involved may be small the issues raised are worrying given that brain damage can have very different consequences for children compared with adults. The issue of informed consent apart, there are a number of special problems. There are, after all, a number of psychiatric and organic problems observed in children that are improved or even eliminated later on in life. The so-called 'hyperkinetic syndrome' is a case in point. The question of psychosurgery in children has to be viewed together with some estimate of the possibility of spontaneous improvement with age.

Post-operative assessment

Evaluating the effects of surgery is greatly dependent on the reliability, validity and comprehensiveness of the data as they are presented in the literature. One recent literature review (Valenstein, 1977), covering 153 articles published between 1971 and 1976 offers little room for complacency. The majority of reports lacked any objective measurement and relied on clinical acumen and subjective impression. Indeed, only 70 of the 153 mentioned tests at all. Five of the 70 merely mentioned unspecified 'psychometric evaluation' while a further 16 reported using intelligence tests. Frequently, there were declarations to the effect that after psychosurgery there were no or minimal changes in intellectual ability. One neurosurgeon relied for his follow-up assessment on, among other items of information, 'annual Christmas greetings' (Freeman, 1971) while another reported 'no or little change in intellect and discrimination ability' following surgery yet the only evidence provided was a sample of the patient's post-operative knitting! (Winter, 1972). For several years insensitive tests following bilateral destruction of the corpus callosum led to the conclusion that there was no impairment of verbal reasoning and intelligence, motor coordination, long-term memory and personality following surgery. No function at all could be attributed to the corpus cellosum until it was revealed by the use of appropriate testing by Sperry and his colleagues. More recently, additional testing has demonstrated short-term memory deficits and impairment in transfer of learning between sensory modalities (Zaidel and Sperry, 1974; Goldstein *et al.*, 1975).

The post-operative effects of psychosurgery are usually reported in terms of categories based on patient interviews, information sought from relatives, employment record, marital and family stability and general information concerning the patient's personality and adjustment. May and Van Putten (1974) have suggested a rating scale of scientific merit whereby psychosurgery reports can be judged. The scale ranges from a rating of 1 to 6. A rating of 1 is applied only to those studies that have matched controls, use objective tests, evaluate patients for an adequate pre- and post-operative period, employ independent raters, analyse data statistically and do not confound any variables (e.g. drug treatment, psychotherapy, etc.). A rating of 6, on the other hand, is applied to reports that provide only descriptive information on the patients and have no comparison group. When Valenstein (1977) applied these criteria to the 153 papers included in his review, most of them received a rating of 5 or 6. Almost 90% of the articles from the US received ratings between 4 and 6. Valenstein (1977) points out that 'it is important to note that a rating of 4 would be given only to articles of low scientific value'. 'It is unlikely' he adds, 'that an animal study with such a low rating would be accepted for publication by the editors of a respected experimental journal.'

The possibility of a placebo effect of psychosurgery is difficult to dismiss. Ethical restraints against performing 'sham' operations militate against any kind of controlled trial along such lines. Livingston (1953) did report on four patients who only underwent a skin incision while believing they had undergone complete surgery. Balasubramaniam and his colleages (1973), in a deliberate attempt to eliminate the possibility of a placebo effect, submitted three drug addicts to burr holes alone. In neither instance were post-operative improvements noted. However, neither study was double-blind and there was inadequate or no matching of the patients.

The most consistent post-operative findings on objective tests concern those symptoms most commonly presented by psychosurgical patients. With few exceptions depression, anxiety, tension, somatic complaints, phobias and obsessional symptoms are reportedly reduced post-operatively. Deficits reported are primarily evident in tests of abstract reasoning, learning and memory and language ability. Deficits have also been reported on tests, such as the Wisconsin Card Sorting and the Goldstein-Scheerer Colour-Form Tests, which require the categorizing of information. Similar deficits have been reported in block design and picture arrangement tests. Language test deficits have been reported following thalamic operations. Learning and memory deficits have also been reported after amygdalectomies. Given that the post-operative follow-up reported can vary from a matter of weeks to several years, it is not wise to assume that the question of possible brain damage following surgery has been properly assessed in even the best reports.

Despite the variation in the nature and length of follow-up, overall post-operative ratings by neurosurgeons and psychiatrists appear favourable. Of the patients reported on between 1971 and 1976 who had received a pre-operative diagnosis of neurotic depression, 96% were regarded as cured or much improved following frontal lobe surgery compared with 72% treated by cingulotomy (Valenstein, 1977). Amygdalectomies for aggression were less impressive with only 28% of patients judged to have improved significantly. Low success rates were reported for patients diagnosed as schizophrenic and for those addicted to drugs.

Caution has to be exercised in interpreting these reports which are based after all on studies already criticized by Valenstein (1977) for various shortcomings. In most cases, the neurosurgeons and psychiatrists responsible for the patients assigned the post-operative ratings. In addition, it has been argued that overall ratings pay excess attention to the alleviation of outstanding symptoms particularly those that bother others, and lay less emphasis on the quality of life that remains possible. This is not always a reasonable objection in that in many instances the criteria for an excellent result seem to have been defined quite broadly and include factors such as the quality of adjustment to the family, social situations and work and whether or not the patients display any loss of initiative.

Post-operative complications

Physical complications of surgery include haemorrhages and infections which are for the most part unrelated to the specific operation. In addition, complications such as seizures, paralysis, dyskinesias, weight changes, anosmia, bladder or bowel incontinence and endocrine changes that may be the result of surgical destruction of a specific brain structure have been reported. Emotional and behavioural complications include loss of motivation, blunting of affect, disinhibition, lowered personal standards, immature behaviour, carelessness, irritability, aggressiveness, alterations in libido and inability to work. The phrase 'frontal lobe syndrome' refers to a cluster of symptoms occurring post-operatively and including either lethargy or disinhibition in addition to seizures, incontinence and some loss in capacity for abstract thinking. It is generally agreed that the incidence of complications following psychosurgery has been significantly reduced since 1965. The most common physical complication had been the occurrence of epileptic seizures, estimates of the incidence during the 1945–1965 period ranging from 10 to 50%. Summaries of post-operative seizures since 1965 on average indicate an incidence of approximately 2% for surgery performed with the aid of stereotactic instruments (Goktepe *et al.*, 1975). The incidence of seizures following the more recent non-stereotactic surgery may still be as high as 10% (Scoville and Bettis, 1976). The incidence of the commonest emotional complications, disinhibition and lethargy, is about 5–10%. In a recent report of thalamic surgery for intractable pain, the incidence of disinhibited behaviour or lethargy post-operatively was approximately 50% (Rodriquez-Burgos et al., 1976).

During the early days of psychosurgery, mortality attributable to operation has been estimated at around 5%. Current estimates of post-operative deaths following stereotaxic procedures are near to zero. Summaries of large patient populations that had undergone stereotaxic frontal or cingulum procedures showed a mortality rate of 0% for 345 operations (Ballantine et al., 1976), 0% for 204 operations (Brown, 1972) and 0·2% for 660 operations (Knight, 1973).

Current status

It is generally accepted that psychosurgery should be performed only on patients for whom other less drastic treatments have proven ineffective. In their detailed study of the effects of stereotactic limbic leucotomy in 16 patients, Mitchell-Heggs et al (1976) revealed that all but seven of these patients had previously received at least one course of ECT, 35 had undergone formal psychotherapy or psychoanalysis while the majority had received 'supportive, non-interpretative psychotherapy' throughout the greater part of their illnesses. Only four, however, had been treated with behaviour therapy although the sample included 27 patients suffering from obsessional neurosis. Yet, several reports (Hodgson and Rachman, 1974; Hodgson et al., 1972; Rachman et al., 1973) have appeared which suggest that considerable success may be obtained using behavioural techniques with the type of obsessive-compulsive and phobic patients often described as among the most suitable candidates for psychosurgery. Behaviour therapists report improvement rates of up to 75% in the case of quite seriously crippled obsessional patients, a rate which compares favourably with the 85% reported by Mitchell-Heggs and her colleagues. It may be that patients referred for surgery are more seriously ill than those referred for behavioural modification. It may also be, however, that at least some of them are referred for surgery by psychiatrists who are unaware of such alternative methods of treatment or who are especially favourable towards psychosurgery. It is in this situation that properly consituted review committees can play an important role (see below).

Ethical issues

Many of the ethical issues relating to psychosurgery, such as the question of informed consent, the conflict between research goals and patient safety and the adequacy of review procedures, are issues of general medical ethics. In the area of psychosurgery, however, the dispute has been particularly acrimonious and bitter (Clare, 1976). Critics tend to portray surgery as 'mutilation' and insist that it blunts, or as one vociferous opponent puts it, 'partially kills' the individual (Breggin, 1972). The situation is not helped by proponents of the procedure asserting or implying that all those who express reservations concerning the use of psychosurgery are ideologically motivated cranks.

Public concern in the United States concerning the possible use of brain surgery in the repression of minorities and the control of prison inmates has resulted in two States, Oregon and California, enacting restrictive legislation concerning the regulation of psychosurgery. In response to this concern, the US National Commission for the Protection of Human Subjects of Biomedical and Behavioural Research was directed to investigate and recommend policies that should govern the use of psychosurgery. In Australia, a Committee of Inquiry into Psychosurgery was established by the New South Wales Minister of Health early in 1977 following the publication of a series of allegations concerning the manner in which psychosurgical procedures had been carried out in that State. In the United Kingdom there have been a number of representations made by interested bodies, including the National Association for Mental Health (MIND) concerning the use of psychosurgery in the case of involuntarily committed psychiatric patients and there have been discussions, hitherto unfruitful, concerning a possible multi-centred, controlled trial of such operations.

At the time of writing, the use of psychosurgery in Britain is regulated by the usual restrictions on any medical treatment including the Mental Health Act (1959). Bridges and Bartlett (1977) have made clear the policy at one British unit, the Geoffrey Knight Unit at the Brook Hospital in South London, concerning informed consent. The Unit does not accept patients for limbic leucotomy who are the subject of an order under the 1959 Mental Health Act. These authors advocate that psychosurgery should be carried out at a few specialized centres where the procedures can be monitored, where research can be undertaken and experience can accumulate. They are critical of the American practice of direct referral to a neurosurgeon preferring instead that all patients be assessed by a psychiatrist and neurosurgeon working closely together. They make no mention of any need for a supervisory Psychosurgery Review Board along the lines suggested in the American and Australian reports quoted above, preferring to see psychosurgery governed by the regulations and restrictions of ordinary clinical practice. They end their review with the expressed hope that with advances in psychopharmacology and other forms of non-surgical treatments psychosurgery will no longer be needed.

Electroconvulsive therapy

History

The roots of electrical treatment lie buried deep in the history of psychiatry. That electricity can stun was known to Hippocrates and his colleagues by way of their familiarity with the electric torpedo fish found in Mediterranean waters. In an address delivered to the Royal Society in 1774, Sir John Pringle described how before the days of Galen the torpedo fish was applied to affected parts of the body and was particularly effective in easing persistent headaches. Earlier, in 1756, John Wesley procured an apparatus that could deliver electric shocks and found the treatment so effective that he declared 'hundreds, perhaps thousands, have received unspeakable good'. John Birch, a surgeon at St Thomas's Hospital, was one of the first dedicated advocates of electricity as a therapeutic agent and in 1792 he explained how he administered the treatment to a porter suffering from a melancholic state for almost a year. Six small shocks were passed through the brain in different directions on each of three successive days, following which the patient regained his spirits, went back to his work and remained perfectly well for seven years (Birch, 1792).

In his 'Treatise on Madness', published in 1758, William Battie noted that 'one species of spasm, however occasioned, seldom fails to put an end to that other which before subsisted'. At this time the belief that massive excitation or exposure to some form of physical stress might have a beneficial effect on mental distress flourished. In 1785, Dr W. Oliver published an account of the results of administering the epileptogenic agent, camphor, in a case of melancholia. The patient promptly recovered, subsequently relapsed, had a further treatment and regained his health. Interest in camphor-induced fits waxed and waned throughout the following two centuries. However, it was a slow and unreliable method of inducing fits and was superseded early in the 1930s by the Hungarian psychiatrist Meduna's discovery that intravenous injections of metrazol produced more reliable convulsions. At about the same time, Ugo Cerletti, a psychiatric research worker in Rome, was investigating changes in brain tissue produced by convulsions in animals. When Cerletti read Meduna's preliminary reports of metrazol-induced convulsions, it occurred to him that electrical methods of inducing convulsions might be technically more acceptable and therapeutically more effective in man.

The rationale for the use of convulsive treatment at this time remained as crude as the treatment itself. Several investigators, including Meduna, believed that there was a sort of biological antagonism between schizophrenia and epilepsy which meant that the courses of the two conditions were either mutually exclusive or weakened each other in their mutual effects. Cerletti, in common with most of his contemporaries, accepted this hypothesis and in 1938 administered the first electrically induced convulsion to a catatonic vagrant found wandering in a Rome railway station. As described by Impastato (1960), the first shock was too weak and it required a second one at a higher voltage to bring about a full-scale convulsion.

Over the following twenty years ECT gradually became established as the major physical treatment in psychiatric practice. The development of muscle-relaxant drugs, such as curare, gallamine and succinylcholine, and of short-acting anaesthetic agents such as thiopental and methohexital, have meant that the treatment can now be administered with reasonable safety, few side-effects and a minimum of discomfort. For details of how ECT is currently administered, the reader is referred to a number of texts devoted to a consideration of the role of physical treatments in psychiatry (Sargant and Slater, 1972; Kalinowsky and Hippius, 1969).

Efficacy

Despite a wealth of research into convulsive therapy (one review conducted by Ridell revealed over 200 studies during the years 1955–1960 alone) there is still disagreement over its efficacy as a treatment. The difficulty is that most studies make no use at all of a control group. Admittedly, it is not as easy to design a suitably controlled trial of ECT as it is to set up a properly controlled drug trial. For a valid trial of ECT to be undertaken, the control group of patients would need to receive exactly the same treatment as the treatment group except the shock; that is to say, the control group would have to receive the anaesthetic, the muscle relaxant and the oxygen and all the care and attention given to the treatment group. However, the ethical implications of giving patients an anaesthetic and a muscle relaxant as part of an experiment and of withholding a treatment that empirically appears to be effective have to date deterred psychiatrists from mounting an adequately controlled trial. However, a number of studies incoporate a form of 'simulated' ECT within their design (see below).

Studies of the efficacy of ECT can broadly be divided into four main groups:

(1) Studies in which the control group patients are anaesthetized but do not receive any electric shock
(2) Studies in which the control group patients receive no treatment at all

(3) Studies in which different methods of administering ECT are compared
(4) Studies in which ECT is compared to other treatment methods

1   Studies with an anaesthetized control group ('Simulated ECT')

The relatively few studies conducted with an anaesthetized control group
have not clarified the question of ECT's therapeutic efficacy. One of the
first studies (Miller *et al.*, 1953) assigned 30 seriously disturbed patients to
three treatment groups: (1) orthodox electrical treatment; (2) thiopental
sodium anaesthesia; (3) thiopental sodium plus non-convulsive electrical
stimulation. None of the three groups showed any change in the state of
their psychoses which were categorized by the authors as schizophrenic.
A somewhat similar approach (Brill *et al.*, 1959) attempted to determine
the role played by each of the major components of ECT in its alleged
therapeutic effect. Patients were randomly assigned to one of five treatment groups: (1) orthodox ECT; (2) ECT with sufficient muscular relaxation to abolish the contraction; (3) ECT under anaesthesia; (4) anaesthesia
alone; (5) nitrous oxide alone. There were 97 patients involved, of whom
about two-thirds were diagnosed as schizophrenics and the remainder as
suffering from a variety of depressive and neurotic conditions. This study
also failed to show that ECT was significantly more effective than anaesthesia alone. A third study (Ulett *et al.*, 1956) did suggest that electroconvulsive and photoconvulsive shock achieved very much better results
than either subconvulsive shock or sedation with barbiturates.

In 1960, Robin and Harris attempted to evaluate the antidepressive
effect of phenelzine. Their study was so designed that suitably depressed
patients were given either a course of ECT or of 'conservative' treatment
and were then compared. 'Conservative' treatment consisted of two
weeks treatment with phenelzine followed by two weeks treatment with
matched placebo tablets. Cases selected for ECT were given either twice
weekly ECT and placebo tablets, twice weekly injections of anaesthetic
plus phenelzine tablets or twice weekly anaesthetic injections plus
placebo tablets. Little antidepressant effect was found with phenelzine.
In contrast, patients treated with ECT responded well whereas those who
received the anaesthetic plus placebo or the anaesthetic plus phenelzine
did relatively poorly. Unfortunately, the clinicians rating the patients'
responses knew which patients received 'true' and which received 'simulated' ECT and hence this portion of the study cannot be considered to be
truly blind.

A recent preliminary report on the efficacy of ECT compared with
placebo suggests that the treatment may not be grossly superior to

placebo. Lambourn and Gill (1977) assigned patients suffering from psychotic depression randomly to one of two groups, matched for age and sex. Psychoactive medication was stopped and all received a standardized intravenous anaesthetic regime plus the application of right unilateral electrodes (Lancaster's position) thrice weekly. This constituted the placebo while the active group also received a brief pulse stimulus and exhibited a bilateral modified convulsion every time. Change was rated blind in four ways. Hamilton ratings showed only a trend in favour of ECT (improvement of 53% against 43%). Leeds self-assessment scores corrected for side-effects showed ECT and placebo equally effective on the depression ratings but ECT was significantly superior on the anxiety ratings. One month follow-up produced comparable outcome for days in hospital, Hamilton ratings, additional ECT and antidepressant medication. The authors conclusion that ECT was shown neither to be grossly superior to placebo nor worthless may seem cautious but the design of the study, and particularly the fact that patients in both groups had already been in receipt of antidepressant medication prior to the trial, makes such caution mandatory.

A second study comparing ECT with a simulated version (Freeman *et al.*, 1978) found ECT to be 'significantly superior' in the treatment of depressive illness but in this study the simulated ECT was restricted to just two applications followed by real ECT in the control group. The authors felt that it was 'ethically unjustified to withold for a complete course a treatment generally regarded to be effective and to submit patients to perhaps unnecessary general anaesthetic'.

2   Studies using a no-treatment control group

Some controlled drug trials make use of a drug group, an ECT group and a placebo group and it is possible in these cases to regard the placebo group as a 'no treatment' group and compare it with the ECT group. One of the most important of such studies is that of the Medical Research Council in 1965.

> The MRC study compared ECT (a course of 4–8 treatments), imipramine (in doses of 200 mg/day), phenelzine (in doses of 60 mg/day) and an inert placebo in the treatment of in-patients suffering from depression. The patients, aged between forty and sixty-nine, had suffered from illnesses of less than eighteen months duration and had not been in receipt of adequate treatment before the trial. Treatments were randomly allocated and were maintained for a minimum of four weeks. If the rater deemed the response to a particular treatment to be satisfactory, it was continued. Otherwise patients failing to respond to ECT were switched to tablets and those failing to respond to tablets were switched to ECT.

At four weeks, 71% of the patients receiving ECT had few or no symptoms compared with 53% for imipramine, 30% for phenelzine and

39% for placebo. ECT was easily the quickest effective treatment in cases of severe depression. More long-term evaluation over a six-month period did not affect these results except to show that most of the patients who had been switched from phenelzine to ECT responded remarkably well.

A large number of other studies (Greenblatt *et al.*, 1964; Kristiansen, 1961; Kiloh *et al.*, 1960; Carney *et al.*, 1965) all support the claims of ECT in the treatment of depression and particularly severe depression. The major methodological defect inherent in simple studies of comparison between ECT, drugs and/or placebo, however, is that they are not blind, that is to say the researchers know which patients receive the drug/placebo and which receive ECT.

3   Studies comparing different types of ECT

Orthodox electroconvulsive treatment has been given in an *unmodified* form (i.e. without an anaesthetic or musle relaxant), in a *modified* form, with an *anticonvulsant*, using a *subconvulsive* stimulus (using an electrical current too weak to induce a fit), and *unilaterally* (both electrodes being applied to one side of the head only). These various methods of administration have been compared with each other, and consequently it has been possible to clarify which of the many factors in ECT appears to exert the claimed therapeutic effect.

In a number of studies, Seager reported that modified and unmodified ECT produced similar results and he concluded that those factors modified by the anaesthetic and muscle relaxant were not crucial to its beneficial therapeutic effects. Two Scandinavian workers, Cronholm and Ottosson, artificially shortened the duration and the extent of the epileptic discharge induced by ECT by administering an anticonvulsant, lidocaine, and found that this did not reduce the therapeutic efficacy. These workers have shown that the memory disturbances reported with ECT and the treatment's antidepressant effect arise, at least in part, via *different* mechanisms; whereas the memory defect is mainly determined by the amount of electrical current and partly by the seizure, the antidepressant effect is bound to the cerebral seizure activity induced by the electrical stimulation. The methodology of this work, however, has been criticized and particularly the randomization procedure employed yet it has been seen by many to lend support to the clinical impression that the seizure is of fundamental importance.

> Ottosson compared the relief of depression and the performance on formal memory tests of three groups of patients in a double-blind trial. The first group was given the *minimum* shock necessary to produce a fit. The second group was given a shock *well above* the convulsive threshold. The third group had their fits *modified* by a previous injection of lidocaine, which shortens the

epileptic discharge without affecting the convulsive threshold. The patients in the first two groups showed a similar response to ECT but the group receiving the larger shock showed more severe post-treatment memory impairment. The third group showed a much poorer treatment response.

Alterations in the nature of the electrical stimuli (from diphasic sinusoidal wave-form pulses to unidirectional fractionated ones) have reduced the energy needed to induce fits and reduced the associated memory disturbances. The replacement of electricity by the chemical, flurethyl, has not caught on and has languished. With unilateral electrode placement, however, a considerable reduction of side-effects, without any loss of therapeutic efficacy has been claimed.

In 1957, Lancaster and his colleagues introduced the *unilateral* technique whereby both electrodes are placed on the non-dominant side of the head. They noted that such application resulted in much less post-treatment disorientation and memory impairment than occurred with bilateral treatment yet there did not appear to be any diminution in therapeutic effect. Subsequently, a very large number of studies (Cannicott and Waggoner, 1967; Gottlieb and Wilson, 1965; Martin *et al*., 1965; Zamora and Kaelbling, 1965) gave support to this claim. Levy (1968) in a careful double-blind study failed to find a significant difference on the Weschler Memory Test or on a paired associate learning test between unilaterally and bilaterally treated nor any difference in the relief of depression achieved. He criticized earlier studies for failing to carry out assessments on a double-blind basis, for not adhering to a proper randomization procedure, for a lack of standardization of anaesthetic and ECT technique and for inadequate assessments of memory functions and depressive symptoms.

A recent review of 29 studies of unilateral versus bilateral ECT by d'Elia and Raotma (1975) does, however, conclude that whereas both types of treatment appear to produce the same antidepressive effect with few exceptions the unilateral form produces less and shorter post-treatment confusion, disorientation for time, agitation, restlessness and automatism. They emphasize, in common with Dornbush (1972), that an indiscriminate study of memory impairment after unilateral ECT is no longer sufficient to increase our insight into the intricate and varying problem of memory functions and their functional localization. For example, it is necessary to consider such factors as the time of administration (anterograde and retrograde designs), modality of input (auditory and visual), content of the tasks (verbal and non-verbal), method of testing (recognition, relearning and recall) and type of memory variable (learning and retention). It is also probable that responses differ not only with the hemispheres stimulated but also with different placements on the same hemisphere.

4   Studies comparing ECT with other treatment methods

Numerous studies have compared ECT with other physical treatments and these include the MRC trial of antidepressant quoted earlier in this chapter. Despite the development of a large number of tricyclic antidepressants and monoamine oxidase inhibitors, ECT is still regarded as marginally more potent, especially in the more severe forms of depression (Klein and Davis, 1969; Greenblatt *et al.*, 1964; Robin and Harris, 1962).

Indications

It has been said that the quick and predictable effect of ECT in certain forms of *depression* represents one of 'the most spectacular results obtainable in psychiatry' (Kalinowsky and Hippius, 1969). The proportion of patients showing a good response to ECT is usually reported as 70–80%. However, not all depressed patients are helped by ECT. Hobson (1953) constructed a check list based on an analysis of the history and clinical state of 127 depressives treated with ECT and identified six items associated with a good response to ECT and nine items associated with a poor response (Table I). He scored one point for the *absence* of each favourable

Table I   *Prediction of response to ECT (Hobson, 1953)*

favourable features (score 1 for each feature absent)	Unfavourable features (score 1 for each feature present)
1 Sudden onset	1 Hypochondriasis
2 Good insight	2 Depersonalization
3 Obessional previous personality	3 Emotional lability
4 Self-reproach	4 Childhood neurotic traits
5 Duration of illness less than one year	5 Adult neurotic traits
6 Pronounced retardation	6 Hysterical attitude to illness
	7 Above average intelligence
	8 Fluctuating course since onset
	9 Ill-adjusted or hysterical previous personality

item and one for the *presence* of each unfavourable one; the higher the total score, the less likely the patient is to respond. Carney *et al.* (1965) assessed 35 individual aspects of depressive illness affecting 108 patients treated with ECT and found that 10 items correlated significantly with the mental state six months after completion of the treatment (Table II). Such attempts to predict response have not been wholly successful. For example, of the 44 patients included in the Carney *et al.* study who showed a

Table II *Prediction of response to ECT (Carney et al., 1965)*

Feature	Score[a]
Weight loss	+3
Pyknic body build	+3
Early wakening	+2
Somatic delusions[b]	+2
Paranoid delusions	+1
Self-pity	−1
Anxiety	−2
Worse in evenings	−3
Hysterical features or attitudes	−3
Hypochondriasis[c]	−3

[a] Score only if feature present. Ignore features which are absent.
[b] Delusions of body change or disease, usually of a bizarre nature.
[c] Excessive or morbid preoccupation with bodily sensations that have a little or no organic basis.

good response to ECT, nine would have been predicted by these researchers' guidelines as having a poor response while of 64 patients showing a poor response, eight would have been predicted to be good responders. Even among patients presenting with the typical features of so called 'endogenous' depression, there are still approximately 15–25% that fail to respond to ECT (Lehmann, 1967; Kielholz, 1973; Stromgren, 1973). It has been suggested (Hobson, 1953; Hamilton and White, 1960) that the response to ECT is worse in patients who have been ill for a lengthy period. Recently, Kukopulos and his colleagues (1977) have proposed that ECT is only effective when given within six months of the spontaneous end of the depression.

Electroconvulsive therapy is sometimes used in the management of *manic illnesses* but there are no satisfactory controlled studies of its use. In a retrospective comparison of groups of patients matched for various clinical features and treated in the same institution before and after the use of ECT, McCabe (1976) found that the group of ECT-treated patients spent less time in hospital, were significantly better on discharge and appeared to have shown a better social response than those not treated with ECT. Both unipolar and bipolar affective illness exhibit a similar response (Abrams and Taylor, 1974).

The value of ECT in the treatment of *schizophrenia* is even more questionable. One prominent textbook on physical treatments asserts that 'all recently ill schizophrenic patients should receive combined drug and convulsive therapy as early as possible' (Sargant and Slater, 1972) whereas another (Shepherd *et al.*, 1968) sees ECT as having been replaced by the phenothiazines. One large study of treatment efficacy in recently diagnosed schizophrenic patients (May, 1968) reported that on a wide variety of indices ECT was shown to be more effective than milieu therapy or psychotherapy alone but consistently less effective than either drug therapy or drugs plus psychotherapy. The common clinical view that certain specific features of schizophrenia, such as catatonic excitement or stupor or affective symptoms, respond to ECT is not supported by the literature and seems to be an area for further enquiry. In the meantime, the overall view expressed by Cawley concerning the role of ECT in schizophrenia to the effect that 'the superiority of modified ECT to pentothal anaesthesia alone has never been satisfactorily demonstrated' remains pertinent.

Side-effects and contraindications

The risk of death with ECT appears to be negligible. In 1953, Maclay reported that he could find only 62 deaths associated with the treatment in the mental hospitals of England and Wales during the period 1947–1952. In 1959, Barker and Baker conducted a questionnaire survey of 259,000 treatments and identified nine deaths probably related to ECT. The absolute number of ECT deaths has declined over the past twenty years so that whereas 34 patients died in 1954–1956 and 11 in 1957–1958 only 25 died during 1959–1966. Perrin (1961) summarized a number of predominantly American studies involving more than 40,000 patients and found that one patient in 950 died, one treatment in 12,500 was fatal and that 50% of the deaths were due to adverse effects on the cardio-vascular system. Cardiac arrest consequent on vagal inhibition and coronary thrombosis are the commonest causes of death (Tewfik and Wells, 1957; Barker and Baker, 1959) but other causes included cerebral haemorrhage, pulmonary embolism and pneumonia. Non-fatal complications include dislocations, fractures and fat embolism, peptic ulcer bleeds and perforation (Perrin, 1961). A recent three-year follow-up of 519 patients with depression found that a group of patients treated with ECT had a significantly lower mortality than a group of patients who had received neither ECT nor antidepressants (Avery and Winokur, 1976).

Adverse psychological effects include mania, which may occasionally be precipitated in manic-depressive subjects, confusion and memory impairment. Assessment of memory impairment following ECT is complicated by the finding that memory functions are impaired in depression and improve with improvements in mental state (Sternberg and Jarvik, 1976). Williams (1966) has shown that the nature of the memory disorder following ECT resembles that seen following a mild head injury. There is a short and rapidly dwindling amnesia for the time-period preceding each treatment (retrograde amnesia) and a longer post-shock (antero-grade) amnesia. The most obvious defect is in the patient's ability to retain recently learned material. This defect outlasts the short (20–40 minutes) post-ECT confusional period and has been shown to affect information presented to the patient either just prior to the shock or during recovery from it. Squire and Miller (1974) have shown how the ability to learn new material is initially impaired and then recovers in the hours after shock treatment. The ability to retain material for 24 hours is more impaired following the fourth than after the first shock treatment. Squire (1975) has further demonstrated that following a course of five treatments there is an impairment of ability to recall events from the remote past and that this impairment has not changed in the 24 hours following the last treatment. It is still not clear how persistent this memory impairment may be following completion of a course of treatment. Cronholm and Molander (1957) examined 28 patients and found no evidence of memory impairment one month after an ECT course had finished. Squire and Chace (1975) could find no objective impairment of memory using a battery of tests of delayed and remote memory six to nine months after ECT. However, patients in their study who had received bilateral ECT rated their memory as impaired significantly more often than those who had received unilateral ECT or who had been treated in other ways. Squire (1977) has concluded, on the basis of a review of the current literature on the relationship between ECT and memory loss, that even when memory is assessed with tests known to be particularly sensitive to dysfunction of the right cerebral hemisphere, bilateral ECT is associated with greater anterograde amnesia than right unilateral ECT.

Some critics of ECT have claimed that it produces gross brain damage (Friedberg, 1977). Brain tissues have been reported to show increased gliosis (Ebaugh *et al.*, 1942), diffuse degeneration (Gralnick, 1944), petechial haemorrhages in the brain stem with fat embolism (Meyer and Teare, 1945) and oedema and subarachnoid haemorrhage (Alpers and Hughes, 1942; Karsen, 1953; Liban *et al.*, 1951). In 1957, Impastato summarized 254 electroshock fatalities. Brain damage was implicated in many and nearly one-fifth of all cerebral deaths were haemorrhagic. Friedberg (1977) refers to 21 reports of neuropathology in patients who had undergone ECT but 20 of these reports concerns treatment administered before 1956 when seizures were generally induced without succinylcholine, oxygen or barbiturates. In such cases, the cerebral damage noted may well have been a consequence of the induced seizure or of an associated anoxia, trauma, hypoglycaemia, hyperpyrexia or impaired cerebral perfusion.

Meldrum and his colleagues have attempted to evaluate the effects of seizure activity in primates. In one study (Meldrum *et al.*, 1973) the presence of peripheral motor paralysis and artificial respiration greatly reduced the severity of the systemic changes and modified the pattern of epileptic brain damage seen after precipitation of status epilepticus in eight baboons. In a subsequent study (Meldrum *et al.*, 1974), 13 baboons were submitted to similar experiments using the convulsant allylglycine. Five animals developed status epilepticus, and in the other eight animals, between six and 63 seizures occurred in a period of 2–11 hours. Post-mortem examination revealed that in those animals that had had between six and 26 seizures over a period of several hours *no* pathological sequelae were found whereas in those that had had more than 26 seizures or status epilepticus, varying degrees of ischaemic cell change and neuronal loss with gliosis in the neocortex and in the hippocampus were seen. Such evidence does not support the belief that ECT, in the manner and frequency with which it is commonly administered to patients, produces brain damage as a matter of course.

How does ECT work?

There is no single explanatory theory of how ECT might exert its therapeutic effect which is widely accepted. Some psychoanalysts have argued that the treatment is effective because it fulfils the patient's repressed desire for pain and punishment, his unconscious hope for death and rebirth and his need to be a passive and helpless recipient of the therapist's power and fantasies (Goode, 1940; Brill *et al.*, 1959; Dies, 1969). Others have attributed the therapeutic effect to damage inflicted by ECT on sensitive nerve cells (Morgan, 1940; Freeman and Watts, 1949; Friedberg, 1977). However, findings such as that lidocaine-modified seizures are less effective than seizures not so modified are difficult to reconcile with such explanatory theories and, so far as one researcher is concerned, it is clear that 'a therapeutically active component is contained in the convulsion' and 'it is unnecessary to waste words on theories which do not take this fact into account' (Ottosson, 1974). Interest has recently switched to more biological explanations such as the possible effect of ECT on neurotransmitter availability in the brain (Schildkraut and Draskoczy, 1974), on altering membrane permeability (Rosenblatt *et al.*, 1960; Angel and Roberts, 1966), on cyclic 3' 5'-adenosine monophosphate (Hamadah *et al.*, 1972) and on protein synthesis (Essman, 1974). The possibility that ECT works by affecting the movement of certain ions, such as sodium, chloride and potassium, across neuronal membranes is supported by the work of Arneson and his colleagues (1965) and by the reports that in severely depressed patients electrolyte metabolism is abnormal and returns to normal on recovery (Coppen, 1970).

    However, the most intriguing hypothesis is that of Grahame-Smith *et al.* (1978) who gave daily electroshock to rats and found an increase in the sensitivity of post-synaptic receptors to monoamines. These authors suggest that ECT produces its antidepressant effects by potentiating the actions of 5HT, dopamine, and perhaps noradrenaline, transmitters which may be depleted in depression (Chapter 12).

Ethical aspects of ECT

Ethical questions concerning the use of ECT are closely related to many of the points already discussed, including the questionable reputation ECT has acquired due to earlier, unmodified treatment methods, its potential for distressing side-effects and the fact that it is a crude treatment applied to a highly sensitive and sophisticated organ, the brain. In addition, some enthusiastic advocates of ECT have tended to over-sell it as a panacea for a wide range of psychiatric disturbances with the inevitable result that there are many articulate patients available to testify to the fact that ECT did not help their particular problems. However, as Salzman has pointed out (Salzman, 1977), such problems must be separated from the ethical concerns that attend the legitimate use of ECT. He identifies these concerns as (1) the right to receive ECT, (2) the right to refuse ECT, and (3) the nature of informed consent about ECT and its potential hazards.

The right to receive ECT, like the right to receive any therapy, hinges on the view that ECT is an effective, reasonably safe and rapid treatment. The right to treatment is often associated with involuntary hospitalization and in at least one American legal case (Wyatt v. Stickney, 1971) the courts ruled that a patient cannot be confined involuntarily if he/she is not offered treatment. The Royal College of Psychiatrists, commenting on a consultative document on the 1959 Mental Health Act, prepared by the Department of Health and Social Security (1976), insisted that the primary purpose of all compulsory procedures must be for treatment 'using the definition of treatment to include medical/nursing treatments, care and training' (Royal College of Psychiatrists, 1977). Indeed, one commentator (Beresford, 1971) has gone so far as to suggest that 'involuntary patients who are not offered ECT for their psychotic depression may later contend that the hospital was negligent in omitting this medically indicated and highly effective treatment'.

The problem becomes even more complicated when a patient's right to refuse ECT is considered. Such a right, like the right to refuse surgery, medication or other medical treatment, is a civil liberty which must ordinarily be protected. The peculiar dilemma which confronts all psychiatrists is due to the fact that a patient's ability to make a rational decision about his or her own well-being may be seriously impaired by the nature of the disorder for which the treatment is indicated. Given that in certain circumstances, the right to refuse treatment is overridden by the decision to treat, what should the procedural controls over such a course of action be? Stone (1975) has suggested that a full judicial hearing in the presence of a judge is necessary before ECT is administered to a protesting patient. He adds that 'other third parties such as guardians, relatives, patient rights committees or other physicians not on the hospital staff will not insure the patient's civil liberties'. The Royal College of Psychiatrists takes quite a contrary view. It supports the basic principle of two medical recommendations by two doctors unrelated in practice, one of whom should be specially approved 'as expert in the appropriate field of mental disorder', the other being, if possible, the patient's regular general practitioner. The College supports making it easier for patients to appeal against compulsory procedures to independent tribunals which have the power to direct discharge if they see fit. Between these two positions, one of which sees ECT as a particularly hazardous and invasive form of treatment, the other of which sees ECT as an effective and useful treatment, no more hazardous than any treatment involving an anaesthetic and muscle relaxant, there is room for various modifications whereby those seriously ill psychiatric patients who refuse ECT and who thereby directly jeopardize their own lives can be treated subject to some form of legal control and possibly even legal supervision.

The issue of informed consent is a further complication. A recent memorandum published by the Royal College of Psychiatrists insisted that consent is a matter between the patient and doctor and it is a medical responsibility to ensure that the patient has been given an explanation 'of the procedure, benefits and dangers of ECT' (Royal College of Psychiatrists, 1977a). The memorandum also recommended that the nearest relative should always be consulted and again the procedure should be explained and approval in writing obtained. In practice, it suggested that patients unable to understand the nature and purpose of the treatment proposed and therefore 'unable to give consent' should be treated as 'unwilling' and the procedure adopted in the case of compulsorily detained patients applied.

This memorandum refrained from being explicit about what it believed constitutes 'informed consent'. How much information must be given to ensure that consent is 'informed' without scaring away the patient? How much information can be handled by patients whose cognitive functioning may be seriously disturbed? Is there sufficient information available concerning the precise risks associated with ECT to enable psychiatrists to be confident that they have properly informed their patients concerning all aspects of the treatment? These issues are not limited to psychiatry (Clare, 1976) but it is in psychiatric practice that they have acquired particular bite. A question left begging in most discussions of informed consent is what is the degree of statistical frequency of a risk which determines that a psychiatrist would be negligent in not mentioning it to a patient? Salzman (1977) observes that it is difficult to imagine that any patient who has been fully informed of the possiblity of permanent, near-total memory loss would consent to ECT. Stone (1975) has compounded the problem by drawing attention to the fact that very large doses of powerful, potentially toxic medication, restraints or maximum security measures may be required to protect the life of an acutely suicidal, psychotic patient who refuses ECT. These difficulties are reflected in the wide variation in court decisions in the United States about how much information is helpful to patients facing ECT (Krouner, 1975).

Spencer (1977) has recently drawn attention to the fact that psychiatrists do not always inform patients about the more mundane and practical aspects of ECT. In a study of 50 patients in Australia, he found that the principal areas of concern relating to ECT were found to be associated with the accompanying anaesthesia, fear of pain, anxiety over possible memory loss and above all the discomfort associated with waiting for the treatment. In an earlier British study, the degree to which the patients understood or, more accurately, failed to understand what was happening to them was commented upon (Spencer, 1968). 'Most surgical patients have the rudiments of their treatment explained to them,' declared Spencer, 'so why not those who are having ECT.' The rise in public concern over the use of ECT coupled with reviews of its place in contemporary psychiatric practice should contribute to a situation in which patients are not given it without the basic information concerning its application being explained to them.

References

Abrams, R. and Taylor, M. A. (1974). Unipolar and bipolar depressive illness. Phenomenology and response to electroconvulsive therapy. *Arch. Gen. Psychiat.* **30**, 320–321.

Alpers, B. J. and Hughes, J. (1942). The brain changes in electrically induced convulsions in the human. *J. Neuropathol. Exp. Neurol.* **1**, 173.

Angel, C. and Roberts, A. J. (1966). Effect of electroshock and antidepressant drugs on cerebrovascular permeability to cocaine in the rat. *J. Nerv. Ment. Dis.* **142**, 375–380.

Arneson, G. A. and Ourso, R. (1965). Bromide intoxication and electroshock therapy. *Am. J. Psychiat.* **121**, 1115–1119.

Avery, D. and Winokur, G. (1976). Mortality in depressed patients treated with electroconvulsive therapy and antidepressants. *Arch. Gen. Psychiat.* **33**, 1029–1137.

Balasubramaniam, V., Kanaka, T. S. and Ramanujam, P. B. (1973). Stereotaxic cingulotomy for drug addiction. *Neurol. India* **21**, 63–66.

Ballantine, H. T., Jr., Cassidy, W. L., Flanagan, N. B. and Marino, R. Jr. (1967). Stereotaxic anterior cingulotomy for neuropsychiatric illness and intractable pain. *J. Neurosurg.* **26**, 488–495.

Ballantine, H. T., Levy, B. S., Dagi, T. S. and Giriunas, I. B. (1976). Cingulotomy for psychiatric illness: Report of 13 years experience. *In* 'Neurosurgical Treatment in Psychiatry' (Ed. W. H. Sweet). University Park Press, Baltimore, Maryland.

Barker, J. C. and Baker, A. A. (1959). Deaths associated with electroplexy. *J. Ment. Sci.* **105**, 339–348.

Battie, W. (1758). 'A Treatise on Madness'. L. Whiston and White, London.

Beresford, H. R. (1971). Legal issues relating to electro-convulsive therapy. *Arch. Gen. Psychiat.* **25**, 100–102.

Birch, J. (1792). *In* 'An Essay on Electricity, Explaining the Principles of that Useful Science and Describing the Instruments' (Ed. G. Adams) (4th edn). London.

Breggin, P. R. (1792). The return of lobotomy and psychosurgery. *Congressional Record* **118** (26) Feb. 24, 5567–5577.

Brill, N. Q., Crumpton, E., Edisun, S., Grayson, H. M., Hillman, L. I. and Richard, R. A. (1959). Relative effectiveness of various components of electro-convulsive therapy. *Arch. Neurol. Psychiat.* **81**, 627–635.

Bridges, P. K. and Bartlett, J. R. (1977). Review article: psychosurgery: yesterday and today. *Br. J. Psychiat.* **131**, 249–260.

Bridges, P. K., Goktepe, E. D. and Maratos, J. (1973). A comparative review of patients with obsessional neurosis and depression treated by psychosurgery. *Br. J. Psychiat.* **123**, 663–674.

Brown, B. S., Wienckowski, L. A. and Bivens, L. W. (1973). Psychosurgery: perspective on a current issue. *DHEW Publ.* (HSM) 73–9119, Washington, D.C.

Brown, M. H. (1972). The changing role of cingulate surgery. *In* 'Transactions of the Symposium on Cingulotomy' (Ed. G. S. Mathews). Hahneman Medical College and Hospital, Philadelphia.

Cannicott, S. M. and Waggoner, R. W. (1967). Unilateral and bilateral electro-convulsive therapy. A comparative study. *Arch. Gen. Psychiat.* **16**, 229–232.

Carney, M. W. P., Roth, M. and Garside, R. F. (1965). The diagnosis of depressive syndromes and the prediction of ECT response. *Br. J. Psychiat.* **111**, 659–674.

Cawley, R. C. H. (1967). The present status of physical treatments in schizophrenia. *In* 'Recent Developments in Schizophrenia' (Eds A. Coppen and A. Walk). *British Journal of Psychiatry* Special Publication No. 1. Headley Bros, Ashford, Kent.

Clare, A. (1976). 'Psychiatry in Dissent'. Tavistock, London.

Coppen, A. (1970). 'The Chemical Pathology of Affective Disorders'. Scientific Basis of Medicine Annual Review, 189–210.

Cronholm, B. and Molander, L. (1957). Memory disturbances after electroconvulsive therapy. 1. Conditions 6 hours after electroshock treatment. *Acta Psychiat. Neurol. Scand.* **32**, 280–306.

d'Elia, G. and Raotma, H. (1975). Is unilateral ECT less effective than bilateral ECT? *Br. J. Psychiat.* **126**, 83–89.

Department of Health and Social Security (1976). 'A Review of The Mental Health Act, 1959'. HMSO, London.

Dieckmann, G. and Hassler, R. (1975). Unilateral hypothalamotomy in sexual delinquents. *Confin. Neurol.* **37**, 177–186.

Dies, R. R. (1969). Electroconvulsive therapy: a social learning theory interpretation. *J. Nerv. Ment. Dis.* **146**, 334.

Dornbush, R. L. (1972). Memory and induced ECT convulsions. *Seminars in Psychiatry*, **4**, 4, 47–54.

Essman, W. B. (1974). Effects of electroconvulsive shock on cerebral protein synthesis. *In* 'Psychobiology of Convulsive Therapy' (Eds M. Fink, S. Kety, J. McGaugh and T. Williams). Wiley, Chichester.

Ebaugh, F. G., Barnacle, C. H. and Neubuerger, K. T. (1942). Fatalities following electric convulsive therapy. A report of 2 cases with autopsy findings. *Trans. Am. Neurol. Assoc.* June, p. 36.

Ferrier, D. (1875). The Croonien Lecture. Experiments on the brain of monkeys (2nd Ser.). *Philos. Trans. Roy. Soc. Lond.* **65**, 433–488.

Foltz, E. L. and White, L. E. (1962). Pain 'relief' by frontal cingulotomy. *J. Neurosurg.* **19**, 89.

Freeman, C. P. L., Basson, J. V. and Crighton, A. (1978). Double-blind controlled trial of electroconvulsive therapy (ECT) and simulated ECT in depressive illness. *Lancet* **i**, 738–740.

Freeman, W. (1971). Frontal lobotomy in early schizophrenia: long follow-up in 415 cases. *Br. J. Psychiat.* **119**, 621–624.

Freeman, W. and Watts J. W. (1949). Psychosurgery in the treatment of mental disorders and intractable pain. *In* 'Psychosurgery' (Eds W. Freeman and J. W. Watts). Thomas, Springfield, Illinois.

Friedberg, J. (1977). Shock treatment, brain damage and memory loss: a neurological perspective. *Am. J. Psychiat.* **134**, 9, 1010–1014.

Gildenberg, P. L. (1975). Survey of stereotactic and functional neurosurgery in the United States and Canada. *Appl. Neurophysiol.* **38**, 31–37.

Goktepe, E. D., Young, L. G. and Bridges, P. K. (1975). A further review of the results of stereotactic subcaudate tractotomy. *Br. J. Psychiat.* **126**, 270–280.

Goldstein, M. N., Joynt, R. J. and Hartley, R. B. (1975). The long-term effects of callosal sectioning. Report of a second case. *Arch. Neurol.* **32**, 52–53.

Goode, R. (1940). Some observations on the psychological aspects of cardiazol therapy. *J. Ment. Sci.* **86**, 491.

Gottlieb, G. and Wilson, I. (1965). Cerebral dominance: Temporary disruption of verbal memory by unilateral electroconvulsive shock treatment. *J. Comp. Physiol. Psychol.* **60**, 368–372.

Gralnick, A. (1944). Fatalities associated with electric shock treatment of psychoses.: report of two cases, with autopsy observations in one of them. *Arch. Neurol. Psychiat.* **51**, 397.

Grahame-Smith, D. G., Green, A. R. and Costain, D. W. (1978). Mechanism of the antidepressant action of ECT. *Lancet* **1**, 254.

Greenblatt, M., Grosser, G. H. and Weschler, H. (1964). Differential response of depressed patients to somatic therapy. *Am. J. Psychiat.* **120**, 935.

Hamadah, K., Holmes, H., Barker, G. B., Hartmen, G. C. and Parke, D. V. W. (1972). Effect of electric convulsion therapy on urinary excretion of 3′ , 5′-cyclic adenosine monophosphate. *Br. Med. J.* **iii**, 439–441.

Hamilton, M. and White, J. M. (1960). Factors related to the outcome of depression treated with ECT. *J. Ment. Sci.* **106**, 1031–1041.

Hitchcock, E., Ashcroft, G. W., Cairns, V. M. and Murray, L. C. (1972). Pre-operative and post-operative assessment and management of psychosurgical patients. *In* 'Psychosurgery' (Eds E. Hitchcock, L. Laitinen and K. Vaernet) pp. 164–176. Charles Thomas, Springfield, Illinois.

Hobson, R. F. (1953). Prognostic factors in electric convulsive therapy. *J. Neurol. Neurosurg. Psychiat.* **16**, 275–281.

Hodgson, R. and Rachman, S. (1974). *11* Desynchrony in measures of fear. *Behav. Res. Ther.* **12**, 319–326.

Hodgson, R., Rachman, S. and Marks, I. M. (1972). The treatment of chronic obsessive-compulsive neurosis: Follow-up and further findings. *Behav. Res. Ther.* **10**, 181–189.

Impastato, D. (1960). The story of the first electroshock treatment. *Am. J. Psychiat.* **116**, 1113–1114.

Kalinowsky, L. and Hippius, H. (1969). 'Pharmacological, Convulsive and Other Somatic Treatments in Psychiatry'. Grune and Stratton, New York.

Kalinowsky, L. and Hoch, P. H. (1961). 'Somatic Treatments in Psychiatry'. New York.

Kelly, D. (1976). Psychosurgery in the 1970s. *Br. J. Hosp. Med.* 165–174.

Kelly, D., Richardson, A. and Mitchell-Heggs, N. (1973). Stereotactic limbic leucotomy: Neurophysiological aspects and operative techniques. *Br. J. Psychiat.* **123**, 133–140.

Keilholz, F. (1973). Chronische endogene Depressionen. *In* 'Chronische endogene Psychosen' (Eds H. Kraus and K. Heinrich) Vol. 6, p. 5. Bad Kreuznacher Symposium, 1972. Thieme, Stuttgart.

Kiloh, L. G., Child, J. P. and Latner, G. (1960). A controlled trial of iproniazid in the treatment of endogenous depression. *J. Ment. Sci.* **106**, 1425–1428.

Kim, Y. K. and Umbach, W. (1973). Combined stereotactic lesions for treatment of behaviour disorders and severe pain. *In* 'Surgical Approaches in Psychiatry' (Eds L. Laitinen and K. Livingston), Ch. 26, pp. 182–188. Medical and Technical Publishing Co., Lancaster.

Klein, D. F. and Davis, J. M. (1969). 'Diagnosis and Drug Treatment of Psychiatric Disorders'. Williams and Wilkins, Baltimore.

Knight, G. C. (1969). Stereotactic surgery for the relief of suicidal and severe depression and intractable psychoneurosis. *Postgrad. Med. J.* **45**, 1–13.

Knight, G. C. (1973). Additional stereotactic lesions in the cingulum following failed tractotomy in the subcaudate region. *In* 'Surgical Approaches in Psychiatry' (Eds L. V. Laitinen and K. Livingston), Ch. 14, pp. 101–106. Medical and Technical Publishing Co, Lancaster.

Kristiansen, E. S. (1961). A comparison of treatment of endogenous depression with electric-convulsive therapy and imipramine. *Acta Psychiat. Scand., Suppl.* 162, 179.

Krouner, L. W. (1975). Shock therapy and psychiatric malpractice: the legal accommodation to a controversial statement. *J. Forensic Sci.* **20**, 404–415.

Kukopulos, A., Reginaldi, D., Tondo, L., Bernabei, A. and Galiari, B. (1977). Spontaneous length of depression and response to ECT. *Psychol. Med.* **7**, 4, 625–629.

Laitinen, L. V. (1972). Stereotactic lesions in the knee of the corpus callosum in the treatment of emotional disorders. *Lancet* **1**, 472–475.

Lambourn, J. and Gill, D. (1977). Is ECT Effective? Preliminary results of a controlled trial. *Br. J. Psychiat.* **131**, 317.

Larsen, E. G. and Vraa-Jansen, G. (1953). Ischaemic changes in the brain following electroshock therapy. *Acta Psychiat. Neurol. Scand.* **28**, 75–80.

Lancaster, N., Steinert, R. and Frost, I. (1958). Unilateral electroconvulsive therapy. *J. Ment. Sci.* **104**, 221–227.

Lehmann, H. E. (1967). Facts v. fallacies in the overall treatment of depression. Winter Symposium on Mental Depression. Washington Psychiatric Society and Department of Psychiatry, Georgetown University School of Medicine, Washington, D.C.

Lehmann, H. E. and Ostrow, D. E. (1973) Quizzing the expert: Clinical criteria for psychosurgery. *Hosp. Physician* **9**, 24–31.

Levy, R. (1968). The clinical evaluation of unilateral electroconvulsive therapy. *Br. J. Psychiat.* **114**, 459–463.

Lewin, W. (1973). Selective Leucotomy: a review. *In* 'Surgical Approaches in Psychiatry' (Eds L. V. Laitinen and K. E. Livingston), Ch. 9, pp. 69–73. Medical and Technical Publishing Co, Lancaster.

Liban, E., Halpern, L. and Rozanski, J. (1951). Vascular changes in the brain in a fatality following electroshock. *J. Neuropathol. Exp. Neurol.* **10**, 309–318.

Livingston, K. E. (1953). Cingulate cortex isolation for the treatment of psychoses and psychoneurosis. *Res. Pub. Assoc. Res. Nerv. Ment. Dis.* **31**, 374–378.

Marshall, J. F. (1974). Stereotaxy for obesity. *Lancet* **2**, 106.

Martin, W. L., Ford, H. D., McDonald, E. C. and Towler, N. L. (1965). Clinical evaluation of unilateral ECT. *Am. J. Psychiat.* **121**, 1087–1090.

May, P. R. A. (1968). 'Treatment of Schizophrenia: A Comparative Study of Five Treatment Methods'. Science House, New York.

May, P. R. A. and Van Putten, T. (1974). Treatment of schizophrenia: 11 A proposed rating scale of design and outcome for use in literature surveys. *Compr. Psychiat.* **15**, 267–275.

McCabe, M. S. (1976). ECT in the treatment of mania: a controlled study. *Am. J. Psychiat.* **133**, 688–690.

Maclay, W. S. (1953). Death due to treatment. *Proc. Roy. Soc. Med.* **46**, 13.

Medical Research Council (1965). Report by Clinical Psychiatry Committee. *Br. Med. J.* **1**, 881.

Meldrum, B. S., Vigoroux, R. A. and Brierley, J. B. (1973). Systemic factors and epileptic brain damage. *Arch. Neurol.* **29**, 82–87.

Meldrum, B. S., Horton, R. W. and Brierley, J. B. (1974). Epileptic brain damage in adolescent baboons following seizures induced by allylglycine. *Brain* **97**, 407–418.

Meyer, A. and Teare, D. (1945). Cerebral fat embolism after electrical convulsion therapy. *Br. Med. J.* **2**, 42.

Miller, D. H., Clancy, J. and Cumming, E. (1953). A comparison between unidirectional current nonconvulsive electrical stimulation given with Reiter's Machine, standard alternating current electroshock (Cerletti Method) and pentothal in chronic schizophrenia. *Am. J. Psychiat.* **189**, 617–620.

Mitchell-Heggs, N., Kelly, D. and Richardson, A. (1976). Stereotactic limbic leucotomy—a follow-up at 16 months. *Br. J. Psychiat.* **128**, 226–240.

Morgan, J. J. B. (1940). Shock as a preparation for readjustment. *J. Psychol.* **10**, 313.

Narabayashi, H., Nagao, R., Saito, Y., Yoshida, M. and Nagahata, M. (1963). Amygdalotomy for behaviour disorders. *Arch. Neurol.* (Chicago) **9**, 11.

Oliver, W. (1785). Account of the effect of camphor in a case of insanity. *London Med. J.* **6**, 120–130.

Ottosson, J. D. (1960). Experimental studies in the mode of action of electroconvulsive therapy. *Acta Psychiat. Scand.* **35** (*Suppl.* 145), 1–141.

Ottosson, J. D. (1974). Comments on induced seizures and human behaviour. *In* 'Psychobiology of Convulsive Therapy' (Eds M. Fink, S. Kety, J. McGaugh and T. Williams). Wiley, Chichester.

Papez, J. W. (1937). A proposed mechanism of emotion. *Arch. Neurol. Psychiat.* (Chicago) **38**, 725–743.

Perrin, G. M. (1961). Cardiovascular aspects of electric shock therapy. *Acta Psychiat. Scand., Suppl.* 152.

Pringle, J. (1774). Discourse on the Torpedo. Lecture delivered at the Royal Society. In 'Three Hundred Years of Psychiatry' (Eds R. Hunter and I. Macalpine). Oxford University Press, Oxford.

Quaade, F. (1974). Stereotaxy for obesity. Lancet 1, 267.

Quaade, F., Vaernet, K. and Larsson, S. (1974). Stereotaxic stimulation and electro-coagulation of the lateral hypothalamus in obese humans. Neurochir. (Wien) 30, 111–117.

Rachman, S., Marks, I. M. and Hodgson, R. (1973). The treatment of obsessive-compulsive neurotics by modelling and flooding in vivo. Behav. Res. Ther. 11, 463–471.

Riddell, S. A. (1963). The therapeutic efficacy of ECT. Arch. Gen. Psychiat. 8, 42–52.

Robin, A. A. and Harris, J. A. (1962). A controlled comparison of imipramine and electroplexy. J. Ment. Sci. 126, 217–219.

Robin, A. and Macdonald, D. (1975). 'Lessons of Leucotomy'. Henry Kimpton, London.

Rodriguez-Burgos, F., Arjona, V. and Rubio, E. (1976). Stereotactic cryothalamotomy for pain. In 'Neurosurgical Treatment in Psychiatry' (Ed. W. H. Sweet). University Park Press, Baltimore, Maryland.

Roeder, F., Orthner, H. and Muller, D. (1972). The stereotaxic treatment of pedophilic homosexuality and other sexual deviations. In 'Psychosurgery' (Eds E. R. Hitchcock, L. V. Laitinen and K. Vaernet). Thomas, Springfield, Illinois.

Rosenblatt, S., Chanley, J. D., Sobotka, H. and Kaufman, M. R. (1960). Interrelationships between electroshock, the blood-brain barrier and catecholamines. J. Neurochem. 5, 172–176.

The Royal College of Psychiatrists' Memorandum on the Use of Electroconvulsive Therapy. (1977a). Br. J. Psychiat. 131, 261–272.

The Royal College of Psychiatrists (1977b). The College's comments on 'a review of the Mental Health Act, 1959'. News and Notes Suppl. Br. J. Psychiat. 130, Jan.

Salzman, C. (1977). ECT and ethical psychiatry. Am. J. Psychiat. 134, 9, 1006–1009.

Sano, K., Sekino, H. and Mayanagi, Y. (1972). Results of stimulation and destruction of the posterior hypothalamus in cases with violent, aggressive or restless behaviours. In 'Psychosurgery' (Eds E. R. Hitchcock, L. Laitinen and K. Vaernet). Thomas, Springfield, Illinois.

Sargant, W. and Slater, E. (1972). 'An Introduction to Physical Methods of Treatment in Psychiatry' (5th edn). Churchill Livingstone, London.

Schildkraut, J. J. and Draskogzy, P. R. (1974). Electroconvulsive shock and norepinephrine turnover. In 'Psychobiology of Convulsive Therapy' (Eds M. Fink, S. Kety, J. McGaugh and T. Williams). Wiley, Chichester.

Scoville, W. B. and Bettis, D. B. (1976). Results of orbital undercutting today: a personal series. In 'Neurosurgical Treatment in Psychiatry' (Ed. W. H. Sweet). University Park Press, Baltimore, Maryland.

Seager, C. P. (1958). A comparison between the result of unmodified and modified electroplexy (ECT). J. Ment. Sci. 14, 206–220.

Seager, C. P. (1959). Controlled trial of straight and modified electroplexy. J. Ment. Sci. 105. 1022–1028.

Shepherd, M., Lader, M. and Rodnight, R. (1968). 'Clinical Psychopharmacology'. English Universities Press, London.

Spencer, D. J. (1968). Some observations on ECT. Medical World 105, 26–29.

Spencer, J. (1977). Psychiatry and convulsant therapy. Med. J. Aust. 1, 844–847.

Squire, L. R. (1975). A stable impairment in remote memory following electroconvulsive therapy. Neuropsychologia 13, 51–58.

Squire, L. R. (1977). ECT and memory loss. *Am. J. Psychiat.* **134**, 9, 997–1001.
Squire, L. R. and Chace, P. M. (1975). Memory functions six to nine months after electroconvulsive therapy. *Arch. Gen. Psychiat.* **32**, 1557–1564.
Squire, L. R. and Miller, P. (1974). Diminution of anterograde amnesia following electroconvulsive therapy. *Br. J. Psychiat.* **125**, 490–495.
Stengel, E. (1951). Intensive ECT. *J. Ment. Sci.* **97**, 139–142.
Sternberg, D. E. and Jarvik, M. E. (1976). Memory functions in depression. *Arch. Gen. Psychiat.* **33**, 219–224.
Stone, A. A. (1975). 'Mental Health and Law: A System in Transition'. National Institute of Mental Health, Rockville, Maryland.
Stromgren, L. S. (1973). Unilateral versus bilateral electroconvulsive therapy. *Acta Psychiat. Scand., Suppl.* 240.
Tewfik, G. I. and Wells, B. G. (1957). The use of Arfonad for the alleviation of cardiovascular stress following electroconvulsive therapy. *J. Ment. Sci.* 103, 636–644.
Tooth, G. C. and Newton, M. P. (1961). Leucotomy in England and Wales 1942–1954. Ministry of Health Reports on Public Health and Medical Subjects, No. 104. HMSO, London.
Turner, E. (1972). Operations for aggression. Bilateral temporal lobotomy and posterior cingulectomy. *In* 'Psychosurgery' (Eds E. R. Hitchcock, L. Laitinen and K. Vaernet). Thomas, Springfield, Illinois.
Ulett, G. A., Smith, K. and Cleser, G. C. (1956). Evaluation of convulsive and subconvulsive shock therapies utilizing a control group. *Am. J. Psychiat.* **112**, 759–802.
US National Commission for the Protection of Human Subjects of Biomedical and Behavioral Research. (1977). *Report and Recommendations: Psychosurgery* US DHEW Publ. No. (OS) 77–0001.
Valenstein, E. S. (1973). 'Brain Control. A Critical Examination of Brain Stimulation and Psychosurgery'. Wiley, New York.
Valenstein, E. S. (1975). 'Persistent Problems in the Physical Control of the Brain'. Forty-Fourth James Arthur Lecture on the Evolution of the Human Brain. The American Museum of Natural History, New York.
Valenstein, E. S. (1977). The practice of psychosurgery: a survey of the literature (1971–1976). *In* 'Psychosurgery', Appendix 1–1–1–143. US National Commission for the Protection of Human Subjects of Biomedical and Behavioral Research. US DHEW Publ. No. (OS) 77–0002.
Wesley, J. (1756). *In* 'Three Hundred Years of Psychiatry' (Eds R. Hunter and I. Macalpine). Oxford University Press, Oxford.
Williams, M. (1966). Memory disorders associated with electroconvulsive therapy. *In* 'Amnesia' (Eds C. M. Whitby and O. L. Zangwill). Butterworth, London.
Winter, A. (1972). Depression and intractable pain treated by modified prefrontal lobotomy. *J. Med. Soc.* **69**, 757–759.
World Health Organization (1976). 'Health Aspects of Human Rights'. WHO, Geneva.
Wyatt v. Stickney, 325 F Supp 781 (MD Ala 1971).
Yakovlev, P. I. (1948). Motility, behavior and the brain: stereodynamic organization and neural coordinates of behavior. *J. Nerv. Ment. Dis.* **107**, 313.
Zaidel, D. and Sperry, R. W. (1974). Memory impairment after commissurotomy in man. *Brain* **97**, 263–272.
Zamora, E. N. and Kaelbling, R. (1955). Memory and electroconvulsive therapy. *Am. J. Psychiat.* **112**, 546–554.

21 Behaviour therapy

Paul Bebbington

Behaviour therapy may be defined as treatment aimed at improving a patient's functioning and well-being by a directed change in his behaviour. This definition casts a wide net and, as we shall see below, it must. Behaviour therapy carries an implied theory of psychiatric disorders; namely, that at least in part they represent inappropriate learned responses and are not to be explained in terms of underlying psychodynamic structures. In modifying behaviour, the therapist draws on principles derived from experimental psychology in general, and from learning theory in particular, although this is changing. In practice, behaviour therapy consists of a body of techniques which are justified empirically, which are sometimes only loosely related to the tenets of learning theory and which are often only placed in a tight conceptual context in retrospect, if at all. Nevertheless, Eysenck (1975) has defended the relationship of behaviour therapy to its conceptual basis.

Behaviour therapy also offers a particular language for the description of human behaviour and it seems that the rapidly increasing acceptance of the behavioural standpoint and the phenomenal growth of behaviour therapy literature in recent years represents a 'paradigm shift' which Kuhn (1971) holds to be the essence of a revolution in scientific thought. Frequent attempts to translate psychodynamic techniques and terminology into behavioural terms can be taken as representing the same process (Mahoney, 1974; Marks, 1974). The hallmark of a 'young' paradigm is that it is intuitively acceptable to its adherents and acceptance goes beyond data; and this seems true of behaviour therapy. Data have been derived from studies both of volunteers and of patients. The use of volunteers who suffer from mild disabilities for which they have not sought treatment (e.g. a snake phobia) is termed an analogue experiment and many of the elements in behavioural techniques have been teased out in this way in well controlled studies. However, extrapolation from these to truly clinical situations may not be justified. For the most part, studies involving patients have reported single cases, or at best a few. Such studies are acceptable if correct single case methodology is used, but this relies on the behaviour change being reversible and some behaviours are inherently irreversible. In addition, there may be ethical difficulties. The studies discussed in this chapter mainly involve patients and are quoted either because of good methodology or because they are particularly suggestive. The whole issue of methodology in this area has been concisely reviewed by Thoresen and Mahoney (1974).

The majority of behaviour therapists have been clinical psychologists although there are distinguished workers in the field who are psychiatrists. Behavioural techniques are not esoteric and can be carried out by specially trained nurses with comparable effectiveness thus extending the availability of this approach (Marks *et al.*, 1975a).

Behaviour therapy may be indicated for perhaps 10% of adult psychiatric patients. It is the treatment of choice in phobic disorders including social phobia and in obsessive compulsive rituals (Marks, 1976). It leads to consistent results in sexual disorders (Chapter 8) although there is some doubt whether these results are better than those obtained with other psychotherapeutic approaches (Bancroft, 1974). The same question hangs over its use in alcoholism (Chapter 10). Behaviour therapy is under evaluation in other areas: obsessive thinking, social skills deficits, habit disorders and appetitive disorders. Operant techniques can. aid in the management of the problem of institutionalization, including those in chronic schizophrenia and techniques are being explored for the treatment of chronic depression. In children (Chapter 5) enuresis and phobic disorders respond best to a behavioural approach as do problems of training in subnormal children (Chapter 6). For appropriate patients, behaviour therapy seems an acceptable method of treatment and dropping out of treatment poses no more of a problem than with other psychiatric therapies.

In theory, the behaviour therapist first negotiates a definition of specific goals of treatment with the patient. Each target response is then analysed in detail as are the circumstances in which it occurs. A plan of approach is formulated and there is usually some attempt at measuring the target response frequency for a period before treatment commences, during treatment and in the follow-up period. This approach puts a considerable advantage in the hands of the behaviour therapist as the patient can see objective benefits of treatment and the therapist can show documented evidence of efficacy: each case constitutes a case study. Moreover, a conscious adherence to a scientific approach makes it possible to refine techniques and eliminate redundant treatment elements.

Recently, attention has been paid to what behaviour therapists actually do in the treatment situation. Staples *et al.* (1975) rated treatment sessions of three behaviour therapists and three traditional psychotherapists and demonstrated that differences between them were not merely of language and technique but also of the basic patterns of interaction. Behaviour therapists talked more, were more directive, more controlling of sessions, were more involved and maintained less of a psychological distance from the patient. Surprisingly, the two types of therapist made similar numbers of interpretations although couched in different languages.

Interestingly, patient assessments of what helped emphasized understanding acceptance and the provision of a rationale with which to understand oneself—although it must be said that this aspect of the study is of only anecdotal value.

Basic learning concepts will be briefly reviewed here although the reader should refer to basic textbooks of psychology for further elaboration (Hilgard *et al.*, 1975).

Classical Conditioning is also known as Pavlovian or respondent conditioning. Any stimulus infallibly eliciting a response, often an autonomic response, may be termed an unconditioned stimulus and the response an unconditioned response.

A stimulus immediately preceding the unconditioned stimulus may itself after several pairings come to elicit the response in the absence of the unconditioned stimulus. This stimulus is said to have been conditioned and the response which may in fact show slight differences from the original unconditioned response becomes known as the conditioned response. Hence, by this procedure a bell (the conditioned stimulus) may come to elicit salivation (the conditioned response) from a dog when it has been rung as a signal for the presentation of food (the unconditioned stimulus). If the bell is then rung on many occasions without being followed by food the dog may cease to salivate in response to it. This is the phenomenon of *extinction*. Extinction is not a permanent state, as, after a time lag, the bell regains its power to make the dog salivate, the phenomenon of *spontaneous recovery*. Stimuli similar to the conditioned stimulus may share its power in proportion to their similarity, so-called *generalization*. It is possible to train *discrimination* between similar stimuli eliciting a conditioned response by associating the unconditioned stimulus with one but not the other. Hence, our dog may be trained to salivate to respond only to one of several similar sounding bells.

Operant or instrumental conditioning is the process by which a response (usually a voluntary response) changes in likelihood as a result of its consequences for the organism. Hence, a rat will be more likely to learn and use a path through a maze if this results in the attainment of food. Operant responses are also under the control of environmental stimuli but the control is *discriminative*; a signal that the response is appropriate, rather than one which automatically elicits the response. Hence, a child may throw a tantrum to obtain sweets with its father but not with its mother—the presence of one or other parent is a discriminative stimulus. Operant conditioning also exhibits the phenomena of extinction, spontaneous recovery, generalization and discrimination. All these phenomena have implications for the treatment of patients.

One can talk of *reinforcement* in the case of both classical and operant conditioning. Reinforcement can be defined as any event the occurrence of which increases the probability that a stimulus will on subsequent occasions evoke a response. In classical conditioning, reinforcement precedes and elicits the response; in operant conditioning, it follows the response. Behaviourists distinguish two types of reinforcement in operant conditioning, *positive reinforcers* such as food and social approval which if they follow a response increase the probability of its recurrence, and *negative reinforcers* such as an electric shock which on being *terminated* increase response probability. Negative reinforcement is the process by which *escape responses* increase in probability, as when an agoraphobic patient runs out of a shop. The negative reinforcer is the fear of the situation and because this stops when the patient escapes in this way, it becomes more likely that she will run away on a following occasion. Reinforcement principles underlie token economies (see below). The *presentation* of a negative reinforcer reduces the likelihood of an ongoing response and is termed punishment: this is the mechanism of aversion therapy.

Withdrawal of a positive reinforcer is also punishment. In practice, these distinctions may be less than clear: the use of a 'time out' room is withdrawal from positive reinforcement, hence punishment. It could also be argued that it involves cessation of reinforcement (extinction) or presentation of a negative reinforcer (a boring grey room)—again punishment.

Negative reinforcers are common in nature, and much of our behaviour is aimed at the removal of irritants or the reasonable avoidance of previously encountered hurt or danger. Hence, it is unlikely that punishment as such should generally have deleterious consequences. As a technique in behaviour modification it has certain drawbacks. It may lead to (1) generalization of inhibition beyond situations in which it is appropriate;

(2) conditioning of fear to the punishment situation; (3) avoidance of the punishment agent and situation; (4) ineffectiveness, if the punished response is maintained by unchanged alternative reinforcement. In addition, staff may dislike administering negative reinforcers. The second and third of these drawbacks only occur with high intensity of aversive stimulation. All the drawbacks are avoidable with skilled application and aversion therapy for sexual deviation has proved both effective and acceptable to the patient.

Reinforcement may be partial or continuous. If a response is partially reinforced, i.e. is reinforced on only a proportion of occasions, as are most responses in everyday situations, it becomes particularly resistant to extinction.

Extreme resistance to extinction distinguishes one class of operant responses, the *avoidance response*. An organism will avoid a situation as a result of an unpleasant experience and this behaviour cannot be maintained by further negative reinforcement by the very nature of the avoidance response. Nevertheless, avoidance responses are very persistent. Mowrer (1939) postulated a two-factor theory to explain this, namely (1) by a process of classical conditioning a negative emotional response including autonomic components (i.e. fear) is attached to the locus of the unpleasant experience; (2) future approach to the situation elicits fear and hence avoidance is reinforced by the cessation of fear, as with an agoraphobic who sets off for the shops and gets no further than the corner of the street before running home. The concept of the conditioned emotional response is central to many behaviour therapy techniques. Desensitization, flooding and related techniques may be formulated as the extinction of a conditional emotional response with consequent abolition of the linked avoidance response, as in a phobic patient.

It should be noted that although this theory was accepted for thirty years and remains a useful framework within which to understand the later departures, it has been refuted by laboratory evidence and provides an inadequate account of human neurosis (Seligman and Johnston, 1973; Eysenck, 1976; Rachman, 1976, 1977). It fails in particular to account for persistence of avoidance when the subject does not approach near enough to experience fear. There are two additional phenomena which may extend the learning theory formulation of human phobias. Preparedness (Seligman *et al.*, 1971) describes the increased potential for certain stimuli of phylogenetic significance to elicit strongly persistent fear reactions. Incubation (Eysenck, 1976) refers to the *enhancement* rather than extinction of fear when the conditioned stimulus is presented without the unconditioned stimulus. This occurs most notably when a conditioned stimulus which has acquired drive properties is presented for a brief period.

Change in human behaviour, in addition to the effects of individual experience outlined above can occur vicariously by *observational learning*—that is by observing the experience of others. We may acquire a fear of dogs by watching *someone else* being bitten—a vicarious conditioned emotional response. Children may learn how to please the teacher by observing compliments paid by others, an example of vicarious positive reinforcement. We may learn an escape response by observing the successful escapes of others, we may learn also from the punishment or non-reward of others (see Bandura, 1969). *Modelling* is the term given to the transfer of response capacity from the observed to the observer and is a rapid means of learning complex responses such as social behaviour—for instance how best to introduce yourself to a girl at a party. Hence, vicarious learning has both contingency and response aspects. Bandura (1969) describes four subprocesses involved in vicarious learning, namely attention, retention, motoric reproduction and motivation.

The characteristics of the model have an effect on the likelihood of response in the observer which correlates with the number of models, model status and similarity to the observer and reinforcement of the observer by the model (see Bandura, 1969).

Behaviour therapy and private events

One of the difficulties which the eclectic psychiatrist meets in understanding behaviour therapy relates to the position of 'private events', of subjective experience. The psychiatrist uses reports of private events as the basis of his diagnostic method and readily accepts their less than perfect reliability. He therefore finds it hard to grasp a theoretical approach which at its toughest appears to deny any usefulness at all to the concept of mental events. He knows with Cartesian certainty that man is a thinking animal and not merely the thoughtless plaything of a whimsical environment. To examine the validity of this judgement on behaviour therapy we must pay a little attention to the history of behaviourism itself.

The word 'behaviourism' belongs to J. B. Watson and his rejection in 1912 of the current mentalistic psychology of Tichener and others: this was concerned with the minute introspection of individual subjective experience and led to a proliferation of theory for which there was no objectifiable test. Watson (1930) states 'Behaviourism . . . holds that the subject matter of human psychology is *the behaviour of the human being*. Behaviourism claims that consciousness is neither a definite nor a useable concept.' The extreme 'metaphysical' behaviourist holds paradoxically that private events are a private illusion. For others, Skinner for instance, behaviourism is a methodological option: we should establish regularities of overt behaviour without reference to private events in so far as this provides an adequate description of data. This approach is justified by appeal to the principle of parsimony, William of Occam's Razor, which states we should opt for the simplest of adequate alternative theories. In fact, the parsimony of the pure behaviourist standpoint is an honourable failure—there are many psychological facts which are not explicable in pure stimulus-response terms (Mahoney, 1974). Many aspects of human behaviour require the inference that there is some thinking occurring between circumstances and the person's response to them. The cognitive process is said to *mediate* between stimulus and response and the inadequacy of a learning theory which avoids inferring such mediation (the clumsily termed 'non-mediational or 'S-R' model) has been reviewed by Mahoney (1974). Major stumbling blocks include the phenomena of vicarious learning and awareness and the fact that human beings are unequivocally self-stimulating creatures whose behaviour is much more likely to be a response to their own private monologue than to external circumstances. Awareness, which may be defined operationally as a subject's ability to describe imposed contingencies, accelerates learning massively.

A further difficulty in the non-mediational approach to human behaviour, and even Skinner's limited mediational approach, is that it relates behaviour to environmental antecedents—in other words, the organism is acted upon. It is not easy for it to accommodate the view that the organism is in *reciprocal* relationship to its environment—a view of man as controlled *and* controlling, an active participant in his own growth (Thoresen and Mahoney, 1974).

In practice, the imagined impurity of inferring private events has rarely disturbed behaviour therapists—after all, Wolpe's (1958) technique of desensitization involved imaginal events—but until recently (Bandura, 1969; Mahoney, 1974; Meichenbaum, 1974) they have avoided being too flagrant in formulating mediational models.

What alternatives are there to the parsimonious but inadequate S-R model? Mahoney (1974) elaborates two cognitive models, one limited, one less so. The first, termed the covert conditioning model, acknowledges the importance of mental or 'covert' events, claiming that they are the covert counterparts of overt events. This is the 'continuity assumption' and there is certainly evidence that covert events can act as stimuli, eliciting, for instance, conditioned emotional responses, as responses and as positive and negative reinforcers. The use of covert events as negative reinforcers is the basis of covert sensitization (Cautela, 1967), a technique of proven efficiency at least in treatment of sexual deviation (Callahan and Leitenberg, 1973). However, this model is undoubtedly simplistic and lacks stringency in some aspects—it is not clear occasionally whether covert processes represent equivalents of classical or operant conditioning. Mahoney (1974) prefers the 'cognitive learning approach' which he develops from information theory and Bandura's (1969) social learning formulation. This model makes more assumptions but is more predictive and puts less of a strain on our common sense models of the mind. Under the model learning is the product of experienced systematic relationships, whether the experience is direct, vicarious or symbolic. Thought is an active process which bridges temporal intervals, organizes experience into (occasionally exaggerated) regularities, anticipates the consequences of action and economizes effort in problem solving. Mahoney (1974) elaborates four origins of behavioural variance, namely (1) attention and perception, (2) relational factors—how situations and performance measure up to the individual's private yardsticks and expectations, (3) response repertoire and (4) feedback. He subsumes certain techniques under the model and indicates further possibilities of treatment derived from it: readers are referred to his very readable book for details.

Learned helplessness

We do not live in a world perfectly organized for behavioural study; it is a world variably predictable and often beyond our control. The meaning of stimuli may change with circumstances and our prior experience of them may affect the appropriateness of our behaviour. One area in which this complex relationship has been studied is that of stimuli associated with aversive events. To a dog, a buzzer may act as a conditioned stimulus indicating the arrival of, say, an electric shock. In the Pavlovian paradigm, the shock is classically unavoidable. In the operant paradigm, the buzzer signals an electric shock from which the dog can escape. A history of unavoidable shock leads dogs to behave unlike 'naïve' dogs when later in an operant escape situation. They fail massively to learn to escape even if they make the escape response incidentally on one occasion, as if they have learned that escape is beyond their powers. For this Seligman (see e.g. Seligman et al., 1971) has coined the term 'learned helplessness'. The experience of helplessness appears to disrupt adaptive operant behaviour over a wide range. The study of the phenomenon has been extended to human subjects and Seligman points out analogous performance between human subjects who have learned helplessness and patients with reactive depression (Seligman, 1974). He bases his analogy on behavioural and physiological symptoms, aetiology, cure and prevention. Although the analogy is skeletal in places the emphasis on the passivity, negative expectations and sense of hopelessness of the depressed patient indicates possible prediction of new treatments of a behavioural type. Seligman's actual analysis of treatments of depression in terms of learned helplessness is interpretative and tentative and his restriction of the model to one portion of a presumed dichotomy between endogenous and reactive depression is perhaps psychiatrically naïve.

Since its delineation, the model has been elaborated considerably. In humans it now involves attribution theory (Kelley, 1973). For a current synthesis, readers are referred to the symposium in the *Journal of Abnormal Psychology* (Feb. 1978).

Phobias and obsessive compulsive disorder

Marks (1977) has suggested six part-models, as yet unintegrated, to account for the clinical features of phobias and obsessions. As clinical aspects imply phylogenetic, genetic, maturational, biochemical and neurophysiological factors, behavioural formulations can only provide an incomplete picture. They do afford a basis for understanding techniques of treatment.

A negative emotion, fear or disgust, attached to a situation, object, idea etc. is not extinguished because the situation is 'avoided', either by physical avoidance or by ritual which reduces anxiety. Hence all widely used behavioural techniques for dealing with neuroses involve exposure to the cause of fear.

The first large report of a behavioural technique in the treatment of these neuroses is that of Wolpe (1958) using '*systematic desensitization*'. He used a neurophysiological explanatory model, namely 'reciprocal inhibition'. This postulated that sympathetic and parasympathetic responses were mutually exclusive but the technique obviously does not stand or fall by the theory. Wolpe's technique involves the elaboration of a hierarchy of fearful situations. The subject is encouraged to carry out a response incompatible with anxiety. This may be an assertive or sexual response but has usually been an easily trained technique of relaxation (Jacobsen, 1938): the subject indicates when he is relaxed and is then asked to imagine increasingly difficult situations whilst maintaining relaxation. Progress is gradually made up the hierarchy. Wolpe reported on 210 adults, mainly with phobic and anxiety responses, of whom 90% were either cured or much improved. The figure was calculated, however, after exclusion of those dropping out of treatment.

Systematic desensitization is a complex treatment package (reviewed by Lipsedge, 1973) and later studies suggest the only necessary condition for change is exposure to the feared object or situation. Muscular relaxation, hierarchical presentation and the interpersonal relationship may be discarded (the last for instance by tape recording the instructions). Benjamin *et al*. (1972) report a controlled trial demonstrating that the active induction of relaxation is unnecessary in treating chronic phobia patients in this way. There is a spectrum of techniques involving exposure, from the gently graded approach of the desensitization hierarychy to the evocation of intense anxiety of *flooding*. Treatment with flooding involves prolonged contact with a maximally feared object. The patient is encouraged to outlast the intense anxiety so aroused. Hence a patient with a spider phobia might be required to remain in close contact with spiders for an hour or more. Marks *et al*. (1971) conducted a controlled trial of flooding versus desensitisation in 16 patients with mixed phobias. Each treatment was given using both fantasized and real life situations. Flooding was shown to be significantly superior on both clinical and physiological measures. It appears to be especially useful in agoraphobia. Watson *et al*. (1971) demonstrated that prolonged *in vivo* exposure produced similar results in six hours to those of eight hours of flooding fantasy and 15 hours of desensitization in fantasy.

The results of flooding appear better with long duration of treatment session (Stern and Marks, 1973) and this accords with animal work which suggests that exposure to a feared situation can be sensitizing or habituating according to the duration of exposure. High arousal during *in vivo* exposure appears to offer no advantage over low arousal (Hafner and Marks, 1976). The effective use of flooding involves considerable clinical skill.

Other techniques have been used to bring about exposure, including modelling and operant methods using social reinforcement. For example, the therapist might show a spider phobic patient that he can allow spiders to run over his hand and that no dire consequences arise. Any progress on the part of the patient will be strongly complimented.

Desensitization in fantasy is largely ineffective in obsessional neurosis for which the most promising results have come from methods which involve sustained exposure *in vivo*. Levy and Meyer (1971) reported the effects of 24 hours prevention of obsessive compulsive rituals. Whenever patients attempted to perform rituals, nursing staff gently but firmly dissuaded them. Total response prevention whilst in graded contact with evoking situations for one to four weeks led to great improvement in nine out of 10 patients. Two patients relapsed slightly in two years of follow-up.

Rachman *et al*. (1971) and Hodgson *et al* (1972) compared a relaxation control procedure with three exposure *in vivo* treatments on a within-subject comparison. All three exposure treatments were superior: they consisted of (1) flooding without modelling, (2) graded exposure with modelling, and (3) flooding with modelling. As an illustration, modelling of exposure for a patient with a fear of dirt involved the therapist touching the floor before getting the patient to imitate him. Patients were treated daily in 15 sessions and were requested to refrain from rituals, but this was not intensively supervised. The majority of patients who did not improve much failed to comply with this request. This work has now been extended and 20 patients *in toto* have been reported (Marks *et al.*, 1975b). At two-year follow-up 14 patients were much improved, one improved and five unchanged. Modelling of exposure conferred no advantage over exposure alone for the total group but was thought to help selected patients.

It would appear that these techniques have much to offer to the obsessional patient with rituals, although the amount of therapeutic effort required varies greatly. Home treatment is of great importance as many obsessionals involve relatives in their rituals.

The status of behavioural techniques in obsessional patients without rituals is less clear. The technique of thought stopping (e.g. Stern *et al.*, 1973) involves the patient inducing an obsessional thought which the therapist then interrupts by shouting 'stop' and making a sudden noise. The patient then interrupts his own thoughts by progressively more internalized commands. However, Stern *et al.* (1973) reported useful gains in only four of 11 patients and it was not clear that even this could be attributed to the thought stopping technique. This treatment flies in the face of the therapeutic package for obsessions with rituals described above. As Rachman (1976b) points out, a more consistent approach would be to get the patient actively to *retain* his ruminative idea, at the same time refraining from any mental 'putting right' of the effects of the rumination. Primary obsessional slowness (Rachman, 1974) seems to respond to prompting, shaping and pacing—a sort of time and motion therapy. Beech (1978) offers a sceptical appraisal of current treatment of obsessional disorders.

Chronic institutionalization

The effects of chronic institutionalization have been well documented (Chapter 11). Operant techniques have been introduced into this situation (1) to improve the quality of life of the patients and (2) to rehabilitate them if possible into the community by restoring lost skills and fostering new ones. In a sense, a description of 'operant techniques' does not involve a separate category, it merely emphasizes a consideration of the therapist's behaviour rather than the patient's situation. Both aspects of course characterize any therapeutic interaction.

One problem in mounting an operant programme for such patients is the temporal characteristic of reinforcement. In classical learning theory it is held that effective reinforcement must occur within a very short time of the response to be reinforced. Most behaviour in most people is controlled by social reinforcement or by a 'cognitive mediator' (e.g. the *expectation* of wages or of a pat on the back). Hence temporal requirements are easily met. Since this is often not so in chronic psychiatric patients two solutions have been used: (1) the introduction of tokens which can be given immediately following the behaviour, (2) the pairing of social approval with the token in the hope of revaluing social reinforcement. The operant use of tokens in the total ward organization is termed a token economy, and was pioneered by Ayllon and Azrin (1968).

Three principles are involved in its establishment. (1) The empirical determination of a pool of reinforcers for the patients. Reinforcers should be *additional to basic ward care* and may include privacy, ground passes, luxuries, interviews with staff, and recreational opportunities. (2) The precise specification of which items of behaviour are to be changed, such as the amount and content of speech, increased socialization and improved regularity of work. (3) The precise establishment of the token-value of behaviours and the token-cost of reinforcers. Once the specification has been agreed, the patients should be told of them, as instruction plus contingent reinforcement is far more effective than reinforcement alone.

Hence a patient will know that if he makes his bed, dresses himself and attends for breakfast on time he will be given, say, 15 tokens towards the 30 he requires to purchase an hour's television time in the evening. It is obvious that such a system may change behaviour in the ward in the direction of self-care but not necessarily in the community or even in another ward. *Weaning* from tokens should be built into the programme and involves planning for the required behaviours to come under control of reinforcement of a type available in the community. Hence reinforcements should eventually be varied in size, consistency and in the temporal delay involved; if possible, reinforcement should be gradually changed in nature from material to social. In some cases close relatives have been trained to apply the programme in the home setting. The aim should be to make the required behaviour self-maintaining.

In some patients, e.g. the mute, there may be a total absence of the behaviour to be reinforced. Absent responses may be elicited by modelling, direct instruction or 'operant shaping'. This involves change in value of reinforcement such that nearer approximation to desired behaviour becomes necessary to maintain a given level of reinforcement. The mute patient may at first be reinforced for grunts but will progressively be reinforced only for words, short sentences and so on.

Recent developments in the technology of the token economy include the application of economic theory to predict the optimal management of reinforcement (Winkler, 1971) and the use of group pressure by making tokens payable to the groups as a whole, whether for the behaviour of all or of one member only. The use of operant techniques has been extended into the classroom.

Results of operant programmes have been assessed in two complementary ways: (1) by within-subject comparisons of contingent versus non-contingent reinforcement; (2) by comparison with a control group under routine hospital management or alternative treatment. Several important questions may be asked of token economies: is it necessary that reinforcement be contingent? Can the reinforced behaviour maintain itself? Does generalization of both situation and response occur? Are tokens essential? How do token economies compare with other treatments?

There seems little doubt from results using single case methodology that effective reinforcement must be contingent. Changes in aspects of behaviour which were not selected for reinforcement have been demonstrated, although it is not always clear whether this represents response generalization or inadvertent contingent reinforcement. Token economies have been remarkably effective in improving even very chronic patients so that they may be considered suitable for discharge (Birky *et al.*, 1971). However, the relapse rate is disappointingly high (e.g. Atthowe and Krasner, 1968). This reflects both failure of behaviour to maintain itself and to generalize to different situations.

An interesting variant of operant techniques is that of Fairweather (1964, 1969) using long-stay, mainly schizophrenic, patients. He set up a programme which differed from a ward control only in the activity within a two-hour period each day. In this period the experimental group met and discussed task objectives, and allocated monetary and pass privilege rewards according to the nature and fulfilment of tasks which had previously been assigned. Patients in this group rapidly developed group cohesiveness, and social reinforcement supplanted material rewards as the main motivato of behaviour. The group gained in decision making and problem solving skills. Fairweather followed up this scheme by transferring the experimental group to a community hostel which became self-regulating and also operated a contract cleaning business. After 35 months in the hostel and seven months in the community, 80% of the experimental group remained out of hospital compared with less than 20% in the control group.

Control groups are necessary to tease out effective components and to establish the superiority of token economies to other treatments. Hence there are some doubts whether tokens are necessary for most patients who seem to do as well with contingent social reinforcement (Baker *et al.*, 1977). The requirements of a suitable control group for overall treatment comparison are not immediately apparent—it can be argued that any treatment would be better than the regimes in the chronic wards of our mental hospitals—but it is difficult to control for attention and enthusiasm. The results of such comparisons are hard to evaluate and no clear picture has yet emerged (Kadzin, 1975). In general psychiatric terms the token economy is essentially a method of creating structure in a rehabilitation programme and in training staff to mount such a programme: its rewards are an unspecified but probably significant increase in efficacy and low investment of effort once established; its costs are the considerable initial investment of effort and expertise. The proliferation of such schemes attest to an increasing willingness and ability to support these costs.

Social skills training

There are two arguments for the attempt to train social performance directly, namely (1) that psychiatric disability may arise from a defect in social performance, (2) that criticism of an inappropriate piece of social behaviour is insufficient unless an alternative is made available. This implies that responses, particularly social responses, occur as complex wholes which themselves require to be learned.

There are two main origins of our present knowledge. The first comes from the work of Argyle (1972) who has studied the communicative value of words, the paralinguistic aspects of speech (e.g. loudness, tone) and the elements of non-verbal communication (gaze, posture, facial expression, sequencing of the interaction, etc.). This in turn led him to propose a model of social interaction, that of a *motor skill*. A motor skill can be broken down into attention to relevant external cues, the characteristic of the response and the use made of feedback in taking corrective action—as for instance, riding a bike in a busy street. Social behaviours can likewise be analysed in terms of cues, response and use of feedback. Interpersonal behaviour differs from a simple motor skill not only in complexity but also in that the object of the skill is capable of independent action and the continuation of the interaction depends on *mutual social rewarding-ness*.

Argyle does not discuss the role of arousal. There is an inverse relation between the degree of skill and arousal as we know, for instance, when learning to drive. At first we are on edge; a short time driving is very tiring. Later our attention to salient features of road and traffic and our response to them is slick and our arousal falls. This appears generally true in the area of social skills. Anxiety is in fact central to the other main derivation of social skills concepts. One pair of incompatibles which

Wolpe used in his treatment by reciprocal inhibition was anxiety and assertiveness and he extended the concept of assertion to include both hostile assertive responses and commendatory assertive responses (Wolpe, 1969). It is obvious that this has become a description of one type of effective social performance. Other workers in the USA took this idea to the point of active training of social skills.

For example, a patient may feel unable to talk to a pretty girl in the office. The therapist may give him *instructions* of what approach to use and what words to say. He may *model*, with a female colleague, what posture to adopt; how to smile appropriately or look interested; how to avoid dropping the gaze. The patient may then *rehearse* the situation either in his mind or in actuality with the co-therapist (the first of these may be of itself desensitizing and has been called *rehearsal desensitization*). The patient's attempt at rehearsal will receive *social reinforcement*—he will be complimented on its good points by the therapist, or by other members, if the therapy is conducted in a group. *Feedback* in which the salient points of the patient's rehearsal receive attention may be verbal; or the therapist may himself imitate the performance; or a video recording may be used. The relative effectiveness of the parts of this treatment package is being worked out in studies with volunteers (reviewed by Hersen *et al.*, 1973) which have vindicated all the elements in the package. The question of application of these results to patient populations again arises. The small controlled trial of Argyle *et al.* (1974) yielded equivocal results. Marzillier *et al.* (1976) reported a controlled trial of systematic desensitization, social skills training and no treatment. Both active treatments produced improvements in the patients' social activity which was maintained at six-month follow-up in the training group. However, there was no significant reduction in anxiety, improvement in social skills or clinical adjustment. Falloon *et al.* (1977) describe a larger trial comparing (a) cohesive group discussion, (b) modelling and role rehearsal and (c) modelling, role rehearsal and daily social 'homework'. All three treatments showed significant but incomplete effects. Role rehearsal and 'homework' seemed independently effective components. However, 20 of the 76 inducted patients dropped out of treatment. Hall and Goldberg (1977) compared systematic desensitization and role-playing-with-feedback in socially anxious psychiatric patients. They found that systematic desensitization reduced anxiety and increased social participation but had little effect on skills. The role playing technique increased skills and also reduced anxiety but did not lead to greater participation. Social skills training has now passed a stage of enthusiastic welcome and is in process of realistic assessment. It is likely to find a permanent if qualified place in the treatment of the socially ineffective patient.

Marital therapy

The recent use of behavioural techniques in marital therapy is based upon the Thibault and Kelley theory of social interaction. This holds that social interaction involves mutual reinforcement and that the outcome of intepersonal relations is the resultant of the reciprocal influence of the partners. Stuart (1969) puts forward three assumptions on which he bases his operant interpersonal treatment for marital discord.

1   The exact pattern of interaction at any point in time is the most rewarding of all available alternatives and represents the best balance which each can achieve between individual and mutual rewards and costs.

2   Spouses expect to enjoy reciprocal relations with their partners. Each party has rights and duties and should dispense social reinforcement at an equitable rate. Whenever one partner unilaterally rewards the other he does so in the expectation of future reinforcement.

3   To modify ineffective marital interactions, it is necessary to develop the power of each partner to initiate rewards for the other. It has been shown that individuals are attracted to each other in proportion to their effectiveness in mutual influence. Failure to influence by positive means leads to 'social bankruptcy' and resort to negative means of control. Successful marriage involves maximization of mutual reward with minimization of cost. Unsuccessful marriage involves minimization of cost with no expectancy of reward which results in two broad alternatives, coercion and withdrawal.

This leads to Stuart's two premises:
   (a) change of behaviour of a partner changes his spouse's perception of him;
   (b) change of interaction in a marriage can only occur if each partner takes the initiative.
Stuart's treatment starts with discussion of the logic of the approach and then each partner lists three positive behaviours which he would most like to increase in the other. Each spouse then records the frequency of the other's compliance in each behaviour. Later on, other behaviours are added. Stuart himself describes four couples treated with success by this approach over 10 weeks.

   To an extent, the Masters and Johnson technique with sexual dysfunction involves a similar 'reciprocity' principle expressed in the watchword 'give to get'. Crowe (1973) includes sexual reciprocity in his variant of Stuart's technique. This worker reports preliminary findings in an intensive study of relative effectiveness of a 'directive' (i.e. behavioural) 'interpretive' and 'general supportive' techniques of marital therapy. His results indicate that interpretive therapies have a higher drop-out rate (possibly because of attention to negative aspects) but with more couples in the categories 'much improved', and that the directive approach is better for specific and sexual problems.

Azrin *et al.* (1973) have reported results of an investigation in which a three-week period of a 'cathartic treatment' was followed by a four-week period of 'reciprocity counselling'. The latter is based on a reciprocal influence operant model of marital interaction although there are considerable differences from the Stuart approach. None of the 12 couples changed during the first period, whilst 96% improved significantly in the second period. Considerable onus is placed upon the couples *to seek out new reinforcers* and hence a flexible strategy is trained. This is borne out in the four-week follow-up period in which gains further increased. Such types of marital therapy would appear to be a hopeful and reasonable area of research with implications for preventive psychiatry.

Combined treatment with behaviour therapy and drugs

This is an area in which advances are likely to be made in the near future. Enhanced responses have been reported in desensitization with methohex tone-induced relaxation (Friedman and Lipsedge, 1971). At one time it was felt that there was enhanced relief of phobias if flooding was carried out during the warming phase of Valium, but it now seems that the role of Valium in flooding is to make the process less strenuous for the patient—it neither helps nor hinders the effect of flooding (Hafner and Marks, 1976). One difficulty with behavioural treatments in the agoraphobic syndrome is the setbacks caused by the occurrence of panic attacks; these may be reduced in frequency and intensity either by tricyclic antidepressants (Klein, 1964) or the monoamine oxidase inhibitors (Tyrer *et al.*, 1973).

It seems likely that the clinical state in obsessional neurosis is intimately tied to affect and the tricyclic antidepressants, in particular clomipramine, may facilitate behavioural treatment (Beech, 1978).

References

Argyle, M. (1972). 'Psychology of Interpersonal Behaviour'. Penguin, London.
Argyle, M., Bryant, B. and Trower, P. (1974). Social skills training and psychotherapy: a comparative study. *Psychol. Med.* **4**, 435–443.
Atthowe, J. M. and Krasner, I. (1968). Preliminary report on the application of

contingent reinforcement procedure (token economy) on a psychiatric ward. *J. Abnorm. Psychol.* **73**, 37–43.

Ayllon, T. and Azrin, N. H. (1968). 'A Motivating Environment for Therapy and Rehabilitation'. Appleton-Century-Crofts, New York.

Azrin, N. H., Naster, B. J. and Jones, R. C. (1973). Reciprocity counsellings: a rapid learning-based procedure for marital counselling. *Behav. Res. Ther.* **11**, 365–382.

Baker, R., Hall, J. N., Hutchinson, K. and Bridge, G. (1977). Symptom changes in chronic Schizophrenic patients on a token economy: A controlled experiment. *Br. J. Psychiat.* **131**, 381–393.

Bancroft, J. H. J. (1974). 'Deviant Sexual Behaviour: Modification and Assessment'. Clarendon Press, Oxford.

Bandura, A. (1969). 'Principles of Behaviour Modification'. Holt, Rinehart and Winston, New York.

Beech, H. R. (1978). Advances in the treatment of obsessional neurosis. *Br. J. Hosp. Med.* **19**, 54–60.

Benjamin, S., Marks, I. M. and Huson, J. (1972). Active muscular relaxation in desensitisation of phobic patients. *Psychol. Med.* **2**, 381–390.

Birky, H. J. Chambliss, J. C. and Wasden, R. (1971). A comparison of residents discharged from a token economy and two traditional psychiatric programmes. *Behav. Ther.* **2**, 46–51.

Callahan, E. J. and Leitenberg, H. (1973). Aversion therapy for sexual deviation. Contingent shock and covert sensitisation. *J. Abnorm. Psychol.* **81**, 60–73.

Cautela, J. R. (1967). Covert sensitisation. *Psychol. Rep.* **20**, 459–468.

Crowe, M. J. (1973). Conjoint marital therapy: advice or interpretation? *J. Psychosom. Res.* **17**, 309–315.

Eysenck, H. J. (1975). Editorial: psychological theories and behaviour therapy. *Psychol. Med.* **5**, 219–221.

Eysenck, H. J. (1976). The learning theory model of neurosis—a new approach. *Behav. Res. Ther.* **14**, 251–267.

Fairweather, G. W. (1964). 'Social Psychology in Treating Mental Illness: An Experimental Approach'. Wiley, New York.

Fairweather, G. W., Sanders, D. H., Maynard, H. and Cressler, D. L. (1969). 'Community Life for the Mentally Ill and an Alternative to Institutional Care'. Aldine, Chicago.

Falloon, I. R. H., Lindley, P., McDonald, R. and Marks, I. M. (1977). Social skills training of outpatient groups. A controlled study of rehearsal and homework. *Br. J. Psychiat.* **131**, 599–609.

Friedman, D. E. and Lipsedge, M. S. (1971). Treatment of phobic anxiety and psychogenic impotence by systematic desensitisation employing methohexitone-induced relaxation. *Br. J. Psychiat.* **118**, 87–90.

Hafner, J. and Marks, I. M. (1976). Exposure *in vivo* of agoraphobics: contributions of diazepam, group exposure, and anxiety evocation. *Psychol. Med.* **6**, 71–88.

Hall, R. and Goldberg, D. (1977). The role of social anxiety in social interaction difficulties. *Br. J. Psychiat.* **131**, 610–615.

Hersen, M., Eisler, R. M. and Miller, P. M. (1973). Development of assertive responses: clinical measurement and research considerations. *Behav. Res. Ther.* **11**, 505–522.

Hilgard, E. R., Atkinson, R. C. and Atkinson, R. L. (1975). 'Introduction to Psychology' (6th Edn). Harcourt Brace Jovanovich, New York.

Hodgson, R., Rachman, S. and Marks, I. M. (1972). The treatment of chronic obsessive-compulsive neurosis: follow up and further findings. *Behav. Res. Ther.* **10**, 181–189.

Jacobsen, E. (1938). 'Progressive Relaxation'. University of Chicago Press, Chicago.

Kadzin, A. E. (1975). Recent advances in token economy research. *In* 'Progress in Behaviour Modification', Vol. 1. (Eds M. Hersen, R. M. Eisler and P. M. Miller), Vol. 1. Academic Press, New York and London.

Kelly, H. H. (1973). The processes of causal attribution. *Am. Psychol.* **28**, 107–128.

Klein, D. F. (1964). Delineation of two drug-responsive anxiety syndromes. *Psychopharmacologia* **5**, 397–408.

Kuhn, T. S. (1971). 'The Structure of Scientific Revolutions' (2nd Edn). University of Chicago Press, Chicago.

Levy, R. and Meyer, V. (1971). Ritual prevention in obsessional patients. *Proc. Roy. Soc. Med.* **64**, 1115–1118.

Lipsedge, M. S. (1973). Systematic desensitisation in phobic disorders. *Br. J. Hosp. Med.* **9**, 657–664.

Mahoney, M. J. (1974). 'Cognition and Behaviour Therapy'. Ballinger Publishing, Cambridge, Mass.

Marks, I. M. (1974). Research in neurosis: A selective review of treatment. *Psychol. Med.* **4**, 89–109.

Marks, I. M. (1976). The current status of behavioural psychotherapy: theory and practice. *Am. J. Psychiat.* **133**, 253–261.

Marks, I. M. (1977). Clinical phenomena in search of laboratory models. *In* 'Psychopathology: Experimental Models' (Eds J. D. Maser and M. E. P. Seligman. Freeman, San Francisco.

Marks, I. M., Boulougouris, J. and Marset, P. (1971). Flooding versus desensitisation in the treatment of phobic patients: a crossover study. *Br. J. Psychiat.* **119**, 353–375.

Marks, I. M., Hallan, R. S. and Philpott, R. (1975a). Nurse therapist in behavioural psychotherapy. *Br. Med. J.* **3**, 144–148.

Marks, I. M., Hodgson, R. and Rachman, S. (1975b). Treatment of chronic obsessive-compulsive neurosis by in-vivo exposure. A two year follow-up and issues in treatment. *Br. J. Psychiat.* **127**, 349–364.

Marzillier, J. S., Lambert, C. and Kellett, J. (1976). A controlled evaluation of systematic desensitisation and social skills training for socially inadequate psychiatric patients. *Behav. Res. Ther.* **14**, 225–238.

Meichenbaum, D. (1974). 'Cognitive Behaviour Modification'. N. J. General Learning Press, Morristown.

Mowrer, O. H. (1939). Stimulus response theory of anxiety. *Psychol. Rev.* **46**, 553–565.

Rachman, S. (1974). Primary obsessional slowness. *Behav. Res. Ther.* **12**, 9–18.

Rachman, S. (1976a). The passing of the two-stage theory of fear and avoidance: fresh possibilities. *Behav. Res. Ther.* **14**, 125–134.

Rachman, S. (1976b). The modification of obsessions: a new formulation. *Behav. Res. Ther.* **14**, 437–443.

Rachman, S. (1977). The conditioning theory of fear-acquisition: a critical examination. *Behav. Res. Ther.* **15**, 375–387.

Rachman, S., Hodgson, R. and Marks, I. M. (1971). Treatment of chronic obsessive-compulsive neurosis. *Behav. Res. Ther.* **9**, 237–247.

Seligman, M. E. P. (1974). Depression and learned helplessness. *In* 'The Psychology of Depression: Contemporary Theory and Research' (Eds R. J. Friedman and M. M. Katz). Wiley, New York.

Seligman, M. E. P., Maier, S. F. and Solomon, R. L. (1971). Unpredictable and uncontrollable aversive events. *In* 'Aversive Conditioning and Learning' (Ed. F. R. Brush). Academic Press, New York and London.

Seligman, M. and Johnston, J. (1973). A cognitive theory of avoidance learning. *In* 'Contemporary Approaches to Conditioning and Learning' (Eds J. McGuigan and B. Lumsden). Wiley, Washington.

Staples, F. R., Sloane, R. B., Whipple, K., Cristol. A. H. and Yorkston, N. J. (1975). Differences between behaviour therapists and psychotherapists. *Arch. Gen. Psychiat.* **32**, 1517–1524.

Stern, R. (1970). Treatment of a case of obsessional neurosis using thought stopping. *Br. J. Psychiat.* **117**, 441–442.

Stern, br. and Marks, I. M. (1973). Brief and prolonged flooding: A comparison in agoraphobic patients. *Erch. Gen. Psychiat.* **28**, 270–276.

Stern, R., Lipsedge, M. and Marks, I. (1973). Obsessive ruminations: a controlled trial of a thought-stopping technique. *Br. J. Psychiat.* **117**, 441–442.

Stuart, R. B. (1969). Operant-interpersonal treatment for marital discord. *J. Consult. Clin. Psychol.* **33**, 675–782.

Thoresen, C. E. and Mahoney, M. J. (1974). 'Behavioural Self-Control'. Holt, Rinehart and Winston, New York.

Tyrer, P. J., Candy, J. and Kelly, D. H. W. (1973). A study of clinical efforts of phenelzine and placebo in the treatment of phobic anxiety. *Psychopharmacologia.* **32**, 237–254.

Watson, J. B. (1930). 'Behaviour sm'. Routledge and Kegan Paul, London.

Watson, J. P., Gaind, R. and Marks, I. M. (1971). Prolonged exposure: a rapid treatment for phobias. *Br. Med. J.* **1**, 13–15.

Winkler, R. C. (1971). The relevance of economic theory and technology of token reinforcement systems. *Behav. Res. Ther.* **9**, 81–88.

Wolpe, J. (1958). 'Psychotherapy by Reciprocal Inhibition'. Stanford University Press, Stanford.

Wolpe, J. (1969). 'The Practice of Behaviour Therapy'. Pergamon, New York.

22 Psychotherapy

I Individual psychotherapy

Warren Kinston and *Rachel Rosser*

Historical introduction

In this part of Chapter 22 the term psychotherapy is used for any treatment in which the doctor–patient relationship is used to change the patient as a person. In its widest sense every doctor does psychotherapy. However, a variety of theories and techniques have been developed which place differing emphasis on cognitive, emotional or behavioural change. We shall be concerned with dynamic and supportive psychotherapies (Wolberg, 1967). Family and other group therapies, behaviour therapy and action therapies are discussed elsewhere (Chapters 21, 22, Parts III and IV). Certain other techniques such as hypnosis and abreaction (Wolberg, 1948; Sargant and Slater, 1972) are not discussed in this book.

The concept of psychotherapy was intrinsic to medicine in early oriental and occidental cultures and remains so in primitive societies (Frank, 1973). However, with the development of the medical model of illness, less attention was directed to the role of psychological factors in the causation and treatment of illness. Psychological treatments, traceable to pre-scientific notions of healing (Veith, 1965; Ellenberger, 1970; Tseng and McDermott, 1975) evolved independently of advances in medical technology. The increasing efficacy of specific biological treatments led to people asking for medical treatment more often with the result that less time was available for the traditional psychotherapeutic approach. But the multifactorial nature of disease is now widely acknowledged and health is again regarded as an aspect of a person's way of life (World Health Organization, 1950; Engel, 1960). The contribution of psychosocial factors to the efficacy of biological treatments has been recognized and psychotherapy is now seen to be relevant to the treatment of people presenting with both psychological and physical disturbances.

Freud's work began with hysteria, which could not be accommodated within the medical model. He developed psychoanalysis not only as a technique of treating patients, but also he believed as a scientific theory and a method of research. His contributions are conventionally divided into three phases: the early period (Stewart, 1967) which ended in 1897 with the discovery of the importance of fantasy, the second period during which the concept of the unconscious was fully developed and the final phase commencing with the introduction of the structural model in 1923. The impact of his work was such that creative schisms and countervailing developments appeared almost from the outset (Brown, 1961; Wyss, 1973).

Patients in psychoanalytic treatment revealed phenomena which had not been noticed in other contexts. The psychoanalyst relied on what he directly experienced with patients. In contrast to physical reality, which is perceived by the senses and detected by instruments, the phenomena of psychoanalysis are attributes of psychic reality perceived by the 'self' and detected only by persons. The principal difficulty in examining the mind by introspection is that the activity of introspection itself becomes the content of the mind. The psychoanalytic method attempted to overcome this by separating the experiencer (the patient or analysand) from the observer (the analyst) who became an empathic participant. The mental events which were perceived in such a situation inevitably centred on the analytic activity itself but this proved useful.

Freud made meaningful such phenomena as dreams (1901a), slips of the tongue (1901b) and neurotic symptoms (1905a). He perceived an order in a person's mental life and the human tendency to introduce order into experience. In addition to psychic determinism and the symbolic mediation of experience, his ideas included the dynamic unconscious and instinctual drives (1911, 1915), infantile sexuality including the early tie to the mother and the Oedipus complex (1905b, 1925), and the importance of conflict, anxiety and defence (1923, 1926). These ideas have a long history (Whyte, 1960) but Freud combined them in a new way with a unique emphasis and purpose. All behaviour could be examined from certain theoretical ('metapsychological') viewpoints. These were the topographical, i.e. the position in the psyche of the event with relation to the conscious and the unconscious; the dynamic, i.e. the particular instinctual drives and non-instinctual wishes involved; the economic, i.e.

the strength of the drives and wishes, and constitutional factors such as tolerance of anxiety; the genetic, i.e. historical and developmental factors; and the adaptational, i.e. the fit between the person and his environment. The acuteness of Freud's psychological observations is more evident in brief clinical vignettes (1916) than in his case histories which served rather to illustrate his theories. He wrote only sparingly on technique (1911–1915, 1937a). In later life he became increasingly pessimistic about the therapeutic value of psychoanalysis as he believed that constitutional (organic) factors severely limited what could be achieved (1937b).

Freud was a complex thinker dealing with intellectually and emotionally taxing issues. He provided some systematic introductions (1916–1917, 1933, 1940) in which he relied on clarity of exposition to convey his ideas. Redlich and Bingham (1953) do this in a cartoon-illustrated version. Aids to understanding the language used by psychoanalysts (including terms used in this chapter with minimal definition) are provided by Rycroft (1972) and Laplanche and Pontalis (1973).

Jung's writing can at times be so obscure as to be unintelligible, but Bennet (1966) and Storr (1973) have extracted the meat of his analytical psychology. Jung outlined some of his ideas in 'Modern Man in Search of a Soul' (1933) and described his personal development in 'Memories, Dreams and Reflections' (1963). His theories reflect his early experience with hospitalized schizophrenics and his notions of archetypal figures and of the innate or collective unconscious have features in common with Fairbairn's and Klein's later object-relations theories. For example, individuation and integration, which he emphasized as goals of therapy, are related to the schizoid dilemmas of loss of boundaries and splitting of the ego. He focused on the current life situation and often treated patients past middle-age who had problems with the meaning of their lives. His therapy was shorter than Freud's and he was the first to insist on the analyst himself being analysed, arguing that the nature of psychotherapy could be understood fully only when its living action had been suffered. His emphasis on the importance of the symbolic function (1964) was the stimulus for the rediscovery in the twentieth century of the therapeutic use of the arts including painting, music, modelling, drama, dancing and writing and of religious practices such as meditation.

Unlike Freud and Jung, Adler neither produced a systematic theory nor formally established a school. He took a rational, common-sense approach to changing a person's life style and the influence of his pragmatic psychology can be widely discerned in practice today. He has been called the inaugurator of modern psychosomatic medicine, the originator of group and family approaches, and a leader in the development of child guidance and social work. In his books, the best known of which is

'Understanding Human Nature' (1927), he restated certain fundamental principles which seem always in danger of being forgotten: that the mind and body are a unity, that aim and purpose matter in psychological disturbance, that the ndividual cannot be understood apart from his surroundings and his family and cultural ties. It is worth noting the similarity of the writings of Adolf Meyer (1957) who like Adler did not develop a theory of the personality but influenced much psychiatric practice. Adler's therapeutic tactic was a face-to-face encounter between patient and therapist in identical chairs. Therapy was intensive at first but he would rapidly reduce the frequency of sessions and was prepared to see members of the family. He confronted his patients with their self-defeating and self-deceptive attitudes, offered explanations of behaviour and pointed out the purposes of symptoms in their current life situation. He believed in a hopeful and encouraging attitude and tried to show kind, consistent interest in the patient.

In the USA, there was a reaction to the biological and instinctual basis of early psychoanalysis and psychotherapeutic theory was widened by an emphasis on the environment. Fromm (1956) and later Reich (Rycroft, 1971) wrote for a popular audience and were concerned with the warping effect of society on personality. Erikson (1950) remained more purely psychoanalytical by demonstrating similarities between the child's early upbringing and his later adjustment to society. Bettelheim (1950) used a residential setting for the application of psychoanalytic principles to the treatment of severely maladjusted children. Sullivan (1953) and Horney (1950) stressed the importance of interpersonal relationships in character formation and the individual's need for security and self-esteem.

Reich (1948) drew attention to the importance of the patient's negative feelings about the analyst and warned against premature deep interpretation. He wrote about the need for and the difficulty of character analysis. Traits are more complex than symptoms and because they are compatible with the person's concept of himself, they are more easily rationalized. Life style and character, consciously accessible to the individual, were used in existential theories which rejected the notion of the unconscious as a dynamic system (May et al., 1958; Laing, 1960; Frankl, 1965).

Within mainstream psychoanalysis, most significant developments have come from analysts working with children (Smirnoff, 1971). Anna Freud at the Hampstead Clinic in London and Heinz Hartmann in the USA became the principal exponents of psychoanalytic ego psychology. In the late 1930s Anna Freud published 'The Ego and the Mechanisms of Defence' and Hartmann 'Ego Psychology and the Problem of Adaption'. A recent summary of Anna Freud's views is available in 'Normality and Pathology in Childhood' (1966). Hartmann (1950) clarified the distinction between the terms 'ego' (a hypothetical mental apparatus) and 'self' (an internal mental representation of the subject). This was part of the elaboration of 'object relations theory' which has become a paradigm in psychoanalytic thinking, displacing the older notions of mental 'forces', 'cathexis' and 'energy'. The concept of 'mental structures' appears to be unavoidable in theories which relate past and present experience and take into account maturation and conflict (cf. Piaget). The individual is conceived as always existing in states of affective relatedness to significant others. The object relation—the 'self', the 'other' and the interactive bond between the two—is susceptible to internalization, the fundamental process in the development of psychic structure and personality.

From his experiences with schizoid patients in whom there is a divorce between emotional and intellectual functions, Fairbairn (1952) developed a pure object relations theory of the personality which was extended by Guntrip (1968). Melanie Klein, who worked with very young children, placed more emphasis on instinctual factors, especially aggression, within an object relations framework (Klein, 1932). Her ideas are set out in a series of popular lectures (Klein and Riviere, 1964) and a fuller account of her work is provided by Segal (1973). Fantasy was elevated to a central position in theory and technique (Isaacs, 1952). She described two personality constellations in psychic development, the paranoid-schizoid and the depressive, which form the basis of a regulatory (i.e. economic) principle of mental functioning. She and her school, mainly in Britain and South America, contributed to the analytical understanding of narcissism, manic states, perversions and the psychoses (Rosenfeld, 1964; Bion, 1967; Meltzer, 1973). Paradoxically the move away from regarding the person as existing in isolation promoted the psychoanalytic investigation of a person's relationship to himself (Jacobson, 1964; Erikson, 1968). Balint and Winnicott stressed the influence of the early environment from studies of deprived patients and were both led to focus on the 'self'. They noted that psychoanalysis required a patient to relate to and to use the analyst in a particular way. When there had been a failure of infant care, their patients had developed a shell or false-self with which they compliantly and rigidly related to the world. They were unable to use analysis for their psychological maturation. According to Balint (1968) the early relationship becomes one in which the self is characterized as weak and bad. Following repression of this relationship a basic fault develops in the character. In Winnicott's model, the true good self becomes buried and unresponsive to the outside world.

Winnicott was a gifted speaker and clinician and an original thinker. He made various theoretical and technical contributions to the nature of dependency, environmental provision, integration of the self, and the holding relationship (Khan et al., 1974) but his most original work was on the transition from object relating to the use of an object. His observations on transitional objects and other transitional phenomena were elaborated in his last book 'Playing and Reality' (1971).

In this brief outline we have avoided focusing on schisms as we think steady progress is discernible. Psychoanalytic concepts began with Freud and they have been elaborated, modified and supplemented with passion and perversity. The origin and fate of new ideas in psychoanalysis is a fascinating study in itself (Greenson, 1969).

The practice of psychotherapy

Psychotherapists aim to change people, but of course people change without therapy. Malan *et al*. (1975), in a study of spontaneous remission, list ways in which improvement is brought about. These include insight, self-analysis, working through feelings in a relationship with the person involved, normal maturing and growth, helpful relationships, taking responsibility for one's own life and breaking vicious circles between the person and his environment. Despite apparent diversity in theory and technique, all psychotherapies aim to open these paths to self-healing. Inevitably there is the risk of making things worse. They may aggravate symptoms and produce new interpersonal problems; they may induce despair by setting the patient inappropriately high goals or even destroy his trust in the value of human relationship (Hadley and Strupp, 1976).

Whatever the apparent differences in techniques or theory, many common factors emerge in practice. Frank (1968) emphasized the importance of optimism and hope. Tseng and McDermott (1975) made cross-cultural comparisons. In all therapy, they said, there must be a socially recognized healer who identifies problems, provides explanations and gives prescriptions for change. The patient must be willing to participate in the procedures. The healer must have a suitable personality and temperament. He defines norms, values and goals and reinforces socially acceptable ways of coping while offering 'cultural time out' within therapy. The purpose of all this is the creation of conditions under which the patient will be amenable to the therapist's influence on his thoughts, feelings and behaviour. Sloane *et al*. (1975) stipulated features in common between analytic and behavioural psychotherapy. In both, the therapist spends specified times with the patient, takes a history and shows an interest in the patient's life and problems; he listens, speaks, avoids technical terms, answers questions, corrects misconceptions, formulates problems, attempts to reconstruct possible original causes and looks for continuing causes.

The treatment or combination of treatments which a patient is offered depends more on the preference of the therapist and the circumstances under which he works than on any specific knowledge about the best match between patient, therapist and technique. Freud (1905c) thought that any convenient method was justified provided there was a prospect of helping the patient.

Psychoanalysis was created 'through and for the treatment of patients permanently unfit for existence' (Freud, 1905c). However, attempts to radically reorganize the personality are rarely realistic. Patients often come to attention at a time of crisis with a transient disturbance or a deterioration in a chronic problem. The therapist has to decide how much to help the patient regain his former equilibrium and how much to help him to learn new ways of solving his personal problems (Caplan, 1964). These two strategies have been called 'supportive' and 'analytic' respectively. This terminology is misleading in that all effective psychotherapy is supportive. In a follow-up study evaluating psychoanalytic group therapy, Malan et al. (1976) found that the therapists' lack of care, consideration and individual attention contributed to a poor outcome.

Supportive psychotherapy

The features of supportive therapy include a sympathetic understanding of the patient and discussion of his personal and social preoccupations and problems. Usually the therapist attempts to prevent or allay anxiety which the patient manifests and encourages him to talk and express his feelings. Client-centred therapy (Rogers, 1951) was one popular attempt in the USA to systematize a supportive technique capitalizing on the beneficial effect of reflecting back to a patient what he is communicating. However, most therapy is unsystematic: the therapist listens attentively, and periodically reflects, advises, explains, reassures, interprets, criticizes, prohibits, sets tasks or challenges the patient, as he deems appropriate. Many patients can take advantage of such efforts and heal themselves within the protective relationship. The Menninger Psychotherapy Research Project (Kernberg et al., 1972) showed that such therapy is more dependent on the skill and experience of the therapist than is analytic therapy. There are few technical guidelines and numerous hazards.

The hazards become more apparent with sicker patients. There is a risk that dependency will be encouraged inappropriately. For example, advice may imply that the patient is unable to think for himself. The role relationship of helper and helped has the advantage of compatibility with the psychiatrist's medical training and public image, but it has the disadvantage of placing the patient in a vulnerable position. (Unfortunately it is often immature patients, considered to be too sick for analytic psychotherapy, who are subjected to the psychic demands entailed by bad organization such as excessive waiting, or interruptions during sessions.) Much of the therapy operates cognitively, and this enhances realistic goals and prevents the patient regressing to infantile behaviour. However, it can result in the psychiatrist denying or avoiding emotional contact with his patient. The therapeutic relationship may be deceptively comfortable if the patient is willing to take the sick role and the therapist treats the patient courteously. The artificiality and lack of emotional understanding in such a relationship lead to misjudgements by the therapist. Clear therapeutic goals, not necessarily made explicit to the patient, counter these hazards and prevent therapy becoming repetitive and stalemated. If this happens therapy becomes a burden to the therapist and does not support the patient.

Although in its wider applicat on the importance of supportive therapy is self-evident, it has been insufficiently explored and it is not surprising that its use and outcome is so dependent on the personality of the therapist.

Analytic psychotherapy

Analytic psychotherapy is characterized by a particular type of relationship, the interpretation of this relationship and the development of a special process within the patient. The qualities of the relationship depend on the personalities of the participants and on their mutual respect. Therapy provides for a normally unattainable degree of intimacy and safe exposure of the self and characteristically the patient recalls and relives past experiences. The personal directness of analytic therapy arises from consistent interpretation of the relationship between the patient and the therapist, especially of the repetitive patterns originating in childhood. This provokes anxiety. The principal aim of analytic therapy is to explore the ways in which a person invests the world with meaning, a process which may be a strange and frightening experience.

Analytic therapy is risky. Not only does it provoke anxiety and other strong feelings in the patient but it is also likely to disrupt his external relationships. This can occur as a result of transient distress or of serious incompatibility between any move towards health and his current life situation. When analytic therapy is going well, both the patient and therapist become deeply involved and bear the tension that inevitably ensues. Certain observations are highly suggestive that things are going wrong. The therapist may feel excessively dedicated, self-doubting, or self-critical; he may find himself emotionally unconcerned or relying on 'deep' interpretations rather than sympathetic understanding, or he may just want to give up. He may make futile efforts to control the patient's behaviour, get trapped in vicious cycles with the patient and become suspicious and perhaps elaborate paranoid fantasies about him. The therapist then needs to look at himself. Is he avoiding his own feelings? Is he colluding with a defensive role relation? Is he obtaining some gratification from the situation? The cause may lie within the patient who may not be suitable for the therapy offered. The criterion for suitability is not only whether a patient needs analytic therapy, but also whether he can use it.

The contract in psychotherapy

Like other medical treatments, psychotherapy depends on the active co-operation of the patient. It takes place within a contract between patient and therapist. This is usually mutually negotiated but may have to be a unilateral statement of intent by the therapist when the patient is too disturbed to enter an agreement or unable to accept his problems. The contract states clearly the therapist's intent, provides limits for the patient and becomes a reference point for assessment of progress. It should include a statement of frequency and duration of sessions, the objectives and rules of the meetings and conditions for alteration and review. A contract for supportive psychotherapy might be:

> We shall meet for six 30-minute sessions at three-weekly intervals and we can discuss your problems at work; in the fifth session we must discuss what further help you might need if matters haven't improved by then.

A pre-therapy contract might be:

> I'll see you next week and the following week, briefly on both occasions, and by then the drugs should be helping you and we can see what else is necessary.

A contract for analytic therapy requires more detail:

> Psychotherapy requires that the two of us meet every week, except for holiday periods, for 45 minutes in this room on Wednesday afternoons at 2 p.m. You can talk about anything you wish and I will comment when I have something to say which might be helpful. As I am leaving the Unit in 10 months we shall have to review the situation a couple of months before this.

The therapist must consider his contract as binding, so it must be realistic. The contract is the most concrete manifestation of the bond between therapist and patient. Bonds imply loyalty and responsibility on both sides. As most patients have been let down in their childhood, these implications of the contract may need to be spelt out. Not uncommonly, the patient subtly or overtly invites the therapist to break the contract. Before a contract is altered, the meanings of the request have to be sorted out and, if they are unclear, the therapist is well advised to adhere to the original commitment.

Starting and ending

Deciding to start therapy is difficult. Even patients who ask for psychotherapy may not know what they are letting themselves in for. Many patients are either not well enough or not informed enough to consider it and it is useful to distinguish a stage of pre-therapy during which patients are assessed and the possibility of psychological treatment can be put to them. When a patient is too ill, the decision as to suitability for psychotherapy has to be postponed while other psychiatric treatments are given. Very disturbed patients may need help in experiencing, recognizing and thinking about themselves. Others may benefit from being seen occasionally over a number of years while they slowly mature.

Patients who are uninformed can be helped to recognize the value of a psychological approach to their problems. For example, one might try to persuade a patient to take responsibility for his life and to realize that he needs to learn new solutions to the stresses he faces. A series of interviews (sometimes ambiguously called a 'trial') can be invaluable preceding therapy proper. These can be used to assess the patient's persistence, his response to interpretation, his ability to use a relationship and his dependence on primitive defence mechanisms. Hasty commitments on both sides can then be avoided. If therapy is contemplated, working through anxieties about it introduces the patient to the ways of analytic therapy. For patients who need to mature, prolonged pre-therapy may be required, e.g. group therapy with its less intense intimacy, or transactional analysis with its focus on the enactment of ego states. Patients who must wait for practical reasons may benefit from periodic contact; lectures and group discussion about therapy have been provided for patients on the waiting list.

The contract should include an agreement on criteria for ending, since this is a potentially disturbing event. Analytic therapists regard work on feelings about termination as crucial to success and Mann (1973) makes it central in his system of brief psychotherapy. Dropping out of therapy may be an assertion of health, a response to external contingencies or a repetition of self-defeating activity. In the last case, the therapist must discuss areas of unfinished work and leave open the option for further help.

Analytic therapeutic strategies

An introduction to the practice of therapy is provided by Colby (1951) and Bruch (1974). Analytic technique may be applied in various ways.

A person in psychosocial transition, for example leaving school, marrying, or losing a spouse by death, does psychological work. When this process is avoided or incomplete, pathological states may result, particularly in previously vulnerable people. The disorganization that accompanies crisis can be exploited by the therapist. At such a time, the patient may be more aware that something is wrong with him, more ready to accept help and more receptive to new ideas. *Crisis therapy* takes place in one or more interviews over a few weeks.

Therapy exceeding six weeks inevitably becomes complicated by problems in the relationship with the therapist. This can be fruitfully used in so-called *brief therapy*, typically lasting up to 12 months. Pathological grief reactions for exemple, often require six to nine months for resolution. The time span may be more crucial than the frequency of sessions, which may be at intervals to suit the patient.

Malan (1976) found that the capacity of neurotics for genuine recovery, involving resolution of internal as well as external problems, is greater than psychoanalysts have previously believed. He claimed that patients can be identified who are suitable for a brief technique and that the more radical the technique, especially in making the transference–childhood link and working through termination, the greater the therapeutic effect. Brief therapy is appropriate in motivated patients with a circumscribed focus of pathology. In recognizing a focus, the therapist should fit evidence from current and past stresses, childhood experience and repetitive life patterns to a minimum of psychodynamic theory. The immediate relevance of the focus and usefulness of focal work can be determined during assessment by the response of the patient to interpretations. As issues surrounding termination must not be insuperable, problems of deprivation and intense dependency are contraindications.

Patients with complex or obscure problems or with difficulties in making contact require *long-term psychotherapy*. The patient is seen for 45 to 60 minutes at least once and up to three times per week, usually over 18 months to two years, but sometimes for much longer. Such therapy is an arduous experience. The therapist must expect the patient to become as unhappy or disturbed as he has ever been in his life. For this reason, a full psychiatric and psychodynamic assessment is essential. The therapist can then obtain an idea of the likely form of the transference and can prepare for contingencies such as the need for hospitalization.

This also applies to *psychoanalysis* which commonly lasts for three to six years with four or more sessions weekly. Practical issues loom large in organizing such a treatment and views are divided as to whether it should be reserved for sicker patients (who may need it more) or healthier patients (who may be able to use it more). For some patients the difference from analytic therapy is largely one of degree, but for others (e.g. narcissistic patients) the increased contact is claimed to be essential.

The aim of all analytic work is to use personal exploration to promote resolution of internal conflicts and to permit maturation through self-understanding. Termination occurs ideally with the acceptance that such a task is potentially endless.

Phenomena of psychotherapy

From their experience of patients, analytic therapists have outlined various phenomena. These are relevant whatever form of therapy is practised although their technical handling will vary. In the following sections we briefly examine some core concepts and aspects of the therapeutic process. These are reviewed by Sandler *et al.* (1973).

Transference

Transference is the patient's transfer into therapy of feelings and expectations derived from childhood. It is most readily recognized when the transfer has a quality of inappropriateness but apparently appropriate feelings such as trust may also be transference based. During therapy, the patient imaginatively or in actuality creates a role-relationship with the therapist. The transference takes the form of either a perception or an action which will produce the wanted perception. For example, the patient may see the therapist as depriving and say so, perhaps adducing as proof a short period of silence (illusory apperception), or the patient may ask the therapist questions which he knows will not be answered, so allowing himself to see that the therapist is depriving him (actualization, acting-in or enactment). In therapy, the neurotic patient relives the past with vivid immediacy. He transfers good experiences which are desired, bad experiences of frustration and environmental failure which are feared and hated, and ways of avoiding experience, i.e. his defences.

Reactivation of childhood experience in adult life is not peculiar to analytic psychotherapy. Non-analytic therapists handle transference phenomena differently. Rational therapists may confront infantile attitudes and attempt to alter such patterns of response by re-education. Behaviour therapists avoid unwanted intrusions of the transference by asking patients to concentrate on the task in hand. Most therapists encourage the development of positive aspects of childhood experience but paradoxical injunctions and challenging techniques activate and then take advantage of the childhood negativism. Supportive therapy allows the therapist to use constructively common manifestations of the transference; for example, over-valuation of the therapist or a tendency to relate by identification can be exploited in modelling techniques.

The central feature of analytic therapy is the use of the transference. Its appearance and recognition is fostered by the analytic attitude. The therapist takes up an observational stance, values what the patient says or does and replaces direct gratification of transference wishes with interpretations.

Countertransference

It is difficult to convey the intensity of a patient's infantile emotions in the transference. When the therapist feels he cannot bear it he will act. When the action is not thought out and takes the form of acceding to unreasonable demands, switching off attention, arriving late to sessions or being unnecessarily clever, it is unlikely to help the patient and becomes a 'countertransference problem'. The countertransference consists of emotions, wishes, fantasies and thoughts which the therapist has about his patient.

The first group of these emanates primarily from the patient and includes responses of the therapist to explicit communications or to manifestations of the transference. Non-verbal communication is the natural language of the emotions and the patient shows the therapist what he cannot tell him in words. To pick up such messages, the therapist's self must be tuned in, i.e. he must be with his patient, be interested in him and attentive to him. In analytic therapy the analyst's attention is suspended and the usual focusing mechanisms such as personal inclination, prejudices and theoretical assumptions are put aside as far as possible so that the therapist can identify empathically. This is called *free floating attention*.

The second group of countertransference experiences consists of intrusion of the therapist's world into therapy. The therapist may respond idiosyncratically to aspects of the patient's style such as his way of speaking or mode of dress. If he is aware of this, no harm should ensue. The patient is protected from intrusions by the therapist's capacity to distinguish between his own thoughts and feelings and those of another person. Under stress this can become difficult and problems arise if the patient becomes confused in the therapist's mind with a figure from his own past (including himself), i.e. if the patient functions as a transference object for the therapist. This will lead the therapist to attribute feelings wrongly, to act irrationally and to mould the patient to meet the therapist's needs. All therapists have blind spots and areas of unresolved conflict about which they have to learn. Early warning signs during therapy include feelings of unease with the patient, dislike of the sessions or unprofessional management of the patient. Personal therapy and supervision are the usual preventive and remedial measures.

Content of the sessions

The patient is invited to talk about his problems and to say whatever comes into his mind, although of course, he tends to be directed by comments, questions and non-verbal indications from the therapist. This is *free association*. He may describe current events, explore his motivations and experiences, recall recent childhood memories and volunteer dreams, day dreams and fantasies. He may directly engage the therapist (e.g. asking personal questions), become unable or refuse to speak at all or feel compelled to do something (e.g. walk around the room). Although skill and experience are invaluable in handling this *material*, psychodynamic theory provides one way of categorizing and dealing with it.

In a predominantly verbal process, action has a special place. Actions reported or performed during therapy serve various functions and must be the subject of therapeutic work. The patient may be unable to communicate something except through an action, he may be using action to control the therapy or the therapist, and he may try to avoid or to get rid of painful states by acting. Impulsive and compulsive repetition of behaviour especially when it is self-defeating is assumed to be indicative of a patient's refusal to acknowledge the transference. Such repetitive action may occur within the session, for example arriving late or ignoring interpretations, or outside therapy, for example marital disputes or losing a job. When it occurs within therapy, it has been called *acting in*, although Freud (in translation) called this *acting out*. The term *acting out* has been so expanded it has become a source of confusion and we prefer to use *action*, rather than 'acting', to indicate overt behaviour and *enactment* to cover actions which derive their principal stimulus from the person's internal world.

The analytic attitude promotes the transference illusion and the patient's material develops the quality of play, a serious activity in a child's life. There are parallels between play in childhood and the dreaming experience in adult life. Both are visual, in both the normal laws of logic are suspended, both permit happenings which would be morally unacceptable in other circumstances, both use symbolization and both are forms of thinking which deal with conflicts.

The patient's capacity to experience and recall a dream cannot be taken for granted and contempt for dreams is not uncommon. The dream content as reported is referred to as *manifest*. From the patient's current situation, his ideas about the manifest content and the material of the session, the therapist infers *latent* content, i.e. the wishes and anxieties that stimulated the production of the dream. The conversion of latent to manifest content is referred to as the *dream work*. Dreams may be produced in overabundance, often without associations, when the patient wishes to unload his experience rather than to understand it.

Resistance

Although patients come to change, many show evidence of opposition to therapy. This non-compliance occurs in numerous forms and has many sources. In analytic therapy it always occurs and is referred to as *resistance*. Patients are used to their symptoms and patterns of adaptation, they feel safe and obtain gratification from them and sometimes they also get secondary gains. People have a natural inertia and fear the unknown. Some patients seem to need to suffer, e.g. they get worse after any successful therapeutic work or feel uneasy when things are going well. Different forms of resistance occur with different therapeutic approaches, so methods of handling resistance are an important part of technique. In analytic therapy, resistance is not avoided or regarded as undesirable, but is a focus of therapeutic activity.

The transference is a major source of resistance because of the patient's compulsion to re-enact rather than recollect and his wish to rebel and take revenge for past hurts. When the patient is in the grip of childhood feelings he is described as *regressed*. A deeply regressed patient in a treatment going well is aware of the 'as if' quality of the experience, knows it is temporary and functions well externally. The term *malignant regression* has been used for regressive behaviour which makes learning impossible, spills over destructively into the patient's outside life, is unaffected by the therapist's explanations, is often not regarded by the patient as inappropriate and is difficult to reverse. It requires active management rather than interpretation.

Interventions

The most characteristic intervention of analytic therapy is *interpretation*.

Interpretation in the sense of explanation and rationalization is used in many therapies. Analytically, an interpretation brings out the hidden meanings in what the patient says and does. It is often preceded by clarification of the relevant details, confrontation with the facts, exploration of associations and drawing together of evidence. The patient's conscious experience may have to be affirmed so that the interpretation does not have an invalidating quality. Nevertheless, interpretative activity provokes anxiety. To counter this, the therapist interprets, not only how the patient feels, but why he is anxious about this feeling coming to light. In other words he gives a 'defence' as well as a 'content' interpretation. Similarly, feelings and wishes should not be interpreted until any associated guilt and shame have been dealt with, as the patient's pride and moral sense should not be offended unnecessarily. Faulty interpretations may at best be useless and are likely to be counterproductive, inducing either pseudo-cooperation or a sense of persecution. Interpretations made prematurely, out of context (wild), or with the wrong tone of voice can produce intense distress. Effective interpretations convey a sense of safety and lead the patient into a close emotional relationship with the therapist.

An interpretation in its classic form links the patient's experience in the transference, his interactions in the external world and his childhood. The external reference buttresses the transference reference, making it more acceptable and more convincing. The interpretation is intended to integrate and give meaning; it conveys information (the 'truth' as it feels to the therapist and patient) about psychic reality. It is an act on the patient and it may be a gesture, question, or brief statement rather than a statement in the full form.

It is commonly held that interpretations arise from deductions based on psychoanalytic theories. However, another point of view with which we agree, is that they are more often a result of an imaginative leap. The therapist responds to the communication of the patient using his perception of emotions or fantasies in himself, his own experience of life and his theoretical knowledge. Of course, this intuitive process is subject to error and, because the laws of logic are not applicable, the therapist may believe an erroneous observation to be correct. Errors are intrinsic to therapy and form part of the material. The patient may be protected by his tendency to keep bringing the same material until it is handled appropriately.

In therapy the same preoccupation or behaviour recurs and must be interpreted repeatedly. The psychoanalytic term for this is *working through*. The same content may recur session after session, in different phases of the therapy and at similar times, e.g. before holidays. The therapist has to observe the repetition, tolerate it and deal with it in a positive way to prevent the therapy becoming futile. Recurrence is a form of analytic evidence from which therapist and patient learn.

Classification of patients for psychotherapy

A classification of patients for the guidance of therapists would consider the nature of intrapsychic structure and maturity in interpersonal relationships rather than focus on observations from a psychiatric interview. Grinker *et al*. (1968) found that a phenomenological approach to a group of patients whose diagnosis seemed to lie between psychosis and neurosis had severe limitations. Psychoanalysts claim that some patients seem to function adequately and are socially well-adapted, and yet reveal paradoxically severe psychopathology during analysis. Despite attempts at classification (Kernberg, 1970) there is no accepted psychodynamic nosology.

Two groups of patients are identifiable principally by their presentation within therapy. *Borderline patients* are defined by their tendency to regress rapidly whenever structure is lacking. In their lives they may show 'stable instability' or superficial normality. In therapy they reveal intense feelings, usually hostile or depressive, impulsive behaviour such as overdoses, self-mutilation and antisocial acts, disturbances of identity and of the boundaries between the self and the other, transient psychotic experiences and vacillation between withdrawal and intense exigency in the relationship. For a review of descriptions of this group see Gunderson and Singer (1975) and for discussion of treatment see Zetzel (1971) and Hartocollis (1977).

Narcissistic patients show better social functioning than borderline patients and sometimes considerable achievement. This is associated with intense ambition, grandiose fantasies, feelings of inferiority and overdependence on admiration and acclaim. Wounds to their pride lead to intense rage and wishes for revenge. Relationship to others is exploitative, paranoid, deficient in empathy and egocentric. These patients are terrified of dependence and deficient in genuine feelings of sadness, and in the transference the analyst is treated as an extension of the patient's self. The problems of pathological narcissism and its treatment have been investigated by Kohut (1971), Kernberg (1975) and Rosenfeld (1964).

Borderline and narcissistic patients, if amenable to psychotherapy, require prolonged treatment. The former are said to benefit more from weekly individual or group therapy both of which serve to contain the regression. However, sharing with others or infrequent contact may be too wounding to the narcissistic patient and full psychoanalysis may be the only treatment which allows him to relate to someone. Narcissistic patients who operate on a borderline level are rarely suitable for psychotherapy.

Maturity

Psychotherapy uses the healing effects of a personal relationship and an assessment of maturity is important. The therapist must adjust his expectations and concentrate on resolving the pathology. Maturation is slow and can only be facilitated so the extent of change may be limited. Maturity has been assessed in two ways, on the basis of the level of the differentiation of the self and on the adaptive style of the person.

Sullivan et al. (1957) drew on the work of Erikson and of Piaget to develop a clinical scale of the self ('I' levels) for use with psychopaths. Bowen (1966) used the concept of self differentiation for his form of individual and family therapy in which the differentiation of members within the family unit is the central focus. At the lowest levels, a person is unaware of the difference between himself and the external world and is inevitably so inadequate or socially disruptive that institutionalization is required. At a slightly higher level, he moves in and out of institutions depending on external stresses and he has a capacity to feel miserable; other people are seen as withholders or givers and he is unaware of the effect on them of his behaviour. Most patients in psychotherapy occupy the next levels. The least differentiated of these live in a feeling world and distort internal reality and manipulate others in an attempt to feel more comfortable. Their use of 'I' is restricted to 'I want', 'I hurt', 'I have my rights'. Above these are people who can function as dependent appendages. They are excessively responsive to the feelings and behaviour of others and may be over-compliant or over-rebellious in an attempt either to obtain love and praise or to react against its absence. With further differentiation, emotional equilibrium is more certain and more energy is available for goal-directed behaviour. The pressure for conformity is still great but a person at this level is far more able to use 'I' for self-affirmation saying 'I am', 'I believe', 'I will do'. Such people break down from time to time under excessive stress. People with greater degrees of self-differentiation can be sympathetic and see the point of view of the other, are equally receptive to criticism or praise, express considered opinions and allow intimacy and temporary fusion with others. They are aware of their dependency and sure of their responsibility to themselves and others and rarely come for psychotherapy.

The second method of assessment is based on adaptive style and uses the concept of defence (A. Freud, 1937; Semrad, 1967) which refers to the way a person copes with his private wishes and emotions, with frustration and loss, with emotional closeness and with the need to maintain a sense of his own worth and a feeling of well-being. Vaillant (1971, 1976) in a 30-year follow-up study of healthy college graduates found that the maturity of defences correlated with other definitions of mental health and with psychosocial adjustment. Significant shifts in the cluster of defences occurred as a person passed through the adult life cycle. This evolution of mature defences was not related to childhood environment but depended on the presence at crucial times of a sustained close relationship, such as a close friend, a spouse or even a psychotherapist.

Mature defences used predominantly by healthy adults to protect against psychic pain include anticipation, suppression, humour, altruism and sublimation. To the user, these integrate conscience, reality, interpersonal relations and private feelings; to others they appear as virtues. *Neurotic* defences, including repression, reaction formation, displacement, rationalization, undoing and dissociation are common in patients in psychotherapy. To others they appear as idiosyncrasies or hang-ups. *Immature* defences present as socially undesirable behaviour and they protect against intimacy and loss. They include projection, schizoid fantasy, hypochondriasis, passive aggression and enactment. *Narcissistic* defences distort reality and the user appears crazy. They include intense denial, projective identification, primitive idealization, omnipotence, splitting and distortion. The appearance of grossly deviant, psychopathic or psychotic behaviour may be prevented at the cost of emotional deadening or of avoiding social situations. When people using predominantly narcissistic and immature defences, whether grossly symptomatic or apparently well adapted, are exposed to the intimacy and lack of structure of the psychotherapeutic relationship, they respond in an extreme, even explosive fashion.

References

Adler, A (1927). 'Understanding Human Nature'. Greenberg, New York.
Balint, M. (1968). 'The Basic Fault: Therapeutic Aspects of Regression'. Tavistock, London.
Bennet, E. D. (1966). 'What Jung Really Said'. Macdonald, London.
Bettelheim, B. (1950). 'Love is Not Enough'. Collier-Macmillan, London.
Bion, W. (1967). 'Second Thoughts—Selected Papers in Psychoanalysis'. Heinemann, London.
Bowen, M. (1966). The use of family theory in clinical practice. *Compr. Psychiat.* 7, 345–374.
Brown, J. A. C. (1961). 'Freud and the Post-Freudians'. Penguin, Harmondsworth.

Bruch, H. (1974). 'Learning Psychotherapy; Rationale and Ground Rules'. Harvard University Press, Cambridge, Mass.

Caplan, G. (1964). 'Principles of Preventive Psychiatry'. Basic Books, New York.

Colby, K. M. (1951). 'A Primer for Psychotherapists'. Ronald Press, New York.

Ellenbeger, H. F. (1970). 'The Discovery of the Unconscious. The History and Evolution of Dynamic Psychiatry'. Allen Lane, The Penguin Press, London.

Engel, G. (1960). A unified concept of health and disease. *Persp. Biol. Med.* 3, 459.

Erikson, E. (1950). 'Childhood and Society'. W. W. Norton, New York.

Erikson, E. (1968). 'Identity: Youth and Crisis'. W. W. Norton, New York.

Fairbairn, W. R. D. (1952). 'Psychoanalytic Studies of the Personality'. Tavistock, London.

Frank, J. D. (1968). The role of hope in psychotherapy. *Int. J. Psychiat.* 5, 383–412.

Frank, J. D. (1973). 'Persuasion and Healing: A Comparative Study of Psychotherapy' (rev. edn). John Hopkins University Press, Baltimore.

Frankl, V. (1965). 'The Doctor and the Soul' (2nd edn). Random House, New York.

Freud, A. (1937). 'The Ego and the Mechanisms of Defence'. Hogarth Press, London, 1968.

Freud, A. (1966). 'Normality and Pathology in Childhood'. Penguin Books, Harmondsworth.

In the following citations 'SE' refers to the appropriate volume and pages in 'The Standard Edition of the Complete Psychological Works of Sigmund Freud' published by Hogarth Press and the Institute of Psychoanalysis, London, 1953–1974. The year indicated is the year of original publication.

Freud, S. (1901a). 'On Dreams'. SE 5, 633–686.

Freud, S. (1901b). 'The Psychopathology of Everyday Life'. SE 6.

Freud, S. (1905a). 'Fragment of an Analysis of a Case of Hysteria'. SE 7, 1–122.

Freud, S. (1905b). 'Three Essays on the Theory of Sexuality'. SE 7, 125–243.

Freud, S. (1905c). 'On Psychotherapy'. SE 7, 257–268.

Freud, S. (1911). 'Formulations on the Two Principles of Mental Functioning'. SE 12, 218–226.

Freud, S. (1911–1915). 'Papers on Technique'. SE 12, 85–174.

Freud, S. (1915). 'Papers on Metapsychology'. SE 14, 105–235.

Freud, S, (1916). 'Some Character-Types Met With in Psychoanalytic Work'. SE 14, 309–333.

Freud, S. (1916–1917). 'Introductory Lectures on Psychoanalysis'. SE 15 and 16.

Freud, S. (1923). 'The Ego and the Id'. SE 19, 3–59.

Freud, S. (1925). 'Some Psychical Consequences of the Anatomical Distinction Between the Sexes'. SE 19, 241–258.

Freud, S. (1926). 'Inhibitions, Symptoms and Anxiety'. SE 20, 75–172.

Freud, S. (1933). 'New Introductory Lectures'. SE 22, 1–182.

Freud, S. (1937a). 'Constructions in Analysis'. SE 23, 257–269.

Freud, S. (1937b). 'Analysis Terminable and Interminable'. SE23, 209–253.

Freud, S. (1940). 'An Outline of Psychoanalysis'. SE 23, 144–207.

Fromm, E. (1956). 'The Art of Loving'. Harper and Row, New York.

Greenson, R. R. (1969). The origin and fate of new ideas in psychoanalysis. *Int. J. Psycho-Anal.* 50, 503–515.

Grinker, R. R. Sr, Werble, B. and Drye, R. C. (1968). 'The Borderline Syndrome: A Behavioural Study of Ego Functions'. Basic Books Inc. New York.

Gunderson, J. G. and Singer, M. T. (1975). Defining borderline patients: an overview. *Am. J. Psychiat.* 132, 1–10.

Guntrip, H. (1968). 'Schizoid Phenomena, Object Relations and the Self'. Hogarth, London.
Hadley, S. W. and Strupp, H. H. (1976). Contemporary views of negative effects in psychotherapy. An integrated account. *Arch. Gen. Psychiat.* 33, 1291–1302.
Hartmann, H. (1950). Comments on the psychoanalytic theory of the ego: introduction. *Psychoanal. Study Child.* 5, 74–96.
Hartmann, H. (1958). 'Ego Psychology and the Problem of Adaptation'. International Universities Press, New York.
Hartocollis, P. (1977). 'Borderline Personality Disorders: The Concept, The Syndrome, The Patient.' International University Press, New York.
Horney, K. (1950). 'Neurosis and Human Growth'. W. W. Norton, New York.
Isaacs, S. (1952). The nature and function of fantasy. *In* 'Developments in Psychoanalysis' (Ed. M. Klein *et al*). Hogarth, London.
Jacobson, E. (1964). 'The Self and the Object World'. Hogarth, London.
Jung, C. G. (1933). 'Modern Man in Search of a Soul'. Routledge and Kegan Paul, London.
Jung, C. G. (1963). 'Memories, Dreams and Reflections'. Routledge and Kegan Paul, London.
Jung, C. G. (1964). 'Man and his Symbols'. Doubleday, New York.
Kernberg, O. F. (1970). A psychoanalytic classification of character pathology. *J. Am. Psychoanal. Ass.* 18, 800–822.
Kernberg, O. F. (1975). 'Borderline Conditions and Pathological Narcissism'. Jason Aronson, New York.
Kernberg, O. F., Burstein, E. D., Coyne, L., Applebaum, A., Horwitz, L. and Voth, H. (1972). Psychotherapy and psychoanalysis. Final report of the Menninger Foundation Psychotherapy Research Project. *Bull. Menninger Clin.* 36, 1–275.
Khan, M. M. R., Davis, J. A. and Davis, M. E. V. (1974). The beginnings and fruition of the self—an essay on D. W. Winnicot. *In* 'Scientific Foundations of Paediatrics' (Eds J. A. Davis and J. Dobbing), pp. 626–640. Heinemann, London.
Klein, M. (1932). 'The Psychoanalysis of Children'. Hogarth, London.
Klein, M. and Riviere, J. (1964). 'Love, Hate and Reparation'. W. W. Norton, New York.
Kohut, H. (1971). 'The Analysis of the Self'. International University Press, New York.
Laing, R. D. (1960). 'The Divided Self'. Tavistock, London.
Laplanche, J. and Pontalis, J. B. (1973). 'The Language of Psychoanalysis'. Hogarth Press, London.
Malan, D. (1976). 'The Frontier of Brief Psychotherapy'. Plenum Press, New York.
Malan, D. H., Heath, E. S., Bacal, H. A. and Balfour, F. H. G. (1975). Psychodynamic changes in untreated neurotic patients II: Apparently genuine improvements. *Arch. Gen. Psychiat.* 32, 110–126.
Malan, D. H., Balfour, F. H. G., Hood, V. G. and Shooter, A. M. N. (1976). Group psychotherapy: a long-term follow-up study. *Arch. Gen. Psychiat.* 33, 1303–1315.
Mann, J. (1973). 'Time-Limited Psychotherapy'. Harvard University Press, Cambridge, Mass.
May, R., Angel, E. and Ellenberger, H. F. (1958). 'Existence—A New Dimension in Psychiatry and Psychology'. Basic Books, New York.
Meltzer, D. (1973). 'Sexual States of Mind'. Clunie Press, Perthshire.

Meyer, A. (1957). 'Psychobiology. A Science of Man'. Thomas, Springfield, Illinois.

Redlich, F. and Bingham, J. (1953). 'The Inside Story. Psychiatry and Everyday Life'. Vintage Books, Alfred A. Knopf, New York.

Reich, W. (1948). Character analysis. In 'The Psychoanalytic Reader' (Ed. R. Fliess), Chapters 1–3, pp. 106–156. International University Press, New York.

Rogers, C. R. (1951). 'Client-Centred Therapy'. Houghton Mifflin, Boston.

Rosenfeld, H. (1964). 'Psychotic States'. Hogarth, London.

Rycroft, C. (1971). 'Reich'. Fontana, London.

Rycroft, C. (1972). 'A Critical Dictionary of Psychoanalysis'. Penguin, Harmondsworth.

Sandler, J., Dare, C. and Holder, A. (1973). 'The Patient and the Analyst: The Basis of the Psychoanalytic Process'. George Allen and Unwin, London.

Sargant, W. and Slater, E. (1972). 'An Introduction to Physical Methods of Treatment in Psychiatry' (5th edn). Churchill Livingstone, Edinburgh.

Segal, H. (1973). 'An Introduction to the Work of Melanie Klein' (2nd edn). Hogarth, London.

Semrad, E. (1967). The organization of the ego defenses and object loss. In 'The Loss of Loved Ones' (Ed. D. M. Moriarty). Thomas, Springfield, Illinois.

Sloane, R. B., Staples, F. R., Cristol, A. H., Yorkston, N. J. and Whipple, K. (1975). 'Psychotherapy Versus Behaviour Therapy'. Harvard University Press, Cambridge.

Smirnoff, V. (1971). 'The Scope of Child Analysis'. Routledge and Kegan Paul, London.

Stewart, W. A. (1967). 'Psychoanalysis—the First Ten Years (1888–1898)'. George Allen and Unwin, Tondon.

Storr, A. (1973). 'Jung'. Fontana, London.

Sullivan, C., Grant, M. Q., and Grant, J. D. (1957). The development of interpersonal maturity—applications to delinquency. Psychiatry 20, 373–385.

Sullivan, H. S. (1953). 'Interpersonal Theory of Psychiatry'. W. W. Norton, New York.

Tseng, W. and McDermott, Jnr., J. F. (1975). Psychotherapy: historical roots, universal elements and cultural variations. Am. J. Psychiat. 132, 378–384.

Vaillant, G. E. (1971). Theoretical hierarchy of adaptive ego mechanisms: a 30 year follow up of 30 men selected for psychological health. Arch. Gen. Psychiat. 24, 107–118.

Vaillant, G. E. (1976). Natural history of male psychological health. V. The relation of choice of ego mechanisms of defense to adult adjustment. Arch. Gen. Psychiat. 33, 535–545.

Veith, I. (1965). 'Hysteria: The History of a Disease'. University of Chicago Press, Chicago.

Whyte, L. L. (1960). 'The Unconscious before Freud'. Basic Books, New York.

Winnicott, D. W. (1971). 'Playing and Reality'. Tavistock, London.

Wolberg, L. (1948). 'Medical Hypnosis', Vols 1 and 2. Grune and Stratton, New York.

Wolberg, L. R. (1967). 'The Technique of Psychotherapy'. Grune and Stratton, New York.

World Health Organization (1950). 'Towards a Definition of Health'. Geneva.

Wyss, D. (1973). 'Psychoanalytic Schools from the Beginning to the Present'. Jason Aronson, New York.

Zetzel, E. (1971). A developmental approach to the borderline patient. Am. J. Psychiat. 128, 867–871.

22 Psychotherapy

II Research in dynamic psychotherapy

Rachel Rosser and Warren Kinston

Historical outline

The length of psychoanalytic treatment and the lack of clear, relevant criteria for classifying patients have caused psychoanalysts, even more than other clinicians, to rely on generalizations from single cases and the gradual accumulation of observations.

The first major systematic study was reported in 1930, when Fenichel published data on 721 cases seen at the Berlin Psychoanalytic Institute during the previous 10 years. Patients were classified by psychiatric diagnosis and by the duration of the analysis, and outcome was rated on a four-point scale between unchanged and cured. This study illustrates some of the problems in interpreting results on the outcome of psychoanalysis. Depending on the logic of the exclusion criteria and the strictness of the definition of improvement, the following percentages of improvement have since been calculated from Fenichel's data: 39% (Eysenck, 1952), 59% (Knight, 1941) and 91% (Bergin, 1971).

The wide use of randomized controlled trials in medicine is relatively recent (Cochrane, 1972) and the extension of such methods to psychotherapy has been complicated by the difficulty in defining type of treatment and type of patient and in building adequate control into the experiment. Controlled evaluation of psychotherapy began with studies of psychosomatic illness in the 1930s and 1940s. During the following two decades, many comparisons were made between different forms of individual therapy, between group and individual therapy, between behaviour therapy and other psychotherapies and between drug treatment and psychotherapy. The effects of various parameters of therapy such as therapist skill and duration of therapy were also investigated. The results were generally ambiguous and inconsistent so that in 1960, Strupp reported that research had had 'little influence on the practical procedures of psychotherapy' and insisted as the decade progressed that he was not fully convinced that it ever would. The history of this phase of research has been described by Malan (1973a). Since no positive results seemed to have emerged from 20 years research, pessimism prevailed. Bergin and Strupp (1972), in a survey of the attitudes of American researchers, reported widespread disillusion with every aspect of psychotherapy research. In England, a comparative study of interpretative psychotherapy at the Maudsley Hospital and Tavistock Clinic was abandoned after reaching the disappointing conclusion that random allocation of patients to the two centres or to a control group was not feasible (Candy et al., 1972).

American researchers countered the general despondency by reviewing the methodological defects which may have obscured positive findings and so prevented firm conclusions from being drawn. The Group for the Advancement of Psychiatry published a report on problems in the measurement of change (1966) and the National Institute of Mental Health sponsored workshops on psychotherapy evaluation (Fiske et al., 1970; Waskow and Parloff, 1975). Strupp and Bergin (1969) set out a conceptual framework for researchers in which they emphasized the importance of specificity and of valid measures of outcome. Luborsky et al. (1971), after searching 166 studies for evidence of factors associated with improvement in psychotherapy, listed 20 important issues which had been neglected in their design. Then a surprising discovery was made, not by experimentation but by a more thorough and systematic review of all published studies: psychotherapy apparently helps people (Meltzoff and Kornreich, 1970)! Their critical review included many types of patients and took into account psychological treatments varying in intensity from five-minute chats to analytic psychotherapy.

In 1971 Bergin and Garfield edited a handbook on the 'state of the art'. Bergin's own paper (Bergin, 1971) re-assessed studies of individual treatment of adult neurotic patients and confirmed Meltzoff and Kornreich's conclusions that psychotherapy is effective. This handbook also covered experimental design, spontaneous remission, client variables, therapist skills, content analysis, placebo effects and psychophysiological methods. Luborsky et al. (1975) classified studies in terms of methodological adequacy and also concluded that the efficacy of psychotherapy had been demonstrated. They pointed out that there was little difference between the outcome of different kinds of psychotherapy, that there were advantages in some combinations of therapy and that being assessed and placed on a waiting list for psychotherapy was therapeutic in itself. Two matches of treatment and patient had been shown to be beneficial: behaviour therapy for specific phobias and dynamic psychotherapy for psychosomatic symptoms. Malan had already pointed out that the efficacy of dynamic psychotherapy had only been demonstrated in psychosomatic conditions (Malan, 1973a). Kellner (1975) surveyed controlled studies of various forms of psychotherapy in psychosomatic disorders and emphasized the advantage of the objective criteria of outcome available in this area of application. His conclusions were that psychotherapeutic techniques were effective in some patients, but specific techniques helped particular patients. In schizophrenia, for which the value of psychotherapy has been most doubted, a review of the five larger studies (Feinsilver and Gunderson, 1972) identified two in which some benefit was detected.

More recently positive results have been reported from two long-term studies: Malan's study of brief focal dynamic psychotherapy (Malan, 1976b) and the study of long-term psychotherapy and psychoanalysis at the Menninger Foundation (Kernberg *et al.*, 1972). Studies conceived and conducted with the knowledge that has accumulated in the past few years have produced further positive and more specific results. For example, the design of Siegel *et al.*'s (1977) study showed that the improvements which did occur in the waiting list control group were limited to patients whose symptoms were of recent onset. Patients in psychotherapy improved whether their complaints were acute or chronic although recent exacerbation was a good prognostic sign.

Process and outcome research

It is customary to distinguish between research into the process and the outcome of psychotherapy. However, this distinction is not without its difficulties since any phenomenon may be considered to be either part of the process of therapy or an intermediate outcome. For example, a patient's silence in a session can be the outcome of work aimed at helping him tolerate being psychologically separate from, but with, another person (Winnicott, 1958); simultaneously the way the silence is used by the therapist is an important part of the psychotherapeutic process. Moreover, a particular phenomenon seen as process has no intrinsic value; its value lies in the extent to which it contributes to a better outcome. If the same outcome could be obtained in a more or less distressing way, one would choose the less painful method. Thus, measures of outcome become more sensitive if they are combined with repeated observations of states during therapy.

The terms exploratory and efficacy research are perhaps more useful. Exploratory research may be hypothesis-seeking or hypothesis-testing. It requires detailed observations of one or a few patients, perhaps of only one or a few sessions. Hypotheses sought may relate to efficacy, i.e. to aspects of the therapeutic process or to psychological functioning, or more broadly to aspects of human nature. The psychotherapeutic situation can provide unique opportunities for testing hypotheses about normal psychological functioning. The field of exploratory research is specialized and limitless. Although it may be unsystematized, it has intuitive appeal to practising psychotherapists when it is written in their own language. Efficacy research, drawing on such exploratory research, is systematic hypothesis-testing and crosses theoretical boundaries. This form of research, which is aimed at establishing general propositions based on evidence and rules of logic, is considered in the rest of this chapter. Even when it has been relevant and conclusive, its effect on current practice has so far been disappointing, and perhaps more work is required on the difficulties of its wider implementation.

Assessment of research studies

In common with other areas of scientific research, psychotherapy research must have the following characteristics:

1 Hypotheses must be clearly stated so as to be testable.
2 Alternative explanations for the results must be ruled out, necessitating adequate controls on the experiment.
3 Measures must be reliable, valid and standardized in normal populations.
4 Researcher bias must be avoided or corrected.
5 The sample must be representative of a defined population.
6 The method must be specified sufficiently to permit replication.
7 The statistical techniques must be appropriate to the data.

Certain issues which have led to classical debates in the natural sciences are still the focus of active controversy in psychotherapy research. Physicists no longer argue about the nature of reality every time they take a measurement although they remain aware of the problems. This is not yet the case in psychotherapy research and in the United Kingdom the debate as to whether dynamic psychotherapy is a science or even fundamentally testable is as lively as ever (Hill, 1970; Rachman, 1971; Slater, 1975; Kelk, 1977; Bebbington, 1977). Gelder (1976) has argued that research into dynamic psychotherapy would progress faster if it followed the lead of behavioural research, integrating the results of many experiments each of which tests hypotheses about one small facet of the work. Others think that the way in which the components of the psychotherapeutic process are combined are critically important and that it is not feasible to study the elements of dynamic psychotherapy piecemeal, since in one session interventions of many kinds may be made, some preparing the ground for others, e.g. clarification preceding interpretation, while some occur together randomly, e.g. non-verbal expression of warmth accompanying a painful interpretation. They are convinced that it is time to accept the complexity of the natural situation and that what is needed is more work on highly specific questions about aspects of naturally occurring therapy (Strupp and Bergin, 1969). The former simplistic position is modelled on the experimental approach; the latter owes more to the methods of social research.

Despite having much in common with other fields of enquiry, certain issues of research design have proved to be peculiarly difficult in psychotherapy research.

Definition of the patient and treatment. The classification of psychopathology, severity of disturbance and suitability of patients for psychotherapy is even more contentious than the classification of formal psychiatric illness. Definition of treatments is equally unsatisfactory but it has been found that therapists who base their techniques on different theories have in practice a great deal in common (Sloane *et al.*, 1975). The least that should be required is a definition by the therapist of precisely what he is trying to do and detailed records of what he remembers doing. As audio and video recordings of therapy become less obtrusive and more acceptable, description of the treatment actually provided can become more objective.

The personal characteristics of the therapist. These are much more important in psychotherapy than in physical treatments. However, studies of the personality traits of therapists (Whitehorn and Betz, 1954, 1960) of particular attributes manifest during therapy (Truax *et al.*, 1966), and of peer ratings (Kernberg *et al.*, 1972), have been unrewarding. The matching of the personality of the therapist to that of the patient has often been postulated and found to be significantly related to outcome (Luborsky *et al.*, 1971).

Sample size. Obtaining a sample of sufficient size for statistical analysis has proved difficult. This is understandable in the longer therapies since in each the therapist can treat only a few patients. The Menninger Group, for example, collected only 42 cases over 15 years. Even with the shorter therapies, the need to stratify the sample and to match or exclude patients on several variables can lead to a shortage of subjects. Rogers *et al.* (1967), for example, took two years to find 18 pairs of schizophrenics matched for age, sex, socio-economic group and chronicity. Use of randomization often leads to subsequent statistical analyses (by type of therapist, type of patient, length of treatment, etc.) with insufficient numbers in each cell. As with drug trials and studies of rare diseases, multi-centre studies could provide a solution, but as yet no one has successfully negotiated the organizational hurdles.

Specification of outcome. This presents complex problems. Outcome can be viewed from various perspectives, e.g. psychodynamic change, symptomatic change or change in social adaptation and various indicators of each of these can be chosen. Differing measures of outcome do not correlate well with one another and conclusions are therefore dependent on valuations of the importance of different aspects of outcome. The distinction between the evidence and its valuation must be maintained as it can have practical importance and the valuations have to be made explicit. For example, May (1968) concluded from his impeccably designed study of the effect of combinations of treatment for schizophrenia, that the treatment of choice in this disorder is drugs alone. This has influenced the current treatment of schizophrenia. Others might value insight more highly than does May and could conclude *from his data* that a combination of drugs and psychotherapy has advantages over drugs alone. A similar problem is posed when data source is considered. Conflicting information and differing views are obtained from the patient, his therapist, an independent judge and 'significant others' in the patient's life. Comparison of global ratings of improvement have tended to reveal the therapist as 'odd man out' (Sloane *et al.*, 1975; Harty and Horwitz, 1976).

Controls. The use of control groups to rule out alternative explanations, though immensely important, is unfortunately only one rather limited method of handling this problem. Usually control groups must be supplemented by detailed collection of relevant data. Typically, there are too many crucial variables requiring too many control groups for the sample size available. A particular concern in psychotherapy research has been to control for the 'non-specific' (usually called, by inappropriate analogy to drug trials, 'placebo') effects of treatment (Rosenthal and Frank, 1956). Factors such as faith and hope in the patient and the personal attention of the therapist are not ancillary to, but an integral part of, any psychotherapy and hence it can be argued that no double or even single blind trial is truly possible. However, evidence as to the feasibility of a 'placebo-effect' control, at least in a group, has been provided by Sil-bergeld *et al*. (1976) studying marital couple group therapy. Four placebo sessions were held prior to 15 therapy sessions. The first session was held in silence and in the next three brief non-interactive informative talks by members were stipulated. On a variety of measures the four sessions were regarded by the patients as similar and moderately effective as therapy.

Research instruments

The researcher's first task is to decide on the relevant and important variables. He then has to consider which data may most directly reflect these variables, i.e. for each variable he must decide on an appropriate indicator. For example, there is a wide choice of indicators of the concept of social class and differing choices may be made according to the circumstances of the study. Only after a particular indicator has been chosen do the issues of reliability, validity, sensitivity, specificity, and other properties of instruments which purport to measure it, arise. If an instrument with these wide and subtle properties cannot be designed or implemented and if measurement is of specific importance, the indicator may have to be discarded in favour of an apparently less appropriate one.

There are many instruments relevant to psychotherapy research —Straus (1969), for example, details 319 techniques for measuring the family—but validation is typically questionable and standardization on normal populations is rare. The use of such a variety of uncertain instruments has made it difficult to compare and coordinate the results of different studies. Very few instruments have been given the crucial test of time and even fewer have survived this test.

When instruments used in psychotherapy research have been developed on an *ad hoc* basis and not submitted to rigorous scrutiny, the critical reader must be left wondering what, if anything, has been demonstrated. An example is the ubiquitous 'global improvement rating scale' which has such an appeal to psychotherapists and researchers. Such scales have a number of points, usually between four and nine, and range from *worse* through *unchanged* to *very much improved*. Reliability for these scales is rarely reported. Bloch *et al*. (1977) asked 42 experienced psychotherapists arranged in 27 teams of three judges to rate the improvement of 27 patients after eight months of therapy. The judges used before and after video-taped interviews. Their agreement on both nine-point scales of target problem resolution and 17-point scales of global outcome was low. The validation of the scales runs into the problem of low correlation amongst outcome measures and of the valuation of change. The value placed on change in a patient appears to depend on the point on the mental health continuum at which the change occurs: a unit of improvement within the healthy ranges is seen and valued as greater than a similar amount at less healthy levels (Mintz, 1972).

The idea of mental health, used as a matter of course in the previous sentence, becomes more complex when the issue of measurement is raised. In 1955, Sir Aubrey Lewis wrote:

> The inherent difficulty of the concept of mental health is underlined when we find the psychoanalyst, so expert in the microscopy of mental happenings, unable to dispense with equivocal and cloudy terms in stating his criteria of recovery.

Matters have altered since then and 'mental health' or 'general adjustment' provides a suitable example for considering problems in the design of instruments specifically for psychotherapy research.

Luborsky's Health-Sickness Rating Scale (HSRS) (Luborsky, 1962) was the first global rating of mental health to be developed. The HSRS is a 100-point scale ranging from imminent death (0) to the ideal state of perfect health (100). Brief definitions are given at 10, 25, 35, 50, 65 and 75. Thirty-four brief case descriptions, fairly evenly distributed over the scale, are also provided. Seven criteria of mental health were used in locating these sample cases on the scale. These were the patient's need to be protected and supported, the seriousness of his symptoms, his subjective discomfort, his effect on his environment, his capacity to use his abilities, the quality of his interpersonal relationships and the breadth and depth of his interests. The user compares his patient with the anchor points to determine the region of the scale in which his case falls. He then turns to the sample cases in that region and assigns a definite score by comparison with these and using the stipulated criteria he also compares the case with previous cases which he has rated.

Ratings have been based on assessment interviews, hospital records, Rorschach tests and transcripts of sessions, and used to compare groups of patients and to measure change with treatment. Inter-observer and test-retest reliability have been demonstrated. Luborsky and Bachrach (1974) report on its use in 18 studies. Despite this repeated use, a number of the properties of the scale, particularly validity and specificity, have not been sufficiently investigated. When used to measure change, the scale is assumed to be equal interval, but this property was not built into its design and, as can be seen from the above description of use, the rating has a large element of ranking. The 100-point Global Assessment Scale (GAS) (Endicott et al., 1976) has been derived from the HSRS but modified to minimize ambiguities, avoid contradictions and reduce the effort of referring to case vignettes, but it is too early to assess its value.

In marked contrast to a single global rating based on information of varying completeness from differing sources is a structured interview which can give a profile of ratings on a variety of objective and subjective indices. This approach to designing a more precise and specific instrument was adopted by Gurland and co-workers (1972a, b) who scaled 60 indicators of adjustment in their Structured and Scaled Interview to Assess Maladjustment (SSIAM). From research and clinical practice they identified five separate areas: work, social and leisure life, family of origin, marriage and sex. Within each of these, five categories referring to deviant behaviour (e.g. social isolation, social nonconformity), three referring to subjective distress (e.g. loneliness, boredom) and one to friction with others were defined. These 45 items are rated on 11-point ordinal scales which have five anchoring definitions. The remaining similar 15 scales are for the rater's subjective assessments. The instrument, which was designed for psychotherapy research, takes about 30 minutes to administer and requires a trained professional. The authors discuss inter-rater reliability and validity but the evidence they quote is insufficient to support their claims that these properties have been adequately demonstrated. The instrument is recent but it has been compared favourably with other measures of social adjustment (Weissman, 1975) and was used by its developers to compare psychotherapy and behaviour therapy (Sloane *et al.*, 1975). Serious limitations in the construction of the test include its bias towards severe disturbance and consequent low sensitivity to change during psychotherapy, its tacit assumption of middle class life style and the irrelevance of some scales to many patients.

The price paid for highly structured formats and quantification may be a loss of credibility and the popular clinic-style guided interview offers an alternative. Thus Brown and Rutter (Brown and Rutter, 1966; Rutter and Brown, 1966) have developed a flexible semi-structured interview using operational definitions and a bank of standardized responses on master tape-recordings to provide information on events, activities, emotions and attitudes in the family life of psychiatric patients. High inter-rater reliability depended on intensive training of interviewers and the only evidence for validity was agreement between the results of interviewing husband and wife separately: often not a satisfactory basis for validation. No independent observations of the family were used as criteria for validation although the low correlation between the amount of warmth reported in an individual interview and that observed in a joint interview suggested this was necessary.

One category of instrument which satisfies many of the problems of measuring dynamic change in the individual, but is less successfully applied to large sample studies, is the repertory grid technique derived from Kelly's personal construct theory. Fransella (1976) has provided an excellent review of the historical development, psychological theory and the various practical applications of the technique. The investigating therapist can derive a grid sensitively related to the patient's way of looking at life, his circumstances and problems. As a technique with wide flexibility and orientated to the individual, rather than a test as such, reliability has little meaning, but where standard forms have been used on samples of patients test-retest reliability can be satisfactorily assessed. Similarly, various studies have shown that repertory grids can be satisfactorily validated. Grids have been used in many individual settings (Fransella, 1976) and as a means of studying interactions between members of a therapeutic group (Watson, 1970). In individual psychotherapy grids can be used to show dynamic changes and investigate transference phenomena (Ryle, 1975). Essentially, the technique allows outcome measurements to integrate with measurements of process and must remain an important tool of psychotherapy research in the future.

Many of the instruments discussed so far largely preclude emotional interaction with the interviewer as a source of data. One alternative is a dynamic interview as developed by Malan (1976a, b) to specifically study the outcome in psychotherapy. Malan's procedure involves obtaining a detailed description of the patient's present problems and current life situation and a psychodynamic history aimed at understanding the events of the patient's psychiatry and social history in emotional terms. The 'dynamic hypothesis' which is formulated becomes a focus for therapy and for establishing criteria of outcome. Evidence for the presence (and later absence if therapy was successful) of the dynamic focus is obtained from interviewer–patient interaction and the response of the patient to dynamic interpretations.

In this framework people are considered to be so diverse and complicated that global scales applying to all are of limited value. Each person's initial state is scored as zero and criteria for each of four points of improvement are laid down, i.e. the scale is tailored to the individual. The scale is ordinal and the intervals are not equal. Towards the lower end the score is mainly based on degree of improvement; at the upper end it measures residual disturbance. Because the zero varies, although a score of four is similar for each person, the statistical problems of measuring gain on an instrument like the HSRS are not encountered (Tucker et al., 1966). Inter-observer reliability in the hands of psychoanalysts is high. Malan dispenses with formal validation and instead publishes full clinical details which allow the reader to draw his own conclusions about the meaningfulness of the ratings.

Malan's technique has contributed to the understanding of so-called 'spontaneous remission' by identifying the various life-events which can result in personality growth (Malan et al., 1975). He has also used it to demonstrate the ineffectiveness of group therapy run along strictly psychoanalytic lines (Malan *et al.*, 1976) and others have modified it for the assessment of family therapy (Kinston and Bentovim, 1978).

Recent studies

We conclude Part II of Chapter 22 by critically discussing three of the more recent studies to which we have already referred.

Sloane: Psychotherapy versus behaviour therapy

Sloane *et al.* (1975) assessed consecutive routine psychiatric out-patient referrals and randomly assigned them to either 14 weekly treatments by analytical psychotherapy or behaviour therapy, or to a waiting list. After the experimental phase all patients were re-assessed and the waiting list patients were offered treatment if it was still desired. Further assessments were made one and two years later. A variety of measures of outcome were used including global change, improvement in target symptoms and some of the SSIAM scales. Outcome was assessed by the therapist, the patient and a friend or relative in addition to the research psychiatrist.

Almost all patients, including those on the wait ng list, improved. The differences in outcome between the groups, though sometimes statistically significant, were nonetheless small. Re-assessment after one and two years contributed little, especially as 50% of the behaviour therapy group, 73% of the waiting list group and 30% of the analytic psychotherapy group received further treatment which was always analytic therapy. A comparison between the two forms of therapy as it was actually given provided few surprises. Although two clearly different therapies were being used, they had many features in common, particularly the qualities of the relationship between patient and therapist. Patients did respond differently to the two approaches and analytic psychotherapy seemed to be more dependent on the match between patient and therapist.

Although the study was carried out painstakingly, certain major defects must be noted. Firstly, while four months of sessions may be a typical contract for behaviour therapy, such a uniformly short contract for unselected patients is not usual analytic psychotherapeutic practice. Thus the two treatments differed in the degree of artificiality in the conditions under which they were offered. The seriousness of this is difficult to determine because, despite details of a large number of in-therapy behaviours of patients and therapists, the reader is left with little feel for either therapeutic process. The reader is even left in doubt as to whether 'truly' analytic, i.e. formal psychoanalytic psychotherapy, was actually provided: no counts of transference interpretations were made and the interpretation of the transference in terms of childhood experience was not examined. The definition of interpretation used was far too broad and it was suggested that the use of 'interpretations' was associated with a poorer outcome. A reader might conjecture that what was offered was supportive-expressive psychotherapy by analytically trained therapists. The applicability of the term 'behaviour therapy' is questionable on similar grounds.

Secondly, the waiting list control group received an intensive initial assessment which took the best part of a day and was partly unrelated to this study. Brown and Bettley (1971) found that patients regard and respond to such interviewing as treatment. The regular telephone support and optional access for urgent therapy meant that this group received a great deal of help. Such intensive assessment also would homogenize the treatment groups as interviewing probably contained dynamic implications and definition of behavioural goals.

Malan: Brief focal psychotherapy

Malan and co-workers (Malan, 1963, 1976a, b) by contrast have no random allocation of patients, or standard units of therapy, and have tended to eschew conventional research design whilst retaining scientific rigour in their common-sense approach to evaluation of brief analytic psychotherapy.

Malan's patients had been referred to his brief psychotherapy workshop and were therefore already a highly selected group. The criteria for subsequent acceptance were complex and were based on psychodynamic interviewing and Rorschach assessment. One requirement was that a specific core conflict should emerge which could be the focus of psychoanalytic work; the resolution of this conflict was then the principal objective of therapy. The aim was to give between 10 and 40 one hour sessions, usually weekly, but the range given was between eight and 500 and some patients attended irregularly.

Two follow-ups have been conducted on the outcome of this therapy. The follow-up, two to 11 years after the end of treatment, consisted of an interview of the patient by his therapist or by a member of the research team. Some patients received more than one follow-up. The sole outcome measure was a rating of the extent of resolution of the focal conflict as described earlier, i.e. symptomatic improvement alone was considered as a failure. Of the 58 patients in his second sample, 19 were rejected as unsuitable for brief therapy and nine of the treated cases failed follow-up. Of the 30 therapies remaining, 19 (33% of the total sample, 49% of the treated group, 63% of those followed up) were successful. Malan's principal conclusions were that successful outcome depended upon the patient's motivation, the ability of patient and therapist to work together, i.e. to dynamically interact on a focus, and the repetitive interpretation of the transference–childhood links.

The claims that the specific effectiveness of psychoanalytic techniques has been demonstrated are put persuasively but, as Malan is himself aware, the arguments are insufficient. Controls for alternative explanations remain essential. For example, the orthodox psychoanalytic view that it is important to link the transference with childhood experience *is* confirmed quantitatively but there are at least three possible explanations of this. Either linking transference and childhood experience could be a technique which has a specific effect on outcome, or patients who take to, or even invite, such interpretations could be those who do well in psychotherapy, or there could be an interaction between these two mechanisms.

Another problem is the limited perspective of assessment. Change which cannot be directly attributed to the resolution of the focal conflict is ignored and symptomatic relief which is achieved at the cost of restricting experience is devalued. This is a therapist's eye view of outcome. Clearly a patient who makes a valuable false solution may experience greater relief of suffering and disability than another who has partially resolved his focal conflict. It is also an individual's eye view and ignores the impact of altered behaviour on the family and wider social network of the patient.

The Menninger Project: Psychoanalysis and psychotherapy

The Menninger Psychotherapy Research Project (Wallerstein *et al.*, 1956; Kernberg *et al.*, 1972) differed from the other two in studying psychoanalysis and longer-term psychotherapy. This is to date the largest, most detailed and important investigation of psychoanalytic psychotherapy as it is customarily practised. A sample of 42 treatments of neurotic and borderline psychotic adults were investigated in a study which lasted 18 years involving 38 investigators, 10 consultants and three project leaders. As this was a study occurring naturally, it was ethical for patients and therapists to be kept in ignorance of their participation. Twenty-one patients received psychoanalysis and the others received psychotherapy of one of three types: expressive, supportive-expressive or supportive. The baseline for the assessment of change was determined from the clinical case notes, the social history and the results of psychological tests. At the end of therapy and at two-year follow-up the patients were sometimes given a research interview to supplement clinical data.

The guiding assumption was that the outcome of treatment depended on the initial characteristics of the patient, on his environment and on the treatment he received. The team's belief, for which they obtained empirical support, that clinical observations and judgement could be sufficiently precise to provide the basis for testing hypotheses was innovative. Three groups of variables, 'patient', 'treatment' and 'environment' were measured using a method in which researchers ranked all patients by taking them in pairs. The patients were also rated on the Health-Sickness Rating Scale and on a five-point rating of global change from 'worse' to 'marked improvement'. Several hundred specific hypotheses were tested by examining the significance of correlations. The data were also examined by the completely different technique of multi-dimensional scaling.

The team's conclusions from their data were not indisputable for a number of reasons (Greenson, 1973; Malan, 1973b; May, 1973). For example, patients were not randomly allocated to treatments, there were no control groups, the possibility of 'spontaneous remission' was not taken into account, no attempt was made to ensure that the treatments were of the intended type and the amounts of other treatments such as nursing care were neither standardized nor recorded. The two statistical techniques did not always produce congruent findings. For example, the paired comparison technique could not distinguish the four types of therapy, identifying only two: psychoanalysis and psychotherapy. Multi-dimensional scaling distinguished the four types, but it is a technique open to varying interpretations, and findings using it cannot be stated within confidence limits. Moreover, some of the inferences, such as those about the importance of environmental factors, were based on data of such low reliability that they can have little meaning. Other data are of either doubtful validity or probably biased, e.g. the assessment of therapist's skill.

Irrespective of the findings, the most important contribution was the systematic scrutiny of psychoanalytic concepts. As a result of this, weaknesses in traditional conceptualizations and observations were identified, observable phenomena were more cleerly defined and concepts were progressively refined. The project paved the way for the major review of psychoanalytic theory which has been undertaken by Kernberg (Kernberg, 1975, 1976).

The substantive findings are summarized below with the study variables italicized. The patient's initial *ego strength* was of overriding importance irrespective of the treatment modality or the therapist's *skill*. Crucial indicators of *ego strength* were *quality of interpersonal relationships* and *anxiety tolerance*. *Motivation* and *psychological mindedness*, in so far as they developed during therapy, were of prognostic significance. Patients with high *ego strength* were helped more by psychoanalysis than by psychotherapy; patients with low *ego strength* were only helped by either in-patient or out-patient expressive psychotherapy focusing on the transference and they did not improve or even deteriorated with either psychoanalysis or supportive psychotherapy. The *skill* of the therapist was significant in all forms of therapy: high *skill* was particularly important in supportive psychotherapy whereas low *skill* was less of an impediment in more analytic work.

This was designed, not as an exercise in hypothesis-testing, but as an exploratory study. The next stage should be a prospective examination of both the positive and negative findings.

General conclusions

Clearly none of these studies is likely to satisfy those who insist on the fullest rigour of experimental methodology. However, within their limitations, they represent a significant step forward from the descriptive and anecdotal chaos of the last fifty years. Many problems clearly remain, but these experimental studies indicate that changes are already taking place: psychoanalysts are using research data to scrutinize and refine their own concepts; the relationship between in-depth analysis and focal psychotherapy is being re-examined; commonalities between behavioural reconstruction and personal growth are beginning to narrow the artificial gulf between behavioural and analytic psychotherapies and integrated techniques, based on experimental evidence, become more than a possibility. In the light of these studies it is not fair to continue insisting that hypothesis testing in dynamic psychotherapy is absolutely impossible, and as more refined instruments are developed, and more psychotherapists become confident in their use and validity, psychotherapy research can eventually earn its own respectability.

References

Bebbington, P. E. (1977). Psychiatry: Science, meaning and purpose. *Br. J. Psychiat.* **130**, 222–228.

Bergin, A. E. (1971). The evaluation of therapeutic outcomes. *In* 'Handbook of Psychotherapy and Behaviour Change' (Eds A. E. Bergin and S. L. Garfield), Chapter 7. Wiley, New York.

Bergin, A. E. and Garfield, S. L. (Eds) (1971). 'Handbook of Psychotherapy and Behaviour Change'. Wiley, New York.

Bergin, A. E. and Strupp, H. H. (1972). 'Changing Frontiers in the Science of Psychotherapy'. Aldine, Chicago.

Bloch, S., Bond, G., Qualls, B., Yalom, I. and Zimmerman, E. (1977). Outcome in psychotherapy evaluated by independent judges. *Br. J. Psychiat.* **131**, 410–414.

Brown, D. G. and Bettley, F. R. (1971). Psychiatric treatment of eczema: a controlled study. *Br. Med. J.* **2**, 729–734.

Brown, G. W. and Rutter, M. (1966). The measurement of family activities and relationships. A methodological study. *Human Relations* **19**, 241–263.

Candy, J., Balfour, F. H. G., Cawley, R. H., Hildebrand, H. P., Malan, D. H., Marks, I. M. and Wilson, J. (1972). A feasibility study for a controlled trial of formal psychotherapy. *Psychol. Med.* **2**, 345–362.

Cochrane, A. L. (1972). 'Effectiveness and Efficiency; Rock Carling Fellowship 1971'. Nuffield Provincial Hospitals Trust, London.

Endicott, J., Spitzer, R. L., Fleiss, J. L. *et al.* (1976). The global assessment scale. *Arch. Gen. Psychiat.* **33**, 766–771.

Eysenck, H. J. (1952). The effects of psychotherapy: an evaluation. *J. Consult. Psychol.* **16**, 319–324.

Feinsilver, D. B. and Gunderson, J. G. (1972). Psychotherapy for schizophrenics—is it indicated? *Schizophrenia Bull.* **6**, 11–23.

Fenichel, P. (1930). 'Ten Years of the Berlin Psychoanalytic Institute, 1920–1930'. German Psychoanalytic Association, Berlin.

Fiske, D. W., Hunt, H., Luborsky, L., Orne, M., Parloff, M., Reiser, M. and Tuma, A. (1970). The planning of research on effectiveness in psychotherapy. *Arch. Gen. Psychiat.* **22**, 22–32.

Fransella, F. (1976). Theory and measurement of personal constructs. *In* 'Recent Advances in Clinical Psychiatry' No. 2 (Ed. K. Granville Grossman). Churchill Livingstone, Edinburgh.

GAP (Group for the Advancement of Psychiatry) (1966). 'Psychiatric Research and the Assessment of Change', Vol. VI, Report No. 63.

Gelder, M. (1976). Research methodology in psychotherapy—why bother? *Proc. Roy. Soc. Med.* **69**, 505–508.

Greenson, R. (1973). A critique of Kernberg's summary and conclusions. *Int. J. Psychiat.* **11**, 91–94.

Gurland, B. J., Yorkston, N. J., Stone, A. R., Frank, J. D. and Fleiss, J. L. (1972a). The Structured and Scaled Interview to Assess Maladjustment (SSIAM) I. Description, rationale and development. *Arch. Gen. Psychiat.* **27**, 259–263.

Gurland, B. J., Yorkston, N. J., Goldberg, K., Fleiss, J. L., Sloane, R. B. and Cristol, A. J. (1972b). The Structured and Scale Interview to Assess Maladjustment (SSIAM) II. Factor analysis, reliability and validity. *Arch. Gen. Psychiat.* **27**, 264–267.

Harty, M. and Horwitz, L. (1976). Therapeutic outcome as rated by patients, therapists, and judges. *Arch. Gen. Psychiat.* **33**, 957–961.

Hill, D. (1970). On the contributions of psychoanalysis to psychiatry: Mechanism and meaning. *Br. J. Psychiat.* **117**, 609–615.

Kelk, N. (1977). Is psychoanalysis a science? A reply to Slater. *Br. J. Psychiat.* **130**, 105–111.

Kellner, R. (1975). Psychotherapy in psychosomatic disorders: A survey of controlled studies. *Arch. Gen. Psychiat.* **32**, 1021–1028.

Kernberg, O. F. (1975). 'Borderline Conditions and Pathological Narcissism'. Jason Aronson, New York.

Kernberg, O. F. (1976). 'Object Relations Theory and Clinical Psychoanalysis'. Jason Aronson, New York.

Kernberg, O. F., Burstein, E. D., Coyne, L., Appelbaum, A., Horwitz, L. and Voth, H. (1972). Psychotherapy and psychoanalysis: Final report of the Menninger Foundation's Psychotherapy Research Project. Bull. Menn. Clin. 36, 3–275.

Kinston, W. and Bentovim, A. (1978).Brief focal family therapy when the child is the referred patient. 2 Methodology and results. J. Child Psychol. Psychiat. 119, 119–144.

Knight, R. P. (1941). Evaluation of the results of psychoanalytic therapy. Am. J. Psychiatry 98, 434–446.

Lewis, A. J. (1955). Health as a social concept. Br. J. Sociol. 14, 109–124.

Luborsky, L. (1962). Clinician's judgements of mental health: a proposed scale. Arch. Gen. Psychiat. 7, 407–417.

Luborsky, L. and Bachrach, H. M. (1974). Factors influencing clinicians' judgements of mental health. Eighteen experiences with the Health-Sickness Rating Scale. Arch. Gen. Psychiat. 31, 292–299.

Luborsky, L., Auerbach, A. H., Chandler, M., Cohen, J. and Bachrach, H. M. (1971). Factors influencing the outcome of psychotherapy. Psychol. Bull. 75, 145–185.

Luborsky, L., Singer, B., and Luborsky, L. (1975). Comparative studies of psychotherapies. Arch. Gen. Psychiat. 32, 995–1008.

Malan, D. H. (1963). 'A Study of Brief Psychotherapy'. Plenum Press, New York.

Malan, D. H. (1973a). The outcome problem in psychotherapy research. Arch. Gen. Psychiat. 29, 719–729.

Malan, D. H. (1973b). Science and psychotherapy. Int. J. Psychiat. 11, 87–90.

Malan, D. H. (1976a). 'The Frontier of Brief Psychotherapy'. Plenum Press, New York.

Malan, D. H. (1976b). 'Towards the Validation of Brief Psychotherapy'. Plenum Press, New York.

Malan, D. H., Heath, E. S., Bacal, H. A. and Balfour, F. H. G. (1975). Psychodynamic changes in untreated neurotic patients. Arch. Gen. Psychiat. 32, 110–126.

Malan, D. H., Balfour, F. H. G., Hood, V. G. and Shooter, A. M. N. (1976). Group Psychotherapy: A long term follow-up study. Arch. Gen. Psychiat. 33, 1303; 1315.

May, P. R. A. (1968). 'Treatment of Schizophrenia. A Comparative Study of Five Treatment Methods'. Science House, New York.

May, P. R. A. (1973). Research in psychotherapy and psychoanalysis. Int. J. Psychiat. 11, 78–86.

Meltzoff, J. and Kornreich, M. (1970). 'Research in Psychotherapy'. Atherton Press, New York.

Mintz, J. (1972). What is 'success' in psychotherapy? J. Abnorm. Psychol. 80, 11–19.

Rachman, S. (1971). 'The Effects of Psychotherapy'. Pergamon, Oxford.

Rogers, C. R., Gendlin, E. G., Kiesler, D. J. and Truax, C. B. (Eds) (1967). 'The Therapeutic Relationship and its Impact: A Study of Psychotherapy with Schizophrenics'. University of Wisconsin Press, Madison, Wisconsin.

Rosenthal, D. and Frank, J. D. (1956). Psychotherapy and the placebo effect. Psychol. Bull. 53, 294–302.

Rutter, M. and Brown, G. W. (1966). The reliability and validity of measures of family life and relationships in families containing a psychiatric patient. *Soc. Psychiat.* **1**, 38–53.

Ryle, A. (1975). 'Frames and Cages: The Repertory Grid Approach to Human Understanding'. Sussex University Press, Brighton.

Siegel, S. M., Rootes, M. D. and Traub, A. (1977). Symptom change and prognosis in clinic psychotherapy. *Arch. Gen. Psychiat.* **34**, 321–329.

Silbergeld, S., Manderscheid, R. W. and Soeken, D. R. (1976). Issues at the clinical research interface: placebo effect control groups. *J. Nerv. Ment. Dis.* **163**, 147–153.

Slater, E. (1975). The psychiatrist in search of a science: III—The depth psychologies. *Br. J. Psychiat.* **126**, 205–224.

Sloane, R. B., Staples, F. R., Cristol, A. H., Yorkston, H. J. and Whipple, K. (1975). 'Psychotherapy versus Behaviour Therapy'. Harvard University Press, Cambridge, Mass.

Straus, M. A. (1969). 'Family Measurement Techniques'. University of Minnesota Press, Minneapolis.

Strupp, H. H. (1960). Some comments on the future of research in psychotherapy. *Behav. Sci.* **5**, 60–71.

Strupp, H. H. and Bergin, A. E. (1969). Some empirical and conceptual bases for coordinated research in psychotherapy. A critical review of issues, trends and evidence. *Int. J. Psychiat.* **7**, 18–90.

Truax, C. B., Wargo, D. G., Frank, J. D., Imber, S. D., Battle, C. C., Hoehn-Saric, R., Nash, E. and Stone, A. (1966). Therapist empathy, genuineness and warmth and patient therapeutic outcome. *J. Consult. Psychol.* **30**, 395–401.

Tucker, L. R., Damarin, F. and Messick, S. (1966). A base-free measure of change. *Psychometrika* **31**, 457–473.

Wallerstein, R. S., Robbins, L. L., Sargent, H. and Luborsky, L. (1956). The Psychotherapy Research Project of the Menninger Foundation: Rationale, method and sample use. *Bull. Menn. Clin.* **20**, 221–278.

Waskow, I. E. and Parloff, M. B. (Eds) (1975). 'Psychotherapy Change Measures'. USGPO, Washington.

Watson, J. P. (1970). A repertory grid method of studying groups. *Br. J. Psychiat.* **117**, 309–318.

Weissman, M. M. (1975). The assessment of social adjustment. *Arch. Gen. Psychiat.* **32**, 357–365.

Whitehorn, J. C. and Betz, B. (1954). A study of psychotherapeutic relationships between physicians and schizophrenic patients. *Am. J. Psychiat.* **103**, 321–331.

Whitehorn, J. C. and Betz, B. J. (1960). Further studies of the doctor as a crucial variable in the outnome of treatment with schizophrenic patients. *Am. J. Psychiat.* **117**, 215–223.

Winnicott, D. W. (1958). The capacity to be alone. *In* 'The Maturational Processes and the Facilitating Environment', pp. 29–36. Hogarth and Institute of Psychoanalysis, London, 1972.

22 Psychotherapy

III Conjoint family therapy

Peter Hill

There is a practice of seeing several members of a family together in order
to involve them jointly in a treatment process. The aim of this is to correct
dysfunction in the family as a natural group and thus achieve change in
individual members. It is associated with certain concepts, the basic one
being that an individual's symptoms are directly related to family dysfunction; and it is, therefore, the family which becomes the 'patient'
rather than the individual symptom-bearer. It is therefore necessary to
construct family formulations to account for the presence of particular
symptoms in particular individuals and to predict aims and goals of
treatment. The language of such formulations derives from three main
sources of influence; psychoanalysis, general systems theory (von Bertalanffy, 1973) and social psychological concepts of role. It is perhaps not.
surprising that there has been a marked tendency for theorists to look
separately to either systems theory or psychoanalysis for inspiration,
rather than attempt to draw from both, though there are no logical
reasons why they should be mutually incompatible. The concern of
systems theory has been the description of family structure, communication patterns, rules and interaction processes, whereas the psychoanalytical approach has been predominantly concerned with relationships,
motivation, meaning and the relevance of the family's history for the
development of individuals.

The construction of a family formulation requires attention to three
areas:

1 *Developmental stage*

Has this family been able to achieve the various tasks involved in its primary function—the healthy development of its members into mature, autonomous individuals? Have the parents (a) separated adequately from their families of origin? (b) established a mutually satisfactory spouse relationship? (c) each established themselves as competent parents?

The characteristic tasks and cycle of family development are reviewed by Solomon (1973).

2 *Historical background*

Are there recurring patterns of relationships, role allocations or allegiances expressed in successive generations? Are the parents bringing the conflicts of their own families of origin to their present family for resolution, e.g. children's antisocial actions vicariously gratifying poorly integrated parental wishes? (Johnson and Szurek, 1952). Is there a myth (Ferreira, 1963), a secret, or other shared assumption that goes unrecognized or unquestioned and which determines identifications and behaviour?

3 *Here-and-now interactions*

Is there clear, unambiguous communication and role allocation, or are verbal instructions countermanded by non-verbal cues? What is the degree of cohesion? What are the precipitants and consequences of particular behaviours?

Indications and contraindications

The preconditions of family therapy are the availability of an intact family unit, the necessity of constructing a relevant family formulation and the acceptance by the family of a whole family treatment approach. Not all individual disturbance is secondary to family dynamics, although where it is not, attention to these may alleviate dysfunction and distress secondary to extra-familial or essentially individual factors.

Consideration of indications and contraindications for whole family treatment is limited to expression of opinion since outcome evaluation has been sparse. Some practitioners are overtly opposed to comparative evaluation because family therapy represents to them a competing metaphor, available to account for psychiatric symptoms in the same way as psychoanalytic or behavioural theory. Thus differing aims and goals are specified, making direct comparison with competing treatment models difficult and unnecessary—only superiority over no-treatment controls need be demonstrated. In my view such a standpoint is arrogant and logically indefensible. Nevertheless, the argument for specifying different goals has some force. Rather than approaching the subject in terms of behavioural syndromes such as school refusal, it seems preferable to talk in terms of situations arising in families: developmental problems such as the failure of a child to achieve age-appropriate individuation or the existence of particular mechanisms like pathological scape-goating. This approach leads to discussion of the necessity for *pieces of therapeutic work*, for instance operational mourning (Paul and Grosser, 1965).

Where discussion has centred on traditional, individual-centred, diagnostic labels, the problem has been that the behaviour or mental state of particular individuals may be seen as the expression of various and different mechanisms operating within the family.

At the other end of the scale, family typologies (e.g. Tseng *et al.*, 1976) are in their infancy and are not yet empirically validated. The general tendency of psychiatry is to classify disorders rather than persons, and it may well be that a typology of *families* will prove less acceptable than a typology of family *disorder*.

Returning to the issue of indications, perhaps all that can be said is that there appears to be a consensus that there are no contraindications to a whole family interview for *assessment* purposes, and that many practitioners agree that the following family situations respond particularly well to a whole family treatment approach. These include:

(a) Pathological scape-goating. One individual persistently carries the blame for all the family woes. Complaints about a child's behaviour frequently serve to camouflage marital difficulties.

(b) Inappropriate or excessive dependency demands by one individual upon another.

(c) Ambiguous communication patterns.

(d) Problems of authority and control.

(e) Vicarious gratification in the deviant behaviour of a member.

(f) Deviant behaviours arising in several members following bereavement.

(g) Successful individual treatment of one family member followed by the appearance of symptoms in another.

There is some agreement, too, upon contraindications, including:

(a) The absence of a family unit as a functioning system with recognizable external psychological boundaries. Family therapy can activate family resources, but cannot provide them in their absence.

(b) A family within which relationships are characterized by sadistic gratification, and cruelty is unmitigated by personal warmth. This is to be differentiated from mere open hostility; certainly no

contraindication. Children exposed to angry words in family sessions have heard them all before at home.
(c) Chronic, widespread dishonesty and deceit within the family.

Procedure

The defining characteristic of family therapy is the attempt to change the system of relationships operating within the family, in order to free individuals from the existing pathological system which promotes symptom formation or persistence. Family members develop settled ways of living with each other which are patterned according to the family's history, especially the families of origin of the parents and the current family developmental tasks. This system of relationships resists imposed changes according to the principle of homeostasis (Jackson, 1957). In order to promote change, the family therapist needs firstly to provide a setting and engage the family in a process of examining the matrix of relationships within the family unit. This requires a high level of therapist activity over and above various specific strategies or interventions employed. Side-taking, or its proscription, commentary, upon the significance of small children's play, pouncing upon ambiguous statements or instructions, fostering empathy and the necessity of maintaining a balance between contributors, are among the active measures required to control the therapeutic process.

The following classification of strategies is an amplification of Feldman's (1976) suggestion that they are derived from paradigms of:
(1) Insight/working through (e.g. Boszormenyi-Nagy and Spark, 1973)
   confrontation, verbal or experimental (e.g. sculpting)
   interpretation: connective, reconstructing
   operational mourning
(2) Behaviour modification (e.g. Liberman, 1976)
   contingency management (reciprocal contracting, formal operant scheme, extinction)
   rehearsal (role play)
(3) Paradox (e.g. Haley, 1963)
   relabelling (e.g. of quarrelling as expression of affection)
   paradoxical injunctions
(4) Systems theory (e.g. Minuchin, 1974)
   establishment of subsystem boundaries, task setting, inclusion/exclusion of members.

Outcome

Whereas there are numerous claims for the potency, speed and economy of whole family treatments, the review by Wells *et al.* (1972) of published evaluation studies located only the work of Langsley (e.g. 1969) which met the usual criteria for scientific acceptance. In this study a random selection of 150 patients who would normally have been admitted to the acute wards of a mental hospital, were treated by out-patient family therapy on a crisis-intervention model. When compared with matched controls (who had been admitted and treated with additional measures) no differences on a variety of measures of social functioning and symptom score could be demonstrated between the two groups. Family therapy was no more effective, but more economical in terms of expenditure and treatment time.

Since Wells' review, matters have not clarified. Alexander and Parsons (1973) found that a behaviourally orientated family treatment approach for families containing juvenile delinquents produced significantly lower reconviction rates at follow-up when compared with a psychodynamic or client-centred family counselling programme. The latter two models were not superior to a no-treatment control group. Ro-Trock *et al.* (1977) found family therapy more effective than individual psychotherapy (without casework with parents) in preventing post-discharge reconviction for hospitalized delinquents.

References

Alexander, J. F. and Parsons, B. V. (1973). Short term behavioural intervention with delinquent families: impact on family process and recidivism. *J. Abnorm. Psychol.* **81**, 219–225.

Boszormenyi-Nagy, I. and Spark, G. (1973). 'Invisible Loyalties'. Harper and Row, Hagerstown.

Feldman, L. B. (1976). Strategies and techniques of family therapy. *Am. J. Psychotherapy* **30**, 14–28.

Ferreira, A. J. (1963). Family myth and homeostasis. *Arch. Gen. Psychiat.* **9**, 457–463.

Haley, J. (1963). 'Strategies of Psychotherapy'. Grune and Stratton, New York.

Jackson, D. D. (1957). The question of family homeostasis. *Psychiat. Q. Suppl.* **31**, 79–90.

Johnson, A. M. and Szurek, S. A. (1952). The genesis of antisocial acting out in children and adults. *Psychoanal. Q.* **21**, 323–343.

Langsley, D. G., Flomenhaft, K. and Machotka, P. (1969). Follow up evaluation of family crisis therapy. *Am. J. Orthopsychiat.* **39**, 753–760.

Liberman, R. (1976). Behavioural approaches to family and couple therapy. *Am. J. Orthopsychiat.* **40**, 106–118.

Minuchin, S. (1974). 'Families and Family Therapy'. Tavistock, London.

Paul, N. L. and Grosser, G. H. (1965). Operational mourning and its role in conjoint family therapy. *Community Hlth J.* **1**, 339–345.

Ro-Trock, G. K., Wellisch, D. K. and Schoolar, J. C. (1977). A family therapy outcome study in an inpatient setting. *Am. J. Orthopsychiat.* **47**, 514–522.

Solomon, M. A. (1973). A developmental, conceptual premise for family therapy. *Fam. Proc.* **12**, 179–188.

Tseng, W. S., Arensdorf, A. M., McDermott, J. F., Hansen, M. J. and Fukunaga, C. S. (1976). Family diagnosis and classification. *J. Am. Acad. Child Psychiat.* **15**, 15–35.

Von Bertalanffy, L. (Ed.) (1973). 'General Systems Theory. Foundations, Development, Applications'. George Braziller, New York.

Wells, R., Dilkes, T. and Trivelli, N. (1972). The results of family therapy. A critical review of the literature. *Fam. Proc.* **11**, 189–207.

22 Psychotherapy

IV Group interaction

John Cobb

'And you really think this crap that went on in the meeting today is bringing about some kinda cure, doing some kinda good?'
McMurphy's comment in 'One Flew Over the Cuckoo's Nest' (Kesey, 1962)

To do justice to McMurphy's pertinent question several subsidiary questions must be considered. Of first importance is *process*. What actually did go on in the meeting? Why were some members silent and others talkative? Why passions aroused at a particular point? Why was the group's attention focused on the problems of one individual? How did the behaviour of the leaders influence what went on in the group? To answer these questions a study of group dynamics is needed. This may lead to an exploration of techniques and strategies and the ways in which group behaviour is determined by the setting, the leadership style and the personal characteristics of the members.

Next, *outcome* must be considered. What were the aims of this group and did it achieve these ends? 'Good' and 'cure' are vague, emotive words which need definition in operational terms. Symptom improvement, an opportunity to air grievances, education, a greater understanding of one's own and others' problems, an attempt to produce profound dynamic change or merely a means of 'warming up' for the activities of the day ahead, are all examples of possible group aims. The aims may be predominantly orientated towards the individual or, as in most ward meetings, be more concerned with the effective running of a unit. Benefit to the group as a whole may mean sacrifices from the individual and thus assessment of the 'value' of the group will depend on the vantage point of the observer.

Finally, there is the problem of *theory*. One of the major problems facing any student of group interaction is the perplexing array of complex theories—psychoanalytic, sociological systems, Gestalt, etc.—often expressed in an erudite language associated with the author's own background, and often only loosely related to the practical techniques advocated. One may well ask what functions a theoretical background serves and whether a sound, coherent theoretical belief is necessary for effectiveness. If, as some evidence suggests (Lieberman *et al.*, 1973), leadership style correlated very poorly with the leader's theoretical beliefs, it may be that most theorizing is of academic and heuristic value rather than practical use.

Historical development of process and theory

Early influences

The first important works were published at the beginning of the twentieth century and consist of a mixture of unsystematic observations of naturally occurring groups, such as various types of crowds together with speculative theories to account for the phenomena described (Anthony, 1971). Le Bon emphasized the changes which occurred in individuals when under the influence of a crowd. He described the heightening of emotion and the reduction of rational control, a combination which could clearly lead to a change in behaviour for better or worse. McDougall contrasted organized and chaotic groups and attempted to identify the components needed if a group meeting was to be constructive; he recognized the importance of continuity of meetings, and the development of traditions. Wilfred Trotter asked, 'Why do people form groups?' and hypothesized the existence of a herd instinct, basing his argument along Darwinian lines and suggesting that the formation of effective groups would lead to an evolutionary advantage. Freud (1922) asked, 'What is a group?' and argued that the sharing of a common bond distinguished a group from a collection of individuals. This was neatly described by Foulkes when he pointed out that individuals on a beach only become a group when someone gets into difficulties in the water. Freud stressed the importance of leaders in the functioning of groups but pointed out that strong, charismatic leadership leads to regression and dependence. Although this has therapeutic potential, it is the opposite of the behaviour that is needed if the group members are to learn to function in an adult, rational way. The difficulty of maintaining a balance between dependency and individual responsibility is the basis of many problems in group interaction.

J. H. Pratt

The first therapeutic application of group methods was described by Joseph H. Pratt (1917) who undertook the home treatment of patients with advanced tuberculosis. He used techniques involving education, group pressure, social rewards and structured weekly meetings, setting homework and encouraging participants to monitor their own progress through keeping detailed diaries. Termed 'confessional-inspirational', this treatment package resembled the approach favoured by modern behaviourally based groups such as Weight Watchers. In several respects Pratt anticipated future development in that he was concerned with the physical debility, social isolation, and the psychological state of the patients in his care. He was aware that the influence of the group helped his patients to gain weight, to meet and share their problems with others and to fight the depression so often associated with tuberculosis. Outcome and, to a lesser extent, process were his fields of interest and in complete contrast to Freud he scarcely mentioned theory.

Psychodrama

Jacob Moreno, an energetic and colourful man, coined the terms 'group therapy' and 'group psychotherapy'. Over a working life which spanned 60 years he acquired a vast experience of group interaction and made major contributions to the area of group process, particularly by drawing attention to the ways in which group interaction may be facilitated. Moreno believed that spontaneity, creativity and open expression of emotions were essential for healthy mental life and that neurosis occurred when these were frustrated (Davies, 1976). He eschewed a purely verbal approach and advocated activity. Thus he introduced warm-up exercises and games to focus the group members' interest and to loosen them up in both a physical and a psychological sense. Then he encouraged the concrete expression of problems through role play and evolved this into systems of therapy known as psychodrama and sociodrama. The techniques used led to a vivid re-enactment of past emotional experiences or present personality styles, sometimes in a cathartic manner. 'Acting out' was a term that was introduced by Moreno to describe a process by which a patient re-enacted his problems within the group setting. This was claimed to be of therapeutic value since it enabled the patient to see the way he behaved and the effect it had on others. The term is to be distinguished from its usage in psychoanalysis where it is applied to undesirable behaviour related to the patient's problems but taking place outside the treatment setting. Groups provide a greater opportunity for acting out than individual sessions and the psychodramatist would see this as a distinct asset (Blatner, 1973). Moreno was primarily attempting to achieve catharsis hoping that understanding and learning would follow, whereas Freud placed primary emphasis on understanding. This difference in approach has never been tested in a properly controlled study, and there is no evidence that encouraging people to be more spontaneous and creative (Moreno's aims) is any more or less beneficial than the resolution of internal, repressed conflicts.

'T' Groups

In 1946 Kurt Lewin, a social psychologist, was asked by the Connecticut Inter-racial Commission to set up a workshop to look at the ways in which community leaders might be trained to help resolve tensions associated with the introduction of a new Fair Employment Practices Act. Lewin adopted a 'here and now' approach and saw group activity not as a product of the personal background of the constituent individuals, as both Freud and Moreno would have done, but as a result of the tensions resulting from the structure of the group at that particular moment. These tensions, according to Lewin's Field Theory, were a product of the conflict between the needs of the individual and the needs of the group. An individual struggles for attention in the group in the same way that an animal struggles for territorial space. The group demands a limitation of these demands but offers mutual support and involvement in return. Lewin argued that the balance of cohesive and disruptive forces at any particular time would depend partially on the way in which the group was organized and integrated and also on the style of the leader which might be either authoritarian, democratic or *laissez-faire*.

Emphasis on the 'here and now' at the famous Connecticut Workshop resulted in a rapid evolution of new techniques. Initially small groups of participants took part in discussion and role play. Observers charted the behaviour of the small group leaders and the sequence of events in the group. Leaders and observers then met in the evenings to share information and experiences. Pressure from the 'ordinary' participants led to their inclusion in feedback meetings which proved highly productive. Lewin died shortly after this workshop but the development of 'T' (Training) groups was continued by his pupils.

The purpose of 'T' groups was essentially educational and was aimed at changing attitudes and behaviour. Emphasis on spontaneous disclosure, focus on the 'here and now' and provision of feedback in an atmosphere of trust were the means of learning. Observation, self-knowledge, awareness, concern for others and the ability to 'learn how to learn' were established as desirable aims.

Encounter

Among those who were so trained was W. C. Schutz (1967), a psychologist, who shifted the aims of the groups he ran to include therapy in the widest sense of the word. By this he implied not only helping patients to overcome psychological problems but also enabling people who appeared to be functioning normally to become more aware of themselves and of others. This increase in sensitivity, Schutz postulated, would lead to an enrichment of experience and a greater sense of fulfilment. Therein lies the basis of the Encounter movement, which though developing into a bewildering variety of subgroups, maintains an emphasis on interpersonal honesty, self-disclosure and feedback. In Schutz's work group dynamics were not emphasized. Focus was on the individuals in the group and though group forces were undoubtedly recognized they were used rather than studied.

Psychoanalysis

A similar statement may be made about the early psychoanalysts who worked in groups. Though very different from Schutz in theory and technique they nevertheless took little or no account of forces resulting from group processes and were initially concerned with applying individual psychoanalytic techniques to more than one patient simultaneously, mainly to save time. They were also interested in showing that phenomena observed in dyadic interaction could also occur in groups.

The realization that the group situation could provide something unique that was absent in one-to-one situations was made by both Slavson and Wolf. Slavson (1940) recognized that the group catalyses individual dynamic, accelerating regression and weakening defences and that transference phenomena were present in the group situation.

Alexander Wolf is known for the way in which he did individual psychoanalysis in groups by focusing on one patient at a time. However, Wolf was not just replicating individual analysis in a group setting. He argued that since a group offered support, individuals could tolerate higher levels of anxiety, allowing for deeper analytic exploration. Furthermore, he allowed other members to act as ancillary therapists.

Bion

Despite the fact that his first experience of groups was when working as a psychiatrist at a military hospital during the Second World War, Bion was initially impressed by the way in which the *modus operandi* of small groups resembled the operation of larger organizations. He saw that an understanding of small group dynamics could lead to a better understanding of the world outside the group room. Later while working at the Tavistock Clinic Bion was asked to 'take' groups comprising either staff or patients. He adopted a reflective approach, trying to feed as little as possible into the groups, other than comments intended to clarify what he thought was going on. From his observations he developed a theory of group dynamics which has had a profound effect on both sides of the Atlantic.

Bion postulated that most of the time a group acts 'as if' it were in the grip of massive, emotional forces beyond its control. Such forces prevent the group from working rationally and effectively on the task in hand. Members avoid reality-testing, they have poor memories, they resist change. They often become disorientated about time and they do not learn from experience in the group. These forces Bion called Basic Assumptions which, in contrast to pressures in a 'work group' situation, operate outside members' awareness.

Dependency, the first of Bion's basic assumptions, causes the group to act *as if* its main aim were to secure security and mutual protection. The therapist is seen as omnipotent and information which undermines this is ignored or misinterpreted. Helplessness and awe of the leader dominate the group. Inevitably disappointment and hostility ensue when the unrealistic, insatiable demands of the group are unsatisfied.

Fight-flight, the second basic assumption, causes the group to act as though its main purpose is self-preservation. Aggressiveness, hostility and fear are the emotions associated with this assumption and the leader is urged to mobilize the group's resources and to recognize (or manufacture) enemies.

Pairing, the third basic assumption, produces the collective fantasy that the group has met for the purposes of reproduction. The 'baby' in this context refers to new ideas and creative efforts but sexually tinged liaisons may be set up which preoccupy the group. Hopeful anticipation and optimism are the prevailing emotions, but, as Bion sagely points out, it is essential that the 'Messiah must be unborn' since a real 'birth' either physical or psychological cannot live up to the group's idealistic expectations.

Bion's classical book 'Experiences in Groups' (1961) is difficult reading but a lucid summary is available (Rioch, 1970).

Bion's ideas can provide a useful model for understanding events in groups which might otherwise appear random or inexplicable. They do not provide an explanation for all that occurs and by focusing attention on the desirability of achieving a reality-based 'working group' they over-look the possible therapeutic work that may be done while the group is in the grip of a 'basic assumption'. Bion, like Lewin, seeks an explanation of individual interaction not in terms of the individual's developmental experiences but as a product of the pressures in the group at that particu-lar moment in time. He is a theorist not a therapist. His primary interest is in what happens in groups rather than in the ways in which groups may effect useful change, though as leader he made interpretations to make the group aware of the basic assumption dominating its interaction, hoping to encourage development of a reality-based 'work' atmosphere. Ezriel was later able to extend Bion's ideas into frankly therapeutic terri-tory.

Focal conflict theory

Whitaker and Lieberman (1965) focused attention on the group as a whole and attempted to balance the contributions made by individual and group pressure to the overall behaviour of the group. Focal conflict theory postulates that an individual's behaviour is an expression of his dealing with current problems which are themselves recapitulations of conflicts originating in early life. It was developed by Thomas French and the Chicago School who were striving to shorten the time needed for classical psychoanalysis. Whitaker and Lieberman suggested that 'Group Focal Conflicts', a concept similar to Bion's 'Basic Assumptions' cause the activities of groups to hang together in such a way that a consistent underlying theme can be detected. Group focal conflicts expose and reactivate individual conflicts and an observer may be able to identify both a *disturbing motive* which leads an individual to act in a particular way and a *reactive motive* which determines the behaviour of the rest of the group. Desire for individual attention is a typical example of a disturbing motive to which the reactive motive might be fear of neglect from the rest of the group. The group as a whole tries to reduce anxiety induced by the difficulty of reconciling two opposing forces, in this case satisfying the need for individual attention, while at the same time allaying the others' fear of neglect. Solutions to such conflict may be *restrictive*, that is aimed at superficial, temporary alleviation of anxiety, or alternatively *enabling*, that is enabling full expression and exploration of underlying motives.

In practice Whitaker and Lieberman provide a flexible approach, which strikes a balance between the extreme group emphasis of Lewin and Bion and the individual emphasis of Fritz Perls and Alexander Wolf. The therapist is less of a 'passive projection screen', and allows focus on the individual as well as the group.

Even though the focal conflict model has an artificial ring about it, it provides the therapist with a useful, theoretical framework (Dick, 1975).

Group analytic school

Foulkes' work (Foulkes and Anthony, 1973) rests on the postulate that an individual can only be understood in terms of the way he interacts with other people. A corollary of this is that the way an individual behaves will be profoundly influenced by the people with whom he is involved. This led Foulkes to an interest in natural networks such as families, extended families and neighbourhoods and to emphasize the important part played by these matrices in the genesis and maintenance of psychiatric disturbance. Foulkes' matrix and Lewin's patterned 'fields' are similar concepts and, just as Lewin argued that each element in the 'field' could not be meaningfully viewed in isolation, Foulkes compared the influences of individual and matrix on determining group interaction to the 'figure'/'ground' phenomenon of Gestalt Psychology. At any moment in time both could be operating and the group leader need only shift focus slightly to see one or the other. Foulkes, whose work was rooted in social psychology rather than in individual psychology, viewed the group as primary. His democratic philosophy was reflected in the way he tried to 'lead from behind'.

Transactional analysis

Eric Berne, a contemporary of Foulkes, has had as much influence on the ways groups are run in North America as Foulkes has in Britain. Berne is chiefly known for the development of transactional analysis which is a practical technique of psychotherapy based on a rigid triadic model of personality function. In its emphasis on the three states in which an individual may function, those of child, parent and adult, it reflects a synthesis of the classical Freudian concepts of three stage development (oral, anal and genital) together with the tripartite structure of the mind (ego, id, super ego).

Berne (1966) attempted to understand and interpret both the currently dominant ego state of individuals and, by shifting his focus to the 'games' that were going on in the group as a whole, understand what social pressures were causing the individual to act the way he did.

The terminology and cultural background of Berne and Foulkes are widely different. Foulkes paid more attention to group dynamics, whereas Berne favoured a more autocratic style of leadership. However, they share emphasis on the way both intrapsychic and extrapsychic factors determine behaviour in groups. They separate the ways in which both the group (the 'matrix' or the 'game') and the individual determine what occurs in a group, and at the same time, ways in which these influences combine.

Eclectism

Irvin Yalom (1975) has drawn on the experience of many schools of theory and practice. Starting from the consensus of agreement concerning group dynamics he has applied objective methods to clarifying and systematizing this knowledge. For example, his studies concerning curative factors—that is those forces which tend to produce beneficial change—concern processes which can be seen in any type of group. Yalom has identified these factors partially from an extensive study of the literature and partially from his own work involving therapist and participant rated questionnaires. Attempts have been made to arrange these in a hierarchy of importance, but it is likely that groups with different purposes differ in the use made of any particular factor. What is true for an intensive small group for mixed neurotic problems is unlikely to be true for a large ward group.

Behavioural

These groups are task-orientated and aimed at highly specific goals such as weight loss, reduction in phobic difficulties or increase in social skills. Structured techniques are usually planned beforehand (e.g. Falloon et al., 1977). Emphasis is placed on careful assessment of change, using a variety of measures, including practical tests if appropriate. Nevertheless, dynamic factors intrude (Liberman, 1970). Falloon (1977) recognized the importance of 'cohesiveness' as a prerequisite for successful work. Hand et al. (1974) showed that while group treatment of agoraphobics is as effective as individiaul treatment, those treated in a group continued to improve at the end of therapy, whereas those in individual treatment did not, thus pointing to some therapeutic influence unique to the group situation.

Table 1   This summarizes distinguishing features of the main schools of group interaction

Approach (originator)	Therapist	Techniques	Focus	Interaction	Aims	Reference
Psychoanalysis in Groups (Wolf and Schwartz)	Reflective Authoritarian	Verbal Interpretive	Individual	Individual ⇆ Leader	Intrapersonal change	Wolf and Schwartz (1962)
Psychodrama (Moreno)	Authoritarian Directive	Role play Exercises Catharsis Empathic identification Sharing	Individual Here and now	Individual ⇆ Leader ↓ Group	Social and emotional growth	Blatner (1973)
Tavistock (Bion and Ezriel)	Reflective (Passive projection screen) Non-authoritarian Consultant	Interpretation of needs rather than gratification	Group	Group ⇆ Leader	Understanding group dynamics and problems of leadership	1 Rioch (1970) 2 Kreeger (1975)
Group Analytic (Foulkes)	Intermediate	Interpretation	Group Individual	Leader ↗↘ Group ↔ Individual	Intrapersonal change Interpersonal change	Foulkes and Anthony (1973)

Gestalt (Fritz Perls)	Authoritarian Directive	Emphasis on body reactions Exercises Catharsis Semantic techniques	Individual	Leader ⇆ Individual (as part of group)	Intrapersonal change Emphasis on self-support	Perls *et al.* (1973)
Behavioural (Lazarus)	Authoritarian Directive	Behavioural techniques) e.g. exposure, modelling desensitization, role rehearsal) Highly structured.	Specific Goals	Individual ⇆ Leader (as part of group)	Relief of symptoms	Shaffer and Galinsky (Chapter 8, 1974)
'T' Group (Lewin)	Teacher Task Setter Consultant	Exercises involving problem-solving tasks Discussion and feedback	Individuals role in team Team's part in social unit.	Individual ⇆ Team Larger social unit	Social and administrative change Attitude and behavioural change	Blumberg and Golembiewski (1976)
Encounter (Schutz)	Leaderless or charismatic, Authoritarian and directive	Awareness games Confrontation Openness	Individual	Individual ⇆ Individual	Intra- and interpersonal change Increased 'awareness' or sensitivity	Rogers (1973)

Structure of groups

'Boundaries' are of great practical importance to group interaction. Consideration of 'Boundaries' must include aims, timing, accommodation, psychological and behavioural factors.

Aims

The particular task of a group should be the ultimate determinant of all other structural variables. Teaching health workers about the problems of leadership requires a different approach to treating agoraphobics. Groups aimed at reducing tension in general psychiatric wards should not be run as though the group was for the intensive psychotherapy of neurotic out-patients. Groups aiming to plan some specific course of action may increase dependence but this may be the antithesis of groups whose aim is to increase the capacity for self-coping.

Timing

Psychotherapeutic groups are usually held regularly on an ongoing basis. For 'orthodox' verbal groups a once a week meeting lasting one and a half hours is usually recommended though more frequent meetings may allow more intensive work. Change may result from interaction outside the group room as well as inside, and it is by no means established that this frequency and length of session is optimal. Timing is more a result of practical considerations and tradition rather than established effectiveness. Leaders favouring a mixed non-verbal and verbal approach usually prefer longer sessions ranging from three hours to a whole weekend, since issues can be worked through in depth as and when they arise. They also argue against a rigid, sudden ending after a set period of time to make it easier to finish on a good note. Setting time limits may, however, help to focus members' attention and it is frequently observed that however long the group, the most intensive interaction often occurs towards the end. Not only does the clock stimulate activity, but it may provide an important protection for a group member who wishes to test the water by introducing a topic, but who does not want to go too deeply in that particular session. Further, there is no evidence that sending people away on a 'good' note facilitates change.

Groups with specific tasks, such as daily ward meetings to 'clear the air', may achieve much in a shorter time, say an hour, whereas groups of agoraphobics undergoing exposure *in vivo* (e.g. travelling on buses and trains together) may meet daily for a week, for sessions lasting several hours. Most encounter leaders would agree that more can be achieved in, say, 12 hours' work held on one weekend, than in four separate sessions of three hours held at weekly intervals, though it must be borne in mind that such groups are usually designed for 'training' rather than 'therapy'.

Apart from the frequency and length of individual sessions, it is important to consider whether the overall number of sessions should be fixed in advance. An indefinite number of sessions allows consideration to be given to individual needs, though lack of planning in advance may allow members to bask in the atmosphere of the group without attempting to achieve their aims. Furthermore, it may postpone that painful but productive stage of group process which is that of facing the ending of the group. Work in behavioural groups tends to support the hypothesis that the slower members accelerate to keep up with the pace of the group rather than the group moving at the pace of its slowest member, and that working towards achieving a target by a fixed deadline increases motivation.

Space

The size, acoustics, privacy and lighting of the room are obvious considerations. Not so obvious is the importance of the setting of the room. Proceedings in a noisy room in the middle of a busy hospital may be quite altered if the same group meets in a secluded room miles from anywhere. Even the arrangement of furniture may be influential. Foulkes maintained that the presence of some object, such as a bare, low table in the centre of the circle, not only helped to focus attention but also reduced anxiety which might otherwise have been aroused by the emptiness. In large groups it may be necessary to arrange chairs so that people may communicate without shouting. One technique is to arrange chairs in concentric circles, another to revert to a traditional lecture hall or theatre arrangement. Leaders favouring action techniques provide a pile of cushions allowing participants to sit wherever they like, encouraging mobility, which is minimized in comfortable armchairs.

Size and duration

Groups in which all members start at the same time and which then, for the life of that particular group, admit no new members are entitled 'closed' groups. This arrangement is particularly suited to time-limited, task-orientated groups since cohesion is rapidly built up and disruption minimized. On the other hand, the group will dwindle in size, particularly over the first 10 sessions when a drop-out rate of about 20% can be expected. Open groups admit new members from time to time, the leader assessing the best moment for topping up numbers and preparing existing members for the change.

The size of a group has an important effect on group process. Small groups of, say, five to eight people tend to discuss personal issues whereas larger groups are more concerned with social matters. However, as Rice (1965) has pointed out, larger groups tend to behave in a primitive 'psychotic' manner. Massive emotions may sweep through a large group causing sophisticated, rational members to behave and think in an irrational manner. Such conflagration is less common in smaller groups. Agenda-less meetings lead to perplexity, anxiety, and irrational behaviour. As these emotions may be magnified by a large group situation the group may be provided with an agenda on which to focus its energies (Pines, 1975). The small group may be seen more as a family situation where people well known to one another sit down together and interact informally. On the other hand, the large group is more like a neighbourhood meeting which if it is not structured by an active chairman may prove to be purposeless or disruptive.

In general, verbal psychotherapy and behavioural groups usually have five to 10 members whereas action groups using non-verbal techniques are slightly larger, say 12 to 18 members. Larger groups than this, usually concerned with training, increase anxiety, reduce cosiness and increase opportunities for avoiding overt involvement. Moving to a small group at the end of a plenary session usually leads to a rebound in the opposite direction, resulting in exaggerated intimacy and involvement.

Composition of group

Groups may be homogeneous, that is composed of people with similar problems and aims, or heterogeneous. In the former, especially if the group is target-orientated and structured, group processes may be less obvious. Several papers describing behavioural groups ignore group dynamics altogether. Whether group phenomena, such as struggle for leadership, establishment of norms, peer envy, scape-goating and anxiety over termination, just did not occur in these groups, or whether they did occur and were ignored by the leader cannot be said. Judging by results obtained this did not impair success. However, it must be borne in mind that these were groups with limited aims. In heterogeneous groups with wider aims group dynamics are unavoidable and are relevant to both personal and social problems. Other arguments in favour of heterogeneous groups are that they more closely resemble the world outside, are less likely to set up conforming and restrictive norms and provide greater opportunity for the development of useful multiple transferences.

Criteria for selection

As far as out-patient dynamic therapy groups are concerned it is easier to cite exclusion criteria rather than to define characteristics of patients likely to benefit from group therapy. Brain-damaged, acutely psychotic, paranoid, extremely narcissistic, severely hypochondriacal, actively suicidal, sociopathic and addicted patients are not only unlikely to benefit from this type of therapy but may prove disruptive to other members.

Yalom (1975) showed that those who drop out in early stages of the group are less likely to benefit than those who stay. Early drop-outs are characterized by: (a) somatization of conflicts; (b) poor motivation; (c) lower IQ and socio-economic class; (d) high denial and (e) seeing their problems as urgent. Addicted and alcoholic patients and those with severe psychosomatic problems are best managed in homogeneous groups, such as those run by Synanon and Alcoholics Anonymous.

On the positive side, patients able to express themselves, able to learn and keen to change are likely to benefit from group situations particularly if their difficulties lie in the realm of interpersonal relations. For such patients, group treatment may be the treatment of choice.

As far as supportive and milieu groups are concerned, such as ward or hostel groups, it is obviously important to include all members of the community irrespective of their particular problems, and the difficulty here lies in how to encourage difficult members to attend rather than in deciding who to exclude.

Various methods of selecting patients for groups have been described and attempts made to correlate behaviour during selection procedure with subsequent behaviour in the group. The traditional intake interview procedure is most commonly used, through habit rather than proven effectiveness. Standard personality description labels have low reliability and standard psychological tests such as the Rorschach and MMPI have failed to yield valid predictions. Specialized procedures may be of value in particular circumstances. For example, the FIRO-B System (Schutz, 1966) is predictive of compatibility on wards and between future room-mates but does not predict behaviour in small interaction groups. Various grids have some value as research tools but are complex and too cumbersome for everyday use (Slater, 1969).

For many years the British Civil Service and German Air Force have used direct sampling of group behaviour to predict future behaviour. Thus, prospective members are placed in trial groups which are matched as near as possible to the future group situation. Some therapeutic groups invite prospective members to meet the group they wished to join. Unfortunately, this not only proves disruptive to the group but is also likely to evoke a display of artificial, interview-orientated behaviour from the applicant. Clearly no method is ideal and Yalom recommends an interview in which the focus is on interpersonal and social aspects. This reflects his style of therapy and a more analytic, intrapersonal-orientated therapist would advocate a style of interview in which the ability to understand and make use of interpretations, together with ability to think in abstract and symbolic terms were made the main focus of interest.

Ground rules and preparation

New members enter groups with a variety of expectations, some valid and some false. The group leader may also want to introduce a number of rules based on his theoretical background, personal whims and anxieties concerning control of the group. Preparation may help to correct some misconceptions, to establish group norms and to encourage early development of cohesion (Bednar et al., 1974). Typical misconceptions are that:

(a) Group therapy is a second rate, diluted form of individual therapy.
(b) The main aim of group therapy is to force members to make public confessions.
(c) Mental contagion will occur, and symptoms be made worse by contact with others rather than better.

Typical leader-imposed rules are:

(1) 'No consorting outside the group' is usually advocated with varying degrees of firmness by analytic, verbal leaders. It is impossible to police this demand and more realistic leaders usually request that interactions between meetings be discussed in the group. Behavioural and encounter leaders usually expect that it is natural for group members to continue to interact outside the group room and may actively encourage this.

(2) 'Inform group if session is to be missed', a maxim which most leaders adhere to since unexpected absence can produce considerable unproductive speculation and disruption.

(3) 'Remember group is for work, not social chit-chat' or 'try to express things here which you would be unable to express outside'.

(4) 'No smoking'. Leaders who are not themselves addicted usually ask members not to smoke. Smoke is offensive to non-smokers in the group. In an action group it can impede the exercises and role

play, and in any group it may provide a convenient screen behind which members may hide when it would be more productive for them to explore less maladaptive means of masking their anxiety.

It is important to decide before the group begins which rules are to be enforced since attempts to change or impose new rules once a group has become established are difficult and disruptive. Means of preparing groups include holding preliminary sessions in which a theoretical framework may be described; plans outlined and didactic discussion encouraged. Some therapists provide audio or video-tape models of well-functioning groups. In practice it is difficult to avoid these sessions becoming full 'therapy' sessions. The more a therapist believes that reality-based interpersonal interaction is the main function of a group, the more he is likely to encourage preparation. On the other hand, those therapists who believe that resolution of neurotic distortions is the crucial factor in group psychotherapy are likely to oppose preparation since enigma, ambiguity and absence of cognitive anchoring lead to maximal transference. After reviewing the literature, Bednar *et al*. (1974a) concluded that 'clients with pre-therapy training responded more appropriately in therapy and achieved more favourable outcome than controls'.

Function of leader

Dispute exists concerning the appropriate title for the person setting up a group. The title chosen reflects the aims and style of that particular person. Encounter group participants are usually looking for 'growth' rather than 'therapy' and thus the leader eschews the title of 'therapist'. Bion claimed that it was the group's collusive fantasy which assumed him to be 'leader' but that he himself made no claims to that title. Leaderless groups at the annual Tavistock Conference are set up by the 'conveners' who retire behind the label of 'consultant'. Foulkes preferred the title 'conductor' since he saw facilitation rather than leadership as his main function in a group.

Be this as it may, there are certain functions which have to be discharged. In the first place the boundaries described above need to be considered, whether or not made explicit to the group, and practical arrangements made. Thereafter the role adopted by the 'leader' (to avoid this term merely adds to semantic confusion) depends on his theoretical background and his aims. Several schools of thought including Wolf, Bion, Moreno, and Fritz Perls argue that the main agent of change is through interaction with the leader. On the other hand, the eclectic therapists such as Yalom argue that peer group interaction is the most important 'curative' factor, a view strongly supported by the encounter movement. Foulkes and the group analysts take the view that both leader–member and member–member interactions are important.

Although the originators of various styles of group leadership tended to be relatively rigid, and advocate a consistent approach, their followers have been more flexible, and many combine elements from totally different techniques.

Group phenomena

Many of the studies describing group development have been American and have involved groups of medical students or psychotherapy trainees. Nevertheless, there is sufficient consensus among different authors describing different groups to anticipate the following main stages.

Introductory stage

During the early sessions trust is established and members develop attachment to the group. Group cohesion, which may be defined as the attractiveness of a group for its members, is built up involving member–member attachment, member–leader attachment and member–group attachment. Few would dispute that this is a necessary prerequisite for effective group function and Yalom has shown a positive correlation between eventual outcome and cohesion measures at six and 12 weeks of five groups meeting at weekly intervals. Anxiety is high during the early sessions and this is the time of high drop-out rate. In this stage, unrealistic beliefs may be apparent, the leader is usually 'deified' and endowed with superhuman powers of understanding and abilities to promote change. In one group (Bennis, 1961) this occurred despite the leader's deliberate efforts to disillusion members. He missed sessions without warning, confined himself to negative comments only, but still he was idolized. Though cohesion builds up whatever the leader does, various techniques may be used to accelerate this process. A review of the literature (Bednar et al., 1974b) suggests that lack of structure in early group sessions not only fails to facilitate early group development, but actually feeds client distortions, interpersonal fears and subjective distress thereby interfering with group development and increasing premature drop-outs. It is therefore advocated that the leader adopt a more active and structuring role in early sessions, becoming less active as cohesion develops. Towards the end of the introductory phase the group settles down, the drop-out rate diminishes, and ideas concerning what the leader can and cannot do have more basis in reality.

Main 'work' stage

Work in the group may refer to achieving understanding of distressing intrapsychic conflicts, altering patterns of interpersonal relationships which have previously led to disaster, overcoming social phobias, controlling desire for alcohol, losing weight and so on. It is possible to separate out a number of components (called by Yalom 'curative factors') which are capable of producing change. These become operative in the 'work stage' of the group and are worth examining in some detail.

1 *Imparting of information.* This refers to advice given either by one member to another or by the leader to the group. In behavioural groups (e.g. treatment of agoraphobics or sexual dysfunction) or supportive groups (Alcoholics Anonymous) it may play an important part. Generally speaking, in heterogeneous groups aiming for 'insight' or 'growth' it is not highly valued, though in the introductory phase members may continually seek advice. Reduction in advice seeking behaviour may be used as an index of maturity in the group. Some patients aptly described as 'help-rejecting complainers' persistently seek out help and advice, only to frustrate the giver by rejecting whatever is offered.

2 *Instillation of hope.* Not only is expectation of success correlated with a positive therapeutic outcome, but anticipation of desired change is likely to keep participants involved in the group situation. This factor may play a major role in some groups, for example, those concerned with increasing self-esteem through assertive training (Liberman, 1970).

3 *Universality.* This has been described as 'welcome to the human race' experience. It disconfirms an individual's feeling of uniqueness, thereby reducing unnecessary anxiety and interpersonal alienation. Confession of guilt-laden preoccupations and ventilation of fears to a receptive and supportive audience are other aspects of this factor.

4 *Altruism.* Jerome Frank (1974) emphasized the importance of the morale-boosting effects that result from members of a group being able to help one another. This factor is reduced if the leader of the group is too charismatic, in that then members look to him rather than to one another for help with their problems. On the other hand, people with authority problems may find it easier to accept comments from their peers than from the leader.

5 *Corrective recapitulation of primary family groups.* Small groups in some respects resemble the family and to leaders may reflect previous attitudes

to parents in the same way that reactions to other members may reflect attitudes to siblings. Recapitulation of these behavioural patterns within the group setting enables maladaptive stereotypes to be recognized and challenged.

6   *Development of socializing techniques.* One of the great advantages of a flexible group situation, allowing movement and encouraging non-verbal as well as verbal interaction is that it permits role-play. Different members of the group are invited to adopt roles which will enable one member to re-enact situations which have proved disastrous in the past. For example, job interviews, dating potential, sexual partners, or practising self-assertive behaviour may all be role-played, allowing the participants not only to become desensitized to the situation, but also to try out alternative approaches. In psychodrama groups, where role-play of an extended type is a major technique, emphasis is placed on the importance of verbal feedback and interaction which takes place after the end of the role-play.

7   *Imitative behaviour* (modelling). It is frequently observed that 'pipe-smoking therapists beget pipe-smoking patients'. In groups, if this is accepted, it is paradoxical to expect that passive, enigmatic, non self-revealing therapists would encourage members of the group to be open, trusting and active. Some leaders, particularly those associated with encounter and psychodrama advocate 'therapist transparancy' by sharing their own personal experiences with the group. Introducing reality in this way reduces transference feelings towards the leader, but what is lost on this particular roundabout may be more than regained on the swings, especially if by considered and partial self-disclosure the leader builds up trust within the group.

8   *Interpersonal learning.* The part played by development of insight in reducing unpleasant emotional states and in changing behaviour remains controversial, though many humans crave 'understanding' of themselves and the world about them. Groups differ in the way that insight is sought. Analytic groups place primary emphasis on the resolution of transference through interpretation. For example, the group analytic approach involves making interpretations which are aimed at helping members understand their interactions with either the leader, the other members, or the group as a whole. As in most groups, emphasis is placed on the 'here and now' rather than the 'there and then'. Comments are referred to events in the group itself rather than to events in an individual member's childhood.

It has been argued that intellectual insight alone is insufficient to produce change and that accompanying reality testing is equally important. In many respects a group provides more opportunities for this than one to one interaction. For example, an individual may have insight into the fact that intense, internal, pent-up feelings of anger are not going to cause catastrophe if released. However, it is only after an emotional explosion in the group and the ensuing exploration of other's reactions that such behaviour may be fully accepted to have positive as well as negative attributes.

Some groups deliberately encourage cathartic experiences, for example by setting up special exercises such as the 'Birth Tunnel'. In this group, members form a tight circle around one member who then is slowly squeezed through a narrow gap. Alternatively, rhythmic chanting, repetition of emotionally laden words with increasing force, or bioenergetic exercises involving stressful body exercises may induce catharsis. Though it produces a short-term feeling of well-being it is not established that cathartic experiences by themselves produce change. However, interwoven with other group 'curative factors' and worked through over a period of time, they may well be the basis of a 'corrective emotional experience'.

9 *Intrapersonal learning.* This factor is considered to be of great importance by both psychoanalysts and by Gestalt therapists. It is a mistake to assume that intrapersonal material can only be dealt with in dyadic interaction. Dream work, symbolism, fantasy exploration and other intrapsychic experiences can be dealt with in the group situation. Scenes chosen for representation in psychodrama may be representations of someone's inner feelings. The group in this situation vividly provides a reflection of the protagonists inner world. Likewise, though in a more academic way, the basic assumptions which rule the behaviour of the verbal, seated group, reflect the basic inner needs which all the group members have in common.

End stage termination

Ending of the group, particularly of an intense, highly cohesive group forces the members back on their own resources. This itself may be profoundly unsettling. In addition, the ending may restimulate memories of previous endings and lead to a type of mourning reaction. Once the end of the group is drawing near, such issues may cloud other events in the group and if the leader is unaware of this, the increasing disturbance may be unexpected and alarming.

To a certain extent, 'ending phenomena' may be observed whenever regular meetings of the group are disturbed by holidays or illness. Acting out may increase, and members may arrive late or unexpectedly miss sessions. Inside the group the work atmosphere may be disrupted by 'scape-goating' and other phenomena.

Special difficulties arising during groups

1   *Tardiness and irregular attendance.* This is disruptive and often signifies resistance to exploring some key issue or expressing strong feelings. Often the behaviour can only be understood and worked through after it has been modified. Although direct interpretation by the leader concerning possible reasons for individual's lateness may sometimes produce change it is usually more effective if other group members can be encouraged to make such comments. Mere observation by the leader may be sufficient to encourage the group to explore the issue, though confrontation may lead the latecomer to become a drop-out.

2   *Subgrouping.* Formation of subgroups is very common and may prove disruptive to both excluded and included members. It is often cited as a cause of drop-outs and one of the reasons for prohibiting extra-group socializing and sexual involvement is to prevent this phenomena. In one study of drop-outs, 31% had left because of problems with subgrouping (Yalom, 1975). There is evidence that an authoritarian, restrictive style of leadership is most likely to be associated with disruptive subgrouping, and that members with strong intimacy, dependency or dominance needs are most likely to be included. The 'conspiracy of silence' or other behaviour adopted by the subgroup, rather than its mere existence, is disruptive. Thus, in order to facilitate progress the leader is better advised to encourage the subgroup to communicate rather than attempting to disband it. The leader should avoid special pledges of confidentiality which are likely to trap him into a subgroup. Most leaders are reluctant to include two members with a special relationship (e.g. husband/wife, room-mates) in an otherwise heterogenous group for similar reasons.

3   *Scape-goating.* When unacceptable emotions are aroused in the group they are often pinned on to one member. It may be sufficient for the leader to clarify the situation and point out the reality of what is happening, but in addition, he may need to give some support to the scape-goat and to explore the need to divert expression of strong emotions and the reasons why one particular individual has been chosen. Alternatively, in an 'action' group an exercise may be set up where each member is encouraged to be as hostile as possible towards the scape-goat. Such exaggeration of emotional feelings may show them to be unrealistic.

4 *Problem individuals.* The monopolist ('I'm like that too . . .'), the inter-rogater, the help-rejecting complainer ('Yes . . . but'), the self-righteous moralist who needs to be right and the leader's assistant who denies problems and blandly offers advice, can all consume time and energy in an unproductive way. Ideally, the rest of the group should deal with an exasperating member. Often, especially in the early stages, this is expect-ing too much. They may be encouraged or goaded by such comments as, 'I wonder why the group is becoming exasperated and cannot do any-thing'. If this fails, the leader may be forced to interrupt a behavioural pattern by an observation or interpretation without totally alienating the individual concerned.

5 *Concurrent individual therapy.* Individual and group approaches may conflict, and the temptation to play one off against the other is great. In special circumstances the leader may wish to see an individual member alone, but to avoid subgrouping this should be done openly and shared with the rest of the group.

6 *Silence.* Silence provokes anxiety and if allowed to persist for too long it may paralyse the group. One of the leader's tasks is to prevent anxiety rising to this point. Particularly in the early stages of the group long silences are unhelpful and most leaders will intervene, the aim being to lower the anxiety and permit interaction to occur. Commenting on the silence, and the discomfort associated with it, may be sufficient, or alternatively, if the leader has some idea what lies behind the reluctance to communicate this may be referred to. Silence may be viewed as the equivalent of resistance in individual therapy and interpreted as such. Alternatively, in 'work' groups simply the question 'Are we working?' may be all that is needed.

In encounter, psychodrama and behavioural groups, special warm-up exercises help to focus attention and to stimulate interaction. The dis-advantages of these techniques in groups without specific targets is that the leader's intervention or the exercise chosen may set the theme for the whole of the ensuing session.

Outcome research

Problems facing the researcher in group psychotherapy are well reviewed by Fielding (1974). First, is the difficulty of defining exactly what package of techniques were being employed. Here one has to bear in mind that it is not only what the group leader does, which may to some extent be controlled, but also what other members of the group do, which can only be observed, that determines the overall therapeutic effect. Second, is the difficulty of running comparison or control groups. Third, is the difficulty of allowing for what occurs outside the group sessions. Fourth, is the difficulty of measurement and of defining what is meant by improvement. Considering these difficulties it is not surprising that the vast majority of work in group psychotherapy has been done on group process and that most of this is highly subjective, a state of affairs described by Malan as 'flight into process'.

Parloff and Dies (1977) in reviewing the previous 10 years outcome research in group psychotherapy found that only 30 studies out of over 100 initially screened matched up to his relatively generous minimum standards of research methodology. Of these only six studies concerned the psychoneuroses which constitute the major target of group therapists' efforts. Taken together these studies fail to show any particular merits of group therapy over other forms of psychosocial intervention. On the basis of the other 32 studies the following conclusions were drawn:

A *In schizophrenics* (as defined in American literature)
  (1) Group therapy probably does not contribute significantly to the usual array of ward milieu treatments.
  (2) Group therapy appears to enhance other specific in-patient psychosocial treatment (such as structured dyadic social interaction and organized ward interaction).
  (3) Group therapy makes patients more acceptable to staff.
  (4) Group therapy failed to enhance post-hospital adjustment of schizophrenic patients.

B *Other categories of patients*
  (1) Two out of seven studies showed positive effects on post-institutional adjustment in juvenile delinquents.
  (2) Only one out of three showed reduction of recidivism in adult offenders, and this was in a study involving sexual offenders.
  (3) As far as treatment of alcoholics and addicts were concerned no clear conclusions could be drawn.

The unimpressive conclusions of this and other reviews of outcome have to be contrasted with the widespread enthusiasm for group therapy, presumably based on clinical impression of value. A simplistic reaction from a supporter of group therapy would be that researchers are hog-tied by methodology and missing the point. Researchers would respond that therapists are blinded by their own enthusiasm. However, there are more subtle factors among which must be included:

(a) 'Group Therapy' is no more a single treatment than 'Pharmacotherapy'. Rather it is a mode of treatment with many constituent parts, each with their own therapeutic indications.

(b) Traditional diagnostic categories may not be the best means of selecting patients for suitability for group therapy (e.g. high anxiety delinquents did better in training groups than those with low anxiety, particularly if stressful elements were minimized—Sarason and Glanzer, 1973).

Three studies provide good examples of the way in which researchers cope with some difficulties but fail to deal with others.

In Barbara Dick's (1975) 10-year study of out-patient analytic group therapy, 93 chronic neurotic or borderline patients were treated for an average of 63 one-and-a-quarter hour sessions. There were no controls, though clinical experience of this type of patient who were 'conditioned to expect failure' suggests that the spontaneous remission rate would be low. A Whitaker and Lieberman model was used and symptom removal was not the primary task of therapy. Seventy-five per cent of patients completed a minimum of 30 sessions, arbitrarily defined 'adequate' treatment. Assessment was made on eight parameters: (a) marital or patient–parent relationship, (b) work, (c) sex, (d) physical health, (e) leisure, (f) self image, (g) self understanding, (h) symptoms; 87% of patients improved on one or more of these criteria, 11% showed no change and 2% became worse. At six-month follow-up 75% still maintained their improvement. Though this study suggests that groups produced change it gives no clue as to which of the many possible ingredients may have been the effective agent of change.

Lieberman et al (1973) compared the effects of 18 groups representing 10 different ideologies. Students aged between 18 and 22 participated in 30 hours of work. This study is often quoted because of the finding that, overall, encounter groups produced less positive change and more negative change than traditional therapy. This conclusion is an artefact produced by averaging since some of the encounter groups were so ineffective that no participants experienced positive change, whereas other encounter groups were so effective that no members underwent negative change. The difference in outcome appeared to be related to the leader's behaviour rather than his theoretical background. 'Providers', giving high positive support and considerable cognitive framework ran high-yield, low-risk groups, while 'Energizers', who were highly charismatic, attacking, active and very personally revealing, ran high-risk, moderate to low-yield groups.

In homogeneous groups with specific aims it is much easier to carry out comparative trials. Thus, Pinick et al. (1971) showed that a series of five-hour group treatment packages, comprising two hours of behavioural treatment, followed by exercise and a low calorie lunch, were more effective in terms of weight loss than traditional discussion groups. However, the range of results was much wider in the first type of group; the very great improvement by two patients improving the average improvement of the group as a whole and masking the fact that some individuals did worse than anyone in the psychotherapy group.

To date, the evidence suggests that the main value of groups lies in the fact that they provide an effective, economic and supportive framework in which a range of specific techniques can operate. Research has indicated that cohesive groups are more likely to do useful work in the fields of therapy, socialization and education and we have some knowledge of the forces that lead to both cohesion and disruption. In the next decade, research is likely to focus on the ways specific techniques may be matched to specific problems.

References

Anthony, E. J. (1971). History of group psychotherapy. *In* 'Comprehensive Group Psychotherapy' (Eds H. E. Kaplan and B. J. Sadock). pp. 4–31. Williams and Wilkins, Baltimore.

Bednar, R. L. *et. al.* (1974b). Empirical guidelines for group therapy; pretraining, cohesion and modelling. *J. Appl. Behav. Sci.* **10**, 2, 149–179.

Bednar, R. L., Melnick, J. and Kaul, T. J. (1974b). Risk, responsibility and structure. A conceptual framework for initiating group counselling and psychotherapy. *J. Counsell. Psychol.* **21**, 1, 31–37.

Bennis, W. G. (1961). Defense against 'Depressive Anxiety' in groups. The case of the absent leader.' *Merrill-Palmer Q.* **7**, 1, 3–30.

Berne, E. (1966). 'Principles of Group Treatment'. Grove Press, New York.

Bion, W. R. (1961). 'Experiences in Groups'. Tavistock, London.

Blatner, H. A. (1973). 'Acting In. Practical Applications of Psychodramatic Methods'. Springfield Publishing, New York.

Blumberg, A. and Golembiewski, R. T. (1976). 'Learning and Change in Groups'. Penguin, Harmondsworth.

Davies, M. H. (1976). The origins and practice of psychodrama. *Br. J. Psychiat.* **129**, 201–206.

Dick, B. M. (1975). A ten year study of out-patients analytic group therapy. *Br. J. Psychiat.* **127**, 365–375.

Falloon, J. H. R. *et al.* (1977). Social skills training of out-patient groups: a controlled study of rehearsal and home-work. *Br. J. Psychiat.* **131**, 599–609.

Fielding, J. M. (1974). Problems of evaluative research into group psychotherapy outcome. *Australian New Zealand J. Psychiat.* **8**, 97–104.

Foulkes, S. M. and Anthony, E. J. (1973). 'Group Psychotherapy. The Psychoanalytical Approach' (2nd edn). Penguin, Harmondsworth.

Frank. J. D. (1974). 'Persuasion and Healing' (revised edn). Schocken Books, New York.

Freud, S. (1922). 'Group Psychology and the Analysis of the Ego'. Hogarth, London.

Hand, I., Lamontagne, Y., and Marks, J. M. (1974). Group exposure (flooding) *in vivo* for agoraphobics. *Br. J. Psychiat.* **124**, 588–602.

Kesey, K. (1962). 'One Flew Over the Cuckoo's Nest'. Methuen, London.

Kreeger, L. (ed.) (1975). 'The Large Group: Dynamics and Therapy'. Constable, London.

Liberman, R. (1970). A behavioural approach to group dynamics. *Behav. Ther.* **1**, 141–175, 312–327.

Lieberman, M. A., Yalom, J. and Miles, M. (1973). 'Encounter Groups. First Facts'. Basic Books, New York.

Parloff, M. B. and Dies, R. R. (1977). Group psychotherapy. Outcome research. 1966–1975. *Int. J. Group Psychother.* **XXVII**, 3, 281–319.

Perls, F. S. Hefferline, R. F. and Goodman, P. (1973). 'Gestalt Therapy'. Penguin Books, Harmondsworth.

Pines, M. (1975). *In* 'The Large Group' (Ed. L. Kreeger). Peacock, California.

Pinick, S. B. *et al* (1971). Behaviour modification in the treatment of obesity. *Psychosom. Med.* **33**, 49–55.

Pratt, J. H. (1917). The tuberculosis class. An experiment in home treatment. *In* 'Group Psychotherapy and Group Function' (Eds M. Rosenbaum and M. Berger). pp. 111–122. Basic Books, New York.

Rice, A. K. (1965). 'Learning for Leadership'. Tavistock, London.

Rioch, M. J. (1970). The work of Wilfred Bion on groups. *Psychiatry* **33**, 55–66.

Rogers, C. (1973). 'Encounter Groups'. Penguin, Harmondsworth.

Sarason, I. G. and Glanzer, V. M. (1973). Modelling and group discussion in the rehabilitation of juvenile delinquents. *J. Counsel. Psychol.* **20**, 422–449.

Schutz, W. C. (1967). 'Joy'. Grove Press, New York.

Schutz, W. C. (1966). The Interpersonal Underworld'. California Science and Behaviour Books, Palo Alto.

Shaffer, K. and Galinsky, M. (1974). 'Models of Group Therapy and Sensitivity Training'. Prentice Hall, New Jersey.

Slater, P. (1969). Theory and technique of the repertory grid. *Br. J. Psychiat.* **115**, 1287–1297.

Slavson, S. (1940). Group therapy. *Mental Hygiene* **24**, 26–49.

Skynner, A. C. R. (1976). 'One Flesh, Separate Persons, Principles of Family and Marital Psychotherapy'. Constable, London.

Whitaker., D. S. and Lieberman, M. A. (1965). 'Psychotherapy through the Group Process'. Atherton Press, New York.

Wolf, A. and Schwartz, E. K. (1962). 'Psychoanalysis in Groups'. Grune and Stratton, New York.

Yalom, I. D. (1975). 'The Theory and Practice of Group Psychotherapy' (2nd edn.). Basic Books, New York.

Subject Index